Biopolymer Networks

Design, dynamics and discovery

Online at: https://doi.org/10.1088/978-0-7503-5037-2

Biophysical Society–IOP Series

About the Series

The Biophysical Society and IOP Publishing have forged a new publishing partnership in biophysics, bringing the world-leading expertise and domain knowledge of the Biophysical Society into the rapidly developing IOP ebooks program.

The program publishes textbooks, monographs, reviews, and handbooks covering all areas of biophysics research, applications, education, methods, computational tools, and techniques. Subjects of the collection will include: bioenergetics; bioengineering; biological fluorescence; biopolymers *in vivo*; cryo-electron microscopy; exocytosis and endocytosis; intrinsically disordered proteins; mechanobiology; membrane biophysics; membrane structure and assembly; molecular biophysics; motility and cytoskeleton; nanoscale biophysics; and permeation and transport.

A full list of titles published in this series can be found here: https://iopscience.iop.org/bookListInfo/iop-series-in-biophysical-society.

Biopolymer Networks

Design, dynamics and discovery

Rae M Robertson-Anderson
Department of Physics and Biophysics, University of San Diego, San Diego, USA

IOP Publishing, Bristol, UK

ISBN 978-0-7503-5037-2 (ebook)
ISBN 978-0-7503-5035-8 (print)
ISBN 978-0-7503-5038-9 (myPrint)
ISBN 978-0-7503-5036-5 (mobi)

DOI 10.1088/978-0-7503-5037-2

Version: 20240801

IOP ebooks

British Library Cataloguing-in-Publication Data: A catalogue record for this book is available from the British Library.

Published by IOP Publishing, wholly owned by The Institute of Physics, London

IOP Publishing, No.2 The Distillery, Glassfields, Avon Street, Bristol, BS2 0GR, UK

US Office: IOP Publishing, Inc., 190 North Independence Mall West, Suite 601, Philadelphia, PA 19106, USA

This journey is dedicated to my husband, Mike, and two boys, Oscar and Ralph, who continue to inspire me every day to dig deeper, question everything, and notice and relish in the wonder of the world around us.

Contents

Part V What now?

Preface

Biopolymer networks are the topic of fervent interdisciplinary research in physics, biophysics, biology, chemistry, engineering, and materials science. Yet, there are very few books available to these communities that are dedicated to this topic, and relevant texts are often narrow in focus and discipline specific. Typically, texts are either (1) largely theoretical and similar to polymer physics books written for a physics audience; (2) written for a narrow chemistry and materials audience with a focus on design and synthesis without discussion of the underlying physics or insights into biology; or (3) focused on a narrow range of biopolymers, for example, polysaccharides. Here, I present a broad and interdisciplinary perspective on research on biopolymer networks, as well as look at the future of the field. One may still ask: *Why are researchers interested in biopolymer networks?* As I will showcase in this monograph, there is a diverse community of researchers who has unique and rich answers to this question and goals for investigating biopolymer networks, including:

1. *Cellular Biology*: Proteins, DNA, RNA, lipids, and polysaccharides are all examples of biopolymers that crowd biological cells. The physical properties of these polymers and their interactions in the densely packed cell drive most processes in living organisms. For example, the cytoskeleton is a dynamic network of filamentous proteins that provide structural support to our cells while allowing for reorganization and fluidity necessary for cell division and motility. Researchers in biology and biophysics design and study biopolymer networks to shed light on biological systems and processes.
2. *Polymer Physics*: Because a multitude of biopolymers naturally exist with a wide range of stiffnesses, sizes, and topologies, they serve as model systems for investigating perplexing problems in polymer physics, such as shortcomings of the reptation model for entangled polymer networks. For example, researchers have used DNA, actin, and microtubules for decades now as model polymer systems to test theoretical predictions regarding the diffusion and relaxation dynamics of entangled flexible, semiflexible, and rigid rod polymers. Biopolymer networks have also been the subject of intense study examining the effect of polymer topology on the rheological properties of polymer networks.
3. *Materials Science*: Biopolymer networks are becoming increasingly important to the materials community seeking to design next-generation biocompatible, tunable materials. Researchers are capitalizing on billions of years of biological evolution to design networks of biopolymers that exhibit emergent material properties not possible with synthetic analogs. The diversity, tunability, versatility, and responsiveness of biopolymers and their networks make them ideal candidates for next-generation materials that are multifunctional, reconfigurable, and autonomous.
4. *Soft and Active Matter*: Biopolymer networks exhibit rich viscoelastic properties that can be precisely tuned by the properties, concentrations,

and interactions of the comprising polymers. This complex viscoelastic behavior continues to be the focus of much research in the soft matter community. The study of biopolymer networks provides insights into other soft matter systems with similar viscoelastic and nonlinear response properties, such as colloids, gels, foams, etc, that are of broad general interest in the physical sciences and engineering communities. Moreover, the soft matter community is increasingly focused on active matter physics, a field of research that was born out of studying motor-driven biopolymer networks. As such, biopolymer networks continue to be the paradigmatic testbed for the design and understanding of active matter.

This book is written with *all of these audiences* and their goals in mind—touching equally on each of these unique perspectives. Topics are grounded in physics but presented at a level accessible to researchers in other fields; and highlight their relevance and applicability to cellular biology and materials science. The text is divided into ten comprehensive chapters that are organized into four main sections. Each chapter may be read in sequence or as a stand-alone chapter, and includes high-level summaries of key points and results, as well as a comprehensive list of references for more in-depth coverage on the topics discussed.

Acknowledgments

First and foremost, I would like to thank my husband, Mike, for watching our boys, Oscar and Ralph, for countless Saturdays and Sundays to give me time to work on this project—and for being an inspiration as a physicist, writer, and parent. I would like to thank Oscar and Ralph for always asking great questions and giving the best hugs. And for my parents who gave me the support and confidence to pursue my passions.

I would also like to thank the many mentors, friends, and collaborators who have supported me, encouraged me, and taught me so much through the years. They have shaped my research interests, how I mentor students and collaborate with others, and what I value most in life and career. Some of these amazing humans include: Doug Smith, Jeff Urbach, David Millar, Jenny Ross, Moumita Das, Megan Valentine, Jacinta Conrad, Mike Rust, Mike Murrell, Richard Weiner, Margaret Gardel, Ken Schweizer, Steve Granick, Ron Larson, Omar Saleh, Pat Doyle, Michael Rubinstein, Andy McCammon, Terry Hwa, David Kleinfeld, and so many more. Your voices decorate the pages of this book.

I would also like to acknowledge the generous support of the funding agencies and program officers that have supported my research through the years, without whom this project would not have been possible: Air Force Office of Scientific Research (FA95550-12-1-0315, FA9550-17-1-0249, FA9550-21-1-0361), National Science Foundation (CAREER DMR-1255446, DBI-1229443, CBET-1603925, CBET-1919429, NSF-CHE-2050846, DMREF DMR-2119663), WM Keck Foundation (Science and Engineering Research Grant), National Institutes of Health (NIGMS R15GM123420-01, R15GM123420-02), Research Corporation for Scientific Advancement (Cottrell College Award 19843, Cottrell Scholars Postbac Award 29203, Scialog Award 4308).

Author biography

Rae M Robertson-Anderson

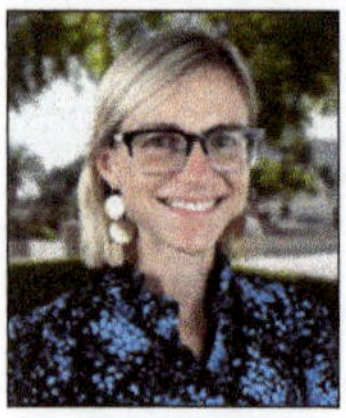

Rae M Robertson-Anderson received her BS in Physics from Georgetown University in 2003, funded by a Clare Boothe Luce Scholarship. She earned her PhD in Physics from University of California, San Diego, in 2007, funded by an NSF Graduate Research Fellowship, after which she was awarded an NIH fellowship to pursue a molecular biology postdoc at The Scripps Research Institute.

In 2009, Robertson-Anderson joined the faculty at the University of San Diego with the goal of engaging undergraduates in cutting-edge research and shaping undergraduate physics programs and research at a national level. She served as department Chair for 8 years, overhauling the physics curriculum and research culture, and establishing an interdisciplinary Biophysics BS that has served as a model for liberal arts institutions nationally. Robertson-Anderson is currently serving as Associate Provost for Engaged Scholarship where she is developing new initiatives to support, promote, and enhance research at University of San Diego.

Robertson-Anderson's research program aims to elucidate microscale mechanics and macromolecular transport in bio-inspired soft and active matter systems. Her lab has pioneered novel optical tweezers microrheology and fluorescence microscopy techniques to probe these systems across decades of spatiotemporal scales. She is also a leading expert in engineering biopolymer networks that leverage biological design paradigms to solve problems in soft and active matter physics.

Robertson-Anderson has been awarded over $5 M to fund her research program, including a Keck Foundation Research Grant, NSF CAREER Award, Air Force Young Investigator Award, and an NSF DMREF grant. In 2022, she was awarded a Research Corporation Cottrell Scholars STAR Award for her excellence in research and teaching, and was named a fellow of the American Physical Society. Robertson-Anderson's 74 publications feature 85 undergraduate co-authors, and in 2023, she received the APS Prize for Faculty Research at an Undergraduate Institution. Robertson-Anderson's notable national service roles include serving on the Executive Committees for the APS Division of Soft Matter and the Beckman Young Investigator Program; and maintaining an active science education TikTok channel, Physics Mama.

Part I

Let's get started

Chapter 1

Introduction to biopolymers and their networks

This chapter covers what biopolymers are and why they are important, introducing the most widely studied biopolymers (nucleic acids, cytoskeleton filaments, proteins, and polysaccharides) and the key physical properties of each. The chapter concludes with a discussion of biopolymer networks, including their importance in biology, physics, and materials science, key features and considerations, and open questions in the field.

1.1 Polymers 101

Modern life as we know it is in large part due to the polymers that are all around us —from plastics and petroleum, to cosmetics and food, to artificial limbs and adhesives (Rubinstein and Colby 2003, Chanda and Roy 2008, Namazi 2017) (figure 1.1(A)). What we think of less often are the polymers that make *life* possible. Biological polymers—**biopolymers**—fill the insides of nearly all biological cells as well as the interstitial space that surrounds them (Maarel 2008, Mathews *et al* 2013, Nelson *et al* 2020) (figure 1.1(B)).

At the most basic level, a polymer is a long chain of repeating subunits, i.e., monomers (figure 1.1(C)). The physical properties of each polymer, as well as the polymeric materials and fluids they comprise, are determined, in large part, by the properties of their monomers as well as the lengths, topologies, and flexibilities of the chains (de Gennes 1979, Doi 1996) (table 1.1).

1.1.1 Non-Newtonian fluid properties

In materials engineering, polymers are used to create materials that are squishy, gooey, stretchy, and deformable and can change their properties depending on the stresses or strains they encounter (Chanda and Roy 2008, Ahmed 2017, Shaw and MacKnight 2018, Brewer 2021). For example, yogurt assumes a solid-like form in steady-state but, when mixed rapidly, becomes more liquid-like and can be poured. Ketchup is a similar 'shear-thinning' fluid, meaning it becomes less viscous the more

doi:10.1088/978-0-7503-5037-2ch1

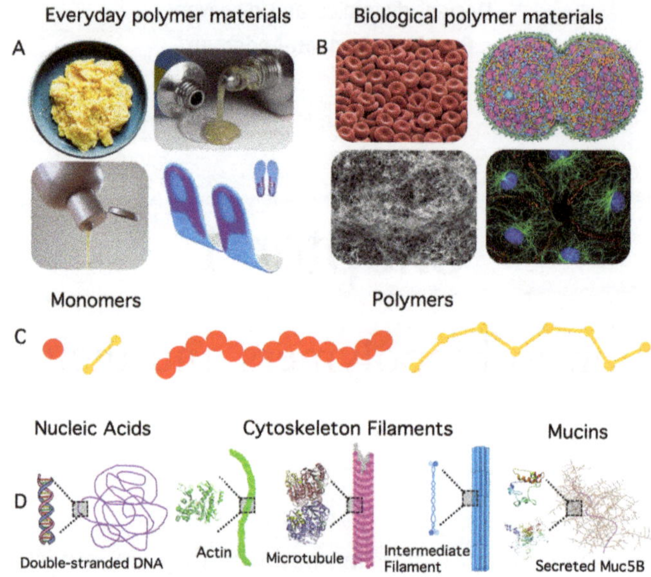

Figure 1.1. Biopolymer basics. (A) Polymers comprise many materials that we encounter in everyday life such as (clockwise): scrambled eggs; glue and other adhesives; shampoo, soap, and other cosmetics; and athletic insoles and protective equipment. Images reproduced from 'Extra-creamy scrambled eggs recipe,' (n.d.), 'Epoxy resin vs. epoxy adhesive—sticky aide,' (2022), 'Pouring shampoo stock illustrations—170 pouring shampoo stock illustrations, vectors & clipart,' (n.d.), 'Amazon.com: envelop gel insoles for men—shoe inserts for walking, running, hiking—insoles for standing all day—cushion soles for heels, arch support, plantar fasciitis flat feet—sneaker boot insoles : health & household,' (n.d.). (B) Polymers are ubiquitous in biology, comprising (clockwise): e.g., red blood cells (Image by DAVID MCCARTHY/Getty Images), dividing cell nuclei (Illustration by David S Goodsell in Somers (2022)), cytoskeleton, and mucus. Images reproduced from 'Learn all about red blood cells,' (n.d.), 'mousefibroblasts.jpg (708 × 512),' (n.d.), 'Mucus,' (n.d.). (C) Polymers are macromolecular chains of repeating subunits, monomers, that can have different structures and sizes. The simplest way to model a polymer is to consider it as a string of connected beads (red) or a chain of rods with freely rotating joints (yellow). (D) Key biopolymers include nucleic acids such as double-stranded DNA; cytoskeleton filaments such as actin, microtubules and intermediate filaments; and mucins such as secreted mucin Muc5B. Adapted from Tong and Gu (2020). CC BY 4.0.

rapidly it is perturbed. If you have ever mixed cornstarch (a polymer) and water together in a bowl, to make the infamous 'ooblek', you know that if you slowly put your hand in the goop it feels like a fluid and you can submerge your hand. But if you try to rapidly pull your hand out, the goop solidifies and traps your hand. This 'shear-thickening' effect is opposite to the thinning of ketchup and yogurt, and is another widely observed phenomenon in polymeric fluids.

While 'Newtonian' fluids can be described by a single intrinsic value of viscosity η, which quantifies their ability to resist flow via frictional drag between the molecules, many polymeric fluids are classified as **non-Newtonian** fluids because their viscosity depends on the nature and rate of the strain or deformation (Chhabra 2010, Brewer 2021). Polymeric materials also often exhibit solid-like or elastic behavior. In fact, ooblek does not just become more viscous when you punch it or run across a swimming pool filled with it—it actually becomes solid-like. Moreover, you can squirt shampoo (often made with the synthetic polymer polyethylene glycol) out of a bottle, like a Newtonian fluid, but you can also elastically stretch a drop of it between your fingers, like a solid. This general property of being able to exhibit both fluid-like (viscous) and solid-like (elastic) behavior—known as **viscoelasticity**—is a hallmark of polymeric materials (Rubinstein and Colby 2003, Shaw and MacKnight 2018).

1.1.2 Newtonian fluids and viscosity

In its most basic form, the stress a fluid exerts to resist strain or deformation is proportional to the rate of the strain, i.e.,

$$F \sim \eta v \tag{1.1a}$$

or

$$\sigma \sim \eta \dot{\gamma} \tag{1.1b}$$

where F or σ are the force or stress (force per unit area) that the fluid exerts to resist a strain applied with a speed or strain rate of v or $\dot{\gamma}$ and a constant η value for any given fluid (Ziegler 2012). A common exact form of the relation between force and speed is the Stokes drag equation that relates the force that a fluid of viscosity η exerts on a submerged sphere of radius R to the speed of the sphere v via

$$F = 6\pi\eta R v \tag{1.2}$$

which is a relation often used in microrheology measurements of polymeric fluids (see chapters 3 and 4) (Squires and Mason 2010, Furst and Squires 2017). Another widely used exact relation between stress and strain rate is the stress exerted by a fluid of viscosity η, sandwiched between two parallel plates of area A that are separated by a distance h, to resist moving one plate relative to the other (i.e., shearing) at a speed v:

$$\frac{F}{A} = \eta \frac{v}{h} \tag{1.3a}$$

or

$$\sigma \sim \eta \dot{\gamma} \tag{1.3b}$$

where

$$\sigma = \frac{F}{A} \tag{1.4}$$

and

$$\dot{\gamma} = \frac{v}{h} \tag{1.5}$$

This general expression is exploited in bulk rheology measurements to determine viscoelastic properties of polymeric materials as described in chapter 3 (Mezger 2006,

Osswald 2015). An important property of fluids is that they *dissipate* or lose all energy put into them from a strain via friction between the molecules, so they are unable to store any memory of their pre-strain state. They cannot 'bounce back', recover, or otherwise move following deformation.

1.1.3 Solids and elasticity

Unlike fluids, the stress a solid exerts to resist strain or deformation is proportional the distance or strain over which the deformation is applied, regardless of its rate, which is most simply captured by Hooke's law for a spring, i.e.,

$$F \sim k\Delta x \tag{1.6}$$

where k is the spring constant, an intrinsic property of the spring that quantifies its ability to resist deformation, and Δx is the displacement over which the spring is stretched. For an extended solid under shear, this relation becomes

$$\frac{F}{A} = G\frac{\Delta x}{h} \tag{1.7}$$

or

$$\sigma = G\gamma \tag{1.8}$$

where G is the intrinsic shear modulus of the solid (analogous to k for a spring) and γ is the strain, or the relative deformation. Like its sister expression for fluid response (equation 1.3b), this relation is also used to characterize the rheological properties of polymeric materials (see chapter 3). Unlike their dissipative fluid counterparts, solids *store* the energy put into them by the strain, so they can return to their pre-strained state. In other words, they maintain 'memory' of their initial state. A spring will always return to its starting point after being stretched as long as it is not stretched past its elastic limit.

1.1.4 Viscoelasticity

The viscoelastic nature of polymeric materials and fluids allows them to both *store* and *dissipate* energy. The relative contributions of each depend on the properties and concentrations of the polymers as well as the nature of the strain. Rather than being solely characterized by an effective viscosity or spring constant, both types of quantities, and how they vary with strain and strain rate, are needed to fully describe the material (Doi 1996, Rubinstein and Colby 2003, Chhabra 2010, Shaw and MacKnight 2018). Viscoelasticity also provides materials with multifunctionality, such that they can serve one mechanical function under small deformations and an entirely different one when subject to large deformations. The most basic model to describe viscoelasticity is the Maxwell model, which treats the viscoelastic fluid as a purely viscous element and purely elastic element in series. This construction results in the relation

$$\eta\dot{\gamma} = G\gamma \tag{1.9}$$

from which a characteristic timescale at which the viscous and elastic contributions are comparable is defined as

$$\tau^* = \eta/G \tag{1.10}$$

(Rubinstein and Colby 2003). For times that are long compared to τ^*, the material behaves as a fluid while for short times $t < \tau^*$ the material behaves as a solid. The exact formalism to describe the viscoelastic properties of polymeric materials, which builds on the Maxwell model, will be discussed in depth in chapters 2–4.

1.1.5 Viscoelasticity in biology

Biology is exquisite in harnessing and exploiting the viscoelastic nature of materials comprising high concentrations of polymers, to allow for myriad mechanical processes and properties of organelles, cells, organs, and tissues, from a finite number of building blocks. For example, the viscoelastic nature of cells, dictated by the network of biopolymers that comprise the cytoskeleton, allows them to be both rigid *and* deformable under different conditions; and enables cell motility, division, and repair (Guilak *et al* 2000, Hoffman and Crocker 2009, Fletcher and Mullins 2010). The viscoelasticity of red blood cells and networks of fibrin regulate blood flow and promote wound healing (Laurens *et al* 2006, Amin *et al* 2007, Puig-de-Morales-Marinkovic *et al* 2007, Barriga and Mayor 2019), and viscoelastic mucin networks (i.e., mucus) allow our lungs to clear toxins from airways while also providing protective coatings to organs (Chen and Dulfano 1978, Georgiades *et al* 2014, Fass and Thornton 2023) (figure 1.1(B)). The broad diversity of properties and processes that networks of biopolymers mediate in living organisms is possible due to the wide range of sizes and stiffness of biopolymers—spanning several orders of magnitude—as well as the many structures, conformations, and topologies that they can assume (Maarel 2008, Mathews *et al* 2013, Burla *et al* 2019) (table 1.1). These properties act in concert to precisely tune the mechanical properties of naturally occurring biopolymer networks.

1.2 Biopolymer basics

The biopolymers that I will primarily focus on in this text, summarized in table 1.1 and selectively depicted in figure 1.1(D), include nucleic acids, cytoskeleton filaments, mucins, and intrinsically disordered proteins (IDPs). Below, I summarize the physical properties of these biopolymers as well as their building blocks and assembly pathways, as detailed in figure 1.2. I also discuss the impact of environmental and chemical conditions, such as salt concentration and temperature, on their structure and function (figure 1.2A, B).

The primary metrics I will use in the following sections to describe the physical properties of biopolymers, which are summarized in table 1.1, include:

Table 1.1. Physical properties of widely studied biopolymers. The principal physical properties that describe each biopolymer or class of biopolymers discussed in this chapter are summarized. The key lengthscales include the persistence length l_p and contour length L. The persistence length values are approximated from multiple sources in the literature and do not consider the effect of ionic conditions or folding, as discussed in section 1.2. The structure and flexibility are categorized as: (structure) random coil, partially extended, or extended; and (flexibility) flexible, semiflexible, or rigid. The different polymer topologies discussed include linear, circular, supercoiled, branched, looped, bottlebrush, or folded. Each polymer is a chain of repeating subunits, i.e., monomers, that are the basic building blocks of the polymers. The italicized entries will not be discussed in subsequent chapters.

Biopolymer	Persistence length (nm)	Contour length (μm)	Structure, flexibility	Topology	Repeating subunits
dsDNA	50	10^{-3}–10^{6}	Random coil, flexible	Supercoiled, linear, relaxed circular	Basepair A–T, G–C
ssDNA	1–4	10^{-3}–10^{6}	Random coil, flexible	Relaxed circular, linear, looped	Nucleotide: A,T,C,G
RNA	2–3	10^{-3}–10^{1}	Random coil, flexible	Linear, hairpin, looped, stacked	Nucleotide: A,U,C,G
Actin filament	10^{4}	1.0–30	Partially extended, semiflexible	Linear	Actin monomer
Microtubule	10^{6}	1.0–40	Extended, rigid rod	Linear	Tubulin dimer
Intermediate filament	50–2000	5.0–20	Random coil, flexible	Linear, branched	Unit length filament
Mucin	3–40	10^{-1}–10^{1}	Random coil, branched	Linear, bottlebrush, branched	Glycoprotein dimer
Intrinsically disordered protein	0.4–12	10^{-2}–10^{-1}	Random coil, folded	Linear, looped, partially folded	Amino acid
Worm-like micelle	10–40	10^{-2}–10^{1}	*Random coil, semiflexible*	*Linear*	*Amphiphile*
Polysaccharide	30–300	10^{-2}–2	*Random coil, flexible*	*Linear*	*Monosaccharide*

Contour length L: the overall length of the fully-extended polymer when entropically stretched to its full extension.

Diameter d: the cross-sectional diameter of the polymeric chain.

Persistence length l_p: the length at which the energetic cost to bend a segment of the polymer exceeds the energy $\sim k_BT$ (where k_B is Boltzmann's constant and T is temperature) from thermal kicks from the surrounding solvent

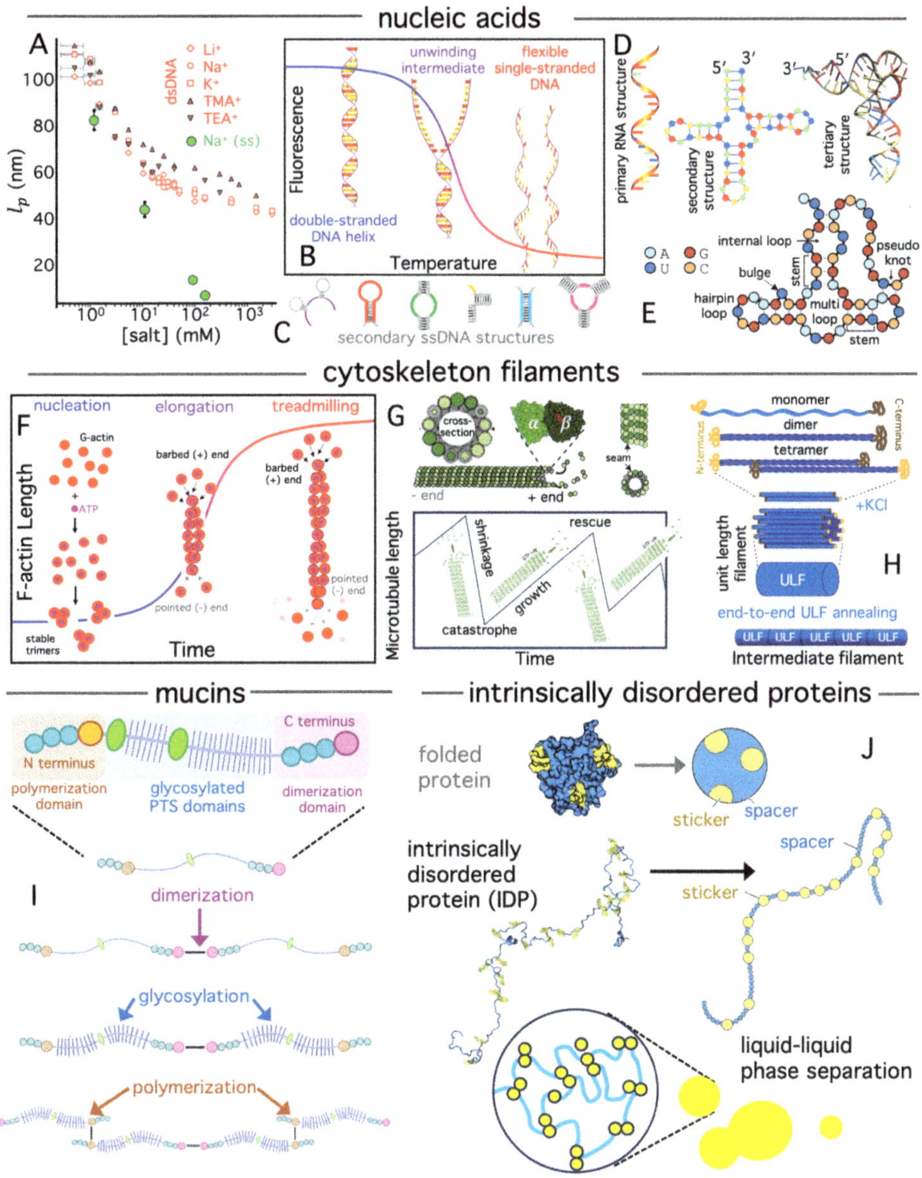

Figure 1.2. Biopolymer building blocks, assembly pathways, and structures. (A–E) Nucleic acids, including DNA (A–C) and RNA (D–E) are flexible polymers that can adopt higher-order structures. (A) The persistence lengths of double-stranded (red data points) and single-stranded (green) DNA decrease with increasing concentration of monovalent salts. The persistence length of ssDNA is much smaller and decreases more rapidly with [salt] as compared to dsDNA. Data is reproduced from Chen *et al* (2012); Guilbaud *et al* (2019). (B) Cartoon depiction of dsDNA melting into two ssDNA strands with increasing temperature. The sigmoidal curve represents the fluorescence signal from dsDNA. At the midpoint melting temperature (purple) half of the DNA is dsDNA and half is ssDNA, as depicted by the intermediate DNA construct that is unwinding. Adapted from Amnuanpol (2016), Copyright (2016), with permission from Springer Nature. (C) ssDNA can adopt higher-order secondary structures such as hairpin loops, internal loops, kinks, ladders, and multiloops.

Adapted from Sullivan *et al* (2019). CC BY 4.0. (D) RNA is typically single-stranded and adopts secondary structures, such as hairpin loops, kinks, and multiloops, that often fold into tertiary structures. Adapted from Zhao *et al* (2021). CC BY 4.0. (E) Many of the types of secondary structures are depicted in a single ssRNA strand. Adapted from Danaee *et al* (2018). Published by Oxford University Press. (F–H) Cytoskeletal filaments assemble from monomers via different pathways to form polymers with varying stiffness and stability. (F) Actin filaments polymerize from monomers via slow nucleation (binding ATP and forming trimers) and fast elongation via monomers binding to either end of the filament. Once steady-state length is reached, actin filaments undergo treadmilling in which monomers continuously bind to the barbed end and dissociate from the pointed end at similar rates. Adapted from Hohmann and Dehghani (2019). CC BY 4.0. (G) Microtubules polymerize from $\alpha\beta$ tubulin heterodimers into protofilaments by elongating from the + end. Thirteen protofilaments then laterally bind and roll up to form a hollow tube. The off-horizontal matching of α and β subunits on neighboring protofilaments creates a helical pattern of dimers with a discontinuity at the seam where the two ends of the protofilament sheet meet. Microtubules do not maintain a steady-state length but instead alternate between phases of shrinkage (catastrophe) and growth (rescue) that is made possible by the GTP cap at the growing end. Adapted from Hawkins *et al* (2010), Copyright (2010), with permission from Elsevier. (H) Intermediate filaments assemble from monomers into polar dimers which then form antiparallel apolar tetrameters. The addition of salt mediates lateral bundling of the tetramers into unit length filaments that serve as the basic building block for intermediate filaments. End-to-end annealing of ULFs creates polymeric intermediate filaments. Cartoon adapted from 'How are intermediate filaments assembled?,' (n.d.). (I) Mucins are the primary structural component of mucus that assemble from glycoproteins that have a central PTS-rich core flanked by a polymerization domain (orange) and dimerization domain (pink). Assembly into mucins proceeds by first forming glycoprotein dimers via linking at the dimerization domain, followed by glycosylation of the PTS regions, after which polymerization into mucin polymers is achieved by antiparallel linking of glycosylated dimers at their polymerization domains. Adapted from McShane *et al* (2021), Copyright (2021), with permission from Elsevier. (J) Intrinsically disordered proteins (IDPs) are distinct from their folded protein counterparts because they lack higher-order folding structure and have long segments of unfolded polypeptide. The unfolded regions (blue) are separated by small hydrophobic patches (yellow) that are prone to sticking together. IDPs can be modeled as chains of stickers (yellow) and spacers (blue). Folded proteins have their hydrophobic 'stickers' hidden in a folded core while the stickers along IDPs are fully exposed. The drive for stickers to 'stick' together makes IDPs prone to undergoing liquid–liquid phase separation (LLPS) and forming liquid-like biomolecular condensates that can coalesce (yellow). Adapted from Choi *et al* (2020). © 2020 by Annual Reviews.

molecules. The persistence length can also be defined and computed as the length over which the direction of two tangent vectors separated by a distance ΔL along the biopolymer remain correlated with one another (Rubinstein and Colby 2003, Maarel 2008), explicitly quantified as $\langle \cos\theta(\Delta L)\rangle = e^{-\Delta L/l_p}$, where θ is the angle between the two tangent vectors.

Monomeric length l_x: the length of the repeating building block, subunit, or monomer, where x signifies the type of subunit (e.g., $x = bp$ for DNA basepairs).

The linear charge density $\frac{Q}{L}$: the charge per unit length along the biopolymer backbone, which is typically negative for biopolymers in aqueous solution.

The relationship between the persistence length and contour length determines how flexible a biopolymer is, which plays a primary role in determining its conformation and/or structure (figure 1.1D), which I discuss in more detail in chapter 2.

Flexible biopolymers ($l_p \ll L$) often adopt random coil configurations which display no orientation or order, and the distributions of tangent vector directions along the chain are completely random at lengthscales beyond $\sim 2l_p$.

Semiflexible biopolymers ($l_p \sim L$) are more extended, with an anisotropic configuration, but exhibit some bending.

Rigid rod biopolymers ($l_p \gg L$) assume straight rod-like conformations with end-to-end distance of L.

Biopolymers can also adopt higher-order structures such as branches, loops, and folds, depending on their flexibility and nature of intrachain interactions (figure 1.2C–E).

1.2.1 Nucleic acids

1.2.1.1 Double-stranded deoxyribonucleic acid (dsDNA)

Double-stranded DNA polymers encode genetic information in long strands of nucleotides (adenine A, cytosine C, guanine G, and thymine T) that are paired together into basepairs (bp) via hydrogen bonding. These torsionally-twisted double-stranded chains of repeating basepairs (A–T or C–G) each have a cross-sectional diameter of $d \simeq 2$ nm and add $l_{bp} \simeq 0.34$ nm to the contour length L of the DNA chain, which can vary over orders of magnitude, from short 'oligos' with $L \approx \mathrm{O(nm)}$ to the human genome that spans meters ($L \approx \mathrm{O(m)}$).

In aqueous solution, dsDNA is negatively charged with a linear charge density of $\frac{Q}{L} = -2e\ \mathrm{bp}^{-1} \simeq -5.9e\ \mathrm{nm}^{-1}$. Electrostatic repulsion between neighboring segments of a dsDNA strand impacts its stiffness, which is quantified by its persistence length l_p. The contribution of electrostatic repulsion to l_p renders it dependent on the ionic conditions of the buffer, with increasing salt concentrations increasingly screening the negative charges thereby increasing the DNA flexibility (and reducing l_p).

The persistence length has been shown to be roughly inversely related to salt concentration (Marko and Siggia 1994, Manning 2006, Guilbaud *et al* 2019) and ranges from $l_p \simeq 110$ nm in the 'low salt' limit (e.g., [NaCl] <1 mM) to $l_p \simeq 45$ nm in the high salt ([NaCl] >100 mM) limit (figure 1.2A). Typical physiological conditions and experimental buffer conditions are in the range [NaCl] ≈10–100 mM, in which $l_p \simeq 50$ nm (Marko and Siggia 1995, Manning 2006, Guilbaud *et al* 2019).

While one typically thinks of a polymer as a linear chain with two free ends and no higher-order structure, and the genomes of eukaryotic cells are linear, DNA also naturally occurs in circular topologies with no free ends, and can adopt loops, sharp bends, and other higher-order structures, essential for, e.g., chromosomal compaction and gene regulation (figure 1.2C) (Matthews 1992, Cloutier and Widom 2004, Chan and Rubinstein 2023). The genomes of prokaryotes, as well as plasmid DNA, are supercoiled circular constructs that have no free ends and have significant torsional stress stored in the form of twist and writhe (Bednar *et al* 1994, Marko and Siggia 1994, 1995). The relative degrees of twist and writhe are dependent on the salt concentration and allow supercoiled constructs to adopt multiple conformations from planar structures to tightly wound superhelices. The supercoils in circular DNA can also be relaxed to form relaxed circular, 'open' circular, or ring topologies that have no stored torsional stress (Marko and Siggia 1994, 1995, Maarel 2008, Regan *et al* 2016).

The untwisting of supercoiled DNA into relaxed circular constructs, via enzymes such as topoisomerases or nicking enzymes, are essential to DNA replication, transcription, and repair (Adams *et al* 2013). Likewise, enzymes such as helicases and gyrases can introduce supercoils into relaxed circles and are essential to the replication process (Lohman and Bjornson 1996). Circular kinetoplast DNA, which make up mitochondrial genomes, are open circular constructs that can concatenate with one another to form large networks that resemble chain mail (Lukeš *et al* 2002, Klotz *et al* 2020).

There are also numerous site-specific restriction endonucleases that cleave both strands of dsDNA at specific sites that have a particular pattern of basepairs. This class of enzymes can linearize ring DNA with a single recognition site, and, with multiple sites, can chop up linear DNA strands into shorter fragments with lengths that depend on the number and placement of recognition sites (Brown *et al* 2001, Espeli and Marians 2004, Seol and Neuman 2016). Finally, there are classes of enzymes known as ligases that can reconnect broken strands and fragments of DNA, which play an essential role in replication of eukaryotic cells and healing DNA lesions from oxidation and radiation (Tomkinson *et al* 2006).

The diverse topologies and their interconversions are critical to processes such as DNA condensation, replication, transcription, repair, and apoptosis (Zhang and Xu 2000, Ohniwa *et al* 2006, Jinek *et al* 2012, Bax *et al* 2019), and can be harnessed to create materials with unique emergent properties that are unattainable with linear polymers (see e.g., Peddireddy *et al* 2020, Khanal *et al* 2022).

1.2.1.2 Single-stranded deoxyribonucleic acid (ssDNA)

Single-stranded DNA chains, simply one strand of a double-stranded DNA (dsDNA) construct, naturally occur during biological processes such as DNA unzipping and melting (figure 1.2B), and are necessary for DNA replication, repair, and synthesis (Crothers *et al* 1965, Alberts 2004, Adams *et al* 2013, Nelson *et al* 2020). These polymers are much more flexible than dsDNA, with reported persistence lengths of $l_p \simeq 1$–4 nm, dependent on the salt concentration (Saleh *et al* 2009, McIntosh and Saleh 2011, Chen *et al* 2012, Chi *et al* 2013, Roth *et al* 2018). However, the length between nucleotides is larger than l_{bp} for dsDNA, presumably due to the lack of twisting, with reported values of $l_{nt} \simeq 0.5$–0.7 nm (Mills *et al* 1999, Chen *et al* 2012, Roth *et al* 2018). Moreover, the nature of ssDNA flexibility has been shown to be more complex than that of linear elastic dsDNA, in part from the enhanced tendency to form loops and folds, exhibiting different regimes of stiffness that depend on the stretching force and ionic conditions (Saleh *et al* 2009, Stevens *et al* 2012).

In eukaryotes and prokaryotes, ssDNA constructs are produced transiently by enzyme-mediated unzipping of DNA, which is essential to, e.g., replication, transcription, and repair. Due to their flexibility, ssDNA are also more prone to form higher-order structures such as loops, hairpins, and folded motifs (figure 1.2C) that assist in, e.g., recombination and gene transfer (Matthews 1992, Bikard *et al* 2010). Finally, the genomic DNA of many viruses is single-stranded, which may facilitate packaging into the capsid head and recombination (Martin *et al* 2011, Speir and Johnson 2012, Stedman 2015).

1.2.1.3 Ribonucleic acid (RNA)

RNA polymers are highly-flexible single-stranded nucleic acid chains comprising four different nucleotides, similar to ssDNA, but with one of the four nucleotides, thymine, replaced by uracil. This substitution leads to key differences between ssDNA and RNA including different persistence lengths, end-to-end distances and lengths between nucleotides (table 1.1) (Conn and Draper 1998, Chen *et al* 2012). For example, RNA has been reported to have a larger persistence length and shorter contour length than a ssDNA chain with the same number of nucleotides, suggested to be due to more efficient stacking of uracil compared to thymine (Chen *et al* 2012). Other differences between ssDNA and RNA include more adoption of secondary and tertiary structures, such as hairpin loops, tetraloops, folds, cross-strand stacks, base triples, zippers, and adenosine platforms (figure 1.2D,E) (Cate *et al* 1996, Conn and Draper 1998). With the exception of very short RNA oligos, most RNA constructs adopt these higher-order structures, which are mediated by base pairing and ion binding. Reported persistence length values for RNA are in the range $l_p \simeq 2$–3 nm but have been shown to be highly dependent on the degree of folding, dropping by a factor of two upon folding (Caliskan *et al* 2005).

Double-stranded RNA constructs also exist in nature, though far less common than single-stranded RNA, and are typically associated with viral infection—serving as the genome of several viruses and generated in host cells during viral replication (Chen and Hur 2022). The relative abundance of single-stranded RNA as compared to double-stranded RNA, opposite to the prevalence of ssDNA and dsDNA, is due to the reduced stability of the base pair bonds as compared to their DNA counterparts. A primary contributing factor to this relative instability is the ribose sugars that replace the deoxyribose sugars in DNA, also rendering RNA more susceptible to degradation. dsRNA adopts helices similar to dsDNA but have been shown to be stiffer than dsDNA with reported persistence length values of $l_p \simeq 70$–80 nm, $\sim$50% larger than dsDNA (Kebbekus *et al* 1995, Hagerman 1997); and length between basepairs of $l_{bp} \simeq 0.28$ nm, $\sim$20% shorter than for dsDNA (Taylor *et al* 1985). These differences are likely due to more efficient inter-strand base stacking of RNA compared to DNA, as well as the formation of higher-order structures.

In nature, there are three main types of RNA—messenger RNA, transfer RNA, and ribosomal RNA—that play critical roles in translation of proteins based on the genetic code from DNA (Speir and Johnson 2012, Adams *et al* 2013, Mathews *et al* 2013). tRNA is rather short with $L \simeq 20$ nm (80 nt), while rRNA and mRNA have a wide range of lengths from $L \simeq 30$ nm to $L \simeq 2$ μm. The genomes of many viruses are also RNA, including SARS-CoV-2 and HIV, and have contour lengths that range from $L \simeq 0.5$ μm (1.7 kilobasepairs (kbp)) to $L \simeq 9$ μm (31 kbp).

1.2.2 Cytoskeleton filaments

The three primary biopolymers that comprise the cytoskeleton of eukaryotic cells include semiflexible actin filaments, rigid microtubules, and the family of flexible intermediate filaments. They each have highly distinct properties and polymerization pathways that dictate and differentiate their biological functions.

1.2.2.1 Filamentous actin (F-actin)

Actin filaments are ubiquitous eukaryotic biopolymers formed by globular actin monomers (G-actin), of molar mass $M_w = 42$ kDa and size $d_{\text{mon}} \simeq 4$–6 nm that polymerize into two inter-twisted polar strands with barbed (+) and pointed (−) ends.

The polymerization process entails an initial conformational change to G-actin, followed by a slow nucleation step, in which stable trimers are formed, then elongation, in which single monomers sequentially bind to the growing filament (figure 1.2F) (Pollard 1986). While monomers can bind to either end, the association/dissociation constants are substantially smaller/larger at the pointed (−) end, resulting in net growth from the barbed (+) end. This process is fueled by ATP hydrolysis and also requires Mg^{2+}, which binds to G-actin to induce the initial conformational change that favors nucleation and elongation (Frieden 1983, Vavylonis *et al* 2005). A critical concentration of monomers, $c_A^* \approx 0.1\ \mu$M in optimal polymerization conditions, is also required to shift the favored equilibrium from G-actin to F-actin (Pollard 1984). Alternatively, Ca^{2+} hinders polymerization and promotes depolymerization by competing with the Mg^{2+} binding site on actin, and thus shifts c_A^* to $\gtrsim 1\ \mu$M (Hartzell *et al* 2016, Ross 1985).

This ATP-fueled process results in filaments that have an actin monomer every $l_{\text{mon}} \simeq 2.7$ nm, diameter of $d \simeq 7$ nm, linear charge density $\frac{Q}{L} \simeq -4e\ \text{nm}^{-1}$, persistence length $l_p \simeq 10\ \mu$m (Gittes *et al* 1993, Pollard *et al* 2001), and typical lengths of $L \simeq 1$–$40\ \mu$m. Unlike DNA, in which the length is controlled by the sequence of basepairs, the actin polymerization process results in a distribution of lengths at any given monomer concentration, and the average length depends on the concentration of actin, Mg^{2+}, and ATP. Moreover, once filaments reach a steady-state distribution of lengths, they do not remain static filaments but instead are continuously depolymerizing at the pointed end and elongating at the barbed end, a process termed treadmilling, that results in constant ATP-fueled exchange or 'turnover' of monomers while maintaining a fixed filament length (figure 1.2F).

There are numerous actin binding proteins (ABPs) that can promote or hinder polymerization to shift steady-state filament length distributions, alter rates of polymerization and turnover, and even promote branching (Khaitlina and Hinssen 1997, Blanchoin *et al* 2000, Vavylonis *et al* 2005). For example, the capping and severing ABP gelsolin can be used to alter the F-actin length at any given c_A by promoting nucleation, the rate limiting step in polymerization (Janmey *et al* 1985, Ermentrout and Edelstein-Keshet 1998). Gelsolin-actin nuclei form much more rapidly than actin trimers without gelsolin such that elongation proceeds nearly entirely from gelsolin-capped nuclei (Khaitlina and Hinssen 1997, Kasza *et al* 2010). In this way, the molarity of gelsolin dictates the resulting molarity of filaments. Specifically, more gelsolin results in shorter filaments according to the relation $L_A \simeq (2.7\ \text{nm})\, c_A/c_G$, where c_G is the molarity of gelsolin. Cofilin is another ubiquitous ABP that enhances actin depolymerization via severing, but at high enough concentrations can also increase actin turnover by nucleating actin assembly (Bamburg 1999, Blanchoin *et al* 2000, Andrianantoandro and Pollard 2006). Another ABP widely used in *in vitro* experiments is the stabilizing ABP phalloidin, which binds to actin filaments to prevent treadmilling and stabilize the filaments against depolymerization. Phalloidin-stabilized filaments do not require a constant supply of ATP due to the suppressed treadmilling, and can more readily survive in suboptimal buffer conditions. Phalloidin stabilization also increases the actin filament persistence length to $l_p \simeq 17\ \mu$m (Gittes *et al* 1993).

In muscle tissue, actin is arranged in organized striated layers, providing the substrate that myosin motors act on to perform muscular function (Pollard 2003, Banerjee *et al* 2020). However, in the cytoskeleton of non-muscle cells, actin filaments arrange into various disordered and dynamic networks of entangled, crosslinked, and bundled filaments to provide cells with tensile strength, while enabling mobility and morphogenesis (Mogilner and Oster 1996, Stricker *et al* 2010. For example, the polymerization of actin filaments at the leading edge of cells drives motility and chemotaxis (Diez *et al* 2005); and actin stress fibers, composed of bundles of crosslinked actin filaments, mediate cell adhesion, morphogenesis, and nuclear stabilization (Tojkander *et al* 2012).

1.2.2.2 Microtubules (MTs)

Microtubules polymerize from tubulin dimers into hollow rigid rods with a diameter $d \simeq 25$ nm, $l_p \approx 1$ mm, and $L \simeq 1$–$40\ \mu$m. Like actin and nucleic acids, microtubules are negatively charged in solution, but with a much larger linear charge density of $\frac{Q}{L} \approx -32.5\mathrm{e\ nm}^{-1}$ (Minoura and Muto 2006), which renders them more electrically conductive and more susceptible to bundling via counterion condensation.

Each tubulin heterodimer, comprising α-tubulin and β-tubulin, has a molecular weight of $M_w = 110$ kDa and size of $d_T \approx 8$ nm. Both monomers bind GTP, which fuels polymerization, but only β-tubulin hydrolyzes GTP into GDP (Desai and Mitchison 1997). The polymerization process proceeds via nucleation followed by head-to-tail (α-to-β) binding of heterodimers to form protofilaments with β-tubulin at the (+) end and α-tubulin at the (−) end (figure 1.2G). These protofilaments then bind laterally to one another in a flat sheet of 13 via α–α and β–β interactions that are slanted at 10°. Following the binding of 13 protofilaments, the flat sheet rolls into a cylindrical tube known as the microtubule, in which α and β tubulin subunits form alternating helical patterns except at the seam where α and β subunits are swapped (figure 1.2G) (Gittes *et al* 1993, Desai and Mitchison 1997, Pegoraro *et al* 2017). Each ring of the microtubule thus comprises 13 tubulin dimers such that each dimer adds $d_T/13$ ($l_{\mathrm{ring}} \simeq 0.6$ nm) to the microtubule length L, which is dictated by the concentrations of tubulin and GTP.

Similar to actin, microtubules are not static structures; however, rather than treadmilling and maintaining a constant length, they undergo continuous growth and shrinkage, referred to as dynamic instability (figure 1.2G) (Desai and Mitchison 1997). During growth, ATP-bound tubulin dimers bind to the (+) end of the microtubule and subsequently hydrolyze their bound ATP, but only once within the microtubule lattice, then release the phosphate. Tubulin at the growing edge thus retains ATP that caps the microtubule and supports subsequent binding of ATP-bound tubulin. In the absence of ATP caps, ADP-bound tubulin subunits, which have a high dissociation constant, reside at the ends of the microtubule and are thus rapidly released from both ends, a process termed 'catastrophe'. One mechanism whereby ADP-bound tubulins at the microtubule ends prevent subsequent binding of additional tubulin dimers is the enhanced curvature of ADP-bound dimers, which causes uncapped protofilaments to peel away from the microtubule core. Following a period of rapid depolymerization, the microtubules begin to polymerize and grow again in a process termed 'rescue' (figure 1.2G). Similar to actin polymerization, Mg^{2+} is required for microtubule assembly and Ca^{2+} promotes depolymerization or shrinkage (Martin *et al* 1987, O'Brien *et al* 1997). However, high Mg^{2+} concentrations (>5 mM) can also inhibit polymerization (O'Brien *et al* 1990). This complex role of counterions on the dynamic instability has been suggested to arise from their impact on the GTP caps at the growing end of microtubules.

The continuous growth and shrinkage, which is largely unique to microtubules, allows them to more rapidly explore the intercellular space and find target sites. This enhanced 'search-capture' is likely necessary for microtubules to locate the kinetochores during mitosis (Blackwell *et al* 2017; Klemm *et al* 2018); and to guide axons during growth cone pathfinding (Tanaka *et al* 1995).

Moreover, myriad microtubule associated proteins (MAPs) can promote polymerization or catastrophe as well as alter the persistence length of microtubules. For example, MCAK and katanin both destabilize microtubules via depolymerization and severing, respectively (Hunter *et al* 2003, Hawkins *et al* 2010). The neuronal MAP, tau, stabilizes microtubules against depolymerization and stiffens their structure, with studies reporting several fold increases in persistence lengths to $l_p \approx$ 2–15 mm (compared to $l_p \approx$ 1 mm without tau) (Mickey and Howard 1995, Felgner *et al* 1997).

Paclitaxel, commonly referred to as Taxol, is a chemotherapy drug that also stabilizes microtubules against dynamic instability and catastrophe, and is widely used in *in vitro* studies owing to the inherent instability of untreated microtubules. Several studies have reported that Taxol stabilization increases microtubule stiffness, reporting values of $l_p \approx$ 3–5 mm, while studies on very short microtubules report decreased persistence lengths as low as $l_p \approx$ 0.1 mm (Kurachi *et al* 1995, Hawkins *et al* 2010). Another common method for maintaining stable microtubules *in vitro* is to use the non-hydrolyzable analog of GTP, GMPCPP, instead of GTP in the polymerization process, which, similar to Taxol, results in $\sim 5\times$ stiffer microtubules ($l_p \approx$ 5 mm) (Mickey and Howard 1995).

The unique rigidity of microtubules allows them to provide compressive strength and shape to cells and serve as tracks for intracellular cargo transport (Stamenović *et al* 2002, Brangwynne *et al* 2006, Hawkins *et al* 2010, Hueschen *et al* 2019, Osunbayo *et al* 2019, Gudimchuk *et al* 2020). This rigidity also supports asymmetric and elongated structures necessary for axonal growth, cilia beating, flagella-based motility, and positioning of the nucleus and other organelles (Haimo and Rosenbaum 1981, Robinson *et al* 1995, Fletcher and Mullins 2010). Moreover, during mitosis, dynamic networks of microtubules form spindles that segregate the daughter chromosomes and orient the plane of division, a process that requires both rigidity and dynamic instability (Gatlin and Bloom 2010, Edozie *et al* 2019). However, given their inability to bend in response to strain, microtubules are more susceptible to buckling than their more flexible cytoskeletal counterparts, actin and intermediate filaments (Kurachi *et al* 1995, Brangwynne *et al* 2006, Ricketts *et al* 2018).

1.2.2.3 Intermediate filaments (IFs)

Intermediate filaments constitute a large family of proteins, such as vimentin, keratin, neurofilaments, lamins, and desmins, that have different physical properties and biological functions (Herrmann *et al* 2007, Köster *et al* 2015, Charrier and Janmey 2016). However, all intermediate filaments are formed from the same basic building block—a central rod-like α-helix subunit comprising three coil domains separated by linkers and flanked on either end by an N terminus and C terminus of variable lengths (figure 1.2H). These extended protein subunits pair up via hydrophobic seams along the α-helix to form parallel coiled-coil dimers of length $l_\alpha \approx 46$–52 nm, which themselves then pair up in an antiparallel fashion to form tetrameters of dimers with opposing N and C termini, overlapping at their first coil domains. These resulting tetrameters, of length $l_{ULF} \approx 65$ nm, are apolar (i.e., no head and tail), due to the antiparallel orientation of dimers; and, upon increasing the ionic strength, they laterally assemble into bundles of the same length termed 'unit length filaments' (ULFs).

The final step in IF assembly is sequential annealing of ULFs to elongate into nonpolar filaments of diameter $d \backsimeq 9$–13 nm (figure 1.2H). The diameter is determined, in large part, by the number of tetramers comprising each ULF, which varies for different intermediate filaments, ranging from 16 monomers for keratins to 47 monomers for desmin (Herrmann *et al* 2007, Block *et al* 2015, Köster *et al* 2015); and can even vary from ULF to ULF along a given intermediate filament such that its mass per unit length is variable. Other assembly pathways for IFs include end-to-end annealing of preformed filaments and subunit exchange in a fully-formed filament.

While the resulting contour lengths of intermediate filaments are similar to their cytoskeletal partners, actin and microtubules, with reported values of $L \approx 5$–$20\ \mu$m, they are substantially more flexible and have more variable charge densities. Specifically, the persistence lengths of intermediate filaments have been reported to range from $l_p \approx 0.05\ \mu$m for neurofilaments (Beck *et al* 2010) to $l_p \approx 2\ \mu$m for vimentin (Nöding and Köster 2012); while linear charge density values ranging from $\frac{Q}{L} \simeq -3e$ nm^{-1} for keratin to $\frac{Q}{L} \simeq -14e$ nm^{-1} for vimentin have been reported (Herrmann *et al* 2007, Block *et al* 2015, Köster *et al* 2015).

These unique properties and diversity of intermediate filaments, as compared to actin and microtubules, are essential for the myriad roles they play in cells, ranging from differentiation and signaling to wound healing and migration. Their increased flexibility renders them more resistant to breakage and buckling than actin and microtubules, so they are expected to act as a 'cushion' that allows cells to absorb stress and provides a scaffold to support actin and microtubules against buckling (Herrmann *et al* 2007, Fletcher and Mullins 2010, Pegoraro *et al* 2017). Intermediate filaments are also uniquely extensible (i.e., they can stretch beyond their steady-state contour length), allowing for cells to stiffen in response to stresses, as needed. Finally, unlike actin and microtubules, which reside largely in the cytoplasm of cells, IFs provide scaffolding and support in the nucleus as well as the extracellular matrix (ECM) required for tissue formation (Herrmann *et al* 2007).

For example, lamins are a class of intermediate filaments that reside in the nucleus and are the primary component of the structural scaffold that supports the inner nuclear membrane and connects it to chromatin, thereby playing essential roles in replication, chromatin organization, nuclear migration, and cell differentiation. Vimentin, perhaps the most widely studied IF *in vitro*, is found in mesenchymal cells and has been shown to play a key role in cell adhesion, signaling, and migration by providing mechanical support and structure and aiding connections between cells via the ECM (Herrmann *et al* 2007). These functions have been shown to be critical to wound healing and other immune responses of cells.

1.2.3 Mucins

The family of mucin proteins are the primary building blocks of mucus that coats nearly all organs and resides in the interstitial space between cells. The polymeric nature of mucins endow mucus with its signature viscoelasticity, which is essential to its biological functions that include lubrication, mechanical protection, and selective passage and trapping of nutrients and toxins (Fass and Thornton 2023). Similar to intermediate filaments, mucins constitute an entire class of proteins that have several unifying features, but can also have different properties depending on their biological function. The two primary types of mucins are those that are membrane-bound, largely interacting with the ECM, and those that are secreted from epithelial cells to coat gastrointestinal, respiratory, and ocular organs, and allow for clearance of toxins and pathogens (Chen and Dulfano 1978, Lai *et al* 2007, McShane *et al* 2021).

The basic building block of a mucin polymer is a chain-like glycoprotein that contains repeating proline-threonine-serine (PTS) domains that have the ability to bind carbohydrates via their oxygen atoms (i.e., O-glycosylation). To allow for polymerization of these PTS-rich mucin subunits, they are flanked on either end by a C terminus dimerization domain and an N terminus polymerization domain. Polymerization proceeds by initial dimerization of two individual subunits via linking of their dimerization domains, followed by O-glycosylation of the PTS domains, giving these proteins a bottlebrush structure. Following glycosylation, the dimers are polymerized into long mucin polymers via linking of their polymerization domains (figure 1.2I) (McShane *et al* 2021, Hughes *et al* 2019).

The resulting linear bottlebrush polymers are considered flexible polymers, similar to nucleic acids, with diameters of $d \simeq$ 1–10 nm and persistence lengths of $l_p \simeq$ 3–40 nm, which are ~3 to 3000 times shorter than their contour lengths of $L \simeq$ 100 nm–10 μm. As such, they are assumed to adopt random coil configurations in solution; however, they can also adopt branched topologies that are suggested to aid in gelation (Celli *et al* 2005, Fass and Thornton 2023). Similar to other biopolymers, glycosylated mucins have an overall negative charge in solution; however, they have alternating sections of varying positive and negative charges along their backbone that depend on the type of mucin (Li *et al* 2013).

The bottlebrush configuration and high degree of glycosylation of mucins, with $\sim$80% of the mucin mass from sugars, allow mucins to swell dramatically in aqueous solution to form viscoelastic hydrogels necessary for lubrication, protection, and toxin clearance (McShane *et al* 2021, Fass and Thornton 2023). Branching and crosslinking of mucins have also been suggested to play important roles in gel formation, cell adhesion, inflammation, and metastasis (Beum and Cheng 2001, Fukuda 2002, Hughes *et al* 2019). The variable charge density of mucins likely facilitates branching and crosslinking, as well as aiding in specific passage and blockage of nutrients and toxins (Li *et al* 2013).

1.2.4 Intrinsically disordered proteins (IDPs)

Unlike the polymeric proteins discussed above, which have extended conformations, the majority of proteins, which are chains of peptides, are small soluble proteins that condense into intricately folded structures to hide their hydrophobic regions and render them similar to compact spheroids (Mathews *et al* 2013, Nelson *et al* 2020). If these soluble proteins are denatured, by, e.g., exposing them to extremely high or low temperature or placing them in an apolar solvent, they unravel into disordered polypeptide chains with similar properties to other flexible biopolymers such as DNA.

Intrinsically disordered proteins (IDPs) are a class of soluble proteins that differ from their ubiquitous folded counterparts by having large sections of polypeptide that do not assume any higher-order structure in native conditions (figure 1.2J). This lack of structure is likely a result of their relatively few hydrophobic residues that are the typical driving force underlying protein folding. IDPs instead primarily comprise charged and polar residues as well as glycine and proline. The overall net charge of IDPs varies between different types and can be positive or negative; and, like mucins, IDPs can have a variable charge profile along their backbone (Forman-Kay and Mittag 2013).

While different types of IDPs have different physical properties and functions, most IDPs can be modeled as flexible or semiflexible polymers with $l_p \simeq 0.4$–12 nm and $L \simeq 10$–100 nm (Choi *et al* 2011, Dyson 2016). However, an important contribution to the conformation and dynamics of IDPs is their hydrophobic patches that are inherently 'sticky' because of the driving force for these patches to come together to hide their hydrophobic regions. This stickiness leads IDPs to exhibit highly dynamic conformations that continuously transition between different conformational states with varying combinations of random coils, loops, and other higher-order structures that arise from the transient linking of the sticky patches along the IDP chain. Models that accurately capture the dynamics of IDPs treat them as chains of stickers separated by flexible chain linkers (figure 1.2J) (Choi *et al* 2011, McCarty *et al* 2019, Zeng *et al* 2020).

Intrinsically disordered proteins are probably most well known for their ability to undergo liquid–liquid phase separation (LLPS) (discussed in chapter 9), which is thought to play a key role in intracellular organization (McCarty *et al* 2019, Shimobayashi *et al* 2021, Abyzov *et al* 2022). Their lack of a shielded hydrophobic core likely facilitates aggregation in crowded conditions to lower the energetic cost of exposed hydrophobic or charged patches. Beyond LLPS, IDPs also form amyloid fibrils, which are ordered β-sheet structures that are hallmarks of amyloid diseases (Harmon *et al* 2017, Abyzov *et al* 2022).

1.2.5 And more…

Numerous other polymers abound in biological matter, including **polysaccharides** and **worm-like micelles (WLMs)**, which I will not cover in this text. Briefly, **polysaccharides**, the most abundant class of biopolymers found in nature, are long chains of monosaccharides polymerized via the action of enzymes with $l_p \simeq 30$–300 nm and $L \simeq 10$ nm–2 μm. They include, e.g., starch, cellulose, and glycogen, and are generally considered flexible polymers; see Dumitriu (2004), Thomas *et al* (2013), Ahmed *et al* (2018) for further reading. **Worm-like micelles** are flexible chains of amphiphiles (i.e., surfactants) that self-assemble in polar solvents, such as water, to protect their hydrophobic tails. While the physical properties of WLMs depend on their amphiphilic building blocks, they can generally be considered flexible polymers, with $d \simeq 1$–10 nm, $l_p \simeq 10$–40 nm and $L \simeq 10$ nm–10 μm; see Buchanan *et al* (2005), Helgeson *et al* (2009), Rogers *et al* (2014), Dreiss (2017), Dreiss and Feng (2017), Rothstein and Mohammadigoushki (2020) for further reading.

While there are far too many biopolymers to cover in this brief monograph, many of the mechanistic principles, experimental approaches, and results I describe in the following chapters can be generally applied to a wide range of biopolymers as well as synthetic polymers.

1.3 Biopolymer networks in biology

In vivo, biopolymers are typically in highly crowded environments and can form percolated networks via chemical and steric interactions and entanglements. These interactions play a principal role in dictating the physical properties and functions of organelles, cells, biofluids, and even organs. In fact, most cellular processes and functions are dictated not by individual biopolymers, but by the diverse and dynamic networks they form (figure 1.3). Sections II and III of this text will focus primarily on *in vitro* realizations of biopolymer networks inspired by biology. I describe a few of these inspirational networks below.

The **cytoskeleton** is quite possibly the most paradigmatic example of an *in vivo* biopolymer network (figure 1.3A). The cytoskeleton comprises actin filaments, microtubules, and intermediate filaments that interact to provide structural support, strength, and viscoelasticity to cells while allowing for motility, growth, division, apoptosis, and morphogenesis (Pollard 2003, Hoffman and Crocker 2009, Fletcher and Mullins 2010, Pegoraro *et al* 2017). Microtubules provide compressive strength, actin filaments provide tensile strength, and intermediate filaments act as shock absorbers, all working

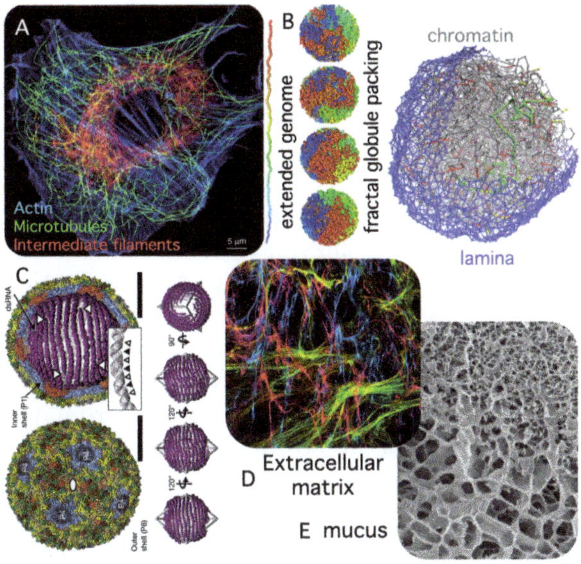

Figure 1.3. Biopolymer networks are ubiquitous in biology. Examples of the networks described in section 1.3 are depicted in the order they are presented in the text. (A) The cytoskeleton is a network of interacting actin, microtubules, and intermediate filaments. Image credit: Harald Herrmann. (B) The cell nucleus contains densely packed chromatin that packs itself in fractal-like patterns that evolve over time (left). Adapted from Mirny (2011), Copyright (2011), with permission from Springer Nature. It is protected by the laminar network (right, purple) comprising the intermediate filament, lamin. Adapted with permission from Liu *et al* (2021), Copyright (2021) by the American Physical Society. Chromatin (grey) is connected along a central chain (green), crosslinked (red), and physically linked to the lamina (orange). (C) dsRNA (purple) is packaged at high density into a viral capsid head (green) with an inner (top, P1) and outer (bottom, P8) shell, as depicted in the cross-sectional slice of the capsid interior (top left). The grey inset shows a zoom-in of the twisted double-stranded RNA structure and the white arrows show where the RNA moves from one layer to the other. Reconstructions of the packaged RNA at different orientations show the organization and tight packing. Adapted from Ilca *et al* (2019), Copyright (2019), with permission from Springer Nature. (D) The extracellular matrix is artistically rendered to show the multiple components and rigidity of the fibrous network. Image from cover of *Nature Reviews Materials*, vol 7, issue 3, 2018 (Image credit: Edna Cukierman). (E) Scanning electron microscopy image of mucus shows the hierarchical structure with a distribution of pore sizes. Adapted from Kirch *et al* (2012), with permission of PNAS.

collectively to provide mechanical integrity to cells. Numerous accessory proteins, crosslinkers, enzymes, and molecular motors allow the cytoskeleton to adopt a wide range of mechanical properties, continuously restructure, and do work, as needed for, e.g., mitosis, mechanosensation, cytoplasmic streaming, and adhesion. I discuss networks of cytoskeleton filaments in chapters 5, 7, and 8.

Steric and chemical interactions between actin, microtubules, and intermediate filaments are also now appreciated as being critical to the multifunctionality of the cytoskeleton. For example, as I describe in chapter 7, vimentin has been shown to stabilize microtubules against catastrophe and enhance rescue rates (Schaedel *et al* 2021). Moreover, cell crawling, while largely attributed to protrusions of polymerizing actin filaments at the leading edge of cells, also requires microtubules and intermediate filaments (Huber *et al* 2015, Dogterom and Koenderink 2019). IFs aid in cell adhesion to the substrate via interactions with the cell membrane, and microtubules provide rigid scaffolding to ensure mechanical integration between the leading edge and the adhesion site. I discuss composites of different cytoskeletal filaments in chapters 7 and 8.

In the nucleus, genomic DNA is condensed into a tightly-packed network of entangled chromatin to protect its genetic information and mediate DNA replication, transcription, looping, and enzyme binding kinetics (figure 1.3B) (Mirny 2011, Liu *et al* 2021). The viscoelastic nature of the chromatin network plays an important role in these processes and allows the nucleus to both resist stresses and deform to preserve its structural integrity (Guilak *et al* 2000, Erdel *et al* 2015, Chan and Rubinstein 2023). Moreover, laminar networks comprising the intermediate filament, lamin, connect the nuclear membrane to the chromatin to provide added mechanical protection and assist in positioning and organizing the chromatin, necessary for mitosis and transcription (Wintner *et al* 2020). I discuss DNA networks and their composites with other biopolymers in chapters 5–8.

Viral packaging of genomic dsRNA into capsids results in a tightly-packed, self-entangled polymer that experiences high osmotic pressure, electrostatic repulsion, and bending costs (figure 1.3C) (Mancini and Tuma 2012, Speir and Johnson 2012, Hesketh *et al* 2015). The motors used to package the genomes require exerting forces that exceed those generated by the dense and confined nucleic acid content in the capsid. The capsid rigidity must also be robust to the forces exerted by the confined genome in efforts to maximize its entropy and lower the energetic costs of bending and electrostatic repulsion. The resulting conformation of the packed genome, the power supplied by the motor, and packaging rates are all dictated by the free-energy minimization of the tightly-packed, self-interacting genome (Berndsen *et al* 2014). I discuss nucleic acids, molecular motors, and effects of confinement in chapters 5–9.

The extracellular matrix (ECM) is a composite network of protein and carbohydrate biopolymers, including collagens, elastins, polysaccharides, and glycoproteins, which structurally supports and connects cells in tissue (figure 1.3D) (Mecham 2011, Tseng *et al* 2012, Yue 2014, Theocharis *et al* 2016). The mechanical properties of the ECM determine the mechanical characteristics of tissues, and play key roles in tissue regeneration, cell migration, polarity, and anchoring (Mecham 2011, Theocharis *et al* 2016). I do not explicitly discuss the ECM in the following chapters as there is little *in vitro* work devoted to their mechanics, but I do discuss their interactions with intermediate filaments in chapters 5 and 7.

Mucus is a hydrated network of mucins that interact via steric entanglements and non-specific crosslinking, branching, and bundling (McShane *et al* 2021, Fass and Thornton 2023). This network is key to the viscoelastic nature of mucus that allows it to effectively coat, lubricate, and protect organs, tissues, and cells; as well as clear toxins from the respiratory pathway. Another notable property of mucus, which allows for its multifunctionality, is its hierarchical structure that allows it to respond primarily viscously at the microscopic level, allowing for passage of nutrients and wetting, while behaving largely elastic-like at macroscopic levels to support its role in mechanical protection and blocking toxins. This feature is due to the flexible nature of mucins and the hierarchical lengthscales over which they form entanglements, crosslinks, and bundles (Chen and Dulfano 1978, Lai *et al* 2009, 2007, Weigand *et al* 2017). I discuss mucus and mucin networks in chapter 5.

Biomolecular condensates or coacervates represent another canonical biopolymer network (Brangwynne *et al* 2015, McCarty *et al* 2019, André and Spruijt 2020, Donau *et al* 2020, Shimobayashi *et al* 2021). These structures form via liquid–liquid phase separation (LLPS) of different species of a network into droplet-like phases of highly-concentrated biopolymers, such as IDPs or RNA, and 'gas' phases that contain the uncondensed solute (Lu and Spruijt 2020, Fonin *et al* 2022). A unique feature of these droplets is that they remain mechanically similar to a fluid rather than exhibiting viscoelastic or elastic properties, despite their high biopolymer content (Ghosh *et al* 2021, Fonin *et al* 2022, Gouveia *et al* 2022). I discuss LLPS and other forms of phase separation and aggregation in chapter 9.

1.4 Biopolymer networks in physics and engineering

1.4.1 Elucidating polymer physics concepts

Beyond their importance to biology, biopolymer networks have been widely investigated as model systems to elucidate the physical principles underlying the dynamics of polymeric fluids and gels (Lin *et al* 2007, Tree *et al* 2013, Dai *et al* 2016, Regan *et al* 2016, Banik *et al* 2021). For example, the widely accepted **reptation model** for entangled polymers, pioneered by de Gennes and extended by Doi and Edwards (de Gennes 1979, 2003, Doi and Edwards 1988), models an entangled polymer as confined to a tube-like region formed by the surrounding entangling polymers (see figure 2.1). This tube potential suppresses motion transverse to the polymer contour such that each polymer diffuses curvilinearly along its backbone, a process termed reptation (see chapter 2 for further discussion).

While the reptation model was introduced in the 1970s and was quite successful in describing the dynamics of entangled polymer systems in the decade that followed, there was no direct evidence of tube-like confinement until 1994, when researchers showed the first direct evidence of reptation by pulling a fluorescent-labeled DNA molecule through an entangled polymer solution using optical tweezers (Perkins *et al* 1994) (see chapter 5, figure 5.1). Since that seminal work, myriad DNA studies have elucidated the dynamics of entangled and semidilute polymer solutions, testing theoretical predictions, connecting macromolecular dynamics to rheological properties, and probing the effects of DNA concentration, size, topology, and buffer conditions on network properties (Pecora 1991, Schroeder *et al* 2004, Robertson and Smith 2007a, 2007b, 2007c, Teixeira *et al* 2007, Chapman and Robertson-Anderson 2014, Pan *et al* 2014, Regan *et al* 2016, Hsiao *et al* 2017, Khan *et al* 2019, Zhou *et al* 2019, Soh and Doyle 2020, Banik *et al* 2021, Kong *et al* 2022).

Networks of semiflexible actin filaments have also been studied as model semiflexible polymers, and used to visualize and characterize the dynamics of polymers in tube confinement (see chapter 5) (Isambert and Maggs 1996, Granick *et al* 2010, Wang *et al* 2010). The reptation model was developed for flexible polymers and extended to rigid rods, but was unable to accurately describe the dynamics of semiflexible polymers with $l_p \sim L$. The extended conformation and slow dynamics of actin filaments allowed researchers to directly visualize single entangled filaments and track their reptation to directly measure the nature of tube confinement (Käs *et al* 1994, 1996, Romanowska *et al* 2009, Wang *et al* 2010). Moreover, armed with the experimentally accessible filament contours and fluctuation timescales, theoretical extensions to the reptation model to describe entangled semiflexible polymers were successfully developed and tested (Isambert and Maggs 1996, Gardel *et al* 2003, Koenderink *et al* 2006).

Finally, understanding the physics underlying the networks of circular polymers, in particular in the entangled regime, has been a topic of fascination and frustration for researchers for decades, and continues to elicit controversy and confusion (Rubinstein 1986, Iyer *et al* 2006, Kapnistos *et al* 2008, McLeish 2008, Habuchi *et al* 2010, Chapman *et al* 2012, Ge *et al* 2016, Michieletto 2016, Regan *et al* 2016, Michieletto *et al* 2017, Smrek *et al* 2019, Zhou *et al* 2019, Papale *et al* 2021, Parisi *et al* 2021, Ubertini *et al* 2022). Several properties of ring polymers and their synthesis complicate the field. First, engineering pure samples of circular synthetic polymers has proven elusive, as the cyclization process to convert linear chains nearly always leaves some linear chains not converted and can also introduce knots and concatenation (Bielawski *et al* 2002, Endo 2008, Kapnistos *et al* 2008). Moreover, experiments have shown that the presence of a small fraction of linear chains dramatically alters the rheological properties of ring polymer networks, exacerbating the problem of incomplete cyclization (McKenna and Plazek 1986, Chapman *et al* 2012, Haque and Grayson 2020, Peddireddy *et al* 2020, Subramanian and Shanbhag 2008). Finally, the reptation framework relies on 'head-first' diffusion of polymers which requires free ends (that rings of course do not have), so there is still debate as to whether or not rings can become entangled and undergo some form of modified reptation (Ge *et al* 2016, Michieletto *et al* 2017, Robertson and Smith 2007d, Shanbhag and Larson 2006, Smrek *et al* 2021). As discussed in section 1.2.1.1., DNA naturally exists in circular topologies, eliminating the need for cyclization, so pure ring samples can be produced. Moreover, because circular DNA molecules can be fluorescent-labeled, their diffusion and relaxation dynamics can be visualized to directly test proposed theoretical extensions to the tube model to account for the end closure of rings (Chapman *et al* 2012, Robertson and Smith 2007b, 2007c, Zhou *et al* 2021, 2019).

1.4.2 Materials applications

The viscoelastic properties of biopolymer networks, which can be tuned across a wide phase space by varying the concentrations and properties of the comprising biopolymers, make them ideal candidates for programmable material platforms (Koch *et al* 2020, McMillan *et al* 2019, Pei *et al* 2021, Thomas *et al* 2013). With lengths and stiffnesses that span many orders of magnitude, distinct assembly pathways, higher-order structures, and novel topologies, biopolymers offer much more diversity than their synthetic polymer counterparts. Moreover, the vast array of accessory proteins, drugs, and chemicals that can alter the structure and mechanics of biopolymers, as well as their interactions with their neighbors, expand the parameter space of tuning knobs many-fold. Further, many biopolymers and their accessory proteins are commercially available, making it easier for researchers without expertise in biology to build materials using biopolymers. For those that are not commercially available, researchers have developed purification protocols to facilitate *in vitro* experiments, e.g., Laib *et al* (2006).

Perhaps even more important than the expansive tunability of biopolymer networks as compared to their synthetic counterparts is their ability to exhibit self-generated non-equilibrium properties and active dynamics, as I describe in chapter 8 (Banerjee *et al* 2020, Burla *et al* 2019, Marfai *et al* 2023, Merindol and Walther 2017). By incorporating motor proteins or enzymes into biopolymer networks, or creating free-energy transduction pathways via chemical gradients or nucleotide hydrolysis, steady-state biopolymer networks can come to life—exhibiting contraction, extension, restructuring, stiffening, and flow; and generating forces, work, and directed motion (Alvarado *et al* 2013, Linsmeier *et al* 2016, Stanhope *et al* 2017, Jahnke *et al* 2020, Chandrakar *et al* 2022, Michieletto *et al* 2022, McGorty *et al* 2023). As such, biopolymer networks are widely studied in the field of active matter research (Lee *et al* 2021, Patteson *et al* 2016, Needleman and Dogic 2017, Voth 2017, Burkholder and Brady 2019, Ross *et al* 2019, Sheung *et al* 2021, Swartz and Camley 2021), and serve as design paradigms for engineering reconfigurable, self-healing, autonomous materials (Merindol and Walther 2017, Burla *et al* 2019, Donau *et al* 2020, Özkale *et al* 2021, Peng *et al* 2023, Wang *et al* 2023).

1.5 What next?

1.5.1 Open questions

The complexity and diversity of biopolymer networks leave many open questions that researchers are actively investigating. One such topic, which I discuss in chapter 6, is the role of polymer topology. Biopolymers are unique in the broad diversity of topologies and conformations they can adopt, including relaxed rings, supercoiled constructs, branched and bottlebrush configurations; and those that contain loops, hairpins, kinks, folds, knots, and sticky patches (Matthews 1992, Blanchoin *et al* 2000, Cloutier and Widom 2004, Espeli and Marians 2004, Bikard *et al* 2010, Honda *et al* 2010, Choi *et al* 2011, Chapman *et al* 2012, Rogers *et al* 2014, Gorczyca *et al* 2015, Li *et al* 2015, Mai and Schroeder 2016, Dong *et al* 2020, Smrek *et al* 2021, Khanal *et al* 2022). Groups of biopolymers can also form higher-order structures such as bundles, sheets and concatemers (Shin *et al* 2004, Krajina *et al* 2018, Klotz *et al* 2020, Lenz 2020, Abyzov *et al* 2022). The effect of these various topologies on the rheology and dynamics of the networks they comprise remains a topic of intense investigation.

Another frontier area of biopolymer network research, as I discuss in chapter 7, is understanding the properties and underlying mechanisms of composite systems composed of two or more distinct biopolymers (Fitzpatrick *et al* 2018, Ricketts *et al* 2018, Dogterom and Koenderink 2019, Francis *et al* 2019, Lopez-Menendez and Gonzalez-Torres 2019, Michieletto *et al* 2019, Shen 2020, Peddireddy *et al* 2021, 2022, Schaedel *et al* 2021, Shen *et al* 2021, Khanal *et al* 2022, Marfai *et al* 2023). Many previous works have shown that composites exhibit emergent mechanical properties that cannot be predicted by the properties of the corresponding single-component systems (Jensen *et al* 2014, Fitzpatrick *et al* 2018, Francis *et al* 2019, Lopez-Menendez and Gonzalez-Torres 2019, Khanal *et al* 2022). However, predicting the parameter space and network designs that give rise to emergent properties, and understanding the underlying physics, remain fervent research questions.

Finally, as I discuss above and in chapter 8, understanding the behavior and properties of non-equilibrium 'active' biopolymer networks is of critical importance to the burgeoning field of active matter research and to understanding the multitude of cellular processes that are driven by various forms of free-energy transduction (Mogilner and Oster 1996, Pollard *et al* 2001, Sanchez *et al* 2012, Needleman and Dogic 2017, Merindol and Walther 2017, Voth 2017, Alvarado *et al* 2019, Burkholder and Brady 2019, Burla *et al* 2019, Banerjee *et al* 2020). Biopolymer networks can be pushed out of equilibrium by, e.g., externally triggered changes to their environment, energy-consuming motors that physically push and pull on the comprising polymers, or enzymatic changes to polymer topology or structure (Lee *et al* 2021, Bertrand *et al* 2012, Nakamura *et al* 2014, Linsmeier *et al* 2016, Nguyen and Saleh 2017, Bacca *et al* 2019, Gurmessa *et al* 2018, 2021, Jahnke *et al* 2020, Ricketts *et al* 2020, Michieletto *et al* 2022, Lemma *et al* 2023, Marfai *et al* 2023, McGorty *et al* 2023). Biopolymer networks are facile systems to engineer and interrogate such non-equilibrium behavior, to reveal new emergent phenomena and test growing theoretical models to describe active matter phenomenon (Lenz 2014, Ronceray and Lenz 2015, Fodor *et al* 2016, Alvarado *et al* 2017, Ramaswamy 2017, Burkholder and Brady 2019).

1.5.2 What to expect

The rest of this monograph, Parts II–IV, builds on the basic framework, concepts, and ideas described in this chapter, layering in complexity and offering new perspectives along the way. I also strive to pay tribute to the diversity of amazing researchers who have helped me to understand and appreciate biopolymer networks. Though I am sure I have overlooked many of you and for that I apologize.

Part II provides the theoretical, experimental, and computational analysis tools needed to interrogate and understand biopolymer networks.

- Chapter 2 provides an overview of polymer physics concepts that we will need to describe and understand the dynamics of biopolymer networks that I discuss in Parts III and IV. It will build on the language and concepts that I introduced here to describe relationships between the physical properties of polymers, such as size, stiffness, and concentration, to the dynamics and rheological properties that the networks exhibit.
- Chapter 3 reviews the key experimental tools used to measure biopolymer network properties. These methods are primarily microscopy based but also include force spectroscopy and rheology.
- Chapter 4 describes computational analysis techniques that can be used to characterize and interpret data collected using the methods described in chapter 3. These techniques can be used to quantify properties such as biopolymer diffusion, structural correlation lengthscales, and network viscoelasticity. I will use

techniques, metrics, methodologies and frameworks discussed in this chapter to describe the properties of networks I discuss in Part III.

Part III discusses our current understanding of steady-state biopolymer networks, focusing on the biopolymers I discussed in section 1.2 of this chapter, with each chapter building in complexity.

- Chapter 5 describes the physical properties of single-component networks of DNA, actin, microtubules, and intermediate filaments. These properties include dynamics, structure, and rheology. I also discuss important considerations for network design and handling to aid those starting out in the field.
- Chapter 6 discusses the properties of networks comprising topologically-novel biopolymers, including DNA and mucins. The topologies discussed include relaxed circular or 'ring' DNA, supercoiled DNA, concatenated DNA rings, branched DNA, and bottlebrush and branched mucins.
- Chapter 7 builds on the results for single-component networks discussed in chapters 5 and 6 to discuss the properties of composites and blends of multiple polymeric species. Some examples include topological DNA blends, actin-microtubule composites, and DNA-actin composites.

Part IV moves the discussion to out-of-equilibrium networks and those that exhibit large-scale temporal and/or spatial heterogeneities not observed in the networks discussed in Part III.

- Chapter 8 discusses non-equilibrium biopolymer networks that incorporate motor proteins or enzymes to drive structural or mechanical changes to the network, or are pushed out of equilibrium by externally modulating the chemical environment. I will devote much real estate to the paradigmatic actomyosin networks that have been studied for decades. I will also discuss motor-driven microtubule networks and cytoskeletal composites, as well as salt-triggered cytoskeleton networks. Finally, I will discuss enzyme-driven topologically active DNA solutions and composites.
- Chapter 9 focuses on biopolymer systems that undergo varying types of phase separation and condensation. The primary discussion will be on liquid–liquid phase separation and biomolecular condensates, in particular, those formed by intrinsically disordered proteins.

Part V closes the monograph by presenting a community-inspired perspective on the open questions and challenges in the field and novel ways we may come together as researchers to advance knowledge and promote collaboration, resource-sharing, and training.

References

Abyzov A, Blackledge M and Zweckstetter M 2022 Conformational dynamics of intrinsically disordered proteins regulate biomolecular condensate chemistry *Chem. Rev.* **122** 6719–48

Adams R L P, Knowler J T and Leader D P 2013 *The Biochemistry of the Nucleic Acids* (Berlin: Springer Science & Business Media)

Ahmed J 2017 Rheological properties of gelatin and advances in measurement ed J Ahmed, P Ptaszek and S Basu *Advances in Food Rheology and Its Applications* (Woodhead Publishing Series in Food Science, Technology and Nutrition) (Woodhead Publishing) ch 15 pp 377–404

Ahmed S, Kanchi S and Kumar G 2018 *Handbook of Biopolymers: Advances and Multifaceted Applications* (Boca Raton, FL: CRC Press)

Alberts B 2004 *Molecular Biology of the Cell* (Garland)

Alvarado J, Cipelletti L and Koenderink G H 2019 Uncovering the dynamic precursors to motor-driven contraction of active gels *Soft Matter* **15** 8552–65

Alvarado J, Sheinman M, Sharma A, MacKintosh F C and Koenderink G H 2017 Force percolation of contractile active gels *Soft Matter* **13** 5624–44

Alvarado J, Sheinman M, Sharma A, MacKintosh F C and Koenderink G H 2013 Molecular motors robustly drive active gels to a critically connected state *Nat. Phys.* **9** 591–7

Amazon.com: envelop gel insoles for men—shoe inserts for walking, running, hiking—insoles for standing all day—cushion soles for heels, arch support, plantar fasciitis flat feet—sneaker boot insoles : health & household [WWW Document] n.d. https://amazon.com/Envelop-Gel-Insoles-Orthotics-Fasciitis/dp/B00L3KYEFS?th=1 (accessed 1 September 2023)

Amin M S, Park Y, Lue N, Dasari R R, Badizadegan K, Feld M S and Popescu G 2007 Microrheology of red blood cell membranes using dynamic scattering microscopy *Opt. Express* **15** 17001

Amnuanpol S 2016 Physical origin of DNA unzipping *J. Biol. Phys.* **42** 69–82

André A A M and Spruijt E 2020 Liquid–liquid phase separation in crowded environments *Int. J. Mol. Sci.* **21** 5908

Andrianantoandro E and Pollard T D 2006 Mechanism of actin filament turnover by severing and nucleation at different concentrations of ADF/cofilin *Mol. Cell* **24** 13–23

Bacca M, Saleh O A and McMeeking R M 2019 Contraction of polymer gels created by the activity of molecular motors *Soft Matter* **15** 4467–75

Bamburg J R 1999 Proteins of the ADF/cofilin family: essential regulators of actin dynamics *Annu. Rev. Cell Dev. Biol.* **15** 185–230

Banerjee S, Gardel M L and Schwarz U S 2020 The actin cytoskeleton as an active adaptive material *Annu. Rev. Condens. Matter Phys.* **11** 421–39

Banik S, Kong D, San Francisco M J and McKenna G B 2021 Monodisperse lambda DNA as a model to conventional polymers: a concentration-dependent scaling of the rheological properties *Macromolecules* **54** 8632–54

Barriga E H and Mayor R 2019 Adjustable viscoelasticity allows for efficient collective cell migration *Semin. Cell Dev. Biol.* **93** 55–68

Bax B D, Murshudov G, Maxwell A and Germe T 2019 DNA topoisomerase inhibitors: trapping a DNA-cleaving machine in motion *J. Mol. Biol.* **431** 3427–49

Beck R, Deek J, Choi M C, Ikawa T, Watanabe O, Frey E, Pincus P and Safinya C R 2010 Unconventional salt trend from soft to stiff in single neurofilament biopolymers *Langmuir* **26** 18595–9

Bednar J, Furrer P, Stasiak A, Dubochet J, Egelman E H and Bates A D 1994 The twist, writhe and overall shape of supercoiled DNA change during counterion-induced transition from a loosely to a tightly interwound superhelix: possible implications for DNA structure *in vivo* *J. Mol. Biol.* **235** 825–47

Berndsen Z T, Keller N, Grimes S, Jardine P J and Smith D E 2014 Nonequilibrium dynamics and ultraslow relaxation of confined DNA during viral packaging *Proc. Natl Acad. Sci.* **111** 8345–50

Bertrand O J N, Fygenson D K and Saleh O A 2012 Active, motor-driven mechanics in a DNA gel *Proc. Natl Acad. Sci.* **109** 17342–7

Beum P V and Cheng P-W 2001 Biosynthesis and function of ß 1,6 branched mucin-type glycans ed A M Wu *The Molecular Immunology of Complex Carbohydrates—2, Advances in Experimental Medicine and Biology* (Boston, MA: Springer) pp 279–312

Bielawski C W, Benitez D and Grubbs R H 2002 An 'endless' route to cyclic polymers *Sci. Sci.* **297** 2041–4

Bikard D, Loot C, Baharoglu Z and Mazel D 2010 Folded DNA in action: hairpin formation and biological functions in prokaryotes *Microbiol. Mol. Biol. Rev.* **74** 570–88

Blackwell R *et al* 2017 Contributions of microtubule dynamic instability and rotational diffusion to kinetochore capture *Biophys. J.* **112** 552–63

Blanchoin L, Pollard T D and Mullins R D 2000 Interactions of ADF/cofilin, Arp2/3 complex, capping protein and profilin in remodeling of branched actin filament networks *Curr. Biol.* **10** 1273–82

Block J, Schroeder V, Pawelzyk P, Willenbacher N and Köster S 2015 Physical properties of cytoplasmic intermediate filaments *Biochim. Biophys. Acta (BBA)—Mol. Cell Res.* **1853** 3053–64

Brangwynne C P, MacKintosh F C, Kumar S, Geisse N A, Talbot J, Mahadevan L, Parker K K, Ingber D E and Weitz D A 2006 Microtubules can bear enhanced compressive loads in living cells because of lateral reinforcement *J. Cell Biol.* **173** 733–41

Brangwynne C P, Tompa P and Pappu R V 2015 Polymer physics of intracellular phase transitions *Nat. Phys.* **11** 899–904

Brewer M 2021 Solid and liquid responses of a non-Newtonian fluid *Phys. Today* **74** 64

Brown S, Lenczycki T and Szamel G 2001 Influence of topological constraints on the statics and dynamics of ring polymers *Phys. Rev. E.* **63** 052801

Buchanan M, Atakhorrami M, Palierne J F and Schmidt c f 2005 Comparing macrorheology and one- and two-point microrheology in wormlike micelle solutions *Macromolecules* **38** 8840–4

Burkholder E W and Brady J F 2019 Fluctuation-dissipation in active matter *J. Chem. Phys.* **ACTV2019** 184901

Burla F, Mulla Y, Vos B E, Aufderhorst-Roberts A and Koenderink G H 2019 From mechanical resilience to active material properties in biopolymer networks *Nat. Rev. Phys.* **1** 249–63

Caliskan G, Hyeon C, Perez-Salas U, Briber R M, Woodson S A and Thirumalai D 2005 Persistence length changes dramatically as RNA folds *Phys. Rev. Lett.* **95** 268303

Cate J H, Gooding A R, Podell E, Zhou K, Golden B L, Szewczak A A, Kundrot C E, Cech T R and Doudna J A 1996 RNA tertiary structure mediation by adenosine platforms *Science* **273** 1696–9

Celli J, Gregor B, Turner B, Afdhal N H, Bansil R and Erramilli S 2005 Viscoelastic properties and dynamics of porcine gastric mucin *Biomacromolecules* **6** 1329–33

Chan B and Rubinstein M 2023 Theory of chromatin organization maintained by active loop extrusion *Proc. Natl Acad. Sci.* **120** e2222078120

Chanda M and Roy S K 2008 *Industrial Polymers, Specialty Polymers, and Their Applications* (Boca Raton, FL: CRC Press)

Chandrakar P *et al* 2022 Engineering stability, longevity, and miscibility of microtubule-based active fluids *Soft Matter* **18** 1825–35

Chapman C D and Robertson-Anderson R M 2014 Nonlinear microrheology reveals entanglement-driven molecular-level viscoelasticity of concentrated DNA *Phys. Rev. Lett.* **113** 098303

Chapman C D, Shanbhag S, Smith D E and Robertson-Anderson R M 2012 Complex effects of molecular topology on diffusion in entangled biopolymer blends *Soft Matter* **8** 9177–82

Charrier E E and Janmey P A 2016 Mechanical properties of intermediate filament proteins ed M B Omary and R K H Liem *Methods Enzymol., Intermediate Filament Proteins* (New York: Academic) ch 2 pp 35–57

Chen H, Meisburger S P, Pabit S A, Sutton J L, Webb W W and Pollack L 2012 Ionic strength-dependent persistence lengths of single-stranded RNA and DNA *Proc. Natl Acad. Sci.* **109** 799–804

Chen T M and Dulfano M J 1978 Mucus viscoelasticity and mucociliary transport rate *J. Lab. Clin. Med.* **91** 423–31

Chen Y G and Hur S 2022 Cellular origins of dsRNA, their recognition and consequences *Nat. Rev. Mol. Cell Biol.* **23** 286–301

Chhabra R P 2010 Non-Newtonian fluids: an introduction ed J M Krishnan, A P Deshpande and P B S Kumar *Rheology of Complex Fluids* (New York: Springer) pp 3–34

Chi Q, Wang G and Jiang J 2013 The persistence length and length per base of single-stranded DNA obtained from fluorescence correlation spectroscopy measurements using mean field theory *Phys.* A **392** 1072–9

Choi J-M, Holehouse A S and Pappu R V 2020 Physical principles underlying the complex biology of intracellular phase transitions *Annu. Rev. Biophys.* **49** 107–33

Choi U B, McCann J J, Weninger K R and Bowen M E 2011 Beyond the random coil: stochastic conformational switching in intrinsically disordered proteins *Structure* **19** 566–76

Cloutier T E and Widom J 2004 Spontaneous sharp bending of double-stranded DNA *Mol. Cell* **14** 355–62

Conn G L and Draper D E 1998 RNA structure *Curr. Opin. Struct. Biol.* **8** 278–85

Crothers D M, Kallenbach N R and Zimm B H 1965 The melting transition of low-molecular-weight DNA: theory and experiment *J. Mol. Biol.* **11** 802–20

Dai L, Renner C B and Doyle P S 2016 The polymer physics of single DNA confined in nanochannels *Adv. Colloid Interface Sci.* **232** 80–100

Danaee P, Rouches M, Wiley M, Deng D, Huang L and Hendrix D 2018 bpRNA: large-scale automated annotation and analysis of RNA secondary structure *Nucleic Acids Res.* **46** 5381–94

de Gennes P-G 1979 *Scaling Concepts in Polymer Physics* (Cornell University Press)

de Gennes P G 2003 Reptation of a polymer chain in the presence of fixed obstacles *J. Chem. Phys.* **55** 572–9

Desai A and Mitchison T J 1997 Microtubule polymerization dynamics *Annu. Rev. Cell Dev. Biol.* **13** 83–117

Diez S *et al* 2005 Subsecond reorganization of the actin network in cell motility and chemotaxis *Proc. Natl Acad. Sci.* **102** 7601–6

Dogterom M and Koenderink G H 2019 Actin–microtubule crosstalk in cell biology *Nat. Rev. Mol. Cell Biol.* **20** 38–54

Doi M 1996 *Introduction to Polymer Physics* (Oxford: Clarendon)

Doi M and Edwards S F 1988 *The Theory of Polymer Dynamics* (Oxford: Clarendon)

Donau C *et al* 2020 Active coacervate droplets as a model for membraneless organelles and a platform towards synthetic life *Nat. Commun.* **11** 5167

Dong Y, Yao C, Zhu Y, Yang L, Luo D and Yang D 2020 DNA functional materials assembled from branched DNA: design, synthesis, and applications *Chem. Rev.* **120** 9420–81

Dreiss C A and Feng Y (ed) 2017 *Wormlike Micelles: Advances in Systems, Characterisation and Applications* (London: Royal Society of Chemistry)

Dreiss C A 2017 Wormlike micelles: an introduction *Wormlike Micelles: Advances in Systems, Characterisation and Applications* (Soft Matter Series) ed C A Dreiss and Y Feng (Cambridge: Royal Society of Chemistry) ch 1 pp 1–8

Dumitriu S (ed) 2004 *Polysaccharides: Structural Diversity and Functional Versatility* 2nd edn (Boca Raton, FL: CRC Press)

Dyson H J 2016 Making sense of intrinsically disordered proteins *Biophys. J.* **110** 1013–6

Edozie B, Sahu S, Pitta M, Englert A, do Rosario C F and Ross J L 2019 Self-organization of spindle-like microtubule structures *Soft Matter* **15** 4797–807

Endo K 2008 Synthesis and properties of cyclic polymers *Adv. Polym. Sci. Adv. Polym. Sci.* **217** 121–83

Epoxy resin vs. epoxy adhesive—sticky aide 2022 https://stickyaide.com/epoxy-resin-vs-epoxy-adhesive/ (accessed 1 September 2023).

Erdel F, Baum M and Rippe K 2015 The viscoelastic properties of chromatin and the nucleoplasm revealed by scale-dependent protein mobility *J. Phys. Condens. Matter* **27** 064115

Ermentrout G B and Edelstein-Keshet L 1998 Models for the length distributions of actin filaments: II. Polymerization and fragmentation by gelsolin acting together *Bull. Math. Biol.* **60** 477–503

Espeli O and Marians K J 2004 Untangling intracellular DNA topology *Mol. Microbiol.* **52** 925–31

Extra-creamy scrambled eggs recipe [WWW Document], NYT Cooking n.d. https://cooking.nytimes.com/recipes/1021931-extra-creamy-scrambled-eggs (accessed 1 September 2023).

Fass D and Thornton D J 2023 Mucin networks: dynamic structural assemblies controlling mucus function *Curr. Opin. Struct. Biol.* **79** 102524

Felgner H, Frank R, Biernat J, Mandelkow E-M, Mandelkow E, Ludin B, Matus A and Schliwa M 1997 Domains of neuronal microtubule-associated proteins and flexural rigidity of microtubules *J. Cell Biol.* **138** 1067–75

Fitzpatrick R, Michieletto D, Peddireddy K R, Hauer C, Kyrillos C, Gurmessa B J and Robertson-Anderson R M 2018 Synergistic interactions between DNA and actin trigger emergent viscoelastic behavior *Phys. Rev. Lett.* **121** 257801

Fletcher D A and Mullins R D 2010 Cell mechanics and the cytoskeleton *Nature* **463** 485–92

Fodor É, Nardini C, Cates M E, Tailleur J, Visco P and van Wijland F 2016 How far from equilibrium is active matter? *Phys. Rev. Lett.* **117** 038103

Fonin A V, Antifeeva I A, Kuznetsova I M, Turoverov K K, Zaslavsky B Y, Kulkarni P and Uversky V N 2022 Biological soft matter: intrinsically disordered proteins in liquid–liquid phase separation and biomolecular condensates *Essays Biochem.* **66** 831–47

Forman-Kay J D and Mittag T 2013 From sequence and forces to structure, function, and evolution of intrinsically disordered proteins *Structure* **21** 1492–9

Francis M L, Ricketts S N, Farhadi L, Rust M J, Das M, Ross J L and Robertson-Anderson R M 2019 Non-monotonic dependence of stiffness on actin crosslinking in cytoskeleton composites *Soft Matter* **15** 9056–65

Frieden C 1983 Polymerization of actin: mechanism of the Mg2+-induced process at pH 8 and 20 degrees C *Proc. Natl Acad. Sci. USA* **80** 6513–7

Fukuda M 2002 Roles of mucin-type O-glycans in cell adhesion *Biochim. Biophys. Acta (BBA)—Gen. Subj.* **1573** 394–405

Furst E M and Squires T M 2017 *Microrheology* (Oxford: Oxford University Press)
Gardel M L, Valentine M T, Crocker J C, Bausch A R and Weitz D A 2003 Microrheology of entangled F-actin solutions *Phys. Rev. Lett.* **91** 158302
Gatlin J C and Bloom K 2010 Microtubule motors in eukaryotic spindle assembly and maintenance *Semin. Cell Dev. Biol.* **21** 248–54
Ge T, Panyukov S and Rubinstein M 2016 Self-similar conformations and dynamics in entangled melts and solutions of nonconcatenated ring polymers *Macromolecules* **49** 708–22
Georgiades P, Pudney P D A, Thornton D J and Waigh T A 2014 Particle tracking microrheology of purified gastrointestinal mucins *Biopolymers* **101** 366–77
Ghosh A, Kota D and Zhou H-X 2021 Shear relaxation governs fusion dynamics of biomolecular condensates *Nat. Commun.* **12** 5995
Gittes F, Mickey B, Nettleton J and Howard J 1993 Flexural rigidity of microtubules and actin filaments measured from thermal fluctuations in shape *J. Cell Biol.* **120** 923–34
Gorczyca S M, Chapman C D and Robertson-Anderson R M 2015 Universal scaling of crowding-induced DNA mobility is coupled with topology-dependent molecular compaction and elongation *Soft Matter* **11** 7762–8
Gouveia B, Kim Y, Shaevitz J W, Petry S, Stone H A and Brangwynne C P 2022 Capillary forces generated by biomolecular condensates *Nature* **609** 255–64
Granick S, Bae S C, Wang B, Kumar S, Guan J A, Yu C Q, Chen K J and Kuo J 2010 Single-molecule methods in polymer science *J. Polym. Sci. Part B-Polym. Phys.* **48** 2542–3
Gudimchuk N B *et al* 2020 Mechanisms of microtubule dynamics and force generation examined with computational modeling and electron cryotomography *Nat. Commun.* **11** 3765
Guilak F, Tedrow J R and Burgkart R 2000 Viscoelastic properties of the cell nucleus *Biochem. Biophys. Res. Commun.* **269** 781–6
Guilbaud S, Salomé L, Destainville N, Manghi M and Tardin C 2019 Dependence of DNA persistence length on ionic strength and ion type *Phys. Rev. Lett.* **122** 028102
Gurmessa B J, Bitten N, Nguyen D T, Saleh O A, Ross J L, Das M and Robertson-Anderson R M 2018 Triggered disassembly and reassembly of actin networks induces rigidity phase transitions *Soft Matter* **15** 1335–44
Gurmessa B J, Rust M J, Das M, Ross J L and Robertson-Anderson R M 2021 Salt-mediated stiffening, destruction, and resculpting of actomyosin network *Front. Phys.* **9** 760340
Habuchi S, Satoh N, Yamamoto T, Tezuka Y and Vacha M 2010 Multimode diffusion of ring polymer molecules revealed by a single-molecule study *Angew. Chem.* **122** 1460–3
Hagerman P J 1997 Flexibility of RNA *Annu. Rev. Biophys. Biomol. Struct.* **26** 139–56
Haimo L T and Rosenbaum J L 1981 Cilia, flagella, and microtubules *J. Cell Biol.* **91** 125s–30s
Haque F M and Grayson S M 2020 The synthesis, properties and potential applications of cyclic polymers *Nat. Chem.* **12** 433–44
Harmon T S, Holehouse A S, Rosen M K and Pappu R V 2017 Intrinsically disordered linkers determine the interplay between phase separation and gelation in multivalent proteins *eLife* **6** e30294
Hartzell C A, Jankowska K I, Burkhardt J K and Lewis R S 2016 Calcium influx through CRAC channels controls actin organization and dynamics at the immune synapse *eLife* **5** e14850
Hawkins T, Mirigian M, Selcuk Yasar M and Ross J L 2010 Mechanics of microtubules *J. Biomech.* Special Issue on Cell Mechanobiology **43** 23–30
Helgeson M, Nettesheim F, Liberatore , Vasquez P, Wagner N, Cook L, Porcar and Hu Y 2009 Microstructure and shear rheology of entangled wormlike micelles in solution *J. Rheol.* **53** 441–58

Herrmann H, Bär H, Kreplak L, Strelkov S V and Aebi U 2007 Intermediate filaments: from cell architecture to nanomechanics *Nat. Rev. Mol. Cell Biol.* **8** 562–73

Hesketh E L, Meshcheriakova Y, Dent K C, Saxena P, Thompson R F, Cockburn J J, Lomonossoff G P and Ranson N A 2015 Mechanisms of assembly and genome packaging in an RNA virus revealed by high-resolution cryo-EM *Nat. Commun.* **6** 10113

Hoffman B D and Crocker J C 2009 Cell mechanics: dissecting the physical responses of cells to force *Annu. Rev. Biomed. Eng.* **11** 259–88

Hohmann T and Dehghani F 2019 The cytoskeleton—a complex interacting meshwork *Cells* **8** 362

Honda S, Yamamoto T and Tezuka Y 2010 Topology-directed control on thermal stability: micelles formed from linear and cyclized amphiphilic block copolymers *J. Am. Chem. Soc.* **132** 10251–3

How are intermediate filaments assembled? [WWW Document] MBInfo n.d. https://mechanobio.info/cytoskeleton-dynamics/what-is-the-cytoskeleton/what-are-intermediate-filaments/how-are-intermediate-filaments-assembled/ (accessed 3 September 2023).

Hsiao K-W, Sasmal C, Ravi Prakash J and Schroeder C M 2017 Direct observation of DNA dynamics in semidilute solutions in extensional flow *J. Rheol.* **61** 151–67

Huber F, Boire A, López M P and Koenderink G H 2015 Cytoskeletal crosstalk: when three different personalities team up *Curr. Opin. Cell Biol.* **32** 39–47

Hueschen C L, Galstyan V, Amouzgar M, Phillips R and Dumont S 2019 Microtubule end-clustering maintains a steady-state spindle shape *Curr. Biol.* **29** 700–708.e5

Hughes G W, Ridley C, Collins R, Roseman A, Ford R and Thornton D J 2019 The MUC5B mucin polymer is dominated by repeating structural motifs and its topology is regulated by calcium and pH *Sci. Rep.* **9** 17350

Hunter A W, Caplow M, Coy D L, Hancock W O, Diez S, Wordeman L and Howard J 2003 The kinesin-related protein MCAK is a microtubule depolymerase that forms an atp-hydrolyzing complex at microtubule ends *Mol. Cell* **11** 445–57

Ilca S L, Sun X, El Omari K, Kotecha A, de Haas F, DiMaio F, Grimes J M, Stuart D I, Poranen M M and Huiskonen J T 2019 Multiple liquid crystalline geometries of highly compacted nucleic acid in a dsRNA virus *Nature* **570** 252–6

Isambert H and Maggs A C 1996 Dynamics and rheology of actin solutions *Macromolecules* **29** 1036–40

Iyer B V S, Lele A K and Juvekar V A 2006 Flexible ring polymers in an obstacle environment: molecular theory of linear viscoelasticity *Phys. Rev.* E **74** 021805

Jahnke K, Weiss M, Weber C, Platzman I, Göpfrich K and Spatz J P 2020 Engineering Light-responsive contractile actomyosin networks with DNA nanotechnology *Adv. Biosyst.* **4** 2000102

Janmey P A, Chaponnier C, Lind S E, Zaner K S, Stossel T P and Yin H L 1985 Interactions of gelsolin and gelsolin-actin complexes with actin. Effects of calcium on actin nucleation, filament severing, and end blocking *Biochemistry* **24** 3714–23

Jensen M H, Morris E J, Goldman R D and Weitz D A 2014 Emergent properties of composite semiflexible biopolymer networks *BioArchitecture* **4** 138–43

Jinek M, Chylinski K, Fonfara I, Hauer M, Doudna J A and Charpentier E 2012 A programmable dual-RNA–guided DNA endonuclease in adaptive bacterial immunity *Science* **337** 816–21

Kapnistos M, Lang M, Vlassopoulos D, Pyckhout-Hintzen W, Richter D, Cho D, Chang T and Rubinstein M 2008 Unexpected power-law stress relaxation of entangled ring polymers *Nat. Mater.* **7** 997–1002

Käs J, Strey H and Sackmann E 1994 Direct imaging of reptation for semiflexible actin filaments *Nature* **368** 226–9

Käs J, Strey H, Tang J X, Finger D, Ezzell R, Sackmann E and Janmey P A 1996 F-actin, a model polymer for semiflexible chains in dilute, semidilute, and liquid crystalline solutions *Biophys. J.* **70** 609–25

Kasza K E, Broedersz C P, Koenderink G H, Lin Y C, Messner W, Millman E A, Nakamura F, Stossel T P, MacKintosh F C and Weitz D A 2010 Actin filament length tunes elasticity of flexibly cross-linked actin networks *Biophys. J.* **99** 1091–100

Kebbekus P, Draper D E and Hagerman P 1995 Persistence length of RNA *Biochemistry* **34** 4354–7

Khaitlina S and Hinssen H 1997 Conformational changes in actin induced by its interaction with gelsolin *Biophys. J.* **73** 929–37

Khan M, Regan K and Robertson-Anderson R M 2019 Optical tweezers microrheology maps the dynamics of strain-induced local inhomogeneities in entangled polymers *Phys. Rev. Lett.* **123** 038001

Khanal P, Peddireddy K R, Marfai J, McGorty R and Robertson-Anderson R M 2022 DNA topology dictates emergent bulk elasticity and hindered macromolecular diffusion in DNA-dextran composites *J. Rheol.* **66** 699–715

Kirch J, Schneider A, Abou B, Hopf A, Schaefer U F, Schneider M, Schall C, Wagner C and Lehr C-M 2012 Optical tweezers reveal relationship between microstructure and nanoparticle penetration of pulmonary mucus *Proc. Natl Acad. Sci.* **109** 18355–60

Klemm A H, Bosilj A, Glunc ic M, Pavin N and Tolic× I M 2018 Metaphase kinetochore movements are regulated by kinesin-8 motors and microtubule dynamic instability *MBoC* **29** 1332–45

Klotz A R, Soh B W and Doyle P S 2020 Equilibrium structure and deformation response of 2D kinetoplast sheets *PNAS* **117** 121–7

Koch J, Gantenbein S, Masania K, Stark W J, Erlich Y and Grass R N 2020 A DNA-of-things storage architecture to create materials with embedded memory *Nat. Biotechnol.* **38** 39–43

Koenderink G H, Atakhorrami M, MacKintosh F C and Schmidt c f 2006 High-frequency stress relaxation in semiflexible polymer solutions and networks *Phys. Rev. Lett.* **96** 138307

Kong D, Banik S, San Francisco M J, Lee M, Robertson Anderson R M, Schroeder C M and McKenna G B 2022 Rheology of entangled solutions of ring–linear DNA blends *Macromolecules* **55** 1205–17

Köster S, Weitz D A, Goldman R D, Aebi U and Herrmann H 2015 Intermediate filament mechanics *in vitro* and in the cell: from coiled coils to filaments, fibers and networks *Curr. Opin. Cell Biol.* Cell architecture **32** 82–91

Krajina B A, Zhu A, Heilshorn S C and Spakowitz A J 2018 Active DNA olympic hydrogels driven by topoisomerase activity *Phys. Rev. Lett.* **121** 148001

Kurachi M, Hoshi M and Tashiro H 1995 Buckling of a single microtubule by optical trapping forces: direct measurement of microtubule rigidity *Cell Motil.* **30** 221–8

Lai S K, O'Hanlon D E, Harrold S, Man S T, Wang Y-Y, Cone R and Hanes J 2007 Rapid transport of large polymeric nanoparticles in fresh undiluted human mucus *Proc. Natl Acad. Sci.* **104** 1482–7

Lai S K, Wang Y-Y, Wirtz D and Hanes J 2009 Micro- and macrorheology of mucus *Adv. Drug Deliv. Rev.* **61** 86–100

Laib S, Robertson R M and Smith D E 2006 Preparation and characterization of a set of linear DNA molecules for polymer physics and rheology studies *Macromol. Macromol.* **39** 4115–9

Laurens N, Koolwijk P and De maat M P M 2006 Fibrin structure and wound healing *J. Thromb. Haemost.* **4** 932–9

Learn all about red blood cells, ThoughtCo. n.d. https://thoughtco.com/red-blood-cells-373487 (accessed 1 September 2023)

Lee G, Leech G, Rust M J, Das M, McGorty R J, Ross J L and Robertson-Anderson R M 2021 Myosin-driven actin-microtubule networks exhibit self-organized contractile dynamics *Sci. Adv.* **7** eabe4334

Lemma L M, Varghese M, Ross T D, Thomson M, Baskaran A and Dogic Z 2023 Spatio-temporal patterning of extensile active stresses in microtubule-based active fluids *PNAS Nexus* **2** pgad130

Lenz M 2020 Reversal of contractility as a signature of self-organization in cytoskeletal bundles *eLife* **9** e51751

Lenz M 2014 Geometrical origins of contractility in disordered actomyosin networks *Phys. Rev.* X **4** 041002

Li L D, Crouzier T, Sarkar A, Dunphy L, Han J and Ribbeck K 2013 Spatial configuration and composition of charge modulates transport into a mucin hydrogel barrier *Biophys. J.* **105** 1357–65

Li Y, Hsiao K-W, Brockman C A, Yates D Y, Robertson-Anderson R M, Kornfield J A, Francisco M J S, Schroeder C M and McKenna G B 2015 When ends meet: circular DNA stretches differently in elongational flows [WWW Document] *Macromolecules* **48** 5997–6001

Lin Y-C, Koenderink G H, MacKintosh F C and Weitz D A 2007 Viscoelastic properties of microtubule networks *Macromolecules* **40** 7714–20

Linsmeier I, Banerjee S, Oakes P W, Jung W, Kim T and Murrell M P 2016 Disordered actomyosin networks are sufficient to produce cooperative and telescopic contractility *Nat. Commun.* **7** 12615

Liu K, Patteson A E, Banigan E J and Schwarz J M 2021 Dynamic nuclear structure emerges from chromatin cross-links and motors *Phys. Rev. Lett.* **126** 158101

Lohman T M and Bjornson K P 1996 Mechanisms of helicase-catalyzed dna unwinding *Annu. Rev. Biochem.* **65** 169–214

Lopez-Menendez H and Gonzalez-Torres L 2019 A theory to describe emergent properties of composite F-actin and vimentin networks *J. Mech. Phys. Solids* **127** 208–20

Lu T and Spruijt E 2020 Multiphase complex coacervate droplets *J. Am. Chem. Soc.* **142** 2905–14

Lukeš J, Lys Guilbride D, Votýpka J, Zíková A, Benne R and Englund P T 2002 Kinetoplast DNA network: evolution of an improbable structure *Eukaryot. Cell* **1** 495–502

Mai D J and Schroeder C M 2016 Single polymer dynamics of topologically complex DNA *Curr. Opinion Colloid Interface Sci.* **26** 28–40

Mancini E J and Tuma R 2012 Mechanism of RNA packaging motor ed M G Rossmann and V B Rao *Viral Molecular Machines, Advances in Experimental Medicine and Biology* (Boston, MA: Springer) pp 609–29

Manning G S 2006 The persistence length of DNA is reached from the persistence length of its null isomer through an internal electrostatic stretching force *Biophys. J.* **91** 3607–16

Marfai J, McGorty R J and Robertson-Anderson R M 2023 Cooperative rheological state-switching of enzymatically-driven composites of circular DNA and dextran *Adv. Mater.* **35** 2305824

Marko J F and Siggia E D 1995 Stretching DNA *Macromolecules* **28** 8759–70

Marko J F and Siggia E D 1995 Statistical mechanics of supercoiled DNA *Phys. Rev.* E **52** 2912–38

Marko J F and Siggia E D 1994 Bending and twisting elasticity of DNA *Macromolecules* **27** 981–8

Martin D P, Biagini P, Lefeuvre P, Golden M, Roumagnac P and Varsani A 2011 Recombination in eukaryotic single stranded DNA viruses *Viruses* **3** 1699–738

Martin S R, Butler F M M, Clark D C, Zhou J-M and Bayley P M 1987 Magnesium ion effects on microtubule nucleation *in vitro Biochim. Biophys. Acta (BBA)—Protein Struct. Mol. Enzymol.* **914** 96–100

Mathews C K, Holde K and van, Appling D 2013 *Biochemistry* (Pearson)

Matthews K S 1992 DNA looping *Microbiol. Rev.* **56** 123–36

McCarty J, Delaney K T, Danielsen S P O, Fredrickson G H and Shea J-E 2019 Complete phase diagram for liquid–liquid phase separation of intrinsically disordered proteins *J. Phys. Chem. Lett.* **10** 1644–52

McGorty R J *et al* 2023 Kinesin and myosin motors compete to drive rich multiphase dynamics in programmable cytoskeletal composites *PNAS Nexus* **2** pgad245

McIntosh D B and Saleh O A 2011 Salt species-dependent electrostatic effects on ssdna elasticity *Macromolecules* **44** 2328–33

McKenna G B and Plazek D J 1986 The viscosity of blends of linear and cyclic molecules of similar molecular mass *Polym. Commun.* **27** 304–6

McLeish T 2008 Polymer dynamics floored by the rings *Nat. Mater.* **7** 933–5

McMillan J R, Hayes O G, Winegar P H and Mirkin C A 2019 Protein materials engineering with DNA *Acc. Chem. Res.* **52** 1939–48

McShane A, Bath J, Jaramillo A M, Ridley C, Walsh A A, Evans C M, Thornton D J and Ribbeck K 2021 Mucus *Curr. Biol.* **31** R938–45

Mecham R 2011 *The Extracellular Matrix: An Overview* (Berlin: Springer Science & Business Media)

Merindol R and Walther A 2017 Materials learning from life: concepts for active, adaptive and autonomous molecular systems *Chem. Soc. Rev.* **46** 5588–619

Mezger T G 2006 *The Rheology Handbook* (Vincentz Network)

Michieletto D 2016 On the tree-like structure of rings in dense solutions *Soft Matter* **12** 9485–500

Michieletto D, Fitzpatrick R and Robertson-Anderson R M 2019 Maximally stiffening composites require maximally coupled rather than maximally entangled polymer species *Soft Matter* **15** 6703–17

Michieletto D, Nahali N and Rosa A 2017 Glassiness and heterogeneous dynamics in dense solutions of ring polymers *Phys. Rev. Lett.* **119** 197801

Michieletto D, Neill P, Weir S, Evans D, Crist N, Martinez V A and Robertson-Anderson R M 2022 Topological digestion drives time-varying rheology of entangled DNA fluids *Nat. Commun.* **13** 4389

Mickey B and Howard J 1995 Rigidity of microtubules is increased by stabilizing agents *J. Cell Biol.* **130** 909–17

Mills J B, Vacano E and Hagerman P J 1999 Flexibility of single-stranded DNA: use of gapped duplex helices to determine the persistence lengths of Poly(dT) and Poly(dA)11Edited by B. Honig *J. Mol. Biol.* **285** 245–57

Minoura I and Muto E 2006 Dielectric measurement of individual microtubules using the electroorientation method *Biophys. J.* **90** 3739–48

Mirny L A 2011 The fractal globule as a model of chromatin architecture in the cell *Chromosome Res.* **19** 37–51

Mogilner A and Oster G 1996 Cell motility driven by actin polymerization *Biophys. J.* **71** 3030–45

mousefibroblasts.jpg (708×512) [WWW Document] n.d. https://people.maths.bris.ac.uk/~matbl/images/mousefibroblasts.jpg (accessed 22 November 2023)

Mucus: It's Snot What You Think n.d. Science Friday https://sciencefriday.com/segments/mucus-snot-human-health/ (accessed 22 November 2023)

Nakamura M, Chen L, Howes S C, Schindler T D, Nogales E and Bryant Z 2014 Remote control of myosin and kinesin motors using light-activated gearshifting *Nat. Nanotech.* **9** 693–7

Namazi H 2017 Polymers in our daily life *Bioimpacts* **7** 73–4

Needleman D and Dogic Z 2017 Active matter at the interface between materials science and cell biology *Nat. Rev. Mater.* **2** 1–14

Nelson P, Chen K and Bromberg S 2020 *Biological Physics: Energy, Information, Life* (Chiliagon Science)

Nguyen D T and Saleh O A 2017 Tuning phase and aging of DNA hydrogels through molecular design *Soft Matter* **13** 5421–7

Nöding B and Köster S 2012 Intermediate filaments in small configuration spaces *Phys. Rev. Lett.* **108** 088101

O'Brien E T, Salmon E d and Erickson H P 1997 How calcium causes microtubule depolymerization *Cell Motil.* **36** 125–35

O'Brien E T, Salmon E D, Walker R A and Erickson H P 1990 Effects of magnesium on the dynamic instability of individual microtubules *Biochemistry* **29** 6648–56

Ohniwa R L, Morikawa K, Kim J, Ohta T, Ishihama A, Wada C and Takeyasu K 2006 Dynamic state of DNA topology is essential for genome condensation in bacteria *EMBO J.* **25** 5591–602

Osswald T A 2015 *Polymer Rheology: Fundamentals and Applications* 1st edn (München: Hanser Publications)

Osunbayo O, Miles C E, Doval F, Reddy B J N, Keener J P and Vershinin M D 2019 Complex nearly immotile behaviour of enzymatically driven cargos *Soft Matter* **15** 1847–52

Özkale B, Sakar M S and Mooney D J 2021 Active biomaterials for mechanobiology *Biomaterials* **267** 120497

Pan S, Nguyen D A, Sridhar T, Sunthar P and Prakash J R 2014 Universal solvent quality crossover of the zero shear rate viscosity of semidilute DNA solutions *J. Rheol.* **58** 339–68

Papale A, Smrek J and Rosa A 2021 Nanorheology of active–passive polymer mixtures differentiates between linear and ring polymer topology *Soft Matter* **17** 7111–7

Parisi D *et al* 2021 Nonlinear shear rheology of entangled polymer rings *Macromolecules* **54** 2811–27

Patteson A E, Gopinath A, Purohit P K and Arratia P E 2016 Particle diffusion in active fluids is non-monotonic in size *Soft Matter* **12** 2365–72

Pecora R 1991 DNA: a model compound for solution studies of macromolecules *Science* **251** 893–8

Peddireddy K R, Clairmont R, Neill P, McGorty R and Robertson-Anderson R M 2022 Optical-tweezers-integrating-differential-dynamic-microscopy maps the spatiotemporal propagation of nonlinear strains in polymer blends and composites *Nat. Commun.* **13** 5180

Peddireddy K R, Lee M, Schroeder C M and Robertson-Anderson R M 2020 Viscoelastic properties of ring-linear DNA blends exhibit nonmonotonic dependence on blend composition *Phys. Rev. Res.* **2** 023213

Peddireddy K R, Michieletto D, Aguirre G, Garamella J, Khanal P and Robertson-Anderson R M 2021 DNA conformation dictates strength and flocculation in dna–microtubule composites *ACS Macro Lett.* **10** 1540–8

Pegoraro A F, Janmey P and Weitz D A 2017 Mechanical properties of the cytoskeleton and cells *Cold Spring Harb. Perspect. Biol.* **9** a022038

Pei Y, Wang L, Tang K and Kaplan D L 2021 Biopolymer nanoscale assemblies as building blocks for new materials: a review *Adv. Funct. Mater.* **31** 2008552

Peng M, Zhao Q, Wang M and Du X 2023 Reconfigurable scaffolds for adaptive tissue regeneration *Nanoscale* **15** 6105–20

Perkins T T, Smith D E and Chu S 1994 Direct observation of tube-like motion of a single polymer chain *Science* **264** 819–22

Pollard T D 2003 The cytoskeleton, cellular motility and the reductionist agenda *Nature* **422** 741–5

Pollard T D 1986 Rate constants for the reactions of ATP- and ADP-actin with the ends of actin filaments *J. Cell Biol.* **103** 2747–54

Pollard T D 1984 Polymerization of ADP-actin *J. Cell Biol.* **99** 769–77

Pollard T D, Blanchoin L and Mullins R D 2001 Cell science at a glance *J. Cell Sci.* **114** 3–4

Pollard T D and Goldman R D 2018 Overview of the cytoskeleton from an evolutionary perspective *Cold Spring Harb. Perspect. Biol.* **10** a030288

Pouring shampoo stock illustrations—170 Pouring shampoo stock illustrations, vectors & clipart [WWW Document]. Dreamstime n.d. https://dreamstime.com/illustration/pouring-shampoo.html (accessed 1 September 2023)

Puig-de-Morales-Marinkovic M, Turner K T, Butler J P, Fredberg J J and Suresh S 2007 Viscoelasticity of the human red blood cell *Am. J. Physiol.-Cell Physiol.* **293** C597–605

Ramaswamy S 2017 Active matter *J. Stat. Mech.* **2017** 054002

Regan K, Ricketts S and Robertson-Anderson R M 2016 DNA as a model for probing polymer entanglements: circular polymers and non-classical dynamics *Polymers* **8** 336

Ricketts S N, Khanal P, Rust M J, Das M, Ross J L and Robertson-Anderson R M 2020 Triggering cation-induced contraction of cytoskeleton networks via microfluidics *Front. Phys.* **8** 596699

Ricketts S N, Ross J L and Robertson-Anderson R M 2018 Co-entangled actin-microtubule composites exhibit tunable stiffening and power-law stress relaxation *Biophys. J.* **115** 1055–67

Robertson R M and Smith D E 2007a Direct measurement of the intermolecular forces confining a single molecule in an entangled polymer solution *Phys. Rev. Lett.* **99** 126001

Robertson R M and Smith D E 2007b Strong effects of molecular topology on diffusion of entangled DNA molecules *PNAS* **104** 4824–7

Robertson R M and Smith D E 2007c Self-diffusion of entangled linear and circular DNA molecules: dependence on length and concentration *Macromol. Macromol.* **40** 3373–7

Robertson R M and Smith D E 2007d Direct measurement of the confining forces imposed on a single molecule in a concentrated solution of circular polymers *Macromolecules* **40** 8737–41

Robinson D R, Sherwin T, Ploubidou A, Byard E H and Gull K 1995 Microtubule polarity and dynamics in the control of organelle positioning, segregation, and cytokinesis in the trypanosome cell cycle *J. Cell Biol.* **128** 1163–72

Rogers S A, Calabrese M A and Wagner N J 2014 Rheology of branched wormlike micelles *Curr. Opin. Colloid Interface Sci.* **19** 530–5

Romanowska M, Hinsch H, Kirchgener N, Giesen M, Degawa M, Hoffmann B, Frey E and Merkel R 2009 Direct observation of the tube model in F-actin solutions: Tube dimensions and curvatures *Epl-Europhys. Lett.* **86** 26003

Ronceray P and Lenz M 2015 Connecting local active forces to macroscopic stress in elastic media *Soft Matter* **11** 1597–605

Ross T 1985 Mechanism of calcium chloride induced actin polymerization *Biochemistry* **24** 4455–60

Ross T D, Lee H J, Qu Z, Banks R A, Phillips R and Thomson M 2019 Controlling organization and forces in active matter through optically defined boundaries *Nature* **572** 224–9

Roth E, Glick Azaria A, Girshevitz O, Bitler A and Garini Y 2018 Measuring the conformation and persistence length of single-stranded DNA using a DNA origami structure *Nano Lett.* **18** 6703–9

Rothstein J P and Mohammadigoushki H 2020 Complex flows of viscoelastic wormlike micelle solutions *J. Non-Newtonian Fluid Mech.* **285** 104382

Rubinstein M 1986 Dynamics of ring polymers in the presence of fixed obstacles *Phys. Rev. Lett.* **57** 3023–6

Rubinstein M and Colby R H 2003 *Polymer Physics* (Oxford: Oxford University Press)

Saleh O A, McIntosh D B, Pincus P and Ribeck N 2009 Nonlinear low-force elasticity of single-stranded DNA molecules *Phys. Rev. Lett.* **102** 068301

Sanchez T, Chen D T N, DeCamp S J, Heymann M and Dogic Z 2012 Spontaneous motion in hierarchically assembled active matter *Nature* **491** 431–4

Schaedel L, Lorenz C, Schepers A V, Klumpp S and Köster S 2021 Vimentin intermediate filaments stabilize dynamic microtubules by direct interactions *Nat. Commun.* **12** 3799

Schroeder C M, Shaqfeh E S G and Chu S 2004 Effect of hydrodynamic interactions on DNA dynamics in extensional flow: simulation and single molecule experiment *Macromol. Macromol.* **37** 9242–56

Seol Y and Neuman K C 2016 The dynamic interplay between DNA topoisomerases and DNA topology *Biophys. Rev.* **8** 101–11

Shanbhag S and Larson R G 2006 Identification of topological constraints in entangled polymer melts using the bond-fluctuation model *Macromol. Macromol.* **39** 2413–7

Shaw M T and MacKnight W J 2018 *Introduction to Polymer Viscoelasticity* (New York: Wiley)

Shen Y 2020 Microrheology of actin-vimentin-microtubule composite cytoskeletal networks *Biophys. J.* **118** 440a

Shen Y *et al* 2021 Effects of vimentin intermediate filaments on the structure and dynamics of *in vitro* multicomponent interpenetrating cytoskeletal networks *Phys. Rev. Lett.* **127** 108101

Sheung J Y *et al* 2021 Motor-driven restructuring of cytoskeleton composites leads to tunable time-varying elasticity *ACS Macro Lett.* **10** 1151–8

Shimobayashi S F, Ronceray P, Sanders D W, Haataja M P and Brangwynne C P 2021 Nucleation landscape of biomolecular condensates *Nature* **599** 503–6

Shin J H, Gardel M L, Mahadevan L, Matsudaira P and Weitz D A 2004 Relating microstructure to rheology of a bundled and cross-linked F-actin network *in vitro PNAS* **101** 9636–41

Smrek J, Garamella J, Robertson-Anderson R and Michieletto D 2021 Topological tuning of DNA mobility in entangled solutions of supercoiled plasmids *Sci. Adv.* **7** eabf9260

Smrek J, Kremer K and Rosa A 2019 Threading of unconcatenated ring polymers at high concentrations: double-folded vs time-equilibrated structures *ACS Macro Lett.* **8** 155–60

Soh B W and Doyle P S 2020 Deformation response of catenated DNA networks in a planar elongational field *ACS Macro Lett.* **9** 944–9

Somers J 2022 A journey to the center of our cells *The New Yorker* https://www.newyorker.com/magazine/2022/03/07/a-journey-to-the-center-of-our-cells

Speir J A and Johnson J E 2012 Nucleic acid packaging in viruses *Curr. Opin. Struct. Biol.* **22** 65–71

Squires T M and Mason T G 2010 Fluid Mechanics of Microrheology *Annu. Rev. Fluid Mech.* **42** 413–38

Stamenović D, Mijailovich S M, Tolić-Nørrelykke I M, Chen J and Wang N 2002 Cell prestress. II. Contribution of microtubules *Am. J. Physiol.-Cell Physiol.* **282** C617–24

Stanhope K T, Yadav V, Santangelo C D and Ross J L 2017 Contractility in an extensile system *Soft Matter* **13** 4268–77

Stedman K M 2015 Deep recombination: RNA and ssDNA virus genes in DNA virus and host genomes *Annu. Rev. Virol.* **2** 203–17

Stevens M J, McIntosh D B and Saleh O A 2012 Simulations of stretching a strong, flexible polyelectrolyte *Macromolecules* **45** 5757–65

Stricker J, Falzone T and Gardel M L 2010 Mechanics of the F-actin cytoskeleton *J. Biomech.* Special Issue on Cell Mechanobiology **43** 9–14

Subramanian G and Shanbhag S 2008 Self-diffusion in binary blends of cyclic and linear polymers *Macromol. Macromol.* **41** 7239–42

Sullivan R, Adams M C, Naik R R and Milam V T 2019 Analyzing secondary structure patterns in DNA aptamers identified via CompELS *Molecules* **24** 1572

Swartz D W and Camley B A 2021 Active gels, heavy tails, and the cytoskeleton *Soft Matter* **17** 9876–92

Tanaka E, Ho T and Kirschner M W 1995 The role of microtubule dynamics in growth cone motility and axonal growth *J. Cell Biol.* **128** 139–55

Taylor P, Rixon F and Desselberger U 1985 Rise per base pair in helices of double-stranded rotavirus RNA determined by electron microscopy *Virus Res.* **2** 175–82

Teixeira R E, Dambal A K, Richter D H, Shaqfeh E S G and Chu S 2007 The individualistic dynamics of entangled DNA in solution *Macromol. Macromol.* **40** 2461–76

Theocharis A D, Skandalis S S, Gialeli C and Karamanos N K 2016 Extracellular matrix structure *Adv. Drug Deliv. Rev.* **97** 4–27

Thomas S, Durand D, Chassenieux C and Jyotishkumar P 2013 *Handbook of Biopolymer-Based Materials: From Blends and Composites to Gels and Complex Networks* (New York: Wiley)

Tojkander S, Gateva G and Lappalainen P 2012 Actin stress fibers—assembly, dynamics and biological roles *J. Cell Sci.* **125** 1855–64

Tomkinson A E, Vijayakumar S, Pascal J M and Ellenberger T 2006 DNA ligases: structure, reaction mechanism, and function *Chem. Rev.* **106** 687–99

Tong J and Gu Q 2020 Expression and clinical significance of mucin gene in chronic rhinosinusitis *Curr. Allergy Asthma Rep.* **20** 63

Tree D R, Muralidhar A, Doyle P S and Dorfman K D 2013 Is DNA a good model polymer? *Macromolecules* **46** 8369–82

Tseng Q, Duchemin-Pelletier E, Deshiere A, Balland M, Guillou H, Filhol O and Théry M 2012 Spatial organization of the extracellular matrix regulates cell–cell junction positioning *Proc. Natl Acad. Sci. USA* **109** 1506–11

Ubertini M A, Smrek J and Rosa A 2022 Entanglement length scale separates threading from branching of unknotted and non-concatenated ring polymers in melts *Macromolecules* **55** 10723–36

van der Maarel J R C 2008 *Introduction to Biopolymer Physics* (Singapore: World Scientific)

Vavylonis D, Yang Q and O'Shaughnessy B 2005 Actin polymerization kinetics, cap structure, and fluctuations *Proc. Natl Acad. Sci.* **102** 8543–8

Voth G A 2017 A multiscale description of biomolecular active matter: the chemistry underlying many life processes *Acc. Chem. Res.* **50** 594–8

Wang B, Guan J, Anthony S M, Bae S C, Schweizer K S and Granick S 2010 Confining potential when a biopolymer filament reptates *Phys. Rev. Lett.* **104** 118301

Wang J, Li Z and Willner I 2023 Dynamic reconfigurable DNA nanostructures, networks and materials *Angew. Chem. Int. Ed.* **62** e202215332

Weigand W J, Messmore A, Tu J, Morales-Sanz A, Blair D L, Deheyn D D, Urbach J S and Robertson-Anderson R M 2017 Active microrheology determines scale-dependent material properties of *Chaetopterus mucus PLoS One* **12** e0176732

Wintner O, Hirsch-Attas N, Schlossberg M, Brofman F, Friedman R, Kupervaser M, Kitsberg D and Buxboim A 2020 A unified linear viscoelastic model of the cell nucleus defines the mechanical contributions of lamins and chromatin *Adv. Sci.* **7** 1901222

Yue B 2014 Biology of the extracellular matrix: an overview *J. Glaucoma.* **Oct.–Nov** S20–3

Zeng X, Holehouse A S, Chilkoti A, Mittag T and Pappu R V 2020 Connecting coil-to-globule transitions to full phase diagrams for intrinsically disordered proteins *Biophys. J.* **119** 402–18

Zhang J H and Xu M 2000 DNA fragmentation in apoptosis *Cell Res.* **10** 205–11

Zhao Q, Zhao Z, Fan X, Yuan Z, Mao Q and Yao Y 2021 Review of machine learning methods for RNA secondary structure prediction *PLoS Comput. Biol.* **17** e1009291

Zhou Y, Hsiao K-W, Regan K E, Kong D, McKenna G B, Robertson-Anderson R M and Schroeder C M 2019 Effect of molecular architecture on ring polymer dynamics in semidilute linear polymer solutions *Nat. Commun.* **10** 10

Zhou Y, Young C D, Lee M, Banik S, Kong D, McKenna G B, Robertson-Anderson R M, Sing C E and Schroeder C M 2021 Dynamics and rheology of ring-linear blend semidilute solutions in extensional flow: single molecule experiments *J. Rheol.* **65** 729–44

Ziegler F 2012 *Mechanics of Solids and Fluids* (Berlin: Springer Science & Business Media)

Part II

Making sense and measuring

IOP Publishing

Biopolymer Networks
Design, dynamics and discovery
Rae M Robertson-Anderson

Chapter 2

Polymer physics for everyone

This chapter covers the theoretical frameworks and tools needed to understand biopolymer network dynamics, structure, and rheological properties. The purpose of the chapter is to provide a high-level overview of theoretical concepts that are necessary to understand polymer networks, but that can be understood by an interdisciplinary audience that may include biologists, chemists, and engineers, as well as advanced physics undergraduates.

2.1 The beauty of polymer physics

Many textbooks have been devoted to detailed derivations and explanations of polymer physics theories, such as de Gennes (1979), Doi and Edwards (1988), Doi (1996), McLeish (2002), Rubinstein and Colby (2003) and van der Maarel (2008). I refer you to these works for a thorough and proper introduction to polymer physics. This chapter is a poor paraphrasing of these foundational texts intended to allow us to speak the same language, to allow you to understand some of the results I discuss in future chapters, and to arm you with the ability to make hypotheses and characterize biopolymer networks of interest to you in the language of polymer physics. We will only consider linear polymers in this chapter and will introduce theories to describe topologically-novel polymers in chapter 6.

2.1.1 Scaling laws

Importantly, various texts and theoretical frameworks include different prefactors in many of the expressions that relate polymer properties to system dynamics. While this discrepancy can lead to slightly different predicted values (of order unity), what is most important for our purposes are the scaling relationships between quantities—how one parameter depends on the other—rather than exact values. Any biologist will tell you that factors of two are rarely significant in biology.

Moreover, due to the fractal nature of polymers, many of these relationships exhibit power-law scaling, and it is the exponent that is the key metric that

doi:10.1088/978-0-7503-5037-2ch2

characterizes the system. This scaling approach also allows us to treat scaling relations as universal across a wide range of different polymer species as long as they are coarse-grained appropriately. In other words, we can ignore the chemical and molecular details of the monomers or subunits of the polymers, and instead only consider the number of monomers in the polymer and the nature of the links between monomers (e.g., freely rotating). This simplification and unification is the true beauty of polymer physics, for which we are indebted to the founding giants of the field—Flory, Zimm, Rouse, de Gennes, Doi, Edwards (Flory 1949a, 1949b, 1953, 1969, Rouse 1953, Zimm 1956, de Gennes 1979, de Gennes and Leger 1982, Doi and Edwards 1988)—for first discovering over half a century ago.

2.1.2 What to expect

Standing on the shoulders of these giants, I will first describe the static properties of single polymer chains, then consider the effect that their interactions with the surrounding solvent and other polymers has on these properties. We will consider different regimes of solvent quality and polymer concentration—starting with the dilute limit and working up to the highly concentrated regime. We will see that the static and dynamic properties of biopolymers and their networks are intricately linked to how the polymer interacts with its surroundings as well as how different segments within a single chain interact with one other. These intrachain interactions are strongly dependent on the stiffness of the polymer. So here is where we start.

2.2 Polymer flexibility

A powerful scaling approach for understanding and comparing the properties of polymers with very different chemical composition is to coarse-grain each polymer to a chain of $2N$ persistence lengths and contour length $L = 2Nl_p$ (figure 2.1). As I describe in chapter 1, the **persistence length l_p** can be understood as the length Δx over which the orientation of two unit tangent vectors $\hat{t}(x)$ and $\hat{t}(x + \Delta x)$ along the polymer becomes decorrelated, which occurs when the thermal energy k_BT surpasses the energetic cost of bending. The correlation between $\hat{t}(x)$ and $\hat{t}(x + \Delta x)$ can be quantified by the expectation value of the cosine of the angle between the two vectors, $\langle\cos\theta(\Delta x)\rangle$, where the average is taken over all x values. This function decays exponentially with the distance between the vectors, and the characteristic decay length associated with this decay is the persistence length l_p:

$$\langle\cos\theta(\Delta x)\rangle = e^{-\Delta x/l_p} \tag{2.1}$$

By comparing L to l_p, we can broadly classify polymers according to their flexibility: flexible ($L \gg l_p$), semiflexible ($L \approx l_p$), or rigid $L \ll l_p$ (figures 2.2(A)–(C)). Table 1.1 categorizes different biopolymers by these three classes. Most of polymer physics theory is devoted to understanding flexible polymers, in part because most synthetic polymers are considered flexible. However, many biopolymers, such as actin and microtubules, are far from flexible, so this classification is important.

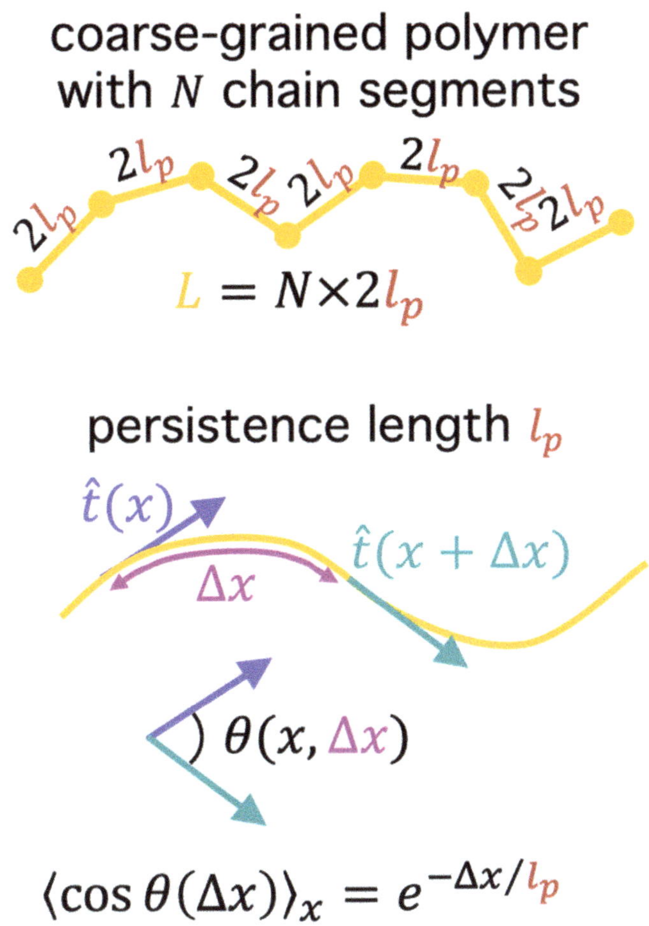

Figure 2.1. Coarse-graining a polymer by its persistence length. (Top) A polymer with contour length L is divided into N segments of length $2l_p$. (Bottom) The persistence length is determined by the characteristic decorrelation lengthscale of tangent vectors along a polymer.

In this chapter, I first focus on the physics of flexible polymers for which the theoretical frameworks are the most mature, then extend to semiflexible and rigid polymers.

2.3 Single polymer conformations

2.3.1 Freely jointed chain model

At the most basic level, a flexible polymer can be modeled as a freely jointed chain (FJC) of rigid segments (figures 2.1, 2.2(A)). The length of each segment, termed the **Kuhn length l_k**, is twice the persistence length, i.e., $l_k = 2l_p$. The orientation of two neighboring Kuhn lengths can be considered completely independent of one another, such that the conformation of a polymer in the FJC framework can be described as a random coil or random walk in space. For a random walk in time, the mean-squared displacement $\langle \vec{r}^2 \rangle$ scales linearly with the number of steps N, such that

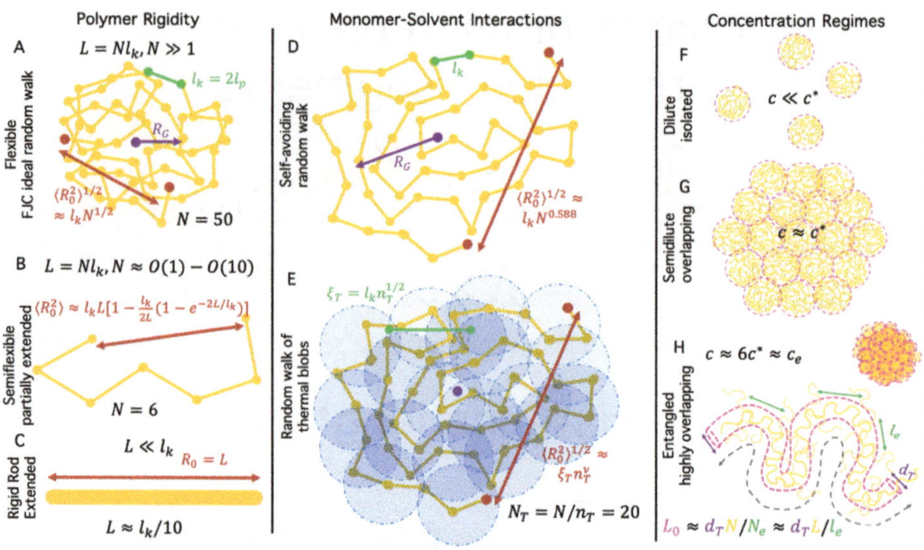

Figure 2.2. Foundational models and metrics that describe networks of biopolymers with different rigidities, solvent conditions, and concentrations. Polymers can be described by their contour length L, persistence length l_p, Kuhn length l_k (green), number of Kuhn lengths N, radius of gyration R_G (purple), and mean end-to-end distance $\langle R_0^2 \rangle^{1/2}$ (red). (A) Most polymers are considered flexible, with contour lengths L that are many times the Kuhn length l_k. Flexible chains can be modeled as freely jointed chains (FJCs) that adopt random coil conformations that can be described as random walks in space. (B) Semiflexible polymers have lengths that are comparable to l_k so they adopt more extended conformations that can be described by the worm-like chain model. (C) Rigid rod polymers have lengths that are shorter than l_k so their end-to-end distance R_0 is equal to L. (D) Because different chain segments of the same polymer cannot occupy the same point in space at the same time, flexible polymer conformations are often more accurately modeled as self-avoiding (random) walks (SAWs), in particular, for long or thick polymers, dilute conditions, and good solvent conditions. (E) Blob theory extends models developed for polymer melts to polymer solutions by replacing l_k as the unit monomer with thermal blobs of polymer and solvent with thermal blob size ξ_T. (F) At concentrations well below c^*, polymers are separated by several R_G so the only polymer–polymer interactions are hydrodynamic interactions that swell the polymers to assume self-avoiding statistics described by Flory theory and the Zimm model. (G) When polymers overlap ($c \approx c^*$), hydrodynamic interactions are screened so polymers collapse to ideal random coils and the Rouse model describes their statistics. (H) When polymers are entangled ($c \approx c_e > c^*$), the reptation tube model describes their conformations and dynamics and the relevant lengthscales become the diameter of the confining tube d_T, the length between entanglements along a chain l_e (or N_e), and the length of the tube, or primitive path length L_0.

$$\langle \vec{r}^2 \rangle = N l_s^2 \tag{2.2}$$

where l_s is the size of each random step and N is a measure of time. Similarly, the **mean-squared end-to-end distance $\langle R_0^2 \rangle$** of an FJC polymer is quantified as:

$$\langle R_0^2 \rangle = N l_k^2 \tag{2.3}$$

where $N = L/l_k$ is the number of Kuhn lengths along the chain (figure 2.2(A)). Taking the square-root of equation (2.3) yields a useful measure of the size of the ideal random coil, its **root mean-squared end-to-end distance**

$$\langle R_0^2 \rangle^{1/2} = l_k N^{1/2} \tag{2.4}$$

(figure 2.2(A)), which scales with the root of the length of the polymer N (in units of l_k). This expression is the first important scaling law we introduce:

$$R_0 \sim N^{\nu} \sim L^{\nu} \tag{2.5}$$

where $\nu = 1/2$ for an ideal chain and R_0 is short-hand for $\langle R_0^2 \rangle^{1/2}$.

A more common and often more useful metric to quantify the coil size is the **radius of gyration R_G**, which is the average distance of a given Kuhn segment from the polymer center-of-mass (COM). R_G is related to R_0 via

$$R_G^2 = \frac{1}{6} \langle R_0^2 \rangle \tag{2.6}$$

such that

$$R_G = \frac{l_k}{\sqrt{6}} N^{1/2} = \frac{l_k^{1/2}}{\sqrt{6}} L^{1/2} \tag{2.7}$$

Note that the same scaling relation between the polymer coil size and its length holds for R_G:

$$R_G \sim R_0 \sim L^{\nu} \tag{2.8}$$

Recall that these expressions are a result of swapping time for space in the random walker problem. However, for a random walk in *time*, the walker can return to a position they previously occupied. It follows that swapping time for space to describe a polymer's conformation means that two different polymer segments can occupy the exact same *space*—which they of course, cannot.

For shorter polymers, in which the probability that two distant Kuhn segments will interact is low, as well as for very thin polymers, in which the lateral space excluded by each Kuhn segment is much smaller than l_k, this 'ideal chain' approximation works relatively well. Beyond these limiting conditions, FJC polymer configurations are more accurately modeled as random **self-avoiding walks (SAWs)** in which the space taken up by each link is excluded from the occupation possibilities of the other links (figure 2.2(D)).

According to Flory theory (Flory 1949a, 1949b), this **excluded volume** effect swells the random coil beyond the ideal limit such that

$$R_0 \approx l_k N^{\nu} \tag{2.9}$$

with $\nu = 3/5$ compared to $\nu = 1/2$ in the ideal case. Refinements to the Flory model based on renormalization group theory predict a slight reduction of the SAW scaling exponent to $\nu \approx 0.588$, in agreement with experimental measurements (Le Guillou and Zinn-Justin 1977, Freed 1987, Rubinstein and Colby 2003, Robertson *et al* 2006). Excluded volume becomes even more important when considering the effect of the surrounding solvent on an FJC polymer, which we explore below.

2.3.2 Polymer–solvent interactions and the Zimm model

The conformation of an individual polymer depends not only on the properties of the polymer itself but also on its interactions with the surrounding solvent, which can be classified as (i) athermal, (ii) good, (iii) theta (θ), and (iv) poor, based on the effect of the solvent on the polymer conformation. Specifically, these solvent conditions are defined by the extent to which the polymer coil swells (athermal, good), behaves as an ideal chain (θ), or collapses (poor).

Swelling arises from the tendency of the polymer chains to want to interact with solvent molecules, which is essentially the self-avoidance criteria (figure 2.2(D)). Conversely, collapse arises from a stronger tendency for polymer chains to interact with each rather than the solvent molecules, which, in extreme cases, can lead to aggregation and phase separation. At the theta point, polymer–polymer and polymer–solvent interactions are equally likely so the polymer conformation is most accurately modeled as an ideal random coil (no self-avoidance, $\nu = 1/2$). Nearly all the systems we will consider in this text can be described as in good solvent or θ-solvent conditions, in which the polymers can be modeled as SAWs ($\nu \approx 0.588$, figure 2.2(D)) or ideal random walks ($\nu \approx 1/2$, figure 2.2(A)), respectively.

The presence of the solvent motivates another empirically accessible measure of the size of a random coil polymer in solution, the **hydrodynamic radius R_H**. R_H can be thought of as equivalent to the radius of a hard sphere R_s with the same diffusion coefficient D as that of the center-of-mass of the polymer. The diffusion coefficient for a sphere in a fluid is related to is radius R_s via the Einstein relation

$$D\zeta = k_B T \tag{2.10}$$

where $\zeta = 6\pi\eta R_s$ is its friction coefficient in a fluid of viscosity η.

By analogy, we can define the hydrodynamic radius for a random coil polymer as

$$R_H = k_B T / 6\pi\eta_s D \tag{2.11}$$

where η_s is the solvent viscosity.

By directly tracking the Brownian motion of individual biopolymers in a solvent of known viscosity, we can measure D and thus determine R_H (Robertson *et al* 2006).

To relate the hydrodynamic radius to the radius of gyration R_G, thereby allowing for testing of theoretical predictions that relate R_G to known parameters of the polymer such as L, N, and l_k, we turn to Zimm theory, first proposed by Bruno Zimm in 1956 (Zimm 1956). The Zimm model successfully describes polymer dynamics in the dilute limit by correctly accounting for **hydrodynamic interactions**, which are long-range forces between polymer segments mediated by the pervading solvent that is dragged by the polymers as they move through the solvent (figure 2.3). Hydrodynamic interaction forces decay slowly with distance ($\sim r^{-1}$), creating a strong, long-range interaction between segments of both the same and different polymers. This effect allows polymer to 'feel' their neighbors, even in the dilute limit, via modified interactions with the solvent. With these considerations, the predicted

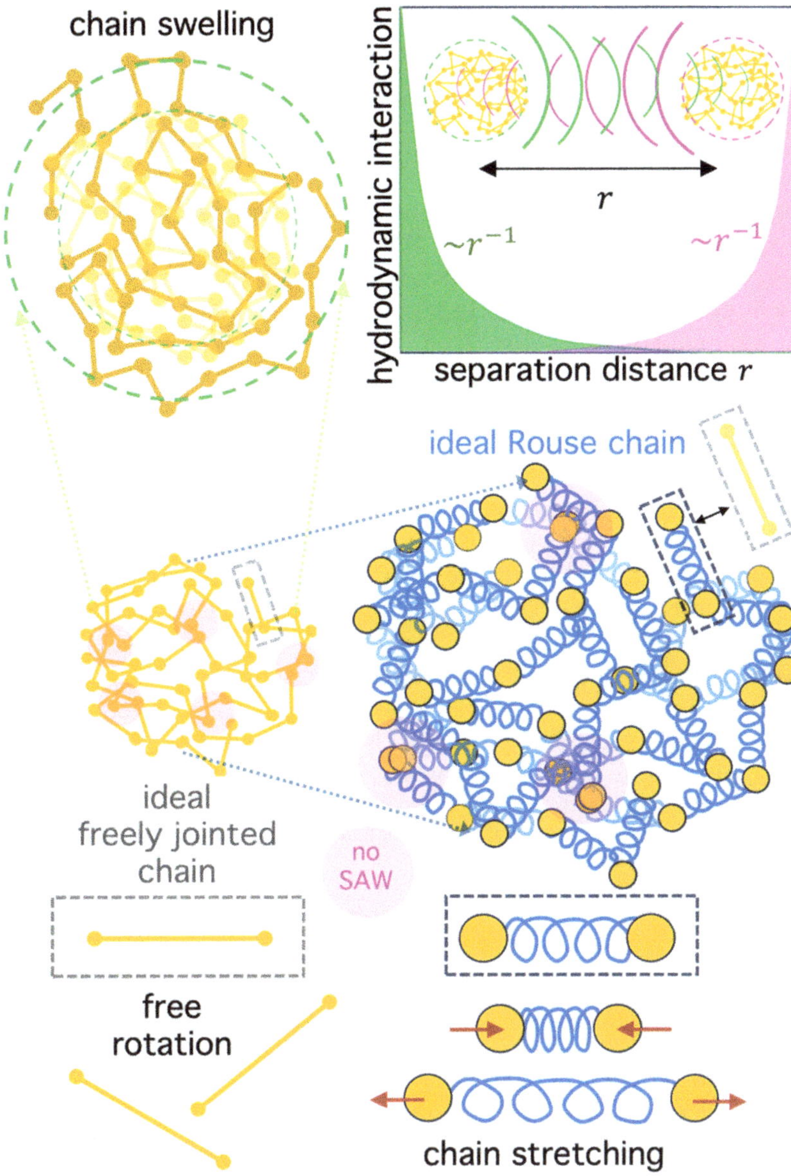

Figure 2.3. Building on the freely jointed ideal chain model to describe polymers in dilute and semidilute regimes. (Top) Long-range hydrodynamics interactions between two polymers, separated by a distance r, are mediated by the fluid between them and cause the polymers to swell from ideal random coils to swollen coils. (left) The translucent chain and green circular periphery depict an ideal FJC coil while the solid counterparts depict a swollen SAW coil. (right) Cartoon depiction of the hydrodynamic interaction and its dependence on the distance between polymers. (Bottom) The Rouse model replaces the rod-like chain links in the FJC model with springs. FJC links only have rotational degrees of freedom, while Rouse chains can relax stress via stretching and compressing. Both models do not consider self-avoidance. Example regions of polymer overlap, that are forbidden in SAW configurations but allowed in FJC and Rouse models, are highlighted in pink.

relations between the hydrodynamic radius and radius of gyration for linear polymers according to the Zimm model are

$$R_G = 1.6R_H \text{ (good solvent)} \tag{2.12}$$

$$R_G = 1.5R_H \ (\theta \text{ solvent})$$

Hydrodynamic interactions that lead to these relations also contribute to the excluded volume effect that leads to SAW conformations. As such, the Flory exponent, $\nu \approx 0.588$, can accurately describe the degree of swelling of polymers in good solvent conditions, even for thin or short polymers that have limited steric intrachain self-avoidance.

2.3.3 Overlapping polymers and the Rouse model

While taking into account hydrodynamic interactions is essential to accurately describe the polymer conformations in dilute conditions, these interactions become less important as the concentration of polymers increases. The neighboring polymers essentially screen out these long-range solvent-mediated hydrodynamic interactions that swell the coils. The concentration at which hydrodynamic interactions are completely screened is comparable to the concentration at which polymer coils begin to overlap with each other. This **coil overlap concentration** c^* can be computed by considering the concentration at which spheres of radius R_G completely fill the volume they occupy, such that every coil is touching another (figure 2.2G). This formulation leads to the following expression for the overlap concentration

$$c^* \simeq (M_W/N_A)/(4\pi/3R_G^3) \tag{2.13}$$

where M_W is the molecular weight of the polymer and N_A is Avogadro's number.

In the **semidilute regime**, where the polymer concentration c is comparable to the overlap concentration, $c \approx c^*$, the screening of hydrodynamic interactions renders the conformation of each polymer more accurately described by an ideal random walk rather than a SAW, with $\nu \approx 1/2$. Ideal chain statistics are captured by the Rouse model, proposed by Prince E Rouse in 1953, that describes the polymer conformations and dynamics in this regime (Rouse 1953).

The Rouse model treats each polymer as a chain of beads connected by springs of length l_k that are subject to thermal forces and frictional drag. This model builds on the FJC model by allowing the chain links (modeled as springs) to stretch and compress, rather than treating them as rigid rods, adding an additional degree of freedom whereby the polymer can relax stress (figure 2.3). Importantly, the Rouse model does not account for hydrodynamic interactions or self-avoidance so the polymers are treated as ideal random coils.

Interestingly, Rouse first developed his model to describe non-interacting polymers in dilute conditions, but his predictions could not accurately describe experimental results in this regime due to hydrodynamic interactions and self-avoidance. However, it was this foundational picture of a polymer as a chain of beads and springs that Zimm built on by incorporating hydrodynamic interactions and self-avoidance to accurately describe experimental observations in the dilute regime.

Quite fortuitously, in the semidilute regime, hydrodynamic interactions and self-avoidance are negligible so the Rouse model elegantly describes the statistics in this regime. It is interesting to note that a more simplified model (Rouse vs Zimm) can be used to describe a seemingly more complex situation (semidilute overlapping polymers vs non-interacting dilute polymers). Sometimes less is more.

The Rouse model also accurately captures the physics of weakly overlapping polymers in 'melts' in which there is no solvent. While synthetic polymers are often found in melt phases, biopolymer networks are nearly always in aqueous solution, so I will focus on the physics and frameworks to describe solutions rather than melts.

2.3.4 Entanglements and the reptation model

As the polymer concentration is increased further, to several times c^*, the polymer chains become entangled with one other (figure 2.2(H)), in which case the **reptation tube model**, first proposed by Pierre de Gennes in 1971 (de Gennes 1979), and later refined by Masao Doi and Sir Samuel Edwards (Doi and Edwards 1988), most accurately describes the physics (figure 2.2(H)). The **critical entanglement concentration** c_e at which entanglements dominate the polymer physics is typically ~4–10 c^* for biopolymers, depending on the polymer type and solvent conditions (Robertson and Smith 2007, Pan *et al* 2014, Banik *et al* 2021).

The Nobel prize-winning reptation theory treats each entangled polymer as confined to a tube-like region, formed by the surrounding polymers, that runs parallel to its contour (figure 2.2(H)). The tube restricts the transverse fluctuations of the polymer to the interior of the tube such that the polymer is forced to diffuse in a curvilinear fashion along its backbone. This one-dimensional 'head-first' diffusion is similar to the slithering motion of a snake, which inspired de Gennes to coin the diffusive process 'reptation', after the French word for slithering, 'reptare'. The beauty of the reptation model is that it reduces an incredibly complex many-body problem down to that of a single mean-field. The entanglements from the many neighboring chains that confine a polymer are reduced to a single hard-wall confining potential—the infamous tube.

2.3.4.1 Entanglement tube properties and scaling relations

With this simplification, the only lengthscales that are needed to predict the system properties are the tube dimensions, which include the diameter d_T and length L_o of the confinement tube. The tube length is also referred to as the **primitive path length**, and is shorter than the contour length L of a flexible polymer due to the fractal nature of polymer conformations. In other words, the polymer is not fully extended within the confining tube, but instead undergoes transverse fluctuations away from the central backbone (not exceeding d_T) that shorten the end-to-end distance of the confined polymer and its tube.

Another important lengthscale, that relates to the tube diameter and can often be empirically inferred, is the polymer length between entanglements N_e (or l_e) in units of Kuhn lengths (or physical length). The relationship between N_e and d_T can be derived in analogy to equation (2.3) by considering the tube diameter to be the mean end-to-end distance of a segment of the polymer that comprises N_e monomers:

$$d_T \approx l_k N_e^{1/2} \tag{2.14}$$

The size of the polymer chain can then be described as an ideal random walk of entanglement segments:

$$R_0 \approx d_T (N/N_e)^{1/2} \approx l_k N^{1/2} \tag{2.15}$$

As described above, due to the fractal nature of the polymer conformation, the primitive path length L_o is smaller than the polymer contour length L by

$$L_o \approx d_T N/N_e \approx d_T L/l_e \approx l_k L/l_e^{1/2}. \tag{2.16}$$

2.3.4.2 Blob theory

The lengthscales given in equations (2.14)–(2.16) were, strictly-speaking, derived for polymer melts, in which there is no solvent and the polymers fill the entire volume. Because of the screening of hydrodynamic interactions above c^*, one may reason that the reptation model may still accurately describe the physics of entangled polymer solutions. However, we cannot ignore the solvent altogether as it takes up considerable volume in the solution, in particular for many biopolymer networks.

Synthetic polymers typically have a much smaller aspect ratio per monomer $L{:}d$ than biopolymers, so they take up substantially more volume for the same degree of polymer overlap. For this reason, it is often difficult to achieve a high degree of entanglement for synthetic polymers unless they are actually in the melt phase. Conversely, a highly entangled solution of dsDNA can occupy less than 1% of the total volume due to very high aspect ratios of ~10^3–10^4 for typical sizes of ~10–100 kbp for DNA used in biopolymer network studies. For this reason, solvent considerations are of heightened importance for understanding networks of biopolymers as compared to their synthetic counterparts.

To extend his celebrated reptation model to concentrated polymer solutions, Pierre de Gennes introduced, and aptly named, **blob theory** (de Gennes 1979), which others have refined (Doi and Edwards 1988, Colby and Rubinstein 1990, Heo and Larson 2005). Blob theory rescales the coarse-graining used in the reptation model to explicitly include polymer *and* solvent in its unit lengthscale, rather than using l_k or l_e, as we have done above for unentangled and entangled polymers, respectively.

Based on this approach, solvent-mediated excluded volume interactions between distinct monomers are only considered important above the **thermal blob size** ξ_T, which is typically larger than the Kuhn length, and is defined as the lengthscale at which the monomer interaction energy is comparable to the thermal energy $k_B T$. For monomers with end-to-end separation distances that are smaller than ξ_T, the excluded volume interaction, and thus the effect of the surrounding solvent, is weak compared to $k_B T$. Based on this criteria, sections of monomers along the polymer with size $R_0 \leqslant \xi_T$ can be treated as ideal (non-swollen) random coils. It follows, in analogy to equation (2.3), that the thermal blob size scales as:

$$\xi_T \approx l_k n_T^{1/2} \tag{2.17}$$

where n_T is the number of Kuhn lengths comprising each blob, which can be determined by considering the following relations:

$$L/\xi_T = N/n_T \tag{2.18}$$

We can now coarse-grain each polymer chain and its surrounding solvent to a Rouse chain of thermal blobs (rather than Kuhn segments) with the following rescaling (figure 2.2(E),(G)):

$$l_k \rightarrow \xi_T$$

$$N \rightarrow N/n_T$$

$$R_0 \approx \xi_T n_T^{\nu} \tag{2.19}$$

Importantly, the volume of each thermal blob contains both monomers and solvent, so the entire system (polymer *and* solvent) can now be considered a melt of thermal blobs and the reptation model predictions are once again valid.

However, in melts there is no polymer concentration to consider, as the entire system is polymer, so the scaling laws to describe melts relate statistics and dynamics solely to the degree of polymerization of the polymer N (i.e., its length in units of l_k). N is the only tuning knob to adjust parameters such as the tube diameter and entanglement density that dictate the dynamics.

For solutions, the polymer concentration c, in relation to c^*, plays an equally important role in the dynamics. Blob theory accounts for the effect of concentration by considering that the number of Kuhn lengths in a thermal blob decreases as concentration increases according to the relation:

$$n_T \sim c^{-1/(3\nu-1)} \tag{2.20}$$

where $\nu \simeq 0.588$ in good solvent conditions.

Therefore, the polymer size depends on concentration as:

$$R_0 \approx \xi_T (N/n_T)^{1/2} \approx l_k N^{1/2} c^{-(2\nu-1)/(6\nu-2)} \tag{2.21}$$

leading to the scaling relations

$$R_0 \sim c^{-0.12} \text{ (good solvent)} \tag{2.22a}$$

$$R_0 \sim c^0 \text{ (}\theta\text{ solvent).} \tag{2.22b}$$

The tube diameter likewise scales with concentration as:

$$d_T \sim c^{-0.76} \text{ (good solvent)} \tag{2.23a}$$

$$d_T \sim c^{-2/3} \text{ (}\theta\text{ solvent).} \tag{2.23b}$$

2.4 Single polymer dynamics

In the previous sections we treated polymers as static entities and focused entirely on their free-energy-minimizing conformations (e.g., ideal random coils, self-avoiding (random) walks). Yet, even in equilibrium, polymers are continuously thermally jiggling—undergoing Brownian motion and relaxing thermal stresses—and the nature of these dynamics is highly dependent on the lengths and concentrations of the polymers. Armed with an understanding of polymer conformations and statistics, we now turn to their dynamics.

Specifically, I will discuss the dynamics of single chains, rather than the bulk dynamics of the network, and derive predictions for center-of-mass diffusion coefficients and relaxation timescales for polymers in the dilute, overlapping, and entangled concentration regimes: $c \ll c^*$, $c^* \lesssim c < c_e$, and $c \gtrsim c_e$ (figures 2.2(F–H)).

2.4.1 Dilute solutions

The center-of-mass diffusion coefficient D_0 for a flexible polymer in the dilute limit ($c \ll c^*$, figure 2.2(F)) can be approximated using the Einstein relation (see equation (2.10)):

$$D_0 = k_B T/\zeta \tag{2.24}$$

where ζ is the friction coefficient that generally scales as the product of the solvent viscosity η_s and particle size, $\mathscr{R}$:

$$\zeta \sim \eta_s \mathscr{R} \tag{2.25}$$

As described in section 2.3.2, for a hard sphere the exact drag coefficient is $\zeta = 6\pi\eta_s R_s$.

The Zimm model couples these relations with modeling of hydrodynamic interactions to predict a dilute limit diffusion coefficient of

$$D_0 \simeq \frac{0.196 k_B T}{\eta_s R_0} \tag{2.26}$$

which can also be expressed as

$$D_0 \simeq \frac{0.196 k_B T}{\eta_s l_k N^\nu} \tag{2.27}$$

using the relation $R_0 \approx l_k N^\nu$, where $\nu \simeq 0.588$ is the Flory exponent (Flory 1949b, Zimm 1956).

Renormalization group theory calculations (Oono and Kohmoto 1983), similar to those used to refine ν from 3/5 to 0.588, refined this prediction for D_0, arriving at the expression:

$$D_0 \simeq \frac{0.230 k_B T}{\sqrt{6}\,\eta_s R_G} \simeq \frac{0.230 k_B T}{\eta_s R_0} \tag{2.28}$$

which has a slightly larger prefactor than equation (2.26).

Another important metric to characterize how 'fast' or 'slow' the polymer dynamics are, relative to, e.g., experimental timescales, is the timescale over which a polymer diffuses a distance R_0. We can assume that after diffusing this distance, the direction of the end-to-end vector $\overrightarrow{R_0}$ of the polymer coil is completely decorrelated from its initial value. The timescale associated with this process can then be considered as the time for the polymer to completely erase all memory of its previous state. This decorrelation timescale, termed the **Zimm time** τ_Z, is predicted by Zimm theory to equate to:

$$\tau_Z \simeq 0.163\, \eta_s R_0^3 / k_B T. \tag{2.29}$$

2.4.2 Semidilute solutions

In the semidilute overlapping regime ($c^* \lesssim c < c_e$,), the polymer dynamics are concentration dependent and can be described by combining the Rouse model with blob theory (figure 2.2(E),(G)).

Within this framework, the diffusion coefficient is predicted to be reduced from the dilute limit value D_0 according to the relation:

$$D \simeq D_0 (c/c^*)^{-(1-\nu)/(3\nu-1)} \tag{2.30}$$

from which it follows that D scales with polymer concentration as

$$D \sim c^{-0.5} \text{ (good solvent)} \tag{2.31a}$$

$$D \sim c^{-1} \text{ (theta solvent)}. \tag{2.31b}$$

Note that equation (2.30) is only valid for concentrations in which $c/c^* \gtrsim 1$ such that the polymers are overlapping. For concentrations below c^* the diffusion coefficient can be approximated as D_0.

Recall that Rouse chains are comprised of springs, so their elastic retraction plays an important role in the stress relaxation of a polymer (figure 2.3). Indeed, the Rouse model predicts that the longest relaxation timescale for a polymer, the **Rouse time** τ_R, is associated with the elastic retraction of its spring-like monomers. In dilute conditions ($c < c^*$), the Rouse time is predicted to be:

$$\tau_{R0} \approx \frac{\eta_s l_k^3 N^2}{k_B T} \tag{2.32}$$

from which it follows:

$$\tau_{R0} \approx 2NR_G^2 / \pi^2 D_0 \tag{2.33}$$

where τ_{R0} denotes the dilute limit Rouse time.

For semidilute solutions, where polymer coils are overlapping, the solvent contribution to each coil needs to be considered. This accounting is accomplished by coupling the Rouse model to blob theory, which leads to the following rescaling of the Rouse time by the polymer concentration relative to its overlap concentration c/c^*:

$$\tau_R \simeq \tau_{R0}(c/c^*)^{(2-3\nu)/(3\nu-1)} \tag{2.34}$$

from which the following solvent-dependent scaling relations are predicted:

$$\tau_R \sim c^{0.31} \text{ (good solvent)} \tag{2.35a}$$

$$\tau_R \sim c^1 \text{ (theta solvent).} \tag{2.35b}$$

2.4.3 Entangled solutions

Once polymers become entangled ($c \gtrsim c_e$), the nature of COM diffusion is distinct from that of the other regimes, and is well-described by the reptation model discussed in section 2.3.4 (figure 2.2(H)). Recall that an entangled polymer does not move isotropically in three dimensions, but instead diffuses 'head-first' in a direction curvilinear to its contour. The snake-like diffusivity, for which de Gennes named his theory, leads to scaling laws that relate the COM diffusion coefficient associated with reptation D_R to the chain length L that are quite distinct from the dilute and semidilute cases (which share similar mechanisms and scalings for COM diffusion between them).

The predicted diffusion coefficient in the melt phase D_{R1} can be written as:

$$D_{R1} \approx k_B T N_e / \zeta N^2 \tag{2.36}$$

yielding the following scaling relations:

$$D_{R1} \sim N^{-2} \sim M_w^{-2} \sim L^{-2}. \tag{2.37}$$

Of note, experiments with synthetic polymer melts report a steeper scaling of $D_{R1} \sim M_w^{-2.3}$ (Lodge 1999), while measurements of solutions of entangled DNA display scaling closer to the classical prediction $D_R \sim L^{-2}$ (Robertson and Smith 2007).

Similar to the semidilute unentangled case, for solutions of entangled polymers, there is an added dependence of the diffusion coefficient D_R on polymer concentration c/c_e that comes from blob theory:

$$D_R \sim c/c_e^{-(2-\nu)/(3\nu-1)} \tag{2.38}$$

This scaling law equates to the following solvent-dependent scaling laws:

$$D_R \sim c^{-7/4} \text{ (good solvent, } \nu \approx 3/5) \tag{2.39a}$$

$$D_R \sim c^{-7/3} \text{ (theta solvent, } \nu \approx 1/2) \tag{2.39b}$$

The tube confinement that dictates the dynamics of entangled polymers elicits longer relaxation timescales compared to the dilute and semidilute cases. The slowest relaxation mechanism for an entangled polymer is predicted by the reptation model to be the diffusion of a polymer out of its initial confining tube and into a new tube. The associated timescale required for a polymer to diffuse the length of its confining tube (i.e., the primitive path length L_0), termed the **disengagement time τ_D**, can be expressed as:

$$\tau_D \simeq 12NR_G^4/\pi^2 d_T^2 D_0. \tag{2.40}$$

τ_D sets the longest timescale associated with the tube confinement of an entangled polymer, such that for times $t > \tau_D$, each polymer retains no memory of its previous confined state, and thus is not constrained by the surrounding entangling chains. In this limit, the network exhibits unconstrained fluid-like behavior.

There is also a short time limit associated with tube confinement, below which the segments of the confined polymer do not 'feel' the tube. The shortest relaxation time, the **entanglement time τ_e**, is the time required for any given segment of an entangled chain to diffuse the width of the confining tube d_T, thereby 'feeling' the constraint it imposes on transverse fluctuations. The expression predicted by the reptation model for the entanglement time is:

$$\tau_e \simeq \frac{d_T^4}{6NR_G^2 D_0} \tag{2.41}$$

which can also be written as

$$\tau_e \simeq d_T^4/N^2 D_0 l_k^2 \tag{2.42}$$

Note the very strong dependence of τ_e on the tube diameter ($\tau_e \sim d_T^4$), as well as the inverse dependence on the free diffusion of the polymer chain.

For $t < \tau_e$ and $t > \tau_D$ the polymer diffuses freely, while for $\tau_e < t < \tau_D$ the polymer is confined to diffuse and relax stress within the confinement tube of diameter d_T. The greater the difference between τ_D and τ_e, the longer the timescales over which entanglements dominate the polymer dynamics. This difference is set by the **number of entanglements per chain Z**, given as:

$$Z = N/N_e \tag{2.43}$$

via the relation:

$$\tau_D/\tau_e \simeq Z^3 \tag{2.44}$$

Note that only in cases in which $Z > 1$, when the length of the chain N is longer than an entanglement segment N_e, will the chain dynamics be influenced by entanglements.

Entangled polymers also undergo elastic Rouse relaxation, just as in the semi-dilute case, over a timescale set by the Rouse time τ_R, defined in equations (2.32)–(2.35). The Rouse time can also be related to τ_e and τ_D via the following relations:

$$\tau_D/\tau_R \cong 3N/N_e = 3Z \tag{2.45}$$

$$\tau_R/\tau_e \simeq Z^2 \tag{2.46}$$

We can see from these relations that for cases in which $Z > 1$, the criterion for being in the entangled state, we have the following hierarchy of timescales: $\tau_e < \tau_R < \tau_D$. This hierarchy requires Rouse relaxation to occur during the time in which the polymer feels the tube confinement. However, this relaxation mode and timescale are unaffected by the confinement as they relate to lateral elastic stretching.

2.5 Beyond the standard tube model

The reptation model has been highly successful in simplifying a very complex problem to make tractable predictions that can describe experimental observations reasonably well. However, while the simplicity of the mean-field tube model is what makes it so powerful, it also leads to discrepancies between experiment and theory in certain cases in which some of the complexities cannot be ignored. For example, the surrounding entangling chains are not static entities, but rather can move themselves. Thus, the idea that the entanglement tube is a single static entity with a single diameter and length is indeed an approximation.

There have been many proposed extensions and variations to the original reptation model that attempt to reconcile predictions with experimental observations by building more complexity into the tube model framework, e.g., (Graessley 1982, des Cloizeaux 1988, Viovy *et al* 1991, Milner and McLeish 1998, Mhetar and Archer 1999, McLeish 2002, Rubinstein and Colby 2003, Haley and Lodge 2005, Shanbhag and Larson 2006, Zhou and Larson 2006, Hinsch *et al* 2007, Larson 2010, Abadi *et al* 2018, Wang *et al*). While most of these extensions are outside the scope of this chapter, three mechanisms that merit discussion are **constraint release, tube dilation,** and **contour length fluctuations.** We will see in the following chapters that these mechanisms play important roles for networks comprising circular polymers (McKenna and Plazek 1986, Chapman *et al* 2012, Regan *et al* 2016, Peddireddy *et al* 2020, Zhou *et al* 2021), those that are subject to nonlinear deformations (Sussman and Schweizer 2013a, Chapman and Robertson-Anderson 2014, Khan *et al* 2019, Peddireddy *et al* 2022), and solutions of polymers with low entanglement densities (Khanal *et al* 2022)—all common occurrences in biopolymer network research.

2.5.1 Constraint release

Constraint release (CR) is the mechanism whereby an entangled polymer can diffuse transverse to its contour over distances larger than d_T—motion that is typically restricted by the confining tube—by the surrounding polymers forming the tube constraint diffusing away and thus releasing their constraints. The relaxation time associated with constraint release can be expressed as:

$$\tau_{CR} \approx \tau_{DT} Z^2 \tag{2.47}$$

where τ_{DT} is the disengagement time of the polymers *forming the tube* rather than that of the *confined polymer* τ_D.

Because the disengagement time of the confined polymer sets the lifetime of the tube confinement, constraint release only contributes appreciably to the relaxation of an entangled polymer when it is faster than that of reptation, i.e., $\tau_{CR} < \tau_D$. Given the requirement that $Z > 1$, it follows that τ_{CR} will only be shorter than τ_D if the disengagement time of the surrounding polymers is likewise shorter than τ_D ($\tau_{DT} < \tau_D$). More exactly, τ_{DT} must be shorter than τ_D by a factor Z^2 ($\tau_{DT}Z^2 < \tau_D$).

This criterion may be met, for example, in the case of a long linear polymer entangled by shorter linear chains (von Meerwall *et al* 2007, Wang and Larson 2008). Because the surrounding chains are shorter than the chain of interest, it follows that their disengagement time is likewise shorter as they have fewer entanglements per chain, so the inequality $\tau_{DT} < \tau_D$ is met.

Constraint release may also play a key role in polymer relaxation in cases in which reptation is completely prohibited or is extremely slow compared to experimental timescales, such that $\tau_D \to \infty$. This situation has been shown to arise in blends of linear and ring polymers due to the threading of rings by linear chains (Michieletto *et al* 2014, Peddireddy *et al* 2020, Zhou *et al* 2021). In this case, the center-of-mass of the threaded or pinned ring cannot move unless the linear polymers that are threading it, pinning it in place, diffuse away and thus release their constraint. Reptation, in this case, is prohibited because the ring has no ends by which to orient 'head-first' curvilinear diffusion. Reptation-like motion would result in the ring moving around in circles, like a dog chasing its tail, without significantly moving its center-of-mass. As such, constraint release (of the threading linear chains) is the only viable way for the ring COM to move.

Previous experiments (Robertson and Smith 2007) have shown that constraint release of ring DNA threaded by linear DNA leads to the diffusion coefficient scaling:

$$D_{CR} \sim c^{-3} \text{ (good solvent)} \tag{2.48}$$

which is steeper than the corresponding reptation scaling $D_R \sim c^{-1.75}$.

This steeper scaling is expected given the very slow process of constraint release as compared to reptation for entangled linear polymers. This relative slowness is also what allows us, in many cases, to not consider constraint release in the relaxation profile of an entangled polymer.

2.5.2 Tube dilation

Tube dilation is the phenomenon whereby the diameter of the entanglement tube d_T expands over time or in response to straining (Zhou and Larson 2006, Rae M. Robertson and Smith 2007, Sussman and Schweizer 2011, 2013a, Chapman and Robertson-Anderson 2014, Peddireddy *et al* 2022, Wang *et al*). In quiescent conditions, tube dilation arises as the confining polymer explores more transverse space over time, which effectively causes the tube diameter to grow, as predicted and seen in experiments with entangled DNA. Notably, these previous works also showed that the confining tube potential is not a hard-wall potential with a discontinuous jump at d_T, but, instead, is better described by a harmonic potential $U_T(y)$ where y is the transverse distance from the central chain backbone. Within this framework, the tube diameter d_T is defined as the transverse distance at which the confining potential energy is equal to the thermal energy:

$$U_T(y = d_T) = k_B T. \tag{2.49}$$

Over time, U_T softens such that the equality in equation (2.49) is met for increasingly larger y values.

The entanglement tube can also be dilated by external straining via forced disentanglement of the surrounding chains that form the entanglement tube of a given polymer (Sussman and Schweizer 2013b, Chapman and Robertson-Anderson 2014, Gurmessa *et al* 2016, Khan *et al* 2019). Forced removal of some of the entangling chains reduces the effective entanglement density Z which increases the tube diameter according to the scaling relation derived from equation (2.14):

$$d_T \sim Z^{-1/2}. \tag{2.50}$$

A similar phenomenon can occur by entangled chains preferentially aligning and stretching in the direction of an applied shear strain. This alignment reduces the effective entanglement density thereby dilating the entanglement tube according to equation (2.50). A similar effect is often what gives rise to shear thinning of entangled polymer solutions, which we will discuss below and in chapters 5–8.

2.5.3 Contour length fluctuations

Contour length fluctuations (CLFs) refer to the phenomenon of the length of the entanglement tube being shortened below the predicted primitive path length L_0. This shrinking arises from chain segments at the two ends of the confined polymer undergoing uncorrelated displacements that are not aligned with the tube contour. The degree to which contour length fluctuations affect the tube length and corresponding polymer dynamics depends on the entanglement density, with fewer entanglements giving rise to more pronounced contour length fluctuations. Taking into account CLF, the predicted tube length can be expressed as:

$$L_{CLF} \approx L_0(1 - X/\sqrt{Z}) \tag{2.51}$$

where X is a coefficient of order unity.

The shorter tube results in a shorter disengagement time according to the relation:

$$\tau_{D\_CLF} \approx \tau_D(1 - X/\sqrt{Z})^2 \tag{2.52}$$

We can see from these expressions that L_{CLF} and τ_{D_CLF} approach L_0 and τ_D as the entanglement density grows ($Z \to \infty$), such that CLF only has an appreciable effect on the dynamics when the number of entanglements per chain is modest ($Z \lesssim 10$).

2.6 Rheology

The discussion above has focused solely on the properties of *single* polymers in networks of many polymers. We next turn to understanding how these dynamics give rise to bulk network dynamics. In particular, we aim to describe the rheological properties of polymeric systems. Namely, how the bulk system responds to deformation.

As I describe in chapter 1 (section 1.1), most biopolymer networks are non-Newtonian viscoelastic fluids that exhibit both elastic storage, akin to solids, and viscous dissipation, akin to Newtonian fluids. Let's review.

Recall that at the most basic level, we can model a solid as a spring that exerts a force F to resist being stretched a distance Δx, i.e., Hooke's Law $F = k\Delta x$. It follows that the stress ($\sigma = F/A$) that a solid of volume $A \cdot h$ exerts to resist an applied strain $\gamma = \Delta x/h$ is proportional to the size of the strain γ:

$$\sigma \sim \gamma \tag{2.53}$$

Importantly, the stress that an elastic solid exerts is independent of the strain rate $\dot{\gamma} = \frac{d\gamma}{dt} = v\ /h$, where v is the strain speed.

Conversely, we recall that the force that a purely viscous Newtonian fluid exerts to resist strain is proportional to the strain speed but independent of displacement, in accord with Stokes' drag force $F = \zeta v$. It follows that the stress a fluid exerts to resist a strain scales with the strain rate as:

$$\sigma \sim \dot{\gamma} \tag{2.54}$$

These relations fundamentally tell us that elastic materials store the energy that the strain loads into the system, and can return to their initial position after being strained, while fluids dissipate (or lose) all loaded energy through viscous friction. Most biopolymer networks exhibit both of these features, but the relative degree to which they store or dissipate energy depends both on the nature of the strain and the network properties.

2.6.1 Defining linear viscoelastic moduli

We will focus our discussion on the rheological properties of polymers in the **linear regime**, in which the deformations are small enough that they do not perturb or disrupt the steady-state interactions between polymers. In this linear limit, rheological measurements are used to sense the bulk viscoelastic properties of the system rather than alter them.

As I describe in chapter 3, linear viscoelastic properties of a sample are typically measured by confining the sample between two plates and applying an oscillatory shear by rotating one plate relative to the other. The stress that the sample exerts on the plate to resist the strain can be measured to relate stress to strain and assess the degree of energy storage versus loss that the sample exhibits. Generally speaking, the rotation frequency ω and amplitude γ of the strain dictate the stress–strain relationship. In the linear regime, the stress is predicted to scale linearly with the strain ($\sigma \sim \gamma$) such that the modulus that relates stress to strain, G, is independent of the amplitude of the strain γ and depends solely on the oscillation frequency.

In this linear regime, the viscoelastic properties of polymeric systems are typically characterized by the frequency-dependent storage modulus $G'(\omega)$ and loss modulus $G''(\omega)$ derived from the time-dependent stress relaxation modulus $G(t)$ (figure 2.3(A)). $G'(\omega)$ and $G''(\omega)$ are measures of elastic-like and viscous-like contributions, respectively, to the stress response of the system. In practice, these quantities are determined by evaluating the extent to which the measured stress oscillations are in phase (G') or out of phase (G'') with the strain, as the former is a signature of elasticity ($\sigma \sim \gamma$) while the latter signifies fluidity ($\sigma \sim \dot{\gamma}$). The angular phase lag δ between stress and strain depends on the oscillation frequency, rendering G' and G'' dependent on ω. As I describe below, many of the polymer theories described in the previous sections predict scaling relations that relate the frequency dependence of the moduli to underlying molecular properties and mechanisms, such that G' and G'' can be used to infer said molecular dynamics.

From $G'(\omega)$ and $G''(\omega)$ we can also evaluate the complex viscosity $\eta^*(\omega)$, defined as:

$$\eta^*(\omega) = (G'(\omega)^2 + G''(\omega)^2)^{1/2}/\omega \tag{2.55}$$

which reduces to the zero-shear steady-state viscosity η_0 as $\omega \rightarrow 0$ and is independent of ω for Newtonian fluids (figure 3.2(C)).

The loss tangent $\tan\delta(\omega)$, defined as:

$$\tan\delta(\omega) = G''(\omega)/G'(\omega) \tag{2.56}$$

is another useful metric that evaluates the frequency-dependent phase lag $\delta(\omega)$ to quantify the extent to which the network dissipates or stores energy. Namely, the degree to which $\tan\delta(\omega)$ is greater or less than 1 determines the relative contributions from viscous and elastic mechanisms (figure 3.3(B)):

$$\tan\delta(\omega) > 1 : \text{viscous dissipation} \tag{2.57a}$$

$$\tan\delta(\omega) < 1 : \text{elastic storage} \tag{2.57b}$$

Chapter 3 will go into greater depth regarding how rheological properties are formulated, measured, and interpreted. Here, we summarize the key predicted scaling relations between the viscoelastic moduli and polymer network properties.

2.6.2 Predicted linear viscoelastic scaling laws

2.6.2.1 Dilute limit and terminal regime scaling

In the dilute limit, in which polymeric fluids behave largely as Newtonian fluids, there is minimal in-phase (elastic) contribution to the stress response so the elastic modulus is negligibly small compared to the viscous modulus

$$G'' \gg G',\ G'(\omega) \rightarrow 0 \tag{2.58}$$

In line with a purely viscous response ($\sigma \sim \dot{\gamma}$), the viscous modulus scales linearly with frequency as

$$G''(\omega) \sim \omega^1 \tag{2.59}$$

and the complex viscosity is an intrinsic property of the fluid that is independent of ω and equivalent to the zero-shear limit value:

$$\eta^*(\omega) \simeq \eta_0 \sim \omega^0. \tag{2.60}$$

In the entangled regime, polymers may also exhibit predominantly viscous response at low enough frequencies, i.e., long enough times. Specifically, for timescales longer than the longest relaxation timescale of the system, $t > \tau_D$ for entangled polymers, which equates to $\omega < 2\pi\tau_D^{-1}$ in frequency space, the system will exhibit fluid-like **terminal flow** behavior with the following scalings (figure 2.4, red region):

$$G''(\omega) \sim \omega^1 \tag{2.61a–d}$$

$$G'(\omega) \sim \omega^2$$

$$\eta^*(\omega) \sim \omega^0$$

$$\tan\delta(\omega) \sim \omega^{-1}$$

and relationships:

$$G'' > G' \tag{2.61e,f}$$

$$\tan\delta(\omega) > 1.$$

The onset of the terminal regime is marked by a crossover from $G' > G''$, from the high-frequency end, to $G'' > G'$ from the low-ω end (figure 2.4(A)), which is predicted to occur at the disengagement time, such that the frequency ω_c at which this crossover occurs can be used to determine τ_D:

$$\omega_c = 2\pi\,\tau_D^{-1} \tag{2.62}$$

2.6.2.2 Entangled regime scaling

For frequencies above ω_c (i.e., $t < \tau_D$) the effects of tube confinement dominate the stress response. The entanglements with surrounding chains provide an elastic contribution to the stress response and restrict dissipative relaxation, such that the network response is rubbery or elastic-like:

$$G' > G''$$

$$\tan\delta(\omega) < 1$$

The defining signature of this **rubbery entanglement regime** is a frequency-independent plateau in the elastic modulus:

$$G'(\omega) \simeq G^0 \sim \omega^0 \tag{2.63}$$

The value of this modulus, the **plateau modulus G^0**, is the primary metric used to characterize the system in this regime (figure 2.3(A), yellow region). Specifically, theoretical predictions from the reptation model and blob theory that relate G^0 to network parameters can be used to estimate the entanglement length, N_e or l_e, and tube diameter d_T via the following expressions:

$$G^0 \approx \frac{ck_BT}{l_k^2 l_e} \tag{2.64}$$

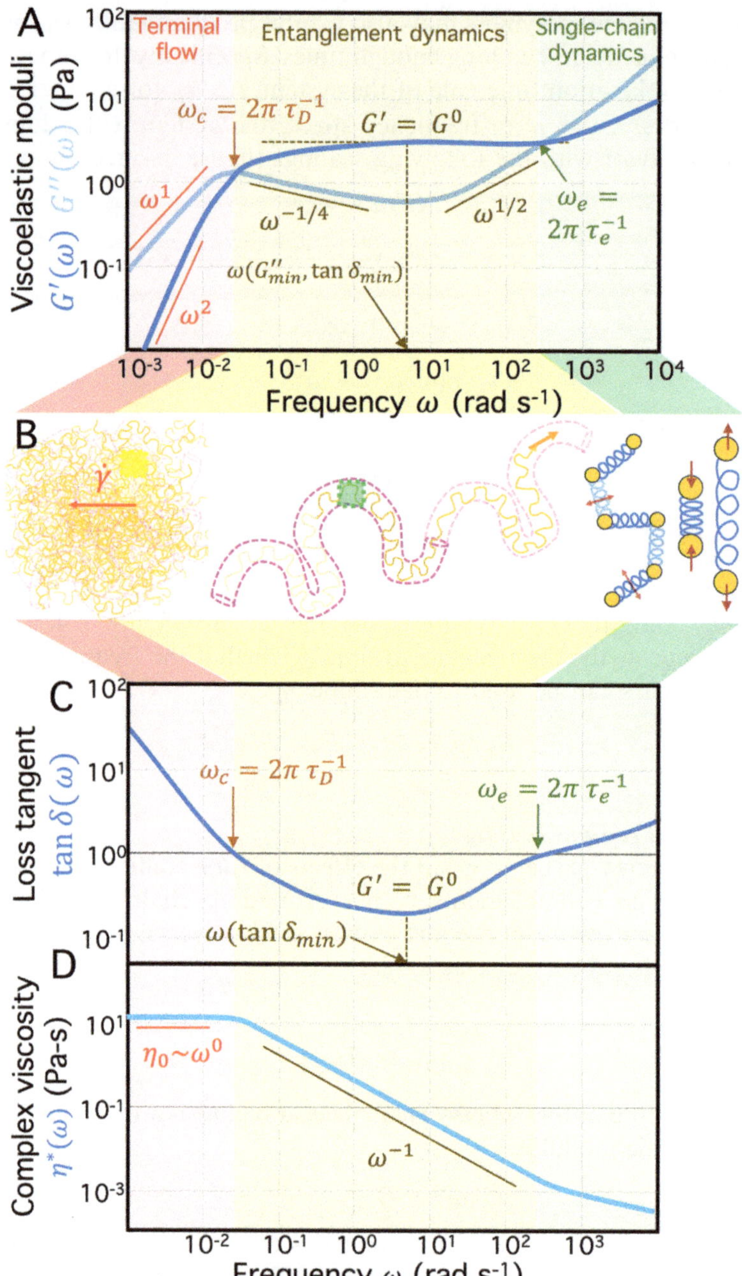

Figure 2.4. Frequency dependent linear viscoelastic properties of entangled polymers. (A) Characteristic elastic and viscous moduli, $G'(\omega)$ (solid blue) and $G''(\omega)$ (translucent blue), for entangled polymers exhibit three distinct scaling regimes that describe the dynamics dominated by terminal viscous flow (red, $\omega < \omega_c$), elastic-like entanglements (yellow, $\omega_c < \omega < \omega_e$) and single-chain Rouse stretching (green, $\omega > \omega_e$). The solid red and dark yellow lines are predicted scaling laws and the dashed lines denote the plateau modulus G^0 and the corresponding frequency ω at which it can be computed. (B) Cartoon depiction of the polymer dynamics that dominate each regime: unencumbered network flow (left), reptation (middle) and Rouse relaxation of isolated

chain segments (right). The yellow and green translucent boxes indicate the scale of the region that is depicted in the subsequent color-coded panels. At higher frequencies, the lengthscales that dominate the dynamics decrease. (C,D) From $G'(\omega)$ and $G''(\omega)$ we can compute the (C) loss tangent $\tan\delta(\omega) = G''(\omega)/G'(\omega)$ and (D) complex viscosity $\eta^*(\omega) = \eta^*(\omega) = \omega^{-1}(G'(\omega)^2 + G''(\omega)^2)^{1/2}$, which are expected to follow distinct scalings in the different frequency regimes as shown. (C) The minimum in $\tan\delta(\omega)$ can be used to determine G^0 and the frequencies at which $\tan\delta(\omega) = 1$ correspond to ω_c and ω_e. (D) Entangled polymers exhibit shear thinning in the entanglement regime (yellow) with $\eta^*(\omega) \sim \omega^{-1}$, and the terminal regime plateau (red) can be used to determine the zero-shear viscosity η_0.

$$l_e \approx l_k n_T d_T^2/\xi_T^2 \tag{2.65}$$

which together yield:

$$G^0 \approx ck_BT\xi_T^2/l_k^3 n_T d_T^2 \tag{2.66}$$

Moreover, l_e is predicted to scale with polymer concentration as:

$$l_e \sim c^{-1/(3\nu-1)} \sim c^{-1.31} \text{ (good solvent)} \tag{2.67a}$$

$$l_e \sim c^{-4/3} \text{ (theta solvent)} \tag{2.67b}$$

Note that the scaling is nearly independent of solvent quality (~1.31 vs ~1.33), unlike many other characteristic quantities.

Combining these relations with the scaling from equation (2.64)

$$G^0 \sim cl_e^{-1} \tag{2.68}$$

yields the predicted concentration scalings of G^0:

$$G^0 \sim c^{-3\nu/(3\nu-1)} \sim c^{2.31} \text{ (good solvent)} \tag{2.69a}$$

$$G^0 \sim c^{7/3} \text{ (theta solvent)} \tag{2.69b}$$

which, as required by equation (2.67), are remarkably similar for the two different solvent conditions.

Unlike the elastic modulus, which exhibits no frequency dependence in the rubbery entanglement regime, the viscous modulus exhibits two phases of power-law scaling, first decreasing as:

$$G''(\omega) \sim \omega^{-1/4} \tag{2.70}$$

then increasing with scaling

$$G''(\omega) \sim \omega^{1/2}. \tag{2.71}$$

The frequency at which G'' is a minimum, ω_0, separating these two scaling regimes, can be used to determine the plateau modulus:

$$G'(\omega_0) \simeq G^0 \tag{2.72}$$

(figure 2.4(A)).

This minimum should also manifest in $\tan\delta(\omega)$ at the same frequency (figure 2.4(B)), offering an alternative method for determining the plateau modulus, i.e., identifying this frequency from the minimum in $\tan\delta$ rather than G''.

Another key feature of the entanglement plateau regime is a power-law scaling of the complex viscosity with frequency (figure 2.4(C)):

$$\eta^*(\omega) \sim \omega^{-x}. \tag{2.73}$$

The predicted asymptotic value for well-entangled polymers ($c \gg c_e$, $Z \gg 1$) is $x = 1$, while lower exponent values of $x \approx 0.7-0.9$ have been experimentally observed for several entangled biopolymer systems (Chapman *et al* 2014, Pan *et al* 2014, Banik *et al* 2021, Dakhil *et al* 2021, Peddireddy *et al* 2020).

In the semidilute unentangled regime ($c^* < c < c_e$), the Rouse model predicts $x = 1/2$, in line with experimental observations (Colby *et al* 2007, Chapman *et al* 2014, Pan *et al* 2018, Khanal *et al* 2022). As the polymers begin to lose overlap ($c \lesssim c^*$), the exponent decreases, approaching $x = 0$ in the dilute limit.

This power-law decrease in $\eta^*(\omega)$ with increasing frequency is related to the phenomenon of **shear thinning**, whereby the steady-shear viscosity $\eta(\dot{\gamma})$ decreases with increasing shear rate $\dot{\gamma}$ due to increasingly affine alignment and stretching of entangled polymers in the direction of the strain. This strain alignment reduces the effective entanglement density, thereby accelerating disengagement and reducing the elastic stress that the network exerts to resist the strain.

Shear thinning manifests as power-law scaling

$$\eta(\dot{\gamma}) \sim \dot{\gamma}^{-X} \tag{2.74}$$

in response to steady-shear strains (distinct from oscillatory strains).

Treating the power-law behavior in equations (2.73) and (2.74) as equivalent, thereby assuming $x = X$, is only valid for systems that obey the **Cox–Merz rule**, which states that the frequency-dependent complex viscosity is the same as the rate-dependent steady-shear viscosity when $\omega = \dot{\gamma}$ (Iannirubertoand Marrucci 1996, Pan *et al* 2014). No biopolymer systems that we will discuss in the following chapters have been shown to violate the Cox–Merz rule. As such, for simplification, we will discuss both relations interchangeably in the subsequent chapters without invoking the Cox–Merz criterion.

2.6.2.3 High-frequency relaxation

As described in section 2.4.3, for times shorter than the entanglement time $t < \tau_e$, an entangled polymer does not feel its surrounding entanglements because there is not enough time for its transverse fluctuations to reach a distance d_T and thus feel the confinement. Likewise, we can expect that the stress response of an entangled polymer network at frequencies faster than the entanglement rate τ_e^{-1}:

$$\omega > \omega_e = 2\pi\tau_e^{-1} \tag{2.75}$$

will be dominated by the free relaxation of entanglement segments (figure 2.4, green regions), rather than the confined motion of the polymer chain, which dominates in the frequency range $\omega_c < \omega < \omega_e$ (figure 2.4, yellow regions).

This entanglement frequency ω_e, from which the entanglement time can be deduced via equation (2.74), is demarcated by a crossover from $G'' < G'$ to $G'' > G'$. In this viscous-dominated $\omega > \omega_e$ regime, contributions to the elastic modulus from tube confinement are frozen out. The primary contribution to G' is instead elastic Rouse retraction, which scales with frequency as:

$$G'(\omega) \sim \omega^{1/2}. \tag{2.76}$$

The viscous modulus likewise exhibits power-law increase with frequency

$$G''(\omega) \sim \omega^{\varepsilon} \tag{2.77}$$

but the exact value of the scaling exponent ε is still debated. The classical Rouse model predicts $\varepsilon = 1/2$, matching the scaling for G', while experiments and refinements to the Rouse model give a range of higher values $0.5 < \varepsilon < 7/8$ (Ferry 1980, Doi and Edwards 1988, Mohamed *et al* 2018, Zhong *et al* 2022). The higher exponent values are typically derived by considering the retraction and relaxation of the chain ends differently than the rest of the chain, mechanistically similar to contour length fluctuations described in section 2.5.3.

2.7 Semiflexible polymers

The scaling laws and theoretical frameworks I presented in the previous sections are excellent for describing the experimentally-measured conformations and dynamics of flexible polymers with $L \gg l_k$. However, they begin to break down as $L \rightarrow l_k$, when polymers are considered semiflexible. In particular, the freely jointed chain and bead-spring models (figure 2.3) fail because the orientation of two neighboring segments can no longer be considered to be completely decorrelated. In this section, we discuss approaches to account for this added layer of complexity.

2.7.1 Worm-like chain model

The **worm-like chain (WLC)** model is perhaps the most widely-invoked and successful theory to describe the conformations of semiflexible chains (Aragon and Pecora 1985, Bouchiat *et al* 1999, Rubinstein and Colby 2003, Maarel 2008). The WLC model treats each polymer as a continuously flexible isotropic rod rather than a FJC model chain of discrete rigid rods. The defining lengthscale in the model is the persistence length, defined as in figure 2.1, rather than the Kuhn length. The mean-squared end-to-end distance of a worm-like chain is predicted to depend on l_p and L as:

$$\langle R_0^2 \rangle = 2 l_p L \left[1 - \frac{l_p}{L}\left(1 - e^{-L/l_p}\right) \right]. \tag{2.78}$$

We can see that in the flexible limit, $L \gg l_p$, the second term becomes negligible and we recover the FJC result (see equations (2.3)–(2.6)) using the relation $l_k = 2 l_p$:

$$\langle R_0^2 \rangle = \left(2 l_p\right) L = l_k^2 N \rightarrow R_0 = l_k N^{\nu} \ \ (L \gg l_p) \tag{2.79}$$

where $\nu = \frac{1}{2}$ is the ideal chain exponent.

From R_0, we can determine R_G, R_H, and D using the same relations outlined in section 2.3.

In the opposite limit of $L \ll l_p$, in which the polymer can be considered a rigid rod, we expect the end-to-end distance to be equal to the polymer contour length, i.e. $R_0 = L$, as bending or rotating of segments along the chain relative to each other are prohibited. By expanding the exponential term in equation (2.77):

$$e^{-L/l_p} \approx 1 - \frac{L}{l_p} + \frac{1}{2}\left(\frac{L}{l_p}\right)^2 \tag{2.80}$$

we can see that the WLC expression for $\langle R_0^2 \rangle$ indeed recovers the expected rigid rod result in the $L \ll l_p$ limit:

$$\langle R_0^2 \rangle \simeq 2 l_p L \frac{l_p}{L}\left[\frac{1}{2}\left(\frac{L}{l_p}\right)^2\right] = L^2. \tag{2.81}$$

The worm-like chain model accurately describes the entropic stretching profile of DNA, as well as the dynamics of semiflexible biopolymers such as short DNA chains ($L \sim O(10)l_p$) (Aragon and Pecora 1985, Marko and Siggia 1995, Bouchiat *et al* 1999).

The WLC model has been incorporated into the tube model framework to make several key scaling predictions that differ from those for flexible chains. Importantly, the critical entanglement concentration c_e, that separates the semidilute unentangled and entangled regimes, is predicted to be nearly two orders of magnitude larger than the overlap concentration c^*

$$c_e \simeq 60c^* \tag{2.82}$$

which is an order of magnitude larger than the flexible polymer result $c_e \simeq (4-10)c^*$.

The predicted scalings for the plateau modulus G^0 and entanglement length l_e with concentration also differ from that for flexible polymers. Specifically, the scaling of G^0 depends on the relative lengthscales of transverse bending undulations of the polymer $R_\perp$ and the network mesh size ξ, which are defined in terms of the system parameters as (Kroy and Frey 1996):

$$R_\perp^2 \simeq 2L^3/3l_p \tag{2.83}$$

$$\xi \simeq 1/\sqrt{c_N a} \tag{2.84}$$

where a is the monomer size and c_N is the monomer number density (Isambert and Maggs 1996). Note that $R_\perp^2$ depends only on the properties of each individual polymer while the mesh size ξ depends only on how many monomers are in the volume.

For networks in which $R_\perp^2 < \xi$, bending is expected to contribute negligibly to entanglement dynamics, so the chains can be considered straight (but not rigid) rods. Conversely, for $R_\perp^2 > \xi$, bending is appreciable and the chains adopt curved 'snake-like' conformations. These different cases result in the scaling laws:

$$G^0 \sim c^{5/3} \; (R_\perp^2 > \xi, \text{ snake}) \tag{2.85a}$$

$$G^0 \sim c^2 \; (R_\perp^2 < \xi, \text{ rod}) \tag{2.85b}$$

Moreover, in the snake-like case, the entanglement length is predicted to relate to the mesh size as:

$$l_e \simeq (l_p \xi^2)^{1/3} \tag{2.86}$$

from which it follows:

$$l_e \sim c^{-1/3}. \tag{2.87}$$

2.7.2 Cooperativity

Another approach to account for non-zero correlations between neighboring chains is to include a cooperativity parameter that accounts for said correlations (Wiggins and Nelson 2006, Nelson *et al* 2020). This model starts with a freely jointed chain but treats each link as having a length equivalent to the persistence length of the chain rather than the Kuhn length:

$$l_k \rightarrow l_p(= l_k/2) \tag{2.88}$$

A cooperative interaction term between neighboring chains is then incorporated so that neighboring chains incur an energetic cost of not being aligned. This model is primarily used to understand the entropic stretching behavior of an individual polymer subject to an external stretching force. Because the focus of this text is on networks of biopolymers rather than single-chain dynamics, we will leave the interested reader with the following suggested texts that discuss this model in detail (Khokhlov *et al* 1994, Marko and Siggia 1995, Wiggins and Nelson 2006, Nelson *et al* 2020).

2.7.3 When semiflexible polymers are stiffer

The above treatments of semiflexibility have been successful in describing chains with $l_p < L$, such as short dsDNA chains with $L \approx O(10)l_p$. For stiffer biopolymers that are still classified as semiflexible because they are far from the $l_p \gg L$ limit, but have persistence lengths comparable to their contour lengths, $l_p \sim L$, further modifications to these foundational theories are necessary to accurately describe their dynamics (figure 2.2(B)). Actin filaments are a quintessential example of such polymers, and have served as primary inspiration for developing theoretical understanding of this regime. Below, I summarize key concepts from these theoretical extensions that describe the $l_p \sim L$ case, focusing on the entangled regime (Isambert and Maggs 1996, Käs *et al* 1996, Hinsch *et al* 2007).

For entangled polymers with $l_p \sim L$, each entanglement segment of length l_e can be approximated as a rigid rod, owing to the fact that $l_e < l_p$, such that the tube diameter and entanglement length can be considered to be comparable:

$$d_T \approx l_e \tag{2.89}$$

This relation is in contrast to that of the flexible chain in which each entanglement segment is treated as a random coil, yielding the relation

$$d_T \approx (l_k l_e)^{1/2} \tag{2.90}$$

as determined from equation (2.14).

It follows from equation (2.89) that the primitive path length is comparable to the polymer contour length (in contrast to equation (2.16)):

$$L_0 \approx L \tag{2.91}$$

The mesh size of the network ξ, defined in equation (2.84), becomes another important lengthscale in this limit, in contrast to the case of flexible polymers, as does the persistence length l_p.

Specifically, the tube dimensions can be expressed as:

$$d_T \approx \xi^{6/5} l_p^{-1/5} \tag{2.92}$$

$$l_e \approx \xi^{4/5} l_p^{1/5} \tag{2.93}$$

where ξ and l_p are properties of the system and the polymer, respectively. Considering the relation $\xi \sim c^{-1/2}$ (equation (2.84)), the scaling of these dimensions with concentration are:

$$d_T \sim c^{-3/5} \tag{2.94}$$

$$l_e \sim c^{-2/5}, \tag{2.95}$$

both steeper than the scalings predicted for flexible polymers in good ($d_T \sim c^{-0.76}$, $l_e \sim c^{-0.38}$) and theta ($d_T \sim c^{-2/3}$, $l_e \sim c^{-1/3}$) solvent conditions.

The plateau modulus has a similar scaling with concentration and entanglement length as the flexible case (see equation (2.68)), which can be seen from the expression:

$$G^0 \approx k_B T/\xi^2 l_e \approx k_B T a c_N l_e^{-1}$$

which, combined with equation (2.95), provides the predicted scaling:

$$G^0 \sim c^{7/5}. \tag{2.96}$$

Finally, predicted expressions for the entanglement time τ_e and disengagement time τ_D, which flank the entanglement regime, are

$$\tau_e \approx (\zeta/k_B T)\, \xi^{16/5} l_p^{-1/5} \tag{2.97}$$

$$\tau_D \approx (\zeta/k_B T) L^3 \tag{2.98}$$

where ζ is the friction coefficient that is expected to be independent of concentration and $\zeta/k_B T \approx 2-4$ s μm^{-3} (Isambert and Maggs 1996, Gurmessa *et al* 2016). These expressions lead to concentration scalings:

$$\tau_e \sim c^{-8/5} \tag{2.99}$$

$$\tau_D \sim c^0 L^3 \tag{2.100}$$

Rouse modes are considered negligible for semiflexible polymers that are neither entropically coiled nor inextensible, so there is minimal entropic or energetic stretching to relax. However, bending plays an important role in relaxation; and, as described above, depends on the relative lengthscales of bending and polymer crossings (i.e., entanglements). This dependence leads to several additional relaxation modes available to semiflexible polymers that are associated with relaxation of density fluctuations across different lengthscales, including the mesh size ξ, persistence length l_p, and polymer contour length L.

The fastest of these relaxation timescales is the time it takes for filaments to feel the hydrodynamic effects of neighboring filaments. The defining lengthscale in this process is the mesh size ξ, and the corresponding mesh relaxation time τ_ξ can be written as:

$$\tau_\xi \approx (\zeta/k_BT)\, \xi^4 l_p^{-1} \quad (\tau_\xi \sim c^{-2}) \tag{2.101}$$

Note that this timescale is shorter than τ_e, and thus occurs in the high-frequency regime that is dominated by the dynamics of single chains rather than that of the network.

For times $\tau_e < t < \tau_D$, when the polymers feel the tube confinement, the relaxation of density fluctuations of polymer segments with lengths l_p and L contribute to the overall relaxation on timescales of:

$$\tau_p \approx (\zeta/k_BT)\, \xi^{8/5} l_p^{7/5} \quad (\tau_p \sim c^{-4/5}) \tag{2.102}$$

$$\tau_L \approx (\zeta/k_BT) L^2 \xi^{8/5} l_p^{-3/5} \quad (\tau_L \sim c^{-4/5} L^2), \tag{2.103}$$

Of note, the rubbery plateau regime for semiflexible polymers, where $G'(\omega) \simeq G^0 \sim \omega^0$, spans $\tau_p < t < \tau_D$ rather than $\tau_e < t < \tau_D$ for flexible polymers. This may contribute to the much larger c_e/c^* values for semiflexible polymers as compared to their flexible counterparts (Kroy and Frey 1996).

Bending modes are also predicted to contribute to stress relaxation with predicted timescales of

$$\tau_b \approx (\epsilon/l_p k_B T)(2L/3\pi)^4 \tag{2.104}$$

where

$$\epsilon = 4\pi\eta_s/\ln\,(2\xi/a) \tag{2.105}$$

is the perpendicular drag coefficient.

As described above, semiflexible polymers exhibit a crossover at $t<\tau_e$, similar to flexible polymers, to a high-frequency regime in which $G'' > G'$ and single-chain dynamics dominate. However, rather than following Rouse scaling in this regime, the viscoelastic moduli are predicted to follow steeper scaling than their flexible counterparts due to the relaxation of axial tension (Gisler and Weitz 1999, Gardel *et al* 2003, Koenderink *et al* 2006, Hiraiwa and Ohta 2009):

$$G'(\omega) \sim G''(\omega) \sim \omega^{3/4}. \tag{2.106}$$

2.8 Rigid rod polymers

Rigid rod polymers with $l_p \gg L$ do not assume entropic coil conformations nor do they undergo thermal bending, simplifying the internal relaxation modes and rendering the root mean-squared end-to-end distance simply equal to the contour length of the polymer, $R_0 = L$ (figure 3.2(C)).

The conformations of rigid rods are anisotropic, in contrast to their more flexible counterparts, such that the diffusion of a rigid rod in the dilute limit is distinct in directions parallel and transverse to its major axis. This effect can be understood as arising from a higher drag coefficient associated with motion perpendicular $\zeta_\perp$ versus parallel $\zeta_\parallel$ to the major axis of a rod:

$$\zeta_\parallel = \frac{2\pi\eta_s L}{\ln\left(\frac{L}{d}\right)} \tag{2.107}$$

$$\zeta_\perp = 2\zeta_\parallel \tag{2.108}$$

By invoking the Einstein relation $D\zeta = k_B T$, we can see that the diffusion coefficient parallel to the long axis is twice as fast as that perpendicular:

$$D_{0,\parallel} = 2D_{0,\perp} = k_B T \frac{\ln\left(\frac{L}{d}\right)}{2\pi\eta_s L} \tag{2.109}$$

The corresponding dilute limit COM diffusion coefficient is given by:

$$D_0 \simeq \frac{D_{0,\parallel} + 2D_{0,\perp}}{3} = k_B T \frac{\ln\left(\frac{L}{d}\right)}{3\pi\eta_s L}. \tag{2.110}$$

Once rods begin to entangle with one another, the tube model framework can be applied, which suppresses motion perpendicular to the major axis of the rod (and tube) but allows for free diffusion along the major axis:

$$D_{R,\parallel} \simeq D_{0,\parallel}, D_{R,\perp} = 0 \tag{2.111}$$

from which it follows that

$$D_R \simeq D_0\left(\frac{D_{0,\parallel}}{D_{0,\parallel} + 2D_{0,\perp}}\right) = \frac{D_0}{2} \tag{2.112}$$

The principal relaxation timescales that flank the entanglement regime, τ_e and τ_D, can be expressed in terms of the parallel and perpendicular diffusion coefficients as:

$$\tau_e \simeq d_T^2 D_{0,\perp}^{-1} \tag{2.113}$$

$$\tau_D \simeq L^2 D_{0,\parallel}^{-1} \tag{2.114}$$

Another important scaling relation that we will consider in later chapters is the concentration dependence of the elastic plateau modulus:

$$G^0 \sim c \tag{2.115}$$

which is much weaker than the predicted scaling for flexible and semiflexible polymers (see equations (2.69a), (2.85a) and (2.96)).

Further predictions for rigid rods can be found in Doi and Edwards (1988), Rubinstein and Colby (2003), Sussman and Schweizer (2013b) and will be discussed as needed in subsequent chapters.

2.9 Crosslinked polymer networks

The theoretical frameworks described above only consider steric and hydrodynamic interactions between adjacent and overlapping polymers. However, in many biopolymer networks in biology, the polymers are chemically crosslinked such that the point at which two polymers overlap is fixed and one polymer cannot slide past the other.

Crosslinking suppresses thermal fluctuations and relaxation mechanisms available to entangled polymers and shifts the rheological properties to more elastic-like, as the polymers have less ability to dissipate stress. It is important to note that creating a percolated network of crosslinked polymers requires concentrations above c_e to ensure that there are a sufficient number of overlap nodes that can be physically connected. If the polymers are not entangled then crosslinking results in local bundling or clustering of nearest neighbors that are not connected to one another. As such, I focus the brief discussion below on the $c > c_e$ regime.

To incorporate crosslinking into the models for concentrated flexible polymer networks described above, we need to consider an additional lengthscale and timescale that will impact the dynamics: the length between crosslinkers along a polymer chain l_c and the binding lifetime of the crosslinker τ_c.

In cases in which the crosslinker length is much larger than the entanglement length, i.e., $l_c \gg l_e$, the effect of crosslinking is minimal as very few overlap nodes (i.e., entanglements) are crosslinked. Likewise, when the crosslinker lifetime τ_c is very short compared to the disengagement time, i.e., $\tau_c \ll \tau_D$, the rate of crosslinker detachment and reattachment is much faster than the rate at which the polymer conformationally relaxes via reptation, such that crosslinking does not impact the longest relaxation time, which remains τ_D, and the rheological signatures are similar to an entangled network.

In the opposite extremes, when every node is crosslinked, i.e., $l_c \leqslant l_e$, and the crosslinkers are essentially permanent ($\tau_c \gg \tau_D$), reptation is prohibited and the network can never fully relax or dissipate energy. This is a hallmark of an elastic system—one that stores induced stress indefinitely until that stress is released and the system can return to its starting point. In this limit, the viscoelastic moduli exhibit no frequency dependence, as $\sigma \sim \gamma^1\dot{\gamma}^0$ for a purely elastic system, and the elastic modulus $G' \simeq G^0 \sim \omega^0$ dominates the response, with $G' \gg G''$.

In regimes between these two limits, the viscoelastic response for flexible polymers smoothly transitions from that of entangled to that of crosslinked networks. The effect of crosslinking of entangled *semiflexible* polymers is inherently more complex than the picture painted above owing to the ample contributions of bending to the stress relaxation, which introduces another lengthscale. Namely, the bending lengthscale:

$$l_b \approx \left(\frac{\epsilon_b}{\kappa}\right)^{\frac{1}{2}} \tag{2.116}$$

which compares the bending modulus ϵ_b to the elastic spring constant κ.

Crosslinking can completely suppress bending modes in the limit $l_c \ll l_b$, L but there exists a broad phase space of filament and crosslinker concentrations and filament lengths over which bending is still appreciable. In this region of the phase space, semiflexible polymer networks exhibit **non-affine** deformation in response to shear, meaning the network strain field is not aligned with the shear direction (figure 2.5(A)). As bending modes become increasingly frozen out by, e.g., decreasing l_c, the networks respond affinely, i.e., oriented along the shear direction. The lengthscale that sets the crossover from non-affine to **affine** deformation is the non-affinity lengthscale:

$$\lambda_{NA} \approx l_c\left(\frac{l_b}{l_c}\right)^{\frac{1}{4}} \tag{2.117}$$

Another key parameter to consider in crosslinked networks is the **rigidity percolation** threshold, below which the network cannot elastically store stress due to the loss of percolating crosslinks (figure 2.5(B)). The rigidity percolation phase transition is expected to align with the transition from non-affine to affine deformation, and is set by the relative length of the polymer compared to the crosslinker length.

The polymer length required to achieve rigidity percolation can be expressed as:

$$L_{RP} \simeq \mathrm{P} l_c \tag{2.118}$$

with P being a constant with predicted values of $\mathrm{P} \simeq 2.53-5.9$ that vary depending on the lattice structure and dimension of the model used in the prediction.

The elastic modulus is predicted to exhibit power-law increase with polymer length in the non-affine regime, until reaching L_{RP} and λ_{NA}, after which a constant affine-limit value is reached that reflects that of a completely elastic network (figure 2.5).

2.10 Nonlinear viscoelasticity

In this chapter, we have focused entirely on polymer dynamics and rheological properties in the quiescent and linear deformation regimes. However, in biology as well as materials processing, biopolymer networks are often subject to large stresses and strains that push them far from equilibrium, warranting a nonlinear stress response. In section 2.6.1, we defined the linear regime as that in which the network modulus is independent of the strain amplitude. We can think of this criterion in

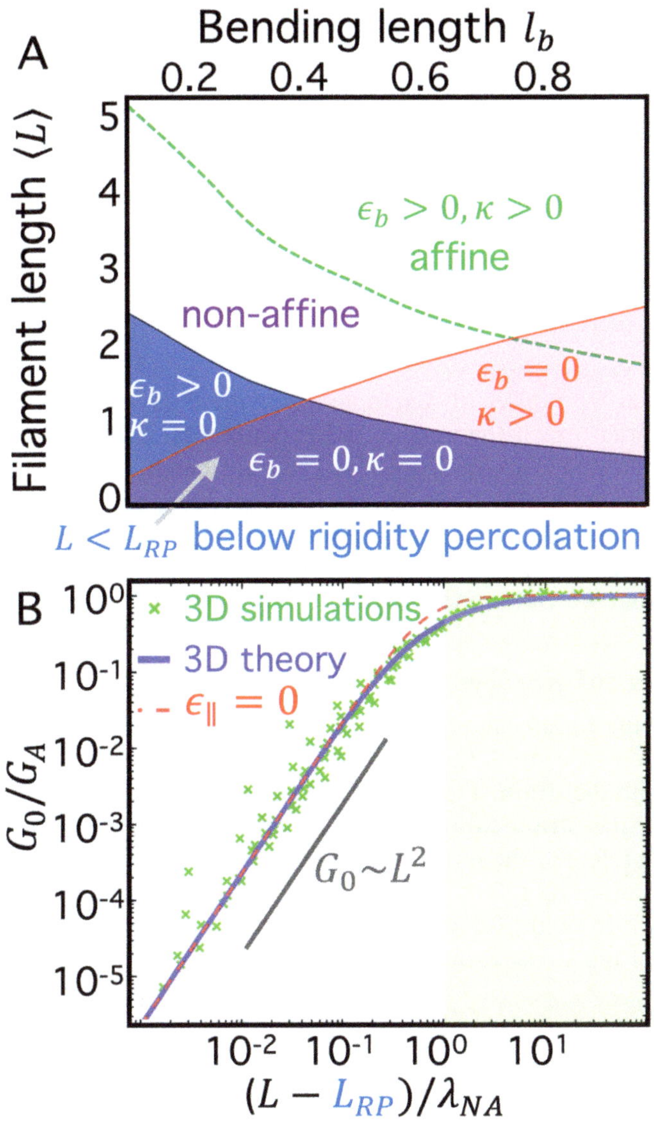

Figure 2.5. Crosslinked semiflexible polymer networks exhibit mechanical phase transitions controlled by bending and stretching. (A) Mechanical phase diagram of crosslinked networks spanned by the average filament length $\langle L \rangle$ and the bending lengthscale l_b. Different regions are marked by different combinations of zero or non-zero bending modulus ϵ_b and elastic constant κ. The blue region marks the region of the phase space that is below the rigidity percolation threshold for a finite shear modulus. The dashed green line separates the non-affine and affine regimes. The red region denotes the region in which there is no resistance to bending, shifting the response towards the non-affine limit. Adapted with permission from Das *et al* (2007), Copyright (2007) by the American Physical Society. (B) The predicted (blue) and simulated (green) elastic shear modulus G_0 scaled by the affine-limit value G_A versus the filament length, shifted by the percolation threshold length L_{RP} and scaled by the non-affinity lengthscale λ_{NA}. The green shaded region denotes the affine limit and the dashed red line is the theoretical result assuming no contributions from longitudinal bending ($\epsilon_\| = 0$), demonstrating that non-affine deformations are dominated by transverse bending ($\epsilon_b \sim \epsilon_\|$) while

longitudinal deformation is dominated by stretching rigidity (κ). The grey scaling line denotes the power-law scaling of the elastic modulus with filament length in the non-affine transition region. This scaling $G_0 \sim L^2$ is also seen for 2D simulations. Adapted with permission from Chen *et al* (2023), Copyright (2023) by the American Physical Society.

analogy to a spring having a single intrinsic spring constant that is invariant to how much the spring is stretched—a property of most elastic materials up until a certain limit, when the structure of the material begins to change, which in turn alters its modulus. This limit is one way to define the nonlinear regime—one in which the elastic properties of the viscoelastic material depend on the nature and size of the strain.

The nonlinear response of entangled polymers is extremely complex and continues to attract much theoretical and experimental debate, which I invite you to explore if interested (Doi and Edwards 1988, Jary *et al* 1999, Mhetar and Archer 1999, Rubinstein and Colby 2003, Semmrich *et al* 2008, Squires 2008, DePuit *et al* 2011, Yao *et al* 2011, Sussman and Schweizer 2013b, Parisi *et al* 2021). Here, I will describe a select few nonlinear features that have been observed in many biopolymer networks and that we will see throughout the remaining chapters.

2.10.1 Stiffening and softening

A hallmark of the nonlinear regime is the emergence of stress-stiffening or stress-softening, whereby the stress the network exerts to resist an applied strain does not scale linearly with the strain. This phenomenon results in a modulus that is no longer independent of the strain amplitude—the defining feature of the linear regime. Stress-stiffening refers to the phenomenon of the modulus increasing with increasing strain whereas softening refers to a decrease with increasing strain.

One approach to quantifying the degree of stiffening or softening, is to evaluate the derivative of the stress with respect to strain:

$$K'(\gamma) = \frac{d\sigma}{d\gamma} \tag{2.119}$$

where K' is termed the differential modulus. In the linear regime, K' is constant and independent of γ, whereas stress-stiffening and softening networks display:

$$\frac{K'}{K_0'} > 1 \text{ (stiffening)} \tag{2.120}$$

$$\frac{K'}{K_0'} < 1 \text{ (softening)} \tag{2.121}$$

where K_0' is the differential modulus in the low strain limit, which should match the linear regime shear modulus G'.

For semiflexible polymer networks, stress-stiffening has been shown to arise from affine deformation and filament stretching, whereas softening emerges for networks that display a non-affine response due to appreciable bending contributions (Das *et al* 2007, Liu *et al* 2007, Yao *et al* 2011, Gurmessa *et al* 2017, Chen *et al* 2023).

2.10.2 Convective constraint release

Section 2.5.1 introduced the concept of quiescent constraint release as a relaxation mode for an entangled polymer that relies on surrounding entangling polymers diffusing away and thus releasing their constraint. When polymer networks are subject to nonlinear strains, that are very fast and/or large compared to the principal relaxation timescales and lengthscales, the applied strain can force polymer chains to disentangle.

This phenomenon arises from the fact that the polymers do not have enough time to configurationally relax to maintain their initial conformation. Instead, they are stretched in the direction of the strain and pulled away from the tube of one polymer by entanglements with another. **Convective constraint release (CCR)** refers to this mechanism whereby the flow field, induced by the strain, forces chains to disentangle from one another (Milner *et al* 2001, Graham *et al* 2003, Ianniruberto and Marrucci 2014).

CCR manifests in rheology measurements as a reduced modulus and/or faster relaxation timescales owing to strain-induced dilation of the entanglement tube i.e., (increasing d_T) and corresponding increase in the entanglement length l_e (Gurmessa *et al* 2017, Peddireddy *et al* 2022).

2.10.3 Power-law force relaxation

In the previous sections, we presented key relaxation modes and corresponding timescales, e.g, the disengagement time τ_D, that were dependent solely on the network properties—not on the strain—a reasonable approximation in the linear regime. For a polymer network that relaxes stress according to multiple timescales that are constant and well-separated in time, we expect that a sum of exponential decays can describe the time-dependent stress profile σ_R following cessation of the strain.

$$\sigma_R(t) = \sum \sigma_i e^{-t/\tau_i} \tag{2.122}$$

These time constants τ_i correlate with the relaxation timescales of the system, as shown in, e.g., Robertson and Smith (2007), Gurmessa *et al* (2016), and Khan *et al* (2019).

However, nonlinear straining can cause the entanglement tube to dilate, stretch, and shrink—all of which impact the relaxation timescales associated with entanglements, τ_e and τ_D. This phenomenon leads to *time*-dependent relaxation timescales $\tau_i(t)$, which we can think of as a spectrum of timescales smeared out in time. The resulting stress decays then adopts power-law scaling with time, rather than exponential decay:

$$\sigma_R(t) \sim t^{-\beta} \tag{2.123}$$

with reported scaling exponents of $\beta \simeq 0.4-0.7$ (Chapman and Robertson-Anderson 2014, Fitzpatrick *et al* 2018, Ricketts *et al* 2018).

2.11 To be continued ...

In this chapter, I have attempted to give a comprehensive yet digestible overview of our current understanding of polymer physics, focusing on concepts and frameworks that we will use in the subsequent chapters. So as to not overwhelm us, I have only considered monodisperse systems comprising identical polymers. As we will see in subsequent chapters, many biopolymer networks are much more complex, and I will discuss the extent to which these foundational theories can be applied to more complex systems as they arise.

Some important concepts that I will discuss include:

- The role of polymer topology, in particular the extent to which reptation theory can be extended to circular, supercoiled, and branched polymers (see chapter 6).
- The impact of mixing polymers of different sizes, stiffness, and/or topologies to create blends and composites (see chapter 7).
- The extent to which theories developed for steady-state systems can be extended to describe non-equilibrium, active networks (see chapter 8).
- The extent to which theories developed for isotropic homogeneous systems can be extended to those that exhibit varying degrees of bundling, clustering, de-mixing, and/or phase separation (see chapters 8 and 9).

References

Abadi M, Serag M F and Habuchi S 2018 Entangled polymer dynamics beyond reptation *Nat. Commun.* **9** 5098

Aragon S R and Pecora R 1985 Dynamics of wormlike chains *Macromolecules* **18** 1868–75

Banik S, Kong D, San Francisco M J and McKenna G B 2021 Monodisperse lambda DNA as a model to conventional polymers: a concentration-dependent scaling of the rheological properties *Macromolecules* **54** 8632–54

Bouchiat C, Wang M D, Allemand J-F, Strick T, Block S M and Croquette V 1999 Estimating the persistence length of a worm-like chain molecule from force-extension measurements *Biophys. J.* **76** 409–13

Chapman C D, Lee K, Henze D, Smith D E and Robertson-Anderson R M 2014 Onset of non-continuum effects in microrheology of entangled polymer solutions *Macromolecules* **47** 1181–6

Chapman C D and Robertson-Anderson R M 2014 Nonlinear microrheology reveals entanglement-driven molecular-level viscoelasticity of concentrated DNA *Phys. Rev. Lett.* **113** 098303

Chapman C D, Shanbhag S, Smith D E and Robertson-Anderson R M 2012 Complex effects of molecular topology on diffusion in entangled biopolymer blends *Soft Matter* **8** 9177–82

Chen S, Markovich T and MacKintosh F C 2023 Nonaffine deformation of semiflexible polymer and fiber networks *Phys. Rev. Lett.* **130** 088101

Colby R H, Boris D C, Krause W E and Dou S 2007 Shear thinning of unentangled flexible polymer liquids *Rheol. Acta* **46** 569–75

Colby R H and Rubinstein M 1990 Two-parameter scaling for polymers in Θ solvents *Macromolecules* **23** 2753–7

Dakhil H, Basu S K, Steiner S, Gerlach Y, Soller A, Pan S, Germann N, Leidenberger M, Kappes B and Wierschem A 2021 Buffered λ-DNA solutions at high shear rates *J. Rheol.* **65** 159–69
Das M, MacKintosh F C and Levine A J 2007 Effective medium theory of semiflexible filamentous networks *Phys. Rev. Lett.* **99** 038101
de Gennes P-G 1979 *Scaling Concepts in Polymer Physics* (Ithaca, NY: Cornell University Press)
de Gennes P G 2003 Reptation of a polymer chain in the presence of fixed obstacles *J. Chem. Phys.* **55** 572–9
de Gennes P G and Leger L 1982 Dynamics of entangled polymer chains *Annu. Rev. Phys. Chem.* **33** 49–61
DePuit R J, Khair A S and Squires T M 2011 A theoretical bridge between linear and nonlinear microrheology *Phys. Fluids* **23** 063102
desCloizeaux J 1988 Double reptation vs. simple reptation in polymer melts *Europhys. Lett.* **5** 437
Doi M 1996 *Introduction to Polymer Physics* (Oxford: Clarendon)
Doi M and Edwards S F 1988 *The Theory of Polymer Dynamics* (Oxford: Clarendon)
Ferry J D 1980 *Viscoelastic Properties of Polymers* (New York: Wiley)
Fitzpatrick R, Michieletto D, Peddireddy K R, Hauer C, Kyrillos C, Gurmessa B J and Robertson-Anderson R M 2018 Synergistic interactions between DNA and actin trigger emergent viscoelastic behavior *Phys. Rev. Lett.* **121** 257801
Flory P J 1969 *Statistical Mechanics of Chain Molecules* (Interscience Publishers)
Flory P J 1953 *Principles of Polymer Chemistry* (Ithaca, NY: Cornell University Press)
Flory P J 1949a The configuration of real polymer chains *J. Chem. Phys.* **17** 303–10
Flory P J 1949b Statistical mechanics of dilute polymer solutions *J. Chem. Phys.* **17** 1347–8
Freed K F 1987 *Renormalization Group Theory of Macromolecules* (New York: Wiley)
Gardel M L, Valentine M T, Crocker J C, Bausch A R and Weitz D A 2003 Microrheology of entangled F-actin solutions *Phys. Rev. Lett.* **91** 158302
Gisler T and Weitz D A 1999 Scaling of the microrheology of semidilute F-actin solutions *Phys. Rev. Lett.* **82** 1606–9
Graessley W W 1982 Entangled linear, branched and network polymer systems—Molecular theories *Adv. Polym. Sci.* **47** 67–117
Graham R S, Likhtman A E, McLeish T C B and Milner S T 2003 Microscopic theory of linear, entangled polymer chains under rapid deformation including chain stretch and convective constraint release *J. Rheol.* **47** 1171–200
Gurmessa B, Fitzpatrick R, Falzone T T and Robertson-Anderson R M 2016 Entanglement density tunes microscale nonlinear response of entangled actin *Macromolecules* **49** 3948–55
Gurmessa B, Ricketts S and Robertson-Anderson R M 2017 Nonlinear actin deformations lead to network stiffening, yielding, and nonuniform stress propagation *Biophys. J.* **113** 1540–50
Haley J C and Lodge T R 2005 Viscosity predictions for model miscible polymer blencils: including self-concentration, double reptation, and tube dilation *J. Rheol.* **49** 1277–302
Heo Y and Larson R G 2005 The scaling of zero-shear viscosities of semidilute polymer solutions with concentration *J. Rheol.* **49** 1117–28
Hinsch H, Wilhelm J and Frey E 2007 Quantitative tube model for semiflexible polymer solutions *Eur. Phys. J E Soft Matter.* **24** 35–46
Hiraiwa T and Ohta T 2009 Viscoelasticity of a single semiflexible polymer chain *Macromolecules* **42** 7553–62
Ianniruberto G and Marrucci G 2014 Convective constraint release (CCR) revisited *J. Rheol.* **58** 89–102

Ianniruberto G and Marrucci G 1996 On compatibility of the Cox–Merz rule with the model of Doi and Edwards *J. Non-Newtonian Fluid Mech.* **65** 241–6

Isambert H and Maggs A C 1996 Dynamics and rheology of actin solutions *Macromolecules* **29** 1036–40

Jary D, Sikorav J L and Lairez D 1999 Nonlinear viscoelasticity of entangled DNA molecules *Europhys. Lett.* **46** 251–5

Käs J, Strey H, Tang J X, Finger D, Ezzell R, Sackmann E and Janmey P A 1996 F-actin, a model polymer for semiflexible chains in dilute, semidilute, and liquid crystalline solutions *Biophys. J.* **70** 609–25

Khan M, Regan K and Robertson-Anderson R M 2019 Optical tweezers microrheology maps the dynamics of strain-induced local inhomogeneities in entangled polymers *Phys. Rev. Lett.* **123** 038001

Khanal P, Peddireddy K R, Marfai J, McGorty R and Robertson-Anderson R M 2022 DNA topology dictates emergent bulk elasticity and hindered macromolecular diffusion in DNA-dextran composites *J. Rheol.* **66** 699–715

Khokhlov A R, Grosberg A Y and Pande V S 1994 *Statistical Physics of Macromolecules* vol 1 (New York: AIP press)

Koenderink G H, Atakhorrami M, MacKintosh F C and Schmidt c f 2006 High-frequency stress relaxation in semiflexible polymer solutions and networks *Phys. Rev. Lett.* **96** 138307

Kroy K and Frey E 1996 Force-extension relation and plateau modulus for wormlike chains *Phys. Rev. Lett.* **77** 306–9

Larson R G 2010 Rheology of entangled polymer melts: recent results from molecular dynamics simulations *Presented at the American Physical Society March Meeting (Portland, Oregon)*

Le Guillou J C and Zinn-Justin J 1977 Critical exponents for the *n*-vector model in three dimensions from field theory *Phys. Rev. Lett.* **39** 95–8

Liu J, Koenderink G H, Kasza K E, MacKintosh F C and Weitz D A 2007 Visualizing the strain field in semiflexible polymer networks: strain fluctuations and nonlinear rheology of *F*-actin gels *Phys. Rev. Lett.* **98** 198304

Lodge T P 1999 Reconciliation of the molecular weight dependence of diffusion and viscosity in entangled polymers *Phys. Rev. Lett.* **83** 3218–21

Marko J F and Siggia E D 1995 Stretching DNA *Macromolecules* **28** 8759–70

McKenna G B and Plazek D J 1986 The viscosity of blends of linear and cyclic molecules of similar molecular mass *Polym. Commun.* **27** 304–6

McLeish T C B 2002 Tube theory of entangled polymer dynamics *Adv. Phys.* **51** 1379–527

Mhetar V and Archer L A 1999 Nonlinear viscoelasticity of entangled polymeric liquids *J Non-Newton. Fluid Mech.* **81** 71–81

Michieletto D, Marenduzzo D, Orlandini E, Alexander G P and Turner M S 2014 Threading dynamics of ring polymers in a gel *ACS Macro Lett.* **3** 255–9

Milner S T and McLeish T C B 1998 Reptation and contour-length fluctuations in melts of linear polymers *Phys. Rev. Lett.* **81** 725–8

Milner S T, McLeish T C B and Likhtman A E 2001 Microscopic theory of convective constraint release *J. Rheol.* **45** 539–63

Mohamed F, Flämig M, Hofmann M, Heymann L, Willner L, Fatkullin N, Aksel N and Rössler E A 2018 Scaling analysis of the viscoelastic response of linear polymers *J. Chem. Phys.* **149** 044902

Nelson P, Chen K and Bromberg S 2020 *Biological Physics: Energy, Information, Life* (Chiliagon Science)

Oono Y and Kohmoto M 1983 Renormalization group theory of transport properties of polymer solutions. I. Dilute solutions *J. Chem. Phys.* **78** 520–8

Pan S, At Nguyen D, Sridhar T, Sunthar P and Ravi Prakash J 2014 Universal solvent quality crossover of the zero shear rate viscosity of semidilute DNA solutions *J. Rheol.* **58** 339–68

Pan S, Nguyen D A, Dünweg B, Sunthar P, Sridhar T and Ravi Prakash J 2018 Shear thinning in dilute and semidilute solutions of polystyrene and DNA *J. Rheol.* **62** 845–67

Parisi D *et al* 2021 Nonlinear shear rheology of entangled polymer rings *Macromolecules* **54** 2811–27

Peddireddy K R, Clairmont R, Neill P, McGorty R and Robertson-Anderson R M 2022 OpTiDDM (Optical Tweezers integrating Differential Dynamic Microscopy) maps the spatiotemporal propagation of nonlinear stresses in polymer blends and composites *arXiv* **2203** 06750

Peddireddy K R *et al* 2022 Optical-tweezers-integrating-differential-dynamic-microscopy maps the spatiotemporal propagation of nonlinear strains in polymer blends and composites *Nat. Commun.* **13** 5180

Regan K, Ricketts S and Robertson-Anderson R 2016 DNA as a model for probing polymer entanglements: circular polymers and non-classical dynamics *Polymers* **8** 336

Ricketts S N, Ross J L and Robertson-Anderson R M 2018 Co-entangled actin-microtubule composites exhibit tunable stiffness and power-law stress relaxation *Biophys. J.* **115** 1055–67

Robertson R M, Laib S and Smith D E 2006 Diffusion of isolated DNA molecules: dependence on length and topology *PNAS* **103** 7310–4

Robertson R M and Smith D E 2007 Self-diffusion of entangled linear and circular DNA molecules: dependence on length and concentration *Macromolecules* **40** 3373–7

Robertson R M and Smith D E 2007 Direct measurement of the intermolecular forces confining a single molecule in an entangled polymer solution *Phys. Rev. Lett.* **99** 126001

Rouse P E 1953 A theory of the linear viscoelastic properties of dilute solutions of coiling polymers *J. Chem. Phys.* **21** 1272–80

Rouse P E and Sittel K 2004 Viscoelastic properties of dilute polymer solutions *J. Appl. Phys.* **24** 690–6

Rubinstein M and Colby R H 2003 *Polymer Physics* (Oxford: Oxford University Press)

Semmrich C, Larsen R J and Bausch A R 2008 Nonlinear mechanics of entangled F-actin solutions *Soft Matter* **4** 1675

Shanbhag S and Larson R G 2006 Identification of topological constraints in entangled polymer melts using the bond-fluctuation model *Macromolecules* **39** 2413–7

Squires T M 2008 Nonlinear microrheology: bulk stresses versus direct interactions *Langmuir* **24** 1147–59

Sussman D M and Schweizer K S 2013a Entangled polymer chain melts: orientation and deformation dependent tube confinement and interchain entanglement elasticity *J. Chem. Phys.* **139** 234904

Sussman D M and Schweizer K S 2013b Entangled rigid macromolecules under continuous startup shear deformation: consequences of a microscopically anharmonic confining tube *Macromolecules* **46** 5684–93

Sussman D M and Schweizer K S 2011 Microscopic theory of the tube confinement potential for liquids of topologically entangled rigid macromolecules *Phys. Rev. Lett.* **107** 078102

van der Maarel J R C 2008 *Introduction to Biopolymer Physics* (Singapore: World Scientific)

Viovy J L, Rubinstein M and Colby R H 1991 Constraint release in polymer melts: tube reorganization versus tube dilation *Macromolecules* **24** 3587–96

von Meerwall E D, Dirama N and Mattice W L 2007 Diffusion in polyethylene blends: constraint release and entanglement dilution *Macromolecules* **40** 3970–6

Wang B, Guan J, Anthony S M, Bae S C, Schweizer K S and Granick S Confining potential when a biopolymer filament reptates *Phys. Rev. Lett.* **104** 118301

Wang Z W and Larson R G 2008 Constraint release in entangled binary blends of linear polymers: a molecular dynamics study *Macromolecules* **41** 4945–60

Wiggins P A and Nelson P C 2006 Generalized theory of semiflexible polymers *Phys. Rev.* E **73** 031906

Yao N Y, Becker D J, Broedersz C P, Depken M, MacKintosh F C, Pollak M R and Weitz D A 2011 Nonlinear viscoelasticity of actin transiently cross-linked with mutant α-actinin-4 *J. Mol. Biol.* **411** 1062–71

Zhong Y, Yu L and Huang Q 2022 Investigating the linear viscoelastic behaviour at high frequencies in the transition to glassy regime for polystyrene melts and solutions *Rheol. Acta* **61** 689–700

Zhou Q and Larson R G 2006 Direct calculation of the tube potential confining entangled polymers *Macromolecules* **39** 6737–43

Zhou Y, Young C D, Lee M, Banik S, Kong D, McKenna G B, Robertson-Anderson R M, Sing C E and Schroeder C M 2021 Dynamics and rheology of ring-linear blend semidilute solutions in extensional flow: single molecule experiments *J. Rheol.* **65** 729–44

Zimm B H 1956 Dynamics of polymer molecules in dilute solution: viscoelasticity, flow birefringence and dielectric loss *J. Chem. Phys.* **24** 269–78

Chapter 3

Measuring mechanics, dynamics, and structure

This chapter discusses some of the key methods currently used to measure dynamics, viscoelastic properties, transport, and structural features of biopolymer networks. Techniques that are covered include: epifluorescence microscopy, multi-spectral confocal microscopy, light-sheet microscopy, optical tweezers force spectroscopy, dynamic light scattering, and bulk rheology. Because nearly all of these methods require imaging biopolymers or embedded probes, I will also discuss considerations for fluorescence labeling and choosing probes for different measurement techniques.

3.1 Direct imaging of biopolymers

Most biopolymers are invisible to white light, so they do not scatter enough light to be imaged with a basic bright-field microscope. However, a quite useful feature of biopolymers, that many of their synthetic counterparts lack, is the ability to fluorescently label them by attaching fluorophore conjugates along their backbone via, e.g., covalent bonding or intercalation. Various fluorophores, versatile attachment methods, and tunable labeling densities allow for direct visualization of a variety of single biopolymers as well as dense networks thereof with the use of fluorescence microscopes.

In this section, I introduce different fluorescence microscopy modalities that you can use to measure dynamical and structural properties of biopolymers. I provide an overview of the key components needed for each modality, the underlying physics of the imaging technology, and important advantages and disadvantages of each. I also discuss the types of networks and measurements that each modality is best-suited for, and how to optimize instrumentation and acquisition parameters for specific measurements and network types.

3.1.1 Epifluorescence microscopy

Epifluorescence microscopy is the simplest and most widely used method for imaging fluorescent-labeled particles. Most other modalities that I discuss in the subsequent sections build on the basic principles and features of epifluorescence to

doi:10.1088/978-0-7503-5037-2ch3

allow for added functionality that a basic epifluorescence microscope lacks. As depicted in figure 3.1(A), the essential components of any epifluorescence microscope include a white light source, an objective lens, a camera, and a filter cube comprising excitation, emission, and dichroic filters.

The most commonly used white light sources have traditionally been mercury arc lamps, but are now being increasingly replaced with LED mimics, such as the Excelitas series of X-Cite Illuminators ('X-cite fluorescence LED illuminators Excelitas,' n.d.) as shown in figure 3.1(A). Using white light rather than a monochromatic laser offers versatility in the fluorophores that can be visualized by incorporating multiple excitation/emission filter cubes into the microscope.

The filter cube is essential for both exciting fluorophores and collecting their Stokes-shifted (lower wavelength) emission. Specifically, the white light from the light source first reaches the excitation filter, which is a bandpass filter that removes all other wavelengths of light except for a narrow band centered near the excitation peak of the excitation spectrum (figure 3.1(B), blue). This quasi-monochromatic light then bounces off of the dichroic filter, angled at 45° from the light path, to direct the light to the objective to illuminate the sample. This illumination excites the fluorophores attached to the biopolymers which then emit a Stokes-shifted spectrum that passes back through the objective and the dichroic before reaching the emission filter. The emission filter, positioned before the camera, removes any stray or scattered light that is not within a narrow band centered near the emission peak (figure 3.1(B), green). The dichroic is an essential component of epifluorescence setups as it reflects light of wavelengths lower than the emission spectra (e.g., the excitation spectrum) and transmits light in the emission range or higher. This feature, along with the 45° orientation of the dichroic, allows the objective to act as both an objective, collecting emitted light and creating an image on the camera, *and* a condenser, collecting light and illuminating the sample.

Excitation/emission filter sets have been designed to optimize the fluorescence signal produced by most standard fluorophores, as summarized in table 3.1. The most commonly used emission/excitation combination is blue/green (480/535) due to the wide range of fluorophores that match that excitation/emission combination, along with their high quantum yield and stability compared to other wavelengths. Green/orange (540/605) fluorophores are also commonly used for similar reasons and can be used together with blue/green fluorophores in experiments requiring two-color imaging (figure 3.1(C)).

The objective is perhaps the most important component of an epifluorescence microscope as it determines the magnification and resolution of the imaging. To resolve single biopolymers (figure 3.1(C)), you typically need submicron diffraction-limited resolution which requires an objective with both a high magnification, such as 60× or 100×, as well as a high numerical aperture of NA = 1.2–1.4. To achieve this high degree of resolution, these objectives require water or oil as the immersion media, due to their higher index of refraction compared to air.

However, if you are interested in observing the larger-scale, mesocopic structure ($\gtrsim 10\ \mu$m) of biopolymer networks (figure 3.1(C)), which is often the case in the field, it may be more appropriate to use lower magnification objectives, e.g., 10× to 40×, to increase the field-of-view while still being able to resolve the mesoscale structure.

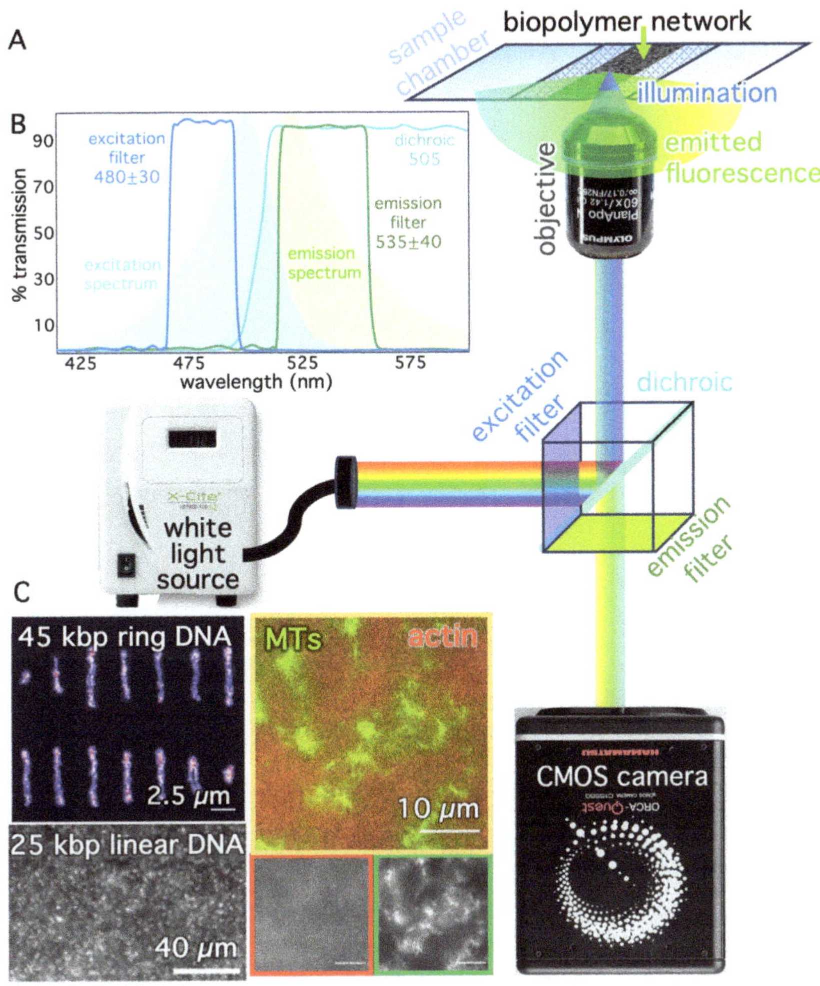

Figure 3.1. Essential components and imaging capabilities of epifluorescence microscopy. (A) Typical epifluorescence microscopes use a **white light source** (image from 'X-cite fluorescence LED illuminators Excelitas,' n.d.) that passes through an **excitation filter** that selectively filters out all wavelengths that are not within a narrow band centered on the desired wavelength, as depicted in B. The light is then redirected by a **dichroic filter** to an **objective** lens (image from 'Olympus PlanApo N 60× oil microscope objective,' n.d.) which focuses the light onto the sample and excites the fluorophores. The lower wavelength light emitted by the fluorophores passes back through the objective, the dichroic, and an **emission filter** that filters out undesired wavelengths, and is then collected by a high-performance camera such as a **CMOS camera** ('Scientific camera Hamamatsu Photonics,' n.d.). (B) Excitation and emission spectra (translucent blue and green) for Alexa488 plotted with spectra for appropriate bandpass excitation (blue) and emission (green) filters with the wavelength bands noted in nm, and dichroic with 50% cutoff wavelength listed in nm. (C) Sample images of biopolymers acquired with epifluorescence: (top left) time-lapse images of ring DNA being stretched and recoiling in a microfluidic device. Adapted from Peddireddy *et al* (2020b) with permission from the Royal Society of Chemistry. (bottom left) 25 kbp linear DNA molecules in a background of unlabeled DNA. Adapted from Khanal *et al* (2022), with the permission of AIP Publishing. (right) A colorized merged image of a network of actin (red) and microtubules (MTs, green), each labeled with different fluorophores and viewed with different filters. Bottom images are the single actin (red) and microtubule (green) images that comprise the composite image. Adapted from Regan *et al* (2018) with permission from the Royal Society of Chemistry.

Table 3.1. Standard filter sets and fluorophores used for imaging and labeling biopolymers. Colors indicate the approximate color corresponding to the wavelength listed. The excitation and emission wavelengths are listed as center/band values and the dichroic value corresponds to the wavelength at 50% transmission. Standard and AlexaFluor (Molecular Probes Trademark) fluorophores listed can be conjugated to monomers or binding proteins associated with biopolymers. The family of Molecular Probes trademarked intercalators listed are fluorophores that intercalate in between the basepairs of double-stranded DNA.

Filter wavelengths (nm)			Fluorophores		
Excitation	Emission	Dichroic	Standard	Intercalator	AlexaFluor
375/28	460/50	415	DAPI	POPO–1	AF350
480/30	535/20	550	Fluorescein, FITC, EFGP, Cy2	YOYO-I	AF488
540/25	605/55	565	Rhodamine, TRITC, Cy3	POPO–3	AF546
569/25	615/40	588	X-rhodamine, Cy3.5	BOBO–3	AF568
620/50	690/50	655	Cy5	TOTO–3	AF647

An advantage to lower magnification objectives, when appropriate, are their reduced cost and lack of a required immersion medium.

Finally, the camera plays a critical role in several image acquisition parameters such as pixel resolution, field-of-view (FOV) size, and frame rate. In most cases, epifluorescence is preferred for tracking the motion of tracer polymers and particles, rather than resolving network structure, due to its lower axial resolution as compared to other modalities that I will discuss below. Tracking applications typically require high spatial resolution (relative to the size of the polymers) as well as fast frame rates (relative to the rate of particle motion) to be able to accurately determine the polymer center-of-mass and not 'freeze out' fast thermal motion. CMOS (Complementary Metal-Oxide Semiconductor) cameras have become the most widely used cameras in these applications due to their combination of fast frame rates, suitable sensitivity, and relatively low cost compared to EMCCDs (Electron Multiplying Charge-Coupled Devices).

An advantage of EMCCDs over CMOS cameras is their increased sensitivity, allowing for single-fluorophore detection. However, this unparalleled sensitivity comes at the cost of frame rate, with most EMCCDs unable to achieve the $\sim10^1$–10^2 frames per second (fps) often required to accurately detect thermal and driven motion of biopolymers. Moreover, because most biopolymer network applications only require detection of biopolymers that are labeled with $\sim10^2$–10^4 fluorophores along their backbones, single-fluorophore detection is typically not necessary.

The primary disadvantage of epifluorescence microscopy is its inability to block out-of-focus light from the field-of-view, which appreciably reduces the signal-to-background ratio of thick and/or densely labeled networks. Because labeled biopolymers above and below the focal plane, as well as laterally beyond the FOV, are excited, they emit fluorescence that contributes to the detected intensity in the focal plane of the FOV. This spurious signal can overwhelm the signal emitted by in-focus elements and dramatically increase the noise floor.

For these reasons, experiments that employ epifluorescence typically dope in a trace amount of labeled biopolymers, each separated by several particle sizes, to serve as representative components of the network and detect the system dynamics. An example is shown in the bottom-left image in figure 3.1(C) in which individually-resolved labeled DNA molecules are diffusing in a network of unlabeled DNA (Chapman *et al* 2012, Khanal *et al* 2022). This imaging approach, combined with the fast frame rates afforded by CMOS cameras, lends itself to single-molecule tracking, in which the center-of-mass (COM) trajectories of individual polymers or tracers are measured to determine dynamic quantities such as mean-squared displacements and diffusion coefficients (see chapter 4 for further discussion) (Manzo and Garcia-Parajo 2015, Regan *et al* 2018).

When computing the COM of polymer coils and extended chains, one typically uses pixel intensity as a proxy for mass, as the local density of fluorophores scales with intrachain polymer density. For this reason, the out-of-focus signal is actually beneficial to accurately measuring the COM of large polymer coils that extend axially beyond the focal plane.

One can also measure the size and shape of polymer coils and their conformational fluctuations over time (Chapman *et al* 2015, Gorczyca *et al* 2015, Garamella *et al* 2020). The radius of gyration tensor can also be evaluated using e.g., normal mode analysis, to determine intra-polymer dynamics and variations in conformational size and shape (Delarue and Sanejouand 2002, Chun *et al* 2009, Rawat and Biswas 2009, Tang *et al* 2010, Liu *et al* 2013, Gong and van der Maarel 2014, Li *et al* 2014). Finally, one can deduce bending dynamics and entanglement tube properties for extended semiflexible filaments, as well as rotational diffusion coefficients for rigid rod microtubules (Käs *et al* 1994, 1996, Wilhelm and Frey 1996, Adami *et al* 2003, Wang *et al* 2010).

In cases in which tracking of the biopolymers themselves is difficult due to small size, photobleaching, ineffective labeling, etc, researchers can instead track the motion of microspheres embedded in the networks to infer system dynamics, as I discuss in chapter 4. In brief, the well-defined size and shape of microsphere probes provide a known Stokes drag coefficient $\zeta = 6\pi\eta R$ from which one can use measured mean-squared displacements and diffusion coefficients to compute the viscosity of biopolymer networks (in the case of Newtonian dynamics) or their elastic and viscous moduli (for viscoelastic systems) using the generalized Stokes–Einstein relation (GSER) (Mason *et al* 1997, Squires and Mason 2010). This basic approach of tracking thermal fluctuations of single diffusing particles to extract local rheological properties of the surrounding material is typically referred to as particle-tracking microrheology or passive microrheology, which I discuss in detail in chapter 4.

3.1.2 Laser scanning confocal microscopy

Laser scanning confocal microscopy (LSCM) builds on the basic framework of epifluorescence microscopy by incorporating pinhole apertures to reduce the intensity of out-of-focus light contributing to an image (figure 3.2(A), (B)). This reduction improves the signal-to-noise and allows for higher-resolution imaging of dense biopolymer networks, as you can see by comparing the images of actin and microtubules in figures 3.1(C) and 3.2(B). LSCM uses monochromatic lasers instead of white light as the illumination source, and most setups include multiple lasers to allow for imaging of multiple spectrally-distinct fluorophores in a single image.

The most important components of any confocal microscope are the pinhole apertures placed in the illumination path and detection path (figure 3.2(A)). The detector pinhole is placed in front of the detector in a focal plane that is conjugate with, or 'confocal' with, the focal plane of the image. This placement allows only in-focus light to pass through the pinhole and reach the detector. Larger pinholes allow for light from more axially shifted planes to reach the detector, serving to set the z thickness of the quasi-2D (x, y) image 'slice'. The illumination pinhole limits the region of sample that is illuminated at any given moment to a point that is roughly the size of a pixel, with the exact size set by the pinhole size, resulting in improved lateral resolution. The intensity of the light emitted from the sample at that point is then collected by a photomultiplier tube (PMT) instead of a camera. For setups with multiple lasers there is a separate PMT for each laser wavelength to allow for multi-color imaging and separation of signals from each fluorophore.

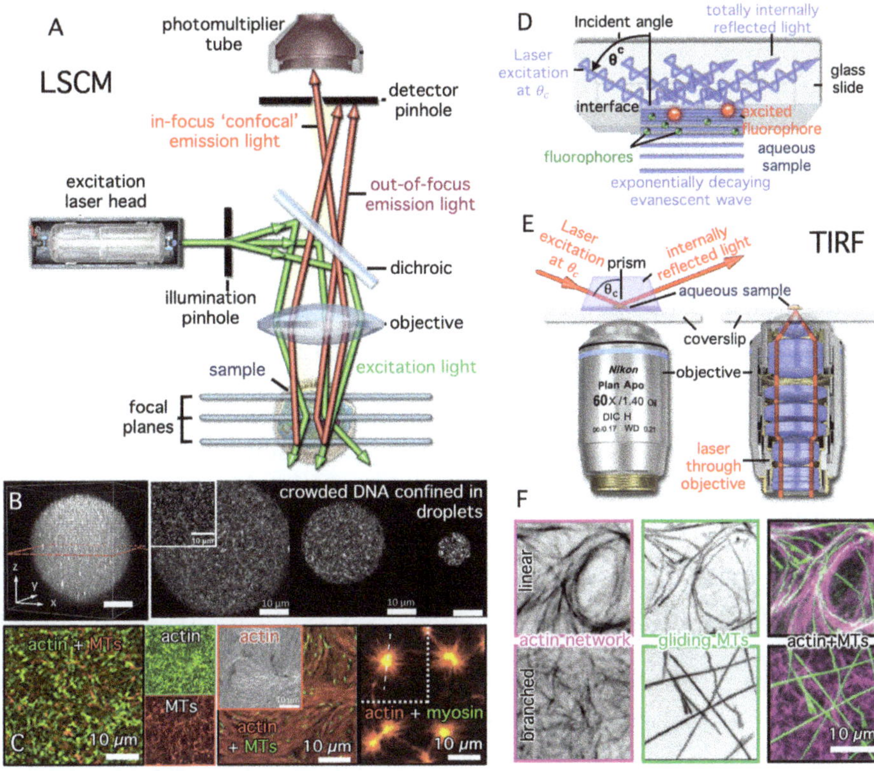

Figure 3.2. Laser Scanning Confocal Microscopy (LSCM) and Total Internal Reflection Fluorescence (TIRF) microscopy allow for imaging of quasi-2D sheets within or at the surface of 3D dense networks. (A–C) LSCM uses illumination and detection pinholes to prevent out-of-focus light from reaching the detector. This advance to epifluorescence microscopy enables imaging 2D planes within thick 3D samples, increases axial and lateral resolution, and allows for multi-spectral imaging. (A) A schematic showing the key components of LSCM and the emission and excitation light paths. Image adapted from 'Nikon's MicroscopyU—The source for microscopy education,' (n.d.). (B) LSCM images of labeled 115 kbp DNA confined in lipid droplets and crowded by (unlabeled) dextran. From left to right: 3D reconstruction, large droplet (inset: no confinement), medium droplet, and small droplet. Adapted from Aporvari *et al* (2022), Copyright (2022), with permission from Elsevier. (C) Left: Two-color image and corresponding single channel images of entangled composite network of actin (green) and microtubules (red) with the same concentrations and conditions as shown in figure 3.1. Note the improved resolution as compared to standard epifluorescence. Right: Two color images of actomyosin networks before and after restructuring of actin (red, greyscale inset) by myosin II minifilaments (green). Adapted from Murrell and Gardel (2012) with permission of PNAS. (D–F) TIRF microscopy uses total internal reflection of excitation light to selectively excite labeled biopolymers bound to or very near to a surface. (D) Cartoon depiction of selective excitation of fluorophores at a glass surface via the evanescent wave produced when light hits a surface at a critical angle θ_C and is totally internally reflected. (E) TIRF can be achieved using a prism (left) or high NA objective (right) to create the evanescent wave via total internal reflection at an interface. Schematics in (D) and (E) are adapted from 'Nikon's MicroscopyU—The source for microscopy education,' (n.d.). (F) TIRF microscopy images of actin (magenta, left) and microtubules (green, middle) on the surface of a sample chamber. Microtubules glide on the surface by binding to surface-bound kinesin motors. Networks of linear (top) and branched (bottom) actin networks are crowded to the surface with a depletant so the actin network can be visualized at the surface and microtubules can glide through the network. Adapted with permission from Kučera *et al* (2022). Copyright (2022) American Chemical Society.

Creating a 2D image of thousands of pixels from point illumination, which provides improved lateral resolution is much more complicated than capturing the entire image at once with a camera. The basis of image formation includes the use of two galvanometer mirrors (fast and slow) to steer the pinhole through all of the point positions comprising a FOV, and then reconstructing the image by mapping each intensity value collected by the PMT to its (x, y) coordinates. Scanning proceeds from the top left to bottom right of the image much like a typewriter (if you are old enough to know what that is): the fast mirror horizontally sweeps left to right across the top row, the slow mirror moves the point down one row, and the process repeats. This horizontal scanning mode produces high resolution images but can take up to several seconds to produce a 512 × 512 pixel image, which is prohibitively long for accurately capturing dynamics of many biopolymer networks. The network can also appear 'smeared out' due to the motion of the polymers that occurs during the scan time. For this reason, standard LSCM is best-suited for static systems or those with correlation timescales on the order of tens of seconds or more.

However, there are multiple approaches to increasing the scan rate of LSCM, which include reducing the size of the scanned FOV or binning squares of pixels together, which may be appropriate if your FOV is much larger than the largest correlation lengthscale of the network or if the smallest relevant lengthscale is large compared to the pixel size, respectively. Another method for increasing the image acquisition rate is to use raster scanning, in which the scan direction alternates between left-to-right and right-to-left instead of 'flying-back' to the left to begin scanning the next row. Raster scanning increases the frame rate but in certain cases can reduce the vertical resolution and introduce misalignment between rows at very fast scan rates.

There have also been several recent advances to laser fluorescence microscopy to improve acquisition rates, including the use of resonant galvanometers in the scanning process. Resonant galvonometers oscillate at fixed high frequencies, typically ~4–8 kHz, that set their scan speed. This is in contrast to traditional galvanometer mirrors that have inertial constraints that limit scan rates to ~100 Hz. A resonant scanner uses a resonant galvanometer for horizontal scanning and two traditional galvanometers to control y-movement. The incorporation of a second vertical scanner increases the rate of vertical scanning to allow for the inertia-limited motion to keep pace with the fast horizontal scanning. This configuration supports frame rates up to ~30 fps for full 512 × 512 images, an order of magnitude faster than traditional LSCM.

Another important advance to confocal microscopy is the use of a Nipkow spinning disk with an array of pinholes to scan through an image. The spiral design of the array allows for scanning an entire image with every disk rotation. This technology offers a major advance in the achievable frame rates—up to 10^3 fps—but rarely can these frame rates be achieved due to the inability of cameras to capture and digitize images at those rates. While spinning disk microscopes are the clear winner when it comes to frame rate, the optical sectioning ability and control over slice thickness is compromised compared to traditional scanning microscopes.

The powerful ability of confocal microscopes to eliminate out-of-focus light from above and below the (x, y) focal plane, allows for optical sectioning of dense and thick 3D samples, into thin sheets with z thickness set by the pinhole size (which is often adjustable). By performing 'z-scans', whereby images in a single planar field-of-view are acquired at increasing z-heights in succession, volumetric 3D reconstruction of a sample can be achieved, as shown in figure 3.2(B). This method allows for imaging biopolymers inside, e.g., droplets (figure 3.2(B)), vesicles, or cells (Bashirzadeh and Liu 2019, Aporvari *et al* 2022, Bashirzadeh *et al* 2022). LSCM is also advantageous for imaging dense biopolymer samples (e.g., entangled, crosslinked, and/or bundled networks of actin and microtubules, figure 3.2(B)) and differentiating and discerning the dynamics and structure of various constituents, labeled with distinct fluorophores, in composite networks (figure 3.2(C)), (Murrell and Gardel 2012, Ricketts *et al* 2018, Lee *et al* 2021, n.d., McGorty *et al* 2023).

3.1.3 Total internal reflection fluorescence microscopy

Total internal reflection fluorescence (TIRF) microscopy uses the principle of total internal reflection to selectively image a quasi-2D layer of a 3D sample on or near the surface of the sample chamber (figures 3.2(D)–(F)). Similar to LSCM, it dramatically reduces the contribution of out-of-focus light to the image to improve lateral and axial resolution, as shown in figure 3.2(F). The thickness of the planar sheet is less than the typical thickness of confocal microscopes, ~100 nm compared to ~500 nm for LSCM, so the axial resolution is even more improved over epifluorescence. Moreover, because there is no point scanning involved, images can be acquired at the frame rate of the camera, which is typically much faster than scanning rates. However, the reduced thickness also reduces the signal intensity, so EMCCDs are often required to capture images.

TIRF microscopy harnesses the phenomenon of total internal reflection to produce an evanescent light wave that only travels ~100 nm into the sample chamber (figure 3.2(D)). Let's unpack this statement. Total internal reflection refers to the phenomenon in which light incident on a surface at an angle $\theta \geqslant \theta_C$ with respect to the normal is completely reflected at the surface, rather than being partially reflected and partially transmitted (as happens for light incident at $\theta < \theta_C$). However, conservation of momentum requires that some light still passes through the interface, which occurs in the form of an exponentially decaying evanescent wave (rather than a conventional oscillating light wave). The intensity of this evanescent wave decays exponentially with axial (normal) z-distance from the surface:

$$I(z) = I_0 e^{-z/\lambda_c} \tag{3.1}$$

where $\lambda_c \approx 100$ nm is the critical decay length which sets the z depth into the sample that fluorophores can be excited and thus imaged.

The traditional method for building a TIRF microscope is to use a prism placed on the opposite side of the sample chamber as the objective to create the internally reflected wave (figure 3.2(E)). In this configuration, a laser is incident on the prism at an angle θ_C and the evanescent wave traverses through the glass slide into the sample chamber. The light emitted by the excited fluorophores travels through the objective which focuses the light onto the camera.

An alternative approach, typically used in commercial setups, is to use a high NA objective to create the TIR (figure 3.2(E)). Here, the emission and excitation light paths both travel through the objective, similar to epifluorescence and confocal microscopes. However, instead of the light path being centered with the objective center, as in these other constructions, it hits the back focal aperture (BFA) of the objective 'off-axis' to allow the objective lens to bend the light rays more than if they were centered, to reach θ_C. Because achieving maximal bending of the incident light is essential for objective-based TIRF, and the extent to which the light can be shifted off-axis is limited by the size of the objective BFA (~6–8 mm) (see figure 3.2(E)), the numerical aperture of the objective typically must be higher than in epifluorescence and LSCM. For example, typical 60× and 100× objectives used in TIRF require NA = 1.5–1.7 as compared to NA = 1.2–1.4 for epifluorescence and LCSM.

The power of TIRF to limit excitation and imaging to very near the surface makes it ideal for investigating interactions between biopolymers and their binding partners, such as motor proteins (Ross and Dixit 2010, Henty-Ridilla 2022). In these studies, the coverslip is treated with, e.g., streptavidin, to allow the associated (e.g., biotinylated) proteins to adhere to it by, e.g. biotin–streptavidin bonding (Vemula *et al* 2021). Non-specific adsorption using substances such as collodion can also be used. The proteins that do not bind to the surface are then washed out and the fluorescent-labeled biopolymers are flown into the sample chamber.

A simple example of this technique is a gliding assay, in which motor proteins such as kinesin or myosin are bound to the surface and microtubule or actin biopolymers are free in solution (Ross and Dixit 2010, Vemula *et al* 2021, Henty-Ridilla 2022). In the presence of ATP, when the biopolymer binds to the motor protein, the motor activity generates 'gliding' of the actin or microtubules, as seen in figure 3.2(F), which shows microtubules being transported by adhered kinesin motors. In the study shown in figure 3.2(F) (Kučera *et al* 2022), actin is also included in the sample chamber and crowded to the surface via a depletant, such as methyl cellulose or polyethylene glycol (PEG). This crowding effect confines the actin network to very near the surface to allow the gliding microtubules to be embedded in the quasi-2D actin network, and the impact of different actin network architectures (linear or branched) on the orientation and organization of the gliding microtubules to be assessed.

TIRF is also widely used to study dynamics of quasi-2D biopolymer networks without direct surface adhesion. In these studies, the network is crowded to the surface, as in the actin network shown in figure 3.2(F), so the entire network is in the evanescent excitation field (Preciado López *et al* 2014, Stam *et al* 2017, Sonal *et al* 2019).

The advantage of this method over confocal microscopy is its lower phototoxicity, higher axial resolution, and faster frame rates.

The primary strengths of TIRF over other methods can also be disadvantages. For example, this method is limited to examining quasi-2D networks near a surface, so the interactions with the surface must be taken into account. Moreover, determining rheological properties from the biopolymer dynamics visualized with TIRF and connecting network properties to polymer physics predictions is not straightforward.

3.1.4 Light-sheet microscopy

Light-sheet microscopy (LSM) is a newer technology, compared to LSCM and TIRF, that allows for similar imaging of quasi-2D sheets in 3D networks (figure 3.3) (Engelbrecht and Stelzer 2006, Gualda *et al* 2013, Girkin and Carvalho 2018, Olarte *et al* 2018, Bishop *et al* 2020). Similar to LSCM, light-sheet microscopes can image planes in varying z-heights throughout the sample to allow for optical sectioning and volumetric 3D image reconstruction. However, rather than using point scanning to illuminate the sample and create an image, LSM uses a second objective to create a plane or 'sheet' of light that illuminates an entire planar FOV at once and captures images at the frame rate of the camera (figures 3.3(A–C)).

Similar to TIRF, by only illuminating a thin layer of the sample at a time, LSM enables reduced photobleaching and phototoxicity, as compared to LSCM and epifluorescence, which both illuminate the 3D volume within the FOV. LSM

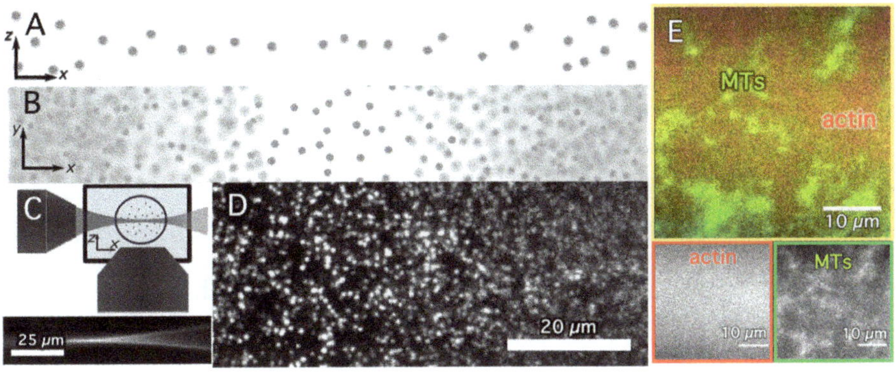

Figure 3.3. Light-sheet microscopy uses a sheet of light to allow for high-speed selective plane illumination. An axial (A) and in-plane (B) image of microspheres in aqueous solution acquired with a light-sheet microscope configured as shown in (C). The horizontally aligned objective creates the plane light (shown below the cartoon) used to illuminate and excite the sample. The vertical objective acts similarly to that in an epifluorescence microscope, capturing emitted light from the excited fluorophores and directing it to a camera. The non-uniform thickness of the light sheet (thicker at the edges than the middle) allows for more focused imaging in the center and more signal at the edges to expand the range of dynamics that can be captured. (D) 115 kbp linear DNA imaged using the light-sheet microscope depicted in (C). (E) LSM images of a composite network of actin and microtubules. The top image is a colorized overlay of images collected with two different filter sets to capture the different fluorophores attached to the actin and microtubules. Bottom images show the separate images. The network conditions are identical to those shown in figures 3.1 and 3.2(C). (A–D) Adapted with permission from Wulstein *et al* (2016) © Optical Society of America. (E) Adapted from Regan *et al* (2018) with permission from the Royal Society of Chemistry.

typically affords faster frame rates compared to LSCM point scanning because the entire FOV is imaged and captured at once by the camera, which is typically a CMOS. This feature of LSM makes it amenable to samples with fast dynamics, such as diffusing colloids and DNA shown in figures 3.3(B) and (D).

Another unique feature of LSM, that has both advantages and disadvantages, is its non-uniform illumination of the FOV due to the non-uniform thickness of the light sheet (figures 3.3(B) and (C)). This effect causes reduced axial resolution and larger depth of field at the edges as compared to the central region of the sheet (figures 3.3(B) and (D)). While this non-uniformity complicates discerning the structure of a sample over a large FOV, it allows for capturing a wider range of dynamics in a single FOV. The central region, with its high axial resolution and low signal-to-noise, is well-equipped to discern structure and dynamics at small spatiotemporal scales, while the thicker edges can capture larger axially-extended features and longer timescale dynamics, as molecules remain in the FOV for longer (Becker *et al* 2013, Wulstein *et al* 2016, Regan *et al* 2018).

Finally, because LSM is still a relatively new and developing technology, there are fewer commercially-available options with suitable functionality, so custom builds are typically required (Engelbrecht and Stelzer 2006, Greger *et al* 2007, Girkin and Carvalho 2018, Glaser *et al* 2020). Other features that commercial LSCM setups are typically outfitted with, that are non-trivial to couple into custom-built LSM setups, include multi-spectral imaging (figure 3.3(E)) (Niedworok *et al* 2012, Girstmair *et al* 2016), and precise rapid z-scanning to allow for accurate 3D reconstruction of thick samples (Duocastella *et al* 2017).

3.2 Direct measurements of force, stress, and dynamics

The microscopy techniques and instrumentation described above are well-suited for imaging diverse biopolymer networks and characterizing dynamics and structure. However, a key characteristic of biopolymer networks, that often dictates their function, dynamics, and structure, is their mechanical response to stress and strain, i.e., their rheological properties.

As described in chapter 1, many biopolymer networks exhibit rich viscoelastic properties that enable their multifunctionality in biology and give insight into the underlying physical interactions and mechanisms that dictate their properties. In many cases, direct visualization of the biopolymers or embedded probes can be used to infer the mechanical properties of the network, as I briefly described in section 3.1 (Keane and Adrian 1992, Mason and Weitz 1995, Mason *et al* 1997, Squires and Mason 2010, Wereley and Meinhart 2010, Chapman *et al* 2014). However, these approaches, which I describe in detail in chapter 4, rely on theoretical assumptions that are often violated in biopolymer networks that are spatially heterogeneous, active, or otherwise time-varying (i.e., aging, coarsening, melting) (Squires and Mason 2010, Zia 2018).

Here, I describe several techniques that been developed to directly measure the mechanics and rheological properties of biopolymer networks subject to thermal forces, as well as linear and nonlinear deformations, on scales ranging from submicron to millimeters.

3.2.1 Optical tweezers

Optical tweezers (OT) is a microscopy-based technique that uses a focused infrared laser beam to trap microspheres embedded in an aqueous medium and measure the forces that the medium exerts on the microsphere (Molloy and Padgett 2002, Moffitt *et al* 2008, Fazal and Block 2011, Jones *et al* 2015, Robertson-Anderson 2018). Optical tweezers has been used extensively over the past several decades to examine the properties of single biopolymers, such as their force-extension profiles and the nature of their interactions with associated binding proteins and motors (Perkins *et al* 1995, Wang *et al* 1997, Block *et al* 2003, Fuller *et al* 2006, Toan and Micheletti 2006, Bianco *et al* 2007, Ferrer *et al* 2008, Guilbaud *et al* 2019). These experiments typically require attaching biopolymers and/or their binding proteins to the trapped microsphere.

3.2.1.1 Paradigmatic applications

DNA stretching experiments that have been used to test predictions from the worm-like chain model (see chapter 2) and measure the salt-dependent persistence length (see figure 1.2) (Tinland *et al* 1997, Wang *et al* 1997, Guilbaud *et al* 2019), rely on adhering one end of the DNA chain to a trapped microsphere and attaching the other end to the surface of the sample chamber or to another trapped microsphere (in setups that have two optical traps). By pulling the trapped probe relative to the chamber surface or the other (fixed) trap, the DNA is entropically stretched and the force that the DNA exerts to resist the stretching is evaluated as a function of stretching distance to determine the characteristic force-extension curve. Similar constructions have been used to determine the strength of RNA hairpins and histone packing (Block *et al* 2003, Bianco *et al* 2007, Ferrer *et al* 2008). Finally, several experiments have used a trapped DNA molecule embedded within an entangled DNA network to demonstrate and characterize the nature of the tube confinement predicted by the reptation (Robertson and Smith 2007). I discuss these experiments further in chapter 5.

Beyond measuring single-molecule properties and interactions, optical tweezers has been demonstrated to be a powerful tool for measuring the rheological properties of biopolymer networks, constituting a class of measurement techniques referred to as Optical Tweezers Microrheology (OTM) (Brau *et al* 2007, Yao *et al* 2009, Tassieri 2016, Robertson-Anderson 2018). OTM measurements use non-interacting microspheres embedded in biopolymer networks to apply local strains to the network and measure the corresponding force response. This approach constitutes the majority of optical tweezers experiments on biopolymer networks and will be the focus of discussion in the subsequent chapters. To design, understand, and optimize OTM measurements, we need to first understand the basic underlying principles and essential components of optical tweezers.

3.2.1.2 Physics of optical trapping

Optical tweezers relies on the principle of momentum conservation to trap microscopic dielectric particles at the focal point of a tightly focused laser beam. Specifically, as light is focused to a point, light rays positioned at different distances from the beam center are bent to varying degrees from parallel with the light path ($\theta_1 = 0$) at the center to a maximum angle $\theta_{1,\max}$ at the edges, determined by the numerical aperture of the objective and laser beam waist at the objective. When a dielectric particle, i.e., one that has a higher index of refraction n_2 than that of the surrounding aqueous medium n_1, is placed at the laser focal point, the light rays hitting the probe at different angles are all bent to varying degrees towards the normal of the interface, according to Snell's law:

$$n_1 \sin\theta_1 = n_2 \sin\theta_2 \tag{3.2}$$

When the light rays pass through the probe back to the medium they bend again, this time away from the normal (figure 3.4(A), (B)). When the probe is centered at the focal point of the laser, the bending directions of the light rays are symmetric about the probe center and the angle that each ray is incident on the probe matches the angle at which it hits the probe-medium interface to exit the probe (figure 3.4(A)). This geometry results in no net change in the direction of the laser light upon passing through the trapped particle, so there is no change in the momentum of the light. No momentum change of the light equates to no change in momentum of the probe, so it stays in the center and experiences no force from the trapping beam. However, when the probe is pushed away from the focal center, by a force exerted by the medium, now the symmetry has broken so there is an overall net change in the direction and thus momentum of the light exiting the probe (figure 3.4(B)). The momentum change is directed away from the trap center, inducing an opposite momentum change to the probe, pushing it back towards the trap center. Newton's Second Law tells us that this momentum change is proportional to the force exerted on the trapped particle to push it back to the center. This restoring force F_{OT} is stronger the further distance Δx that the probe is pulled away from the center, much like a spring, and the strength of the trap can be defined in terms of a trap constant k_{OT} that relates the restoring force to the distance the probe is pulled from the trap:

$$F_{OT} = k_{OT}\Delta x \tag{3.3}$$

Invoking Newton's Third Law tells us that the restoring force is equal to the force that the surrounding medium exerts on the probe to push it out of the trap. From these relations, and proper calibration to determine k_{OT}, we can directly measure the force exerted on a trapped probe by a surrounding biopolymer network.

3.2.1.3 Instrumentation considerations

It is important to note that effective optical tweezers measurements require proper alignment and strong focus of the laser beam as well as accurate measurement of the

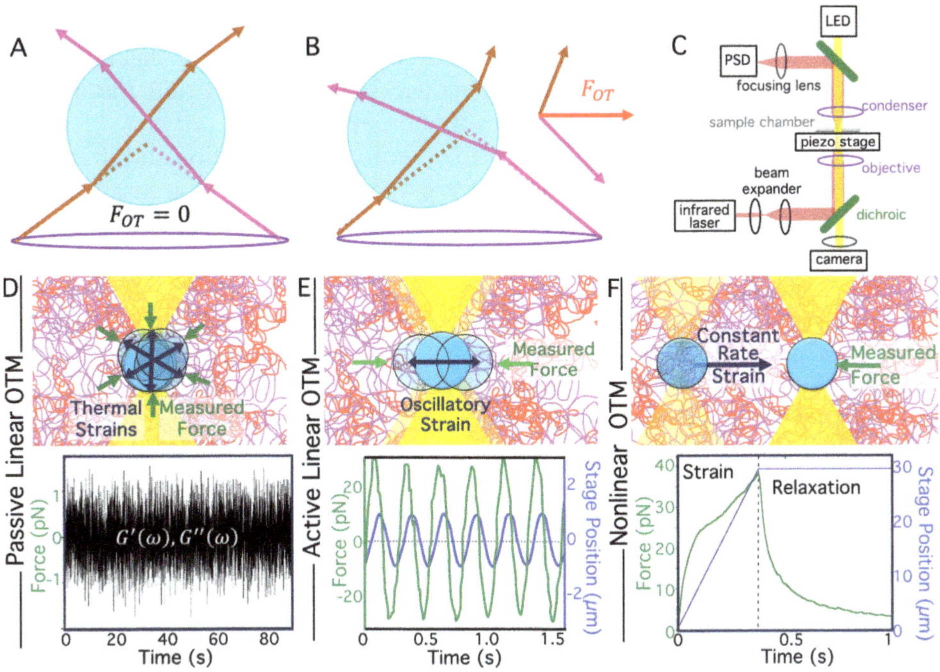

Figure 3.4. Principles and applications of optical tweezers microrheology. (A,B) Optical tweezers uses an objective lens (purple) to tightly focus laser light, as shown by two light rays (magenta and maroon), which acts as a trap for dielectric microsphere probes (cyan). (A) When the probe is positioned in the trap center there is no net change in momentum of the trapping laser light so there is no force F_{OT} exerted on the probe so it remains in the trap center. (B) When an external force pushes the probe out of the trap, there is a net momentum change of the light due to the change in its direction, which induces an equal and opposite change in momentum of the probe, providing the spring-like restoring force F_{OT}. The vector diagram shows the force exerted on the probe due to the momentum change of the magenta and maroon light rays, and the resultant force F_{OT} that is directed back to the center of the trap. (C) A simplified schematic of optical tweezers showing the key components necessary to form the trap and measure force. The translucent red lines depict the trapping laser light path and the yellow lines depict the white light from the LED that is used to image the probes to facilitate trapping. (D–F) Optical tweezers can be used to perform linear (D and E) and nonlinear (F) measurements by trapping a probe and (D) measuring the laser deflection from thermal fluctuations, (E) oscillating the probe at small amplitudes over a range of frequencies, and (F) moving the probe at a constant speed over a large distance and then holding the probe fixed and recording the relaxation of force. Sample measured forces and stage positions (for E and F) versus time for each measurement type are shown below the corresponding cartoon.

probe displacement and/or laser deflection. Strong trapping relies on a very tight focus, i.e., steep bending gradient, of the light rays, which requires a high NA objective (NA $\geqslant$ 1.2). The laser beam must also fill or overfill the objective BFA to maximize the bending gradient. Because typical beam waists are <4 mm, and typical BFAs are ~6–8 mm, this filling requires beam expansion via a pair of lenses with a proper ratio of their focal distances (figure 3.4(C)). The laser needs to also have a Gaussian intensity profile such that the intensity is maximum at the beam center and decreases according to a Gaussian function as the light rays move further off-axis. This profile ensures that the light rays hitting the on-axis side of the probe, which are the ones that create the restoring force, have greater momentum than those off-axis rays that counteract this force. The wide-spread use of infrared lasers in optical trapping is motivated by its reduced photodamage and local heating of the biological molecules being investigated, reduces local heating, and the ability to couple optical tweezers with fluorescence microscopy.

The considerations described above are to optimize trap formation and strength, but another essential component to optical tweezers microrheology is accurate measurement of force. There are multiple ways to measure force, including using image-based tracking of the probe displacement, using a second detection laser, and projecting the trapping laser onto a position-sensing detector (PSD) to measure its deflection (figure 3.4(C)), which scales with the force. I will focus on the latter approach due to its relative ease to construct compared to incorporating a second detection laser and faster data acquisition rates compared to image-based methods. The key components required for this force detection approach are: a condenser that collects the exiting trapping beam after passing through the trapped particle and the sample, a PSD photodiode placed downstream from the condenser to measure the deflection of the laser resulting from the probe displacement, and a data acquisition (DAQ) device that interfaces between the analog PSD and the computer to allow for high-speed data capture.

The condenser should have a higher NA aperture than those typically used to illuminate a FOV in bright-field microscopes, and more closely match that of the objective (NA $\geqslant$1.2) to ensure that large laser deflections can be captured. The PSD is a silicon-based photodiode that converts photons to electrons to convert the position of the projected beam centroid to a voltage, which is then digitized via the DAQ interface. In this construction, the position of the deflected laser is used in equation (3.3) instead of the physical displacement of the probe from the trap center Δx, and the trap constant k_{OT} is quantified in dimensions of force per voltage rather than force per displacement, with typical units of pN V^{-1} and k_{OT} values of $\sim$10–100 pN V^{-1}.

The components described above are sufficient to perform passive OTM that uses thermal fluctuations to determine rheological properties. In this approach, the trap and sample chamber remain fixed and the laser deflection resulting from thermal forces on the trapped probe is measured (figure 3.4(D)). Applying specific strains to the sample, often achieved by moving the trapped probe relative to the sample chamber (figure 3.4(E), (F)), typically requires incorporating a piezoelectric nanopositioning stage that can move the sample relative to the trapped probe with precisely programmed speeds and distances. Alternatively, a piezoelectric mirror can be incorporated to move the trap while keeping the sample fixed. However, for the latter approach the calibration for accurate force measurement is more difficult as the trapping strength can vary with trap position.

3.2.1.4 Passive OTM using GSER

Let's start with the passive case—which is the simplest measurement to make for reasons I just described—but is perhaps the most complex to analyze (figure 3.4(A)). Here, we can determine the linear viscoelastic moduli, $G'(\omega)$ and $G''(\omega)$, from the laser deflections due to thermal forces, measured with the PSD, by using the Generalized Stokes–Einstein Relation (GSER) (Mason and Weitz 1995, Banchio *et al* 1999, Mason 2000, Squires and Mason 2010, Tassieri 2016). GSER starts with the standard Stokes–Einstein relation defined in chapter 2:

$$D = k_B T/\zeta \tag{3.4}$$

where $\zeta = 6\pi R_s \eta$ for a sphere of radius $R$and $D = \frac{\langle(\Delta r)^2\rangle}{6\Delta t}$.

The mean-squared displacement of the particle can then be related to the viscosity of a Newtonian fluid according to

$$\langle(\Delta r(\Delta t))^2\rangle = k_B T \Delta t / \pi R \eta \tag{3.5}$$

We can extend this construction to viscoelastic fluids by generalizing ζ according to the relation:

$$\zeta^* = \frac{\eta}{\eta^*(\omega)}\zeta \tag{3.6}$$

and recognizing that the complex modulus $G^*(\omega)$ that contains $G'(\omega)$ and $G''(\omega)$:

$$G^*(\omega) = G'(\omega) + i\omega G''(\omega) \tag{3.7}$$

is related to the complex viscosity as:

$$G^* = i\omega\eta^*(\omega) \tag{3.8}$$

Combining these relations and taking the Laplace transform of G^* yields the widely used GSER expression:

$$\widetilde{G}(s) = \frac{k_B T}{\pi R s \langle(\Delta \tilde{r}(s))^2\rangle} \tag{3.9}$$

where s is frequency (Squires and Mason 2010). A similar expression can be written in Fourier space (Mason and Weitz 1995).

To incorporate the mean-squared displacements of the measured laser deflections into this framework, we compute the normalized mean-squared displacement:

$$\pi(\Delta t) = \frac{\langle(\Delta r(\Delta t))^2\rangle}{2\langle(\Delta r)^2\rangle} \tag{3.10}$$

which we numerically convert to Fourier space using the following relation:

$$-\omega^2\pi(\omega) = (1 - e^{-i\omega\,\Delta t_1})\frac{\pi(\Delta t_1)}{\Delta t_1} + \dot{\pi}_\infty e^{-i\omega\,\Delta t_N} + \sum_{k=2}^{N}\left(\frac{\pi_k - \pi_{k-1}}{\tau_k - \tau_{k-1}}\right)(e^{-i\omega\,\Delta t_{k-1}} - e^{-i\omega\,\Delta t_k}) \tag{3.11}$$

where Δt, 1, and N represent the lag time and the first and last point of the oversampled $\pi(\Delta t)$, and $\dot{\pi}_\infty$ is the extrapolated slope of $\pi(\Delta t)$ at infinity (Tassieri *et al* 2012, Peddireddy *et al* 2020a).

$\pi(\omega)$ is related to the complex modulus and corresponding viscoelastic moduli via:

$$G^*(\omega) = G'(\omega) + iG''(\omega) = \left(\frac{k_{OT}}{6\pi R}\right)\left(\frac{1}{i\omega\pi(\omega)} - 1\right). \tag{3.12}$$

This approach of extracting viscoelastic moduli from thermal fluctuations using GSER is the same as that used in particle-tracking microrheology (PTM), as I describe in chapter 4. However, the advantage of passive OTM over PTM is that data can be recorded at rates up to $\sim 10^5$ Hz and for durations of 10 s of minutes, limited only by the data acquisition rate and computer random-access memory. Conversely, PTM timescales are bounded below by the camera frame rate, typically limited to $\sim$100 Hz, and above by the time over which the particle remains in focus in the FOV ($\lesssim 10^2$ s). The several orders of magnitude larger range of timescales afforded by OTM translate to decades more frequencies over which $G'(\omega)$ and $G''(\omega)$ can be evaluated. OTM also provides users with precise control over the location of the measurement within the sample to facilitate characterization of spatial heterogeneities, and directly connect local rheological properties to network structure. Finally, localizing the force to a single location provides unambiguous differentiation of spatial and temporal heterogeneities, necessary for networks that exhibit aging, coarsening and other non-equilibrium processes that manifest as time-evolving mechanical properties.

A note of caution when using GSER to determine viscoelastic moduli is that GSER is only strictly valid for systems that can be considered in steady-state and as continuum materials on the spatiotemporal scales of the measurement. These assumptions are often violated in biopolymer networks, in particular, in active matter systems or networks that are highly bundled, de-mixed, or phase-separated.

3.2.1.5 Linear oscillatory OTM

An alternative method to determine $G'(\omega)$ and $G''(\omega)$ using optical tweezers is to apply a small amplitude oscillatory strain and measure the resulting oscillatory force (Brau *et al* 2007, Chapman *et al* 2014, Robertson-Anderson 2018, Zia 2018, Gurmessa *et al* 2019) (figure 3.4(E)), in analogy to the bulk linear oscillatory rheology measurements I describe in chapter 2. Specifically, a trapped probe oscillates relative to the sample, by the sample stage oscillating relative to the fixed trap, over a range of frequencies according to:

$$x(t) = |\, x_0 \,| \sin \omega t \tag{3.13}$$

where $x(t)$ is the stage position and $|\, x_0 \,|$ and ω are the amplitude and frequency of the oscillation (figure 3.4(E)). Simultaneously, the force exerted on the probe by the sample to resist the oscillatory strain is measured by recording the laser deflections with the PSD. This force likewise varies in a sinusoidal fashion:

$$F(t) = |\, F_0 \,| \sin(\omega t + \delta) \tag{3.14}$$

where $|\, F_0 \,|$ and δ are the force amplitude and phase difference between the oscillatory displacement $x(t)$ and force $F(t)$. The in-phase and out-of-phase components of the force with respect to the stage position correlate with $G'(\omega)$ and $G''(\omega)$, respectively, according to:

$$G'(\omega) = \frac{|\, F_0 \,|}{|\, x_0 \,| \, 6\pi R} \cos \delta \tag{3.15}$$

$$G''(\omega) = \frac{|F_0|}{|x_0|\, 6\pi R_s} \sin\delta. \tag{3.16}$$

The validity of these relations is limited to the linear regime in which the moduli are independent of strain amplitude $|G'| \sim |G''| \sim \gamma^0$, which translates to $|G'| \sim |G''| \sim |x_0|^0$ and occurs in the small amplitude limit. In typical OTM experiments this criterion is achieved for $|x_0| \leqslant 1\ \mu\text{m}$ (Chapman *et al* 2014, Gurmessa *et al* 2018, Robertson-Anderson 2018, Francis *et al* 2019). However, the maximum $|x_0|$ in which the system remains in the linear regime should be determined specifically for each system by performing a strain sweep. Because smaller amplitudes result in smaller forces in the linear regime (i.e., $\sigma \sim \gamma$, $|F_0| \sim |x_0|$), the optimal amplitude is one near the upper limit of the linear regime to maximize signal-to-noise.

The advantage of this approach over the passive method described in the previous section is that it does not rely on GSER and makes no assumptions about the relationship between fluctuations and dissipation. Rather, it directly applies a strain and measures a stress. The disadvantage is the reduced range of available frequencies compared to passive OTM. The upper limit is set by the response time of the nanopositioning stage (~kHz), which limits oscillation frequencies to $\omega_{\max} \approx 10^2$ rad s^{-1}, and the lower limit is set by the noise floor (~10^{-1} pN), which typically translates to a lower bound of $\omega_{\min} \approx 10^{-1}$ rad s^{-1} (Chapman *et al* 2014, Weigand *et al* 2017, Gurmessa *et al* 2019, Peddireddy *et al* 2020a).

3.2.1.6 Nonlinear oscillatory OTM

One of the primary advantages of OTM over passive particle-tracking microrheology is that one can precisely program the strain properties (speed, distance, direction, etc) by varying the speed and distance over which the trapped particle is moved through the network (typically by moving the sample stage relative to the trapped particle). This control enables strains that are much faster and/or larger than the relaxation timescales and/or lengthscales of the network to probe the nonlinear regime, in which networks are pushed far from equilibrium (figure 3.4(F)) (Falzone *et al* 2015, Gurmessa *et al* 2016, 2017, 2019, Ricketts *et al* 2018, 2019). Conversely, PTM is limited to the linear steady-state regime dominated by thermal fluctuations.

While there are many different strain profiles that can be designed and applied to a biopolymer network to elicit a nonlinear response, interpreting the measured force is non-trivial as robust theoretical frameworks for describing the nonlinear regime are lacking. With this caveat in mind, strain profiles that are analogous to those used in bulk rheology are the most straightforward to interpret and compare to bulk rheology studies, and there is now a body of literature describing and validating the measurements and analysis methods (Chapman and Robertson-Anderson 2014, Falzone and Robertson-Anderson 2015, Gurmessa *et al* 2016, 2017, Robertson-Anderson 2018, Khan *et al* 2019).

The canonical nonlinear OTM strain profile, shown in figure 3.4(F), is a constant rate strain followed by a relaxation period. The constant rate strain is achieved by moving the stage relative to the trapped probe through a fixed distance from $x = 0$

to $x = x_{\max}$ at a constant speed $v = dx/dt$, with both $x_{\max}$ and v precisely programmed by the user. Following the strain phase, the probe is held fixed at $x_{\max}$ for a set time to measure the decay of the force over time.

The force exerted on the probe during the strain is used to determine the extent to which the network responds elastically or viscously over different lengthscales and timescales, and the degree to which nonlinear stress features, such as stress-stiffening and stress-softening, manifest. Specifically, a purely elastic system would exhibit a linear increase in force as x increases from 0 to $x_{\max}$, i.e., $F \sim x^1$; and the slope of that line would be a measure of the elastic stiffness of the network, $K = dF/dx$, analogous to the spring constant in Hooke's law, which would be independent of the strain speed, i.e., $F \sim v^0$. Conversely, the force exerted by a purely viscous system would instantaneously jump to a non-zero value F_v that would remain constant for the duration of the strain and would be proportional to the strain speed, i.e., $F \sim x^0 v^1$. Most biopolymer networks are viscoelastic, so display combinations of elastic and viscous features that depend on x and v. Typically, the initial (small x) response is stiffer, displayed as a steeper slope K, than that at larger strains in which the force softens to a more viscous-like regime, manifested as a decreasing K or $\frac{dK}{dx} < 0$ (figure 3.4(F)). This terminal regime may be completely viscous, with $K \approx 0$, or retain an elastic component and thus a non-zero slope, K. Beyond these general features, networks can also exhibit initial stress-stiffening, $\frac{dK}{dx} > 0$, at very small strains (short times) as well as at large strains (long times) that are beyond the scales of the subsequent softening phase. These features can be seen in figure 3.4(F) and will appear in many of the networks I discuss in subsequent chapters.

Following the strain, the relaxation of the force exerted on the probe over time can be analyzed to determine stress relaxation timescales and dynamics. For many systems, the force relaxation can be described by a sum of exponential decays resulting from distinct relaxation mechanisms that occur over well-separated timescales, analogous to equation (2.118), with an added residual term F_∞ that accounts for any sustained elasticity, as may arise in crosslinked networks (Francis *et al* 2019, Gurmessa *et al* 2017, 2019).

$$F_R(t) = \sum C_i e^{-\frac{t}{\tau_i}} + F_\infty \tag{3.17}$$

The time constants τ_i correlate to the relaxation timescales of the system, as shown in, e.g., Robertson and Smith (2007), Gurmessa *et al* (2016), and Khan *et al* (2019), and the amplitudes C_i can be evaluated to determine the fraction of the stress relaxation that is driven by each relaxation mechanism. In practice, this relative contribution is evaluated as the fractional amplitude c_i:

$$c_i = C_i / \sum C_i \tag{3.18}$$

where $\sum c_i = 1$ (Peddireddy *et al* 2020a, 2020b).

The fractional dissipation, namely how much of the initial resistive force relaxes versus being elastically sustained, can be expressed as:

$$f_R = F_R(0) - F_\infty / F_R(0) \tag{3.19}$$

where $f_R = 1$ and $f_R = 0$ correspond to purely viscous dissipation and elastic memory, respectively (Gurmessa *et al* 2019, Ricketts *et al* 2019).

In certain cases, as described in chapter 2, the force relaxation does not decay exponentially but instead decays with time according to a power law, similar to equation (2.119) (Chapman and Robertson-Anderson 2014, Falzone *et al* 2015, Ricketts *et al* 2018):

$$F_R(t) \sim t^{-\beta} \tag{3.20}$$

and may also exhibit different phases of power-law scaling over different times during the relaxation, resulting in multiple scaling exponents β_i that depend on the time relative to the end of the strain phase (Fitzpatrick *et al* 2018, Ricketts *et al* 2018).

There are other strain profiles, such as microrheological large amplitude oscillatory straining (mLAOS) (Khan *et al* 2019), and releasing the probe following the strain phase to track its recoil dynamics and creep (Chapman and Robertson-Anderson 2014), that have also been validated to provide important information regarding the nonlinear response of biopolymer networks. Select results of these studies will be discussed in subsequent chapters.

Finally, to more directly compare nonlinear OTM measurements with comparable bulk rheology measurements, we can use the following relations to convert force F to stress σ (Chapman and Robertson-Anderson 2014), stage position x to strain γ (Chapman and Robertson-Anderson 2014, Khan *et al* 2019), and stage speed v to strain rate $\dot{\gamma}$ (Squires 2008, Squires and Mason 2010, Khan *et al* 2019):

$$\sigma = \frac{F}{\pi R^2} \tag{3.17}$$

$$\gamma = \frac{x}{2R} \tag{3.18}$$

$$\dot{\gamma} = \sqrt{18}\frac{v}{R}. \tag{3.19}$$

3.2.2 Magnetic tweezers

Magnetic tweezers have also been employed as active microrheology platforms, in similar fashion to OTM, to measure the stress response of biopolymer networks, as described in (Neuman and Nagy 2008, Lin and Valentine 2012a, 2012b, Yang *et al* 2012a, 2012b, 2012c). Magnetic tweezers employ a magnetic field gradient, created by a combination of magnets, to impart a force on a superparamagnetic bead to drive it through a sample (Strick *et al* 1996, Lipfert *et al* 2009, Rich *et al* 2011, Lin and Valentine 2012a). The magnets can be strong permanent magnets such as neodymium iron boron or electromagnets, with the latter providing more tunability of the magnetic field while the former is cheaper and more stable (De Vlaminck and

Dekker 2012, Sarkar and Rybenkov 2016). The orientation and strength of the magnets determine the trap geometry and strength which dictate how the bead will move through the sample (Lipfert *et al* 2009, Sarkar and Rybenkov 2016).

Magnetic tweezers microrheology has been used extensively to investigate microrheological properties of *in vitro* cytoskeleton networks and live cells, as described in Bausch *et al* (1999), Uhde *et al* (2005), Waigh (2005, 2016), Luan *et al* (2008), Lin and Valentine (2012a, 2012b), Yang *et al* (2012b).

Magnetic tweezers are much simpler and cheaper to build compared to optical tweezers, and they are also able to generate much higher forces, up to $\sim 10^3$ pN, versus $\sim 10^2$ pN that OT can accommodate. However, magnetic tweezers microrheology (MTM) lacks the fine control and tunability of strain profiles that OTM affords such as varying strain speeds, positions, and directions. Moreover, MTM lacks the precision in force measurements and trapped particle displacements that PSDs in optical tweezers provide. For these reasons, MTM is most well-suited for nonlinear strain measurements that can benefit from large force generation and are less susceptible to low signal-to-noise.

Another key difference between OTM and MTM is that magnetic tweezers strains are force-controlled strains while optical tweezers strains are rate-controlled. Namely, in MTM, a user-defined force is applied to the magnetic bead and the motion of the bead is tracked via microscopy. The relationship between the force and bead displacement is evaluated to determine viscoelastic properties. Conversely, as I described above, in OTM, the probe is pulled through the network at a user-defined speed and the force is measured via the laser deflections recorded by the PSD.

3.2.3 Atomic force microscopy

Atomic Force Microscopy (AFM) uses microscale cantilevers to impart a force on the surface of a soft material and determine its stiffness by measuring the cantilever deflection. For cantilevers with a known modulus acting on an elastic substrate, the relationship between the cantilever deflection and force is straightforward. However, when the substrate is viscoelastic, parsing the contributions from elastic and viscous components to the deflection is non-trivial.

One method to overcome this complication is to incorporate piezoelectric actuators to allow the cantilever to oscillate over a range of frequencies, with reported values of $\sim$1–700 Hz. From the measured frequency-dependent deflections, the viscoelastic moduli of biopolymer networks and cells can be determined in a similar fashion to linear oscillatory OTM measurements (see section 3.2.1.5), as first presented in Mahaffy *et al* (2000, 2004).

Following this seminal work, numerous studies have used AFM to characterize the rheological properties of whole cells, intracellular regions, tissues, and biofilms (Alcaraz *et al* 2002, 2003, Miyagi *et al* 2008, Gavara and Chadwick 2010, Wang *et al* 2013, Rebêlo *et al* 2014, Rother *et al* 2014, Martinez-Torres *et al* 2016, Lherbette *et al* 2017). Far fewer studies have been devoted to *in vitro* biopolymer networks (Mahaffy *et al* 2000, Keresztes *et al* 2001, Morris *et al* 2001, Radić *et al* 2011).

3.2.4 Dynamic light scattering

Dynamic Light Scattering (DLS) examines the correlations in scattered light from a sample to discern sizes of microscale and nanoscale particles within the sample, as well as their diffusion coefficients. Moreover, using a GSER approach, similar to passive OTM and particle-tracking microrheology, the viscoelastic moduli G' and G'' can be extracted from the time-dependent correlations. The basic principle of DLS relies on the fact that the intensity of the scattered light fluctuates over time due to constructive and destructive interference that varies as particles thermally fluctuate in solution, such that the autocorrelation of the scattered light intensity decays exponentially with increasing lag time. Because smaller particles fluctuate more quickly, the associated autocorrelation decays more steeply than for larger (slower moving) particles, so the decay time of the correlation function can be used to determine the particle size. Alternatively, if the particle size is known, DLS can be used to determine solution viscosity or viscoelasticity using GSER. Let's unpack this.

DLS is typically performed on a sample placed in a cuvette that requires much larger volumes, of order 10^2–10^3 μL, compared to the $\sim$10 μL needed for microscopy-based techniques. While this sample volume can be prohibitive for many biopolymer samples, there are specialized quartz microcuvettes that can accommodate volumes as low as 20–30 μL (if you can afford spending $\sim$\$10K to purchase one).

To evaluate correlations in scattered light, a monochromatic laser is sent through a polarizer to align it vertically, and then passes through the cuvette window into the sample. The particles in the sample absorb and scatter the light which is collected by another polarizer, typically aligned in the same direction as the first one. Because the light will be scattered in all directions, only a small fraction of that light will still be in the polarized direction and thus pass through the detector polarizer. For this reason, a photomultiplier is typically used to amplify the scattering signal.

If the particles are not moving, then the fraction of scattered light in the polarized direction will be constant so the correlation in the scattered intensity will not decay over time. The scattered light from each particle may constructively or destructively interfere with each other, but this interference will not change over time. However, if the particles are fluctuating over time, then the extent to which they constructively or destructively interfere likewise fluctuates at a rate that mirrors that of the particle fluctuations. By evaluating the correlation in the scattered intensity over time, a characteristic decay time can be determined, which relates to the mean-squared displacement and thus diffusion coefficient and size of the particle. In practice, this decay time is quantified by computing the normalized second-order correlation function g_2 of intensities I, related to a particle's motion, as a function of lag time Δt:

$$g_2(\Delta t) = \frac{\langle (I(t)I(t + \Delta t) \rangle}{\langle I(t) \rangle^2} \tag{3.20}$$

Because the motion of an individual particle cannot be determined with DLS, the first-order correlation function that evaluates the relative correlated motion of particles in also needed, and is determined by computing the correlation in scattered electric fields E:

$$g_1(\Delta t) = \frac{\langle E(t)E(t + \Delta t)\rangle}{\langle E(t)\rangle^2} \tag{3.21}$$

The first- and second-order correlation functions can be coupled as follows:

$$g_2(\Delta t) = B + \beta \mid g_1(\Delta t)|^2 \tag{3.22}$$

where B is a constant background term and β contains information about the detector and sample scattering properties (but not the dynamics). For monodisperse systems, g_1 decays exponentially with increasing lag time:

$$g_1(\Delta t) = e^{-\Gamma\Delta t} \tag{3.23}$$

with a characteristic decay time Γ that relates to the particle diffusion coefficient as:

$$\Gamma = Dq^2 \tag{3.24}$$

where the wave vector q is related to the solvent index of refraction n, the incident light wavelength λ, and detector angle θ via:

$$q = \frac{4\pi n}{\lambda} \sin \frac{\theta}{2} \tag{3.25}$$

By coupling equations 3.22–3.24 we arrive at:

$$g_2(\Delta t) = B + \beta e^{-2\Gamma Dq^2 t} \tag{3.26}$$

from which the particle diffusion coefficient can be determined.

From D we can compute the particle size for systems in which the particles can be approximated as spherical and the solvent is a Newtonian fluid of known viscosity, according to the Stokes–Einstein relation (see equation (3.4)). Alternatively, if the particle size is known then the fluid viscosity can be determined.

For a viscoelastic material with embedded particles of known size, we can use GSER to determine $G'(\omega)$ and $G''(\omega)$ from the diffusion coefficient using a process similar to that described in section 3.2.1.4 (see equations (3.4)–(3.9)).

Of note, because DLS relies on bulk averaging of the scattering signals, it is not well-suited for polydisperse or heterogeneous samples. For a sample with multiple particle types, each particle will contribute a distinct exponential decay to the correlation function. If the number of different particles is low and their size difference is significant then the different signals can be resolved. However, for higher polydispersity, the signal from each contribution is prohibitively weak to resolve. Another important consideration in DLS measurements is the choice of particle size. Larger particles will provide a larger scattering signal, which may be important if embedded in a network of biopolymers that, themselves, scatter light. However, because the sedimentation rate scales with the particle size, larger particles will sediment faster such that drift can contribute to the signal over the measurement timescale. Finally, very small contaminants such as dust can contribute to the scattering signal and complicate the analysis.

3.2.5 Bulk rheology

All of the techniques described above have been designed, in part, to try to mimic traditional bulk rheological measurements, for which there are well-established theoretical frameworks that connect the stress–strain relationships to properties of the network. The simplicity of bulk rheology measurements and our theoretical understanding thereof, make them an elegant way to measure the viscoelasticity of biopolymer networks.

However, bulk rheometers typically require much larger sample volumes of $\sim 10^2$–10^3 μL compared to their microrheology counterparts which require only ~ 10 μl. These volumes can be prohibitive for many biopolymers which require time-intensive purification processes or are costly to purchase. While small geometries and higher sensitivity rheometers have been developed that only require ~ 20–30 μL, often the soft nature of the biopolymer networks render the stress response from these small volumes below the minimum measurable torque limit of the rheometers.

I discuss the general concept of bulk rheology and its deliverables in chapter 2. In brief, traditional bulk rheology applies macroscopic strains to a viscoelastic material and measures the bulk stress response that the material exerts to resist the strain. In practice, samples are typically confined between two parallel plates or a cone and plate, and oscillatory strains are applied to the sample by rotating one plate relative to the other (figure 3.5). The strain amplitude γ, defined as the fractional distance the plate is rotated relative to a full rotation, and the sampled angular frequences of oscillation ω, are programmed by the user; and the stress that the sample exerts on the plate to resist the strain is measured (figure 3.5). The relationship between measured stress σ and applied strain γ, as well as the phase angle δ between the two, determine the elastic and viscous moduli $G'(\omega)$ and $G''(\omega)$ (figure 3.5).

The advantage of bulk rheology measurements over the techniques discussed above is that the strain field is well-characterized and there are well-established theoretical frameworks that relate the viscoelastic properties measured via bulk rheology to the microscopic network properties. For example, as described in chapter 2, the plateau modulus can be used to determine the number of entanglements per chain in linear polymer melts and solutions. Another advantage of bulk rheology is that $G'(\omega)$ and $G''(\omega)$ are determined directly from the frequency and amplitude of the applied strain and its relation to the measured stress, unlike passive microrheology methods which rely on GSER, and the assumptions within, to determine rheological properties. However, similar to DLS, bulk rheology measures a single stress value for the entire sample, so it cannot reliably characterize the mechanical properties of heterogenous networks.

3.3 What's next

There is a growing multitude of advances to microscopy and rheology instrumentation and approaches that build upon the fundamental techniques I discussed in this chapter. For example, methods that couple microscopy-based imaging of biopolymers

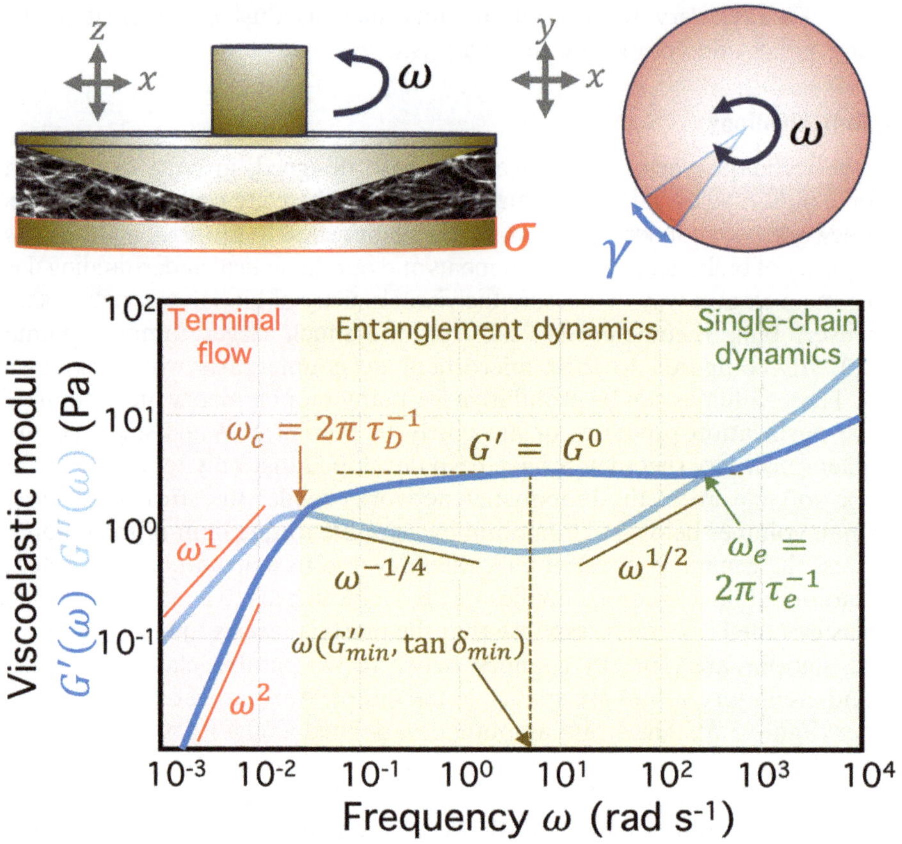

Figure 3.5. Bulk rheology basics and deliverables. To perform bulk rheology, (top) a sample is confined between a cone and plate and the cone is rotated with respect to the bottom plate at set frequencies ω and strains γ. The stress σ that the sample exerts to resist the strain is measured by sensors on the bottom plate (red). (Bottom) From the measured stress and strain, the frequency-dependent linear viscoelastic moduli $G'(\omega)$ and $G''(\omega)$ can be determined and used to characterize the rheological properties of the sample.

with rheology and force measurements have made great strides in directly connecting biopolymer dynamics, structure, and deformation fields to the stress response. For example, optical tweezers, magnetic tweezers, and bulk rheometers have all been outfitted with fluorescence microscopy capabilities, as described, for example, in Rickgauer and Smith (2007), Schmoller *et al* (2010), Dutta *et al* (2013), Shundo *et al* (2013), Arevalo *et al* (2015), Falzone and Robertson-Anderson (2015), Vlijm *et al* (2015), Gurmessa *et al* (2017), Robertson-Anderson (2018), Sheung *et al* (2021), Khanal *et al* (2022), Peddireddy *et al* (2022).

Moreover, there are numerous advanced fluorescence microscopy and force spectroscopy techniques that I did not cover here, as they are not currently widely used in biopolymer network research. However, these techniques may prove to be increasingly useful for investigating biopolymer networks in the near future. I encourage you to think creatively about how different techniques may help overcome some of the shortcomings of the methods I discussed above and the current needs in the field, for example: characterizing heterogeneous and time-varying systems; coupling dynamics and rheology across different spatiotemporal scales; improving upon current limits on spatial resolution, signal-to-noise, and data acquisition rates; and measuring interfacial rheological properties.

Some examples of promising advanced techniques include:

- Stochastic optical reconstruction microscopy (STORM) (Rust *et al* 2006, Endesfelder and Heilemann 2015, Xu *et al* 2017): STORM is a super-resolution imaging technique that evades the optical resolution limit of $\sim$500 nm by using photoswitchable fluorophores that stochastically turn on and off. Through a series of imaging cycles, each one only exciting a fraction of the fluorophores, an image containing signals from all of the fluorophores can be reconstructed with a resolution of $\sim$20 nm.
- Light-field microscopy (LFM) (Levoy *et al* 2006, Prevedel *et al* 2014, Guo *et al* 2019): LFM allows for 3D volumetric imaging from a single camera frame, a major advance over other methods such as LSCM and LSM that reconstruct volumetric images by sequential scanning through z. Typical light-field microscopes incorporate a microlens array into a conventional microscope to simultaneously capture planar and angular information of the incident light, which together contain all of the information necessary to computationally reconstruct a 3D image. This method is ideal for fast-moving and dynamic 3D systems, but is limited by demanding computational post-processing.
- Traction force microscopy (TFM) (Plotnikov *et al* 2014, Style *et al* 2014, Zancla *et al* 2022): TFM measures interfacial forces generated by, e.g., a moving or contracting cell, by adhering the cell (or other biopolymer network of interest) to a soft hydrogel substrate with embedded nanoparticles. By imaging the nanoparticles and tracking their motion, the strain field generated by the sample can be determined. Because the elastic properties of the hydrogel substrate are known, the strains can be mapped to forces.
- Holographic and multiplexed optical tweezers (Curtis *et al* 2002, Hossack *et al* 2003, Montes-Usategui *et al* 2006, Dixon and Reece 2020, Chen and Cheng 2022, Cibula, n.d.): These advanced OT methods are able to generate an array of many traps in a variety of patterns. The ability to trap multiple particles positioned throughout a sample has promise for, e.g., measuring spatially-resolved forces in heterogeneous biopolymer networks.

References

Adami R, Cintio O, Trombetta G, Choquet D and Grazi E 2003 On the stiffness of the natural actin filament decorated with alexa fluor tropomyosin *Biophys. Chem.* **104** 469–76

Alcaraz J, Buscemi L, Grabulosa M, Trepat X, Fabry B, Farré R and Navajas D 2003 Microrheology of human lung epithelial cells measured by atomic force microscopy *Biophys. J.* **84** 2071–9

Alcaraz J, Buscemi L, Puig-de-Morales M, Colchero J, Baró A and Navajas D 2002 Correction of microrheological measurements of soft samples with atomic force microscopy for the hydrodynamic drag on the cantilever *Langmuir* **18** 716–21

Aporvari M S, Dang S, Marfai J, Coursey K, McGorty R and Robertson-Anderson R M 2022 Crowding and confinement act in concert to slow DNA diffusion within cell-sized droplets *iScience* **25** 105122

Arevalo R C, Kumar P, Urbach J S and Blair D L 2015 Stress heterogeneities in sheared type-I collagen networks revealed by boundary stress microscopy *PLoS One* **10** e0118021

Banchio A J, Nägele G and Bergenholtz J 1999 Viscoelasticity and generalized Stokes–Einstein relations of colloidal dispersions *J. Chem. Phys.* **111** 8721–40

Bashirzadeh Y and Liu A P 2019 Encapsulation of the cytoskeleton: towards mimicking the mechanics of a cell *Soft Matter* **15** 8425–36

Bashirzadeh Y, Moghimianavval H and Liu A P 2022 Encapsulated actomyosin patterns drive cell-like membrane shape changes *iScience* **25** 104236

Bausch A R, Möller W and Sackmann E 1999 Measurement of local viscoelasticity and forces in living cells by magnetic tweezers *Biophys. J.* **76** 573–9

Becker K, Jährling N, Saghafi S and Dodt H-U 2013 Ultramicroscopy: light-sheet-based microscopy for imaging centimeter-sized objects with micrometer resolution *Cold Spring Harb. Protoc.* **2013** pdb.top076539

Bianco P, Nagy A, Kengyel A, Szatmári D, Mártonfalvi Z, Huber T and Kellermayer M S Z 2007 Interaction forces between F-actin and titin PEVK domain measured with optical tweezers *Biophys. J.* **93** 2102–9

Bishop K W, Glaser A K and Liu J T C 2020 Performance trade-offs for single- and dual-objective light-sheet microscope designs: a simulation-based analysis *Biomed. Opt. Express* **11** 4627–4650

Block S M, Asbury C L, Shaevitz J W and Lang M J 2003 Probing the kinesin reaction cycle with a 2D optical force clamp *Proc. Natl Acad. Sci. USA* **100** 2351–6

Brau R R, Ferrer J M, Lee H, Castro C E, Tam B K, Tarsa P B, Matsudaira P, Boyce M C, Kamm R D and Lang M J 2007 Passive and active microrheology with optical tweezers *J. Opt. A: Pure Appl. Opt.* **9** S103

Chapman C D, Gorczyca S and Robertson-Anderson R M 2015 Crowding induces complex ergodic diffusion and dynamic elongation of large DNA molecules *Biophys. J.* **108** 1220–8

Chapman C D, Lee K, Henze D, Smith D E and Robertson-Anderson R M 2014 Onset of non-continuum effects in microrheology of entangled polymer solutions *Macromolecules* **47** 1181–6

Chapman C D and Robertson-Anderson R M 2014 nonlinear microrheology reveals entanglement-driven molecular-level viscoelasticity of concentrated DNA *Phys. Rev. Lett.* **113**

Chapman C D, Shanbhag S, Smith D E and Robertson-Anderson R M 2012 Complex effects of molecular topology on diffusion in entangled biopolymer blends *Soft Matter* **8** 9177–82

Chen H-C and Cheng C-J 2022 Holographic optical tweezers: techniques and biomedical applications *Appl. Sci.* **12** 10244

Chun M-S, Kim C and Lee D E 2009 Conformation and translational diffusion of a xanthan polyelectrolyte chain: brownian dynamics simulation and single molecule tracking *Phys. Rev.* E **79** 051919

Cibula M A 2015 Applications of holographic optical tweezers: multiplexed fluorescence spectroscopy and the micromechanics of type-I collagen *PhD Thesis* Oregon State University https://ir.library.oregonstate.edu/concern/graduate_thesis_or_dissertations/6t053j54p

Curtis J E, Koss B A and Grier D G 2002 Dynamic holographic optical tweezers *Opt. Commun.* **207** 169–75

De Vlaminck I and Dekker C 2012 Recent advances in magnetic tweezers *Annu. Rev. Biophys.* **41** 453–72

Delarue M and Sanejouand Y-H 2002 Simplified normal mode analysis of conformational transitions in DNA-dependent polymerases: the elastic network model *J. Mol. Biol.* **320** 1011–24

Dixon T F and Reece P J 2020 Stroboscopic detection of multi-colloidal hydrodynamics using time-multiplexed optical tweezers *Optical Trapping and Optical Micromanipulation XVII. Presented at the Optical Trapping and Optical Micromanipulation XVII, SPIE* pp 31–40

Duocastella M, Sancataldo G, Saggau P, Ramoino P, Bianchini P and Diaspro A 2017 fast inertia-free volumetric light-sheet microscope *ACS Photonics* **4** 1797–804

Dutta S K, Mbi A, Arevalo R C and Blair D L 2013 Development of a confocal rheometer for soft and biological materials *Rev. Sci. Instrum.* **84** 063702

Endesfelder U and Heilemann M 2015 Direct stochastic optical reconstruction microscopy (dSTORM) ed P J Verveer *Advanced Fluorescence Microscopy: Methods and Protocols, Methods in Molecular Biology* (New York: Springer) pp 263–76

Engelbrecht C J and Stelzer E H 2006 Resolution enhancement in a light-sheet-based microscope (SPIM *Opt. Lett.* **31** 1477

Falzone T T, Blair S and Robertson-Anderson R M 2015 Entangled F-actin displays a unique crossover to microscale nonlinearity dominated by entanglement segment dynamics *Soft Matter* **11** 4418–23

Falzone T T and Robertson-Anderson R M 2015 Active entanglement-tracking microrheology directly couples macromolecular deformations to nonlinear microscale force response of entangled actin *ACS Macro Lett.* **4** 1194–9

Fazal F M and Block S M 2011 Optical tweezers study life under tension *Nat. Photonics* **5** 318–21

Ferrer J M, Lee H, Chen J, Pelz B, Nakamura F, Kamm R D and Lang M J 2008 Measuring molecular rupture forces between single actin filaments and actin-binding proteins *PNAS* **105** 9221–6

Fitzpatrick R, Michieletto D, Peddireddy K R, Hauer C, Kyrillos C, Gurmessa B J and Robertson-Anderson R M 2018 Synergistic interactions between DNA and Actin trigger emergent viscoelastic behavior *Phys. Rev. Lett.* **121** 257801

Francis M L, Ricketts S N, Farhadi L, Rust M J, Das M, Ross J L and Robertson-Anderson R M 2019 Non-monotonic dependence of stiffness on actin crosslinking in cytoskeleton composites *Soft Matter* **15** 9056–65

Fuller D N, Gemmen G J, Rickgauer J P, Dupont A, Millin R, Recouvreux P and Smith D E 2006 A general method for manipulating DNA sequences from any organism with optical tweezers *Nucleic Acids Res.* **34** e15

Garamella J, Regan K, Aguirre G, McGorty R J and Robertson-Anderson R M 2020 Anomalous and heterogeneous DNA transport in biomimetic cytoskeleton networks *Soft Matter* **16** 6344–53

Gavara N and Chadwick R S 2010 Noncontact microrheology at acoustic frequencies using frequency-modulated atomic force microscopy *Nat. Methods* **7** 650–4

Girkin J M and Carvalho M T 2018 The light-sheet microscopy revolution *J. Opt.* **20** 053002

Girstmair J, Zakrzewski A, Lapraz F, Handberg-Thorsager M, Tomancak P, Pitrone P G, Simpson F and Telford M J 2016 Light-sheet microscopy for everyone? Experience of building an OpenSPIM to study flatworm development *BMC Dev. Biol.* **16** 22

Glaser A K, Bishop K W, Barner L A, Serafin R B and Liu J T C 2022 A hybrid open-top light-sheet microscope for multi-scale imaging of cleared tissues *Nat. Methods* **19** 613–9

Gong Z and van der Maarel J R C 2014 Translational and reorientational dynamics of entangled DNA *Macromolecules* **47** 7230–7

Gorczyca S M, Chapman C D and Robertson-Anderson R M 2015 Universal scaling of crowding-induced DNA mobility is coupled with topology-dependent molecular compaction and elongation *Soft Matter* **11** 7762–8

Greger K, Swoger J and Stelzer E H K 2007 Basic building units and properties of a fluorescence single plane illumination microscope *Rev. Sci. Instrum.* **78** 023705

Gualda E J, Vale T, Almada P, Feijó J A, Martins G G and Moreno N 2013 OpenSpinMicroscopy: an open-source integrated microscopy platform *Nat. Methods* **10** 599–600

Guilbaud S, Salomé L, Destainville N, Manghi M and Tardin C 2019 Dependence of DNA persistence length on ionic strength and ion type *Phys. Rev. Lett.* **122** 028102

Guo C, Liu W, Hua X, Li H and Jia S 2019 Fourier light-field microscopy *Opt. Express* **27** 25573–94

Gurmessa B, Fitzpatrick R, Falzone T T and Robertson-Anderson R M 2016 Entanglement density tunes microscale nonlinear response of entangled actin *Macromolecules* **49** 3948–55

Gurmessa B, Francis M, Rust M J, Das M, Ross J L and Robertson-Anderson R M 2019 Counterion crossbridges enable robust multiscale elasticity in actin networks *Phys. Rev. Res.* **1** 013016

Gurmessa B, Ricketts S and Robertson-Anderson R M 2017 Nonlinear actin deformations lead to network stiffening, yielding and nonuniform stress propagation *Biophys. J.* **113** 1540–50

Gurmessa B J, Bitten N, Nguyen D T, Saleh O A, Ross J L, Das M and Robertson-Anderson R M 2019 Triggered disassembly and reassembly of actin networks induces rigidity phase transitions *Soft Matter* **15** 1335–44

Henty-Ridilla J L 2022 Visualizing actin and microtubule coupling dynamics *in vitro* by total internal reflection fluorescence (TIRF) microscopy *J. Vis. Exp.* **185** e64074

Hossack W J, Theofanidou E, Crain J, Heggarty K and Birch M 2003 High-speed holographic optical tweezers using a ferroelectric liquid crystal microdisplay *Opt. Express* **11** 2053–9

Jones P H, Maragò O M and Volpe G 2015 *Optical Tweezers: Principles and Applications* (Cambridge: Cambridge University Press)

Käs J, Strey H and Sackmann E 1994 Direct imaging of reptation for semiflexible actin filaments *Nature* **368** 226–9

Käs J, Strey H, Tang J X, Finger D, Ezzell R, Sackmann E and Janmey P A 1996 F-actin, a model polymer for semiflexible chains in dilute, semidilute, and liquid crystalline solutions *Biophys. J.* **70** 609–25

Keane R D and Adrian R J 1992 Theory of cross-correlation analysis of PIV images *Appl. Sci. Res.* **49** 191–215

Keresztes Z, Rigó T, Telegdi J and Kálmán E 2001 Investigation of biopolymer networks by means of AFM *Appl. Phys.* A **72** S113–6

Khan M, Regan K and Robertson-Anderson R M 2019 Optical tweezers microrheology maps the dynamics of strain-induced local inhomogeneities in entangled polymers *Phys. Rev. Lett.* **123** 038001

Khanal P, Peddireddy K R, Marfai J, McGorty R and Robertson-Anderson R M 2022 DNA topology dictates emergent bulk elasticity and hindered macromolecular diffusion in DNA-dextran composites *J. Rheol.* **66** 699–715

Kučera O, Gaillard J, Guérin C, Utzschneider C, Théry M and Blanchoin L 2022 Actin architecture steers microtubules in active cytoskeletal composite *Nano Lett.* **22** 8584–91

Lee G, Leech G, Lwin P, Michel J, Currie C, Rust M J, Ross J L, McGorty R J, Das M and Robertson-Anderson R M 2021 Active cytoskeletal composites display emergent tunable contractility and restructuring *Soft Matter* **17** 10765–76

Lee G, Leech G, Rust M J, Das M, McGorty R J, Ross J L and Robertson-Anderson R M n.d. Myosin-driven actin-microtubule networks exhibit self-organized contractile dynamics *Sci. Adv.* **7** eabe4334

Levoy M, Ng R, Adams A, Footer M and Horowitz M 2006 Light field microscopy *ACM SIGGRAPH 2006 Papers, SIGGRAPH '06* (New York: Association for Computing Machinery) pp 924–34

Lherbette M, dos Santos Á, Hari-Gupta Y, Fili N, Toseland C P and Schaap I A T 2017 Atomic force microscopy micro-rheology reveals large structural inhomogeneities in single cell-nuclei *Sci. Rep.* **7** 8116

Li Y, Kröger M and Liu W K 2014 Dynamic structure of unentangled polymer chains in the vicinity of non-attractive nanoparticles *Soft Matter* **10** 1723

Lin J and Valentine M T 2012a High-force NdFeB-based magnetic tweezers device optimized for microrheology experiments *Rev. Sci. Instrum.* **83** 053905

Lin J and Valentine M T 2012b Ring-shaped NdFeB-based magnetic tweezers enables oscillatory microrheology measurements *Appl. Phys. Lett.* **100** 201902

Lipfert J, Hao X and Dekker N H 2009 Quantitative modeling and optimization of magnetic tweezers *Biophys. J.* **96** 5040–9

Liu S-L, Li J, Zhang Z-L, Wang Z-G, Tian Z-Q, Wang G-P and Pang D-W 2013 Fast and high-accuracy localization for three-dimensional single-particle tracking *Sci. Rep.* **3** 2462

Luan Y, Lieleg O, Wagner B and Bausch A R 2008 Micro- and macrorheological properties of isotropically cross-linked actin networks *Biophys. J.* **94** 688–93

Mahaffy R E, Park S, Gerde E, Käs J and Shih C K 2004 Quantitative analysis of the viscoelastic properties of thin regions of fibroblasts using atomic force microscopy *Biophys. J.* **86** 1777–93

Mahaffy R E, Shih C K, MacKintosh F C and Käs J 2000 Scanning probe-based frequency-dependent microrheology of polymer gels and biological cells *Phys. Rev. Lett.* **85** 880–3

Manzo C and Garcia-Parajo M F 2015 A review of progress in single particle tracking: from methods to biophysical insights *Rep. Prog. Phys.* **78** 124601

Martinez-Torres C, Arneodo A, Streppa L, Argoul P and Argoul F 2016 Passive microrheology of soft materials with atomic force microscopy: a wavelet-based spectral analysis *Appl. Phys. Lett.* **108** 034102

Mason T G 2000 Estimating the viscoelastic moduli of complex fluids using the generalized stokes–einstein equation *Rheol. Acta* **39** 371–8

Mason T G, Ganesan K, van Zanten J H, Wirtz D and Kuo S C 1997 Particle tracking microrheology of complex fluids *Phys. Rev. Lett.* **79** 3282–5

Mason T G and Weitz D A 1995 Optical measurements of frequency-dependent linear viscoelastic moduli of complex fluids *Phys. Rev. Lett.* **74** 1250–3

McGorty R J *et al* 2023 Kinesin and myosin motors compete to drive rich multiphase dynamics in programmable cytoskeletal composites *PNAS Nexus* **2** pgad245

Miyagi A, Tsunaka Y, Uchihashi T, Mayanagi K, Hirose S, Morikawa K and Ando T 2008 Visualization of intrinsically disordered regions of proteins by high-speed atomic force microscopy *ChemPhysChem.* **9** 1859–66

Moffitt J R, Chemla Y R, Smith S B and Bustamante C 2008 Recent advances in optical tweezers *Annu. Rev. Biochem.* **77** 205–28

Molloy J E and Padgett M J 2002 Lights, action: optical tweezers *Contemp. Phys.* **43** 241–58

Montes-Usategui M, Pleguezuelos E, Andilla J and Martín-Badosa E 2006 Fast generation of holographic optical tweezers by random mask encoding of fourier components *Opt. Express* **14** 2101–7

Morris V J, Mackie A R, Wilde P J, Kirby A R, Mills E C N and Patrick Gunning A 2001 Atomic force microscopy as a tool for interpreting the rheology of food biopolymers at the molecular level *LWT—Food Sci. Technol.* **34** 3–10

Murrell M P and Gardel M L 2012 F-actin buckling coordinates contractility and severing in a biomimetic actomyosin cortex *PNAS* **109** 20820–5

Neuman K C and Nagy A 2008 Single-molecule force spectroscopy: optical tweezers, magnetic tweezers and atomic force microscopy *Nat. Methods* **5** 491–505

Niedworok C J, Schwarz I, Ledderose J, Giese G, Conzelmann K-K and Schwarz M K 2012 Charting monosynaptic connectivity maps by two-color light-sheet fluorescence microscopy *Cell Rep.* **2** 1375–86

Nikon's MicroscopyU—The Source for Microscopy Education n.d. Nikon's MicroscopyU https://microscopyu.com/ (accessed 9 July 2023).

Olarte O E, Andilla J, Gualda E J and Loza-Alvarez P 2018 Light-sheet microscopy: a tutorial *Adv. Opt. Photon.* **10** 111–79

Olympus PlanApo N 60× oil microscope objective, Microscope Central n.d. https://microscope-central.com/products/olympus-planapo-n-60x-oil-microscope-objective (accessed 9 July 2023).

Peddireddy K R, Clairmont R, Neill P, McGorty R and Robertson-Anderson R M 2022 OpTiDDM (Optical Tweezers integrating Differential Dynamic Microscopy) maps the spatiotemporal propagation of nonlinear stresses in polymer blends and composites *Nat. Commun.* **13** 5180

Peddireddy K R, Lee M, Schroeder C M and Robertson-Anderson R M 2020a Viscoelastic properties of ring-linear DNA blends exhibit nonmonotonic dependence on blend composition *Phys. Rev. Res.* **2** 023213

Peddireddy K R, Lee M, Zhou Y, Adalbert S, Anderson S, Schroeder C M and Robertson-Anderson R M 2020b Unexpected entanglement dynamics in semidilute blends of supercoiled and ring DNA *Soft Matter* **16** 152–61

Perkins T T, Smith D E, Larson R G and Chu S 1995 Stretching of a single tethered polymer in a uniform flow *Science* **268** 83–7

Plotnikov S V, Sabass B, Schwarz U S and Waterman C M 2014 High-resolution traction force microscopy ed J C Waters and T Wittman *Methods in Cell Biology, Quantitative Imaging in Cell Biology* (New York: Academic) ch 20 pp 367–94

Preciado López M, Huber F, Grigoriev I, Steinmetz M O, Akhmanova A, Dogterom M and Koenderink G H 2014 In vitro reconstitution of dynamic microtubules interacting with actin filament networks *Methods Enzymol.* **540** 301–20

Prevedel R *et al* 2014 Simultaneous whole-animal 3D imaging of neuronal activity using light-field microscopy *Nat. Methods* **11** 727–30

Radić T M, Svetličić V, Žutić V and Boulgaropoulos B 2011 Seawater at the nanoscale: marine gel imaged by atomic force microscopy *J. Mol. Recognit.* **24** 397–405

Rawat N and Biswas P 2009 Size, shape, and flexibility of proteins and DNA *J. Chem. Phys.* **131** 165104

Rebêlo L M, Sousa J S, de, Filho J M, Schäpe J, Doschke H and Radmacher M 2014 Microrheology of cells with magnetic force modulation atomic force microscopy *Soft Matter* **10** 2141–9

Regan K, Wulstein D, Rasmussen H, McGorty R and Robertson-Anderson R M 2018 Bridging the spatiotemporal scales of macromolecular transport in crowded biomimetic systems *Soft Matter* **15** 1200–9

Rich J P, Lammerding J, McKinley G H and Doyle P S 2011 Nonlinear microrheology of an aging, yield stress fluid using magnetic tweezers *Soft Matter* **7** 9933–43

Ricketts S N, Francis M L, Farhadi L, Rust M J, Das M, Ross J L and Robertson-Anderson R M 2019 Varying crosslinking motifs drive the mesoscale mechanics of actin-microtubule composites *Sci. Rep.* **9** 12831

Ricketts S N, Ross J L and Robertson-Anderson R M 2018 Co-entangled actin-microtubule composites exhibit tunable stiffening and power-law stress relaxation *Biophys. J.* **115** 1055–67

Rickgauer J P and Smith D E 2007 Single-molecule studies of DNA: Visualization and manipulation of individual dna molecules with fluorescence microscopy and optical tweezers ed R Pecora and R Borsali *Soft Matter: Scattering, Imaging and Manipulation* (New York: Springer)

Robertson R M and Smith D E 2007 Direct measurement of the intermolecular forces confining a single molecule in an entangled polymer solution *Phys. Rev. Lett.* **99** 126001

Robertson-Anderson R M 2018 Optical tweezers microrheology: from the basics to advanced techniques and applications *ACS Macro Lett.* **7** 968–75

Ross J L and Dixit R 2010 Multiple color single molecule TIRF imaging and tracking of MAPs and motors ed L Wilson and J J Correia *Methods in Cell Biology, Microtubules, In Vitro* (New York: Academic) ch 26 pp 521–42

Rother J, Nöding H, Mey I and Janshoff A 2014 Atomic force microscopy-based microrheology reveals significant differences in the viscoelastic response between malign and benign cell lines *Open Biol.* **4** 140046

Rust M J, Bates M and Zhuang X 2006 Sub-diffraction-limit imaging by stochastic optical reconstruction microscopy (STORM) *Nat. Methods* **3** 793–6

Sarkar R and Rybenkov V V 2016 A guide to magnetic tweezers and their applications *Front. Phys.* **4** 48

Schmoller K M, Fernández P, Arevalo R C, Blair D L and Bausch A R 2010 Cyclic hardening in bundled actin networks *Nat. Commun.* **1** 134

Scientific camera Hamamatsu photonics n.d. <https://camera.hamamatsu.com/jp/en.html> (accessed 9 July 2023)

Sheung J Y *et al* 2021 Motor-driven restructuring of cytoskeleton composites leads to tunable time-varying elasticity *ACS Macro Lett.* **10** 1151–8

Shundo A, Hori K, Penaloza D P and Tanaka K 2013 Optical tweezers with fluorescence detection for temperature-dependent microrheological measurements *Rev. Sci. Instrum.* **84** 014103

Sonal , Ganzinger K A, Vogel S K, Mücksch J, Blumhardt P and Schwille P 2019 Myosin-II activity generates a dynamic steady state with continuous actin turnover in a minimal actin cortex *J. Cell Sci.* **132** jcs219899

Squires T M 2008 Nonlinear microrheology: bulk stresses versus direct interactions *Langmuir* **24** 1147–59

Squires T M and Mason T G 2010 Fluid mechanics of microrheology *Annu. Rev. Fluid Mech.* **42** 413–38

Stam S, Freedman S L, Banerjee S, Weirich K L, Dinner A R and Gardel M L 2017 Filament rigidity and connectivity tune the deformation modes of active biopolymer networks *Proc. Natl Acad. Sci.* **114** E10037–45

Strick T R, Allemand J-F, Bensimon D, Bensimon A and Croquette V 1996 The elasticity of a single supercoiled DNA molecule *Science* **271** 1835–7

Style R W, Boltyanskiy R, German G K, Hyland C, MacMinn C W, Mertz A F, Wilen L A, Xu Y and Dufresne E R 2014 Traction force microscopy in physics and biology *Soft Matter* **10** 4047–55

Tang J, Levy S L, Trahan D W, Jones J J, Craighead H G and Doyle P S 2010 revisiting the conformation and dynamics of DNA in slitlike confinement *Macromolecules* **43** 7368–77

Tassieri M (ed) 2016 *Microrheology with Optical Tweezers: Principles and Applications* (Boca Raton, FL: CRC Press)

Tassieri M, Evans R M L, Warren R L, Bailey N J and Cooper J M 2012 Microrheology with optical tweezers: data analysis *New J. Phys.* **14** 115032

Tinland B, Pluen A, Sturm J and Weill G 1997 Persistence length of single-stranded DNA *Macromolecules* **30** 5763–5

Toan N M and Micheletti C 2006 Inferring the effective thickness of polyelectrolytes from stretching measurements at various ionic strengths: applications to DNA and RNA *J. Phys. Condens. Matter* **18** S269

Uhde J, Ter-Oganessian N, Pink D A, Sackmann E and Boulbitch A 2005 Viscoelasticity of entangled actin networks studied by long-pulse magnetic bead microrheometry *Phys. Rev.* E **72** 061916

Vemula V, Huber T, Ušaj M, Bugyi B and Månsson A 2021 Myosin and gelsolin cooperate in actin filament severing and actomyosin motor activity *J. Biol. Chem.* **296**

Vlijm R, Mashaghi A, Bernard S, Modesti M and Dekker C 2015 Experimental phase diagram of negatively supercoiled DNA measured by magnetic tweezers and fluorescence *Nanoscale* **7** 3205–16

Waigh T A 2016 Advances in the microrheology of complex fluids *Rep. Prog. Phys.* **79** 074601

Waigh T A 2005 Microrheology of complex fluids *Rep. Prog. Phys.* **68** 685

Wang B, Guan J, Anthony S M, Bae S C, Schweizer K S and Granick S 2010 Confining potential when a biopolymer filament reptates *Phys. Rev. Lett.* **104** 118301

Wang B, Lançon P, Bienvenu C, Vierling P, Di Giorgio C and Bossis G 2013 A general approach for the microrheology of cancer cells by atomic force microscopy *Micron* **44** 287–97

Wang M D, Yin H, Landick R, Gelles J and Block S M 1997 Stretching DNA with optical tweezers *Biophys. J.* **72** 1335–46

Weigand W J, Messmore A, Tu J, Morales-Sanz A, Blair D L, Deheyn D D, Urbach J S and Robertson-Anderson R M 2017 Active microrheology determines scale-dependent material properties of chaetopterus mucus *PLoS One* **12** e0176732

Wereley S and Meinhart C 2010 Recent advances in microparticle image velocimetry *Annu. Rev. Fluid mech.* **42** 557–76

Wilhelm J and Frey E 1996 Radial distribution function of semiflexible polymers *Phys. Rev. Lett.* **77** 2581–4

Wulstein D M, Regan K E, Robertson-Anderson R M and McGorty R 2016 Light-sheet microscopy with digital fourier analysis measures transport properties over large field-of-view *Opt. Express* **24** 20881–94

X-cite fluorescence LED illuminators Excelitas n.d. https://excelitas.com/product-category/x-cite-fluorescence-led-illuminators (accessed 9 July 2023)

Xu J, Ma H and Liu Y 2017 Stochastic optical reconstruction microscopy (STORM) *Curr. Protoc. Cytom.* **81** 12.46.1–12.46.27

Yang Y, Bai M, Klug W S, Levine A J and Valentine M T 2012a Microrheology of highly crosslinked microtubule networks is dominated by force-induced crosslinker unbinding *Soft Matter* **9** 383–93

Yang Y, Lin J, Kaytanli B, Saleh O A and Valentine M T 2012b Direct correlation between creep compliance and deformation in entangled and sparsely crosslinked microtubule networks *Soft Matter* **8** 1776–84

Yang Y, Lin J, Kaytanli B, Saleh O A and Valentine M T 2012c Direct correlation between creep compliance and deformation in entangled and sparsely crosslinked microtubule networks *Soft Matter* **8** 1776–84

Yao A, Tassieri M, Padgett M and Cooper J 2009 Microrheology with optical tweezers *Lab Chip* **9** 2568

Zancla A, Mozetic P, Orsini M, Forte G and Rainer A 2022 A primer to traction force microscopy *J. Biol. Chem.* **298** 101867

Zia R N 2018 Active and passive microrheology: theory and simulation *Annu. Rev. Fluid Mech.* **50** 371–405

IOP Publishing

Biopolymer Networks
Design, dynamics and discovery
Rae M Robertson-Anderson

Chapter 4

Analysis methods, algorithms, and deliverables

This chapter discusses various methods for analyzing data acquired using the methods I describe in chapter 3 to determine biopolymer transport properties, single-molecule and ensemble dynamics, and network structure and rheology. Methods for determining single-polymer dynamics and conformations include single-molecule center-of-mass (COM) tracking, single-particle tracking, and single-molecule conformational tracking (SMCT). I will then discuss the use of differential dynamic microscopy (DDM) and particle-image velocimetry (PIV), the generalized Stokes–Einstein relation (GSER) approach to determining linear viscoelastic moduli, and spatial image autocorrelation (SIA) analysis.

4.1 Single-molecule center-of-mass tracking

As I have discussed in previous chapters, most biopolymers can be labeled with fluorescent dyes to enable tracking of individual biopolymers. Uniform labeling of biopolymers, in which fluorophores are attached to every n_L^{th} monomer along the polymer chain, allows pixel intensity to serve as a proxy for mass, to accurately compute COM coordinates and relative sizes of particles (figure 4.1(A)), as I discuss briefly in chapter 3.

4.1.1 Framework and considerations

Typical tracking algorithms ('Introduction to TrackPy,' n.d., 'Matlab particle tracking,' n.d., Weeks and Crocker, n.d.) identify particles in each frame of an image stack (i.e., movie) and determine their in-plane COM coordinates (x, y) via a center-of-intensity computation for each object (e.g., a DNA random coil). After this procedure, trajectories are stitched together by identifying a particle COM position in each consecutive frame that is in close proximity to a particle COM in the previous frame, categorizing these positions as being occupied by the same particle, and computing the frame-to-frame displacement (Δx, Δy) of the particle (figure 4.1(A)).

doi:10.1088/978-0-7503-5037-2ch4

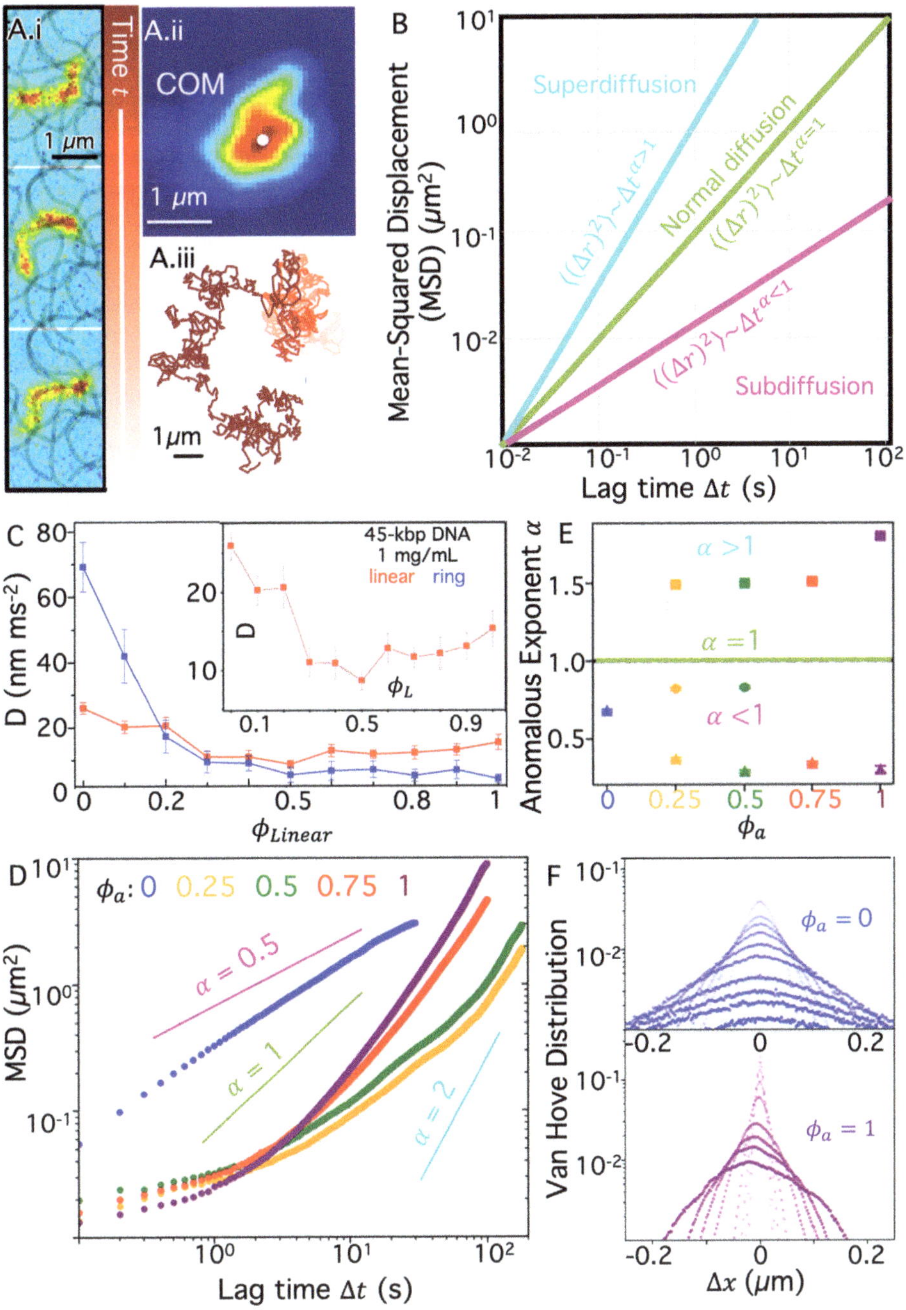

Figure 4.1. Single-molecule tracking to determine mean-squared displacements, diffusion coefficients, and anomalous transport characteristics. (A) Single biopolymers at tracer concentrations are mixed with unlabeled molecules (i) and their center-of-mass positions are identified (ii) and tracked to reconstruct their frame-to-frame trajectories (iii). (i–ii) Heat intensity images of fluorescent-labeled 45 kbp DNA, with pixel intensity values increasing from blue to red, show the Brownian motion of the molecule over time (i), with grey lines representing unlabeled chains, and the identified COM position (ii). (A.iii) Adapted from Michieletto *et al* (2022). CC BY 4.0.

(B) From the trajectories (A.iii), the mean-squared displacement (MSD, $\langle(\Delta\vec{r})^2\rangle$) as a function of lag time Δt can be evaluated to determine the scaling relation $\langle(\Delta\vec{r})^2\rangle \sim (\Delta t)^\alpha$. The exponent α categorizes motion into: normal Brownian diffusion (olive, $\alpha = 1$), subdiffusion (magenta, $\alpha < 1$) or superdiffusion (cyan, $\alpha > 1$). (C) For polymers exhibiting normal diffusion ($\alpha = 1$), deduced from (x, y) COM positions, the diffusion coefficient D can be computed from the relation $\langle(\Delta x)^2\rangle = \langle(\Delta y)^2\rangle = 2D\Delta t$. Shown are the diffusion coefficients for linear (red) and ring (blue) 45 kbp DNA embedded in entangled blends of linear and ring DNA with varying mass fractions of linear DNA ϕ_{Linear}. Adapted from Chapman *et al* (2012) with permission from the Royal Society of Chemistry. (D) MSDs for myosin-driven actin-microtubule composites with varying molar fractions of actin ϕ_a and tubulin ($\phi_T = 1 - \phi_a$), denoted by the color-coded legend, show dynamics that range from subdiffusive ($0.5 \lesssim \alpha < 1$) to superdiffusive ($1 < \alpha \lesssim 2$) depending on the lag time Δt and actin fraction ϕ_a. (E) The anomalous scaling exponents determined via power-law fits of the MSDs over different ranges of Δt shown in (D): short (triangles), intermediate (circles) and long (squares) lag times. The olive horizontal line denotes normal diffusion ($\alpha = 1$). (F) van Hove probability distributions of particle displacements Δx and Δy determined from the same trajectories that were used to determine MSDs in (D) for $\phi_a = 0$ (top) and $\phi_a = 1$ (bottom). Both distributions show non-Gaussian tails and peaks. $\phi_a = 1$ distributions are not centered at $\Delta x = \Delta y = 0$, indicating directed (non-Brownian) motion. (D)–(F) Adapted from Sheung *et al* (2022). CC BY 4.0.

To improve the accuracy of COM localization beyond the resolution of a single pixel, methods have been developed that fit the intensity distribution of each particle to a function, such as a Gaussian, and equate the peak with the COM position (Rogers *et al* 2007, Parthasarathy 2012, Liu *et al* 2013, Manzo and Garcia-Parajo 2015, Vallotton *et al* 2017, Rose *et al* 2020). Super-resolution microscopy methods have also been developed that use patterned illumination or photoswitchable fluorophores to evade the optical resolution limit of ~500 nm, enabling localization at the scale of nanometers (Betzig *et al* 2006, Rust *et al* 2006, Sharonov and Hochstrasser 2006, Huang *et al* 2010, Hu *et al* 2014, Jaques *et al* 2019). Finally, microscopy methods and post-processing algorithms to track particles in three dimensions (i.e., adding z) have enabled tracking within volumetric images and improved accuracy of COM measurements of three-dimensional extended objects (Toprak *et al* 2007, Quirin *et al* 2012, Liu *et al* 2013, Memmolo *et al* 2015, Schröder and Schanz 2023).

4.1.2 Characterizing transport

Typically, the motion of biopolymers and other microscopic particles is thermally-driven Brownian motion, which is quantified by the mean-squared displacement (MSD, $\langle(\Delta\vec{r})^2\rangle$) and the corresponding diffusion coefficient D. As such, standard single-molecule tracking algorithms compute MSDs in the x and y direction ($\langle(\Delta x)^2\rangle$, $\langle(\Delta y)^2\rangle$) from the stitched-together trajectories (figure 4.1(B)). The computed MSDs can be evaluated to determine the diffusion coefficient (figure 4.1(C)) via the Einstein relation

$$\langle(\Delta x)^2\rangle = \langle(\Delta y)^2\rangle = \langle(\Delta z)^2\rangle = 2D\Delta t. \tag{4.1}$$

However, this relation only holds for conventional Brownian motion, which is an ergodic, Gaussian process in which the MSD scales linearly with lag time, i.e.,

$$\langle(\Delta\vec{r})^2\rangle \sim \Delta t. \tag{4.2}$$

Particle motion that is more accurately described by

$$\langle(\Delta\vec{r})^2\rangle \sim (\Delta t)^\alpha \tag{4.3}$$

where $\alpha \neq 1$, is termed anomalous diffusion with $\alpha > 1$ and $\alpha < 1$ indicating superdiffusion and subdiffusion, respectively (figure 4.1(D), (E)) (Sokolov 2012, Shin *et al* 2017, Sheung *et al* 2022).

Subdiffusion is a common feature in crowded and entangled biopolymer networks (Amblard *et al* 1996, Sokolov 2012, Chapman *et al* 2015, Gorczyca *et al* 2015, Sentjabrskaja *et al* 2016, Mardoum *et al* 2018, Regan *et al* 2019, Wulstein *et al* 2019, Garamella *et al* 2020, Aporvari *et al* 2022) and superdiffusion may arise in motor-driven or otherwise active networks (figure 4.1(D), (E)) (Metzler *et al* 1998, Reverey *et al* 2015, Shin *et al* 2017, Cherstvy *et al* 2018, Lee *et al* 2021a, 2021b, Sheung *et al* 2022).

The distribution of particle displacements for a given lag time Δt, termed the van Hove distribution $G(\Delta x, \Delta t)$ (figure 4.1(F)), can also be evaluated to determine the diffusion coefficient and identify possible deviations from standard Brownian diffusion. Specifically, the displacements Δx of a homogenous ensemble of particles undergoing normal Brownian motion are expected to be described by a Gaussian distribution:

$$G(\Delta x, \Delta t) = G_1 \exp\left(-\frac{(\Delta x)^2}{4D\Delta t}\right) \tag{4.4}$$

with a width that increases with increasing Δt. However, distributions for highly confined particles may exhibit a larger than expected value of the distribution peak G_1, which should be centered at $\Delta x = 0$ (figure 4.1(F)). This non-Gaussian feature is often indicative of caging or trapping of particles within the biopolymer mesh for extended periods of time, leading to more near-zero displacements than expected for a Gaussian process (Stuhrmann *et al* 2012, Michieletto *et al* 2017, Burla *et al* 2020, Garamella *et al* 2020, Anderson *et al* 2021).

Another common non-Gaussian feature of van Hove distributions is a large displacement 'tail' that extends beyond displacements expected for a Gaussian distribution, suggestive of large discrete events such as 'hopping' from one pocket of a network to another or athermal (driven) network dynamics (Brangwynne *et al* 2008, Toyota *et al* 2011, Stuhrmann *et al* 2012, Chechkin *et al* 2017) (figure 3.1(F)). These tails often follow an exponential dependence on Δx, such that the van Hove distribution is better described by a sum of a Gaussian and exponential

$$G(\Delta x, \Delta t) = G_1 \exp\left(-\frac{(\Delta x)^2}{4D\Delta t}\right) + G_2 \exp\left(-\frac{|\Delta x|}{\lambda_{NG}(t)}\right) \tag{4.5}$$

where λ_{NG} is the characteristic decay length, or lengthscale of hopping events or other non-Gaussian processes. This lengthscale has been shown to follow a power-law relation with lag time:

$$\lambda_{\mathrm{NG}}(\Delta t) \sim (\Delta t)^{\Omega} \tag{4.6}$$

indicative of heterogenous transport (Chechkin *et al* 2017, Michieletto *et al* 2017, Garamella *et al* 2020), with reported values of $\Omega \approx 0.2$–0.4 for particles diffusing in dense biopolymer networks (Wang *et al* 2009, 2012, Burla *et al* 2020, Singh *et al* 2020).

Finally, COM trajectories can be evaluated to determine the extent to which the particle motion is ergodic (as is the case for Brownian motion), such that the time-averaged MSD can be equated to the ensemble-averaged MSD. For example, the ergodicity-breaking parameter EB, defined as

$$\mathrm{EB}(\Delta t) = \frac{\left\langle \left(\overline{(\Delta x)^2(\Delta t)} \right)^2 \right\rangle - \langle (\Delta x)^2 \rangle^2}{\langle (\Delta x)^2 \rangle^2} \tag{4.7}$$

in which $\overline{(\Delta x)^2(\Delta t)}$ is the time-averaged (but not ensemble-averaged) MSD, indicates the degree to which the motion is non-ergodic, with $\mathrm{EB} = 0$ indicative of ergodic motion while $\mathrm{EB} > 0$ indicates heterogeneous and subdiffusive processes (Chapman *et al* 2015, Garamella *et al* 2020, Anderson *et al* 2021).

The non-Gaussianity parameter NG, defined as

$$\mathrm{NG}(\Delta t) = \frac{\overline{\langle (\Delta x)^4(\Delta t) \rangle}}{3\langle (\Delta x)^2 \rangle^2} - 1 \tag{4.8}$$

where $(\Delta x)^4(\Delta t)$ is the 4th moment of the displacement, is another indicator of non-ergodic transport with $\mathrm{NG} \to 0$ for an ergodic process and $|\ \mathrm{NG}\ | > 0$, indicative of anomalous non-Gaussian transport.

4.1.3 Conformational analysis

Because biopolymers are extended objects with internal degrees of freedom and fluctuations, the conformations and sizes of the polymers can vary across an ensemble and fluctuate over time. Quantifying conformational shapes, sizes, and fluctuations, and pairing with COM motion, can provide a much richer picture of the physics underlying the observed transport.

One approach for determining conformation dynamics is single-molecule conformational tracking (SMCT), which computes the major and minor axis vectors, $\vec{R}_{max}$ and $\vec{R}_{min}$, of a spheroidal particle in each frame of a video (figure 4.2(A)) (Chapman *et al* 2015, Gorczyca *et al* 2015, Mardoum *et al* 2018, Wulstein *et al* 2019, Garamella *et al* 2020). From the vector lengths, R_{max} and R_{min}, an average coil size R_{coil} (figures 4.2(A) and (B)), can be computed as

$$R_{coil} = \frac{1}{2}(R_{max}^2 + R_{min}^2)^{1/2} \tag{4.9}$$

The conformational heterogeneity in an ensemble of particles can be determined by evaluating the ensemble distributions of R_{max}, R_{min}, and R_{coil} (figures 4.2(A.ii) and (B)). Distributions with broader widths, multiple peaks, or extended tails, are indicative of dynamic heterogeneity, as seen in figure 4.2(Bii).

SMCT can also determine the extent to which polymer conformations deviate from random coils or spherical particles by computing the distribution of eccentricity parameters E, defined as

$$E = \left| \frac{R_{max}}{R_{min}} \right| - 1 \tag{4.10}$$

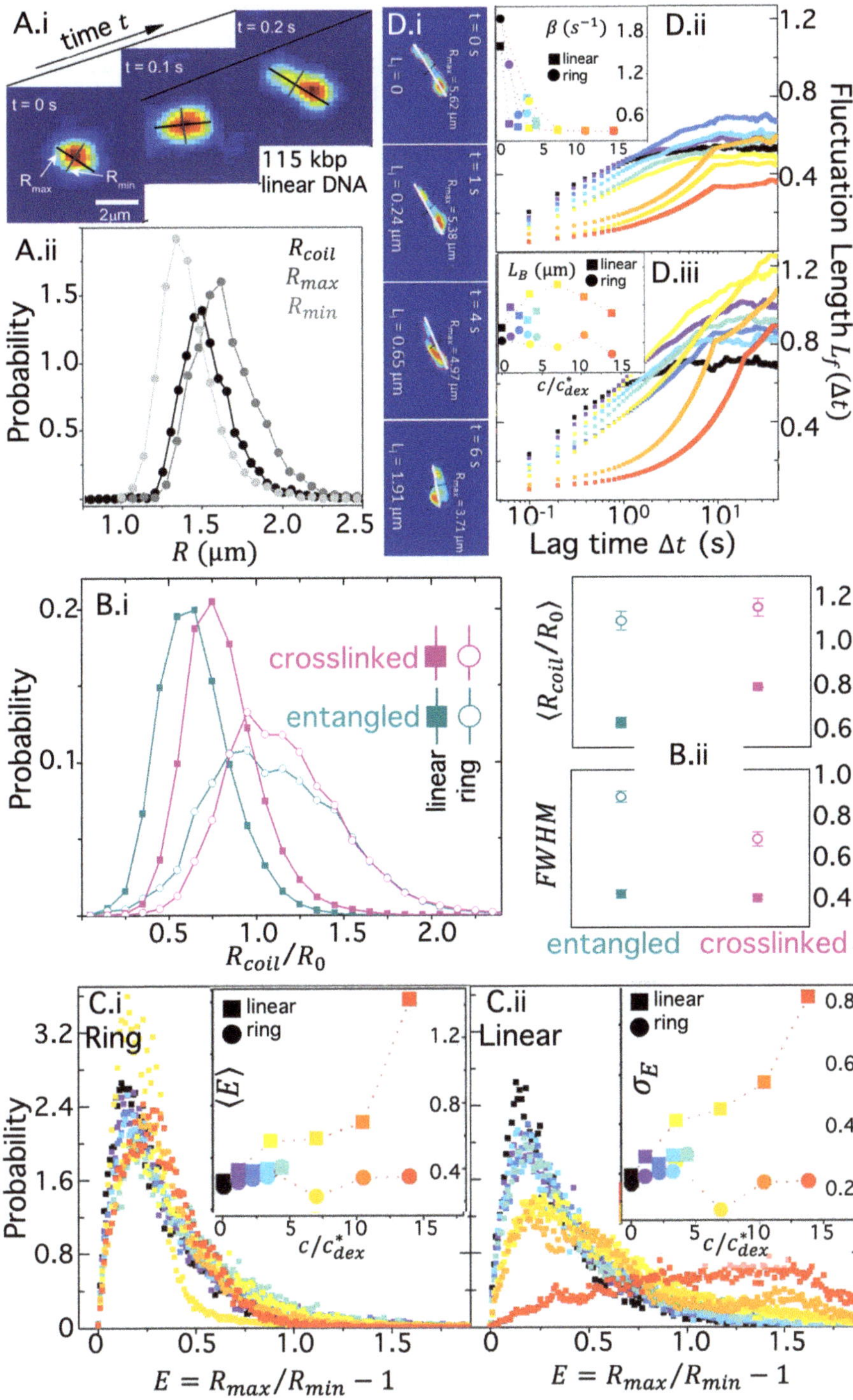

Figure 4.2. Single-molecule conformational tracking (SMCT) measures size, shape, and conformational fluctuations of biopolymers. (A) SMCT measures the major and minor axes vectors $\vec{R}_{\max}$ and $\vec{R}_{\min}$ of a diffusing

biopolymer in (i) each frame of a video; and this process is carried out on the entire ensemble of tracked biopolymers to determine (ii) probability distributions of the axes lengths $|R_{max}|$ (dark grey) and $|R_{min}|$ (light grey) and the resulting coil size $R_{coil} = \frac{1}{2}(R_{max}^2 + R_{min}^2)^{1/2}$ (black). Data shown are for 115 kbp DNA diffusing through a crowded medium of (i) dextran polymers and (ii) actin filaments. Images are false-colored to represent pixel intensity. Adapted from Regan *et al* (2019) with permission from the Royal Society of Chemistry. (B) Coil size distributions (i) and corresponding metrics (ii) for linear (filled squares), and ring (open circles) DNA diffusing in entangled (teal) and crosslinked (magenta) composite networks of actin ($c_A = 2.9\ \mu$M) and microtubules ($c_T = 2.9\ \mu$M). (i) R_{coil} is scaled by the predicted end-to-end distance of the DNA random coil R_0 in dilute conditions, such that $R_{coil}/R_0 > 1$ and $R_{coil}/R_0 < 1$, indicating swelling and compaction, respectively. The distributions show that rings are swollen with broadly distributed coil sizes whereas linear DNA is compacted and has much narrower distribution of conformational sizes. (ii) The average coil size $\langle R_{coil}/R_0\rangle$ and full width at half maximum (FWHM) determined from the distributions in (i) show that crosslinking has little effect on the conformational statistics while DNA topology plays an important role. Modified from Wulstein *et al* (2019). © The Authors, some rights reserved; exclusive licensee AAAS. (C) Eccentricity distributions for ring (i) and linear (ii) DNA crowded by varying concentrations c of dextran polymers relative to their overlap concentration c^*_{dex}, with colors indicating increasing c/c^*_{dex} from purple to red. Insets show average eccentricity values $\langle E\rangle$ (i) and standard deviations σ_E (ii) determined from the distributions shown. Linear DNA (squares) exhibit pronounced elongation that increases with c/c^*_{dex} while rings show slight reduction in $\langle E\rangle$ suggestive of a transition from random coil to compacted more spherical conformations. (D) Time-dependent fluctuation lengths are measured by (i) evaluating differences in R_{max} values of a single polymer over varying lag times Δt and (ii, iii) analyzing the ensemble-averaged $L_f(\Delta t)$ curves to determine the fluctuation rate $\tau_f^{-1} = \beta$ (ii, inset) and steady-state breathing length $L_f = L_B$ (iii, inset) as a function of c/c^*_{dex}. $L_f(\Delta t)$ curves in (ii) and (iii) are computed from the same data analyzed in C.i (ii) and C.ii (iii) with matching colors and symbols. (C, D.iii) Adapted from Gorczyca *et al* (2015) with permission from the Royal Society of Chemistry. (D.i) Adapted from Chapman *et al* (2015), Copyright (2015), with permission from Elsevier.

where $E = 0$ defines a spherical particle and $E \approx 0.3$ describes a random coil (figure 4.2(C)) (Chapman *et al* 2015, Regan *et al* 2019, Wulstein *et al* 2019).

However, because the distributions described above contain values from each frame and from each molecule in the ensemble, without differentiation, the temporal and ensemble heterogeneities are convolved.

To parse these different contributions, SMCT algorithms also compute the lengthscale of conformational fluctuations L_f as a function of lag time (figure 4.2(D)),

$$L_f(\Delta t) = \langle | R_{max}(0) - R_{max}(\Delta t) | \rangle \tag{4.11}$$

which can often be described as an exponential rise to a maximum plateau value L_B

$$L_f(\Delta t) = L_B\left(1 - e^{-\frac{\Delta t}{\tau_f}}\right) \tag{4.12}$$

where the characteristic decay time τ_f is a measure of the timescale over which the polymer conformation decorrelates from its previous conformational state, and τ_f^{-1} is the corresponding fluctuation rate (figure 4.2(D.ii)). The plateau value L_B is a measure of the steady-state lengthscale over which the polymers fluctuate, providing a metric for how much the conformational size of the polymer changes as it 'breathes' between different states (figure 4.2(D.iii)).

Alternative approaches to characterizing conformational fluctuations are to compute the autocorrelation of the coil size $g_R(\Delta t) = \langle R_{coil}(0) \cdot R_{coil}(\Delta t)\rangle$, which decays exponentially with Δt, giving a similar decay rate as L_f. However, g_R does not provide a steady-state fluctuation lengthscale. The normal modes of the radius of gyration tensor can also be computed, and their decay with Δt can be evaluated to characterize conformational relaxation dynamics. In particular, the zeroth order mode equates to the COM motion while higher-order modes provide the dynamics of internal fluctuations (Delarue and Sanejouand 2002, Chun *et al* 2009, Rawat and Biswas 2009, Liu *et al* 2013, Gong and van der Maarel 2014, Li *et al* 2014).

Finally, from the orientations, $\theta_{\max}$ and $\theta_{\min}$, the rotational diffusion coefficient D_θ can be determined via:

$$\langle(\Delta\theta_{\max})^2\rangle = \langle(\Delta\theta_{\min})^2\rangle = 2D_\theta\Delta t. \tag{4.13}$$

4.2 Single-particle tracking (SPT)

In certain cases, the biopolymers cannot be fluorescent-labeled or are too small, too dim, or move too fast to accurately track. An alternative, in such cases, is to embed tracer particles, such as microsphere probes, into the network. In this widely used approach that I discuss in chapter 3, all of the metrics that can be derived from the COM trajectories of diffusing polymers, described in section 4.1.2, can also be derived from the displacements of spherical probes, include MSDs, diffusion coefficients, anomalous scaling exponents, ergodicity-breaking metrics, and van Hove distributions (figures 4.3(A) and (B)).

Moreover, by tracking and characterizing the motion of the probes with a well-defined size R_s and shape (sphere), the Stokes–Einstein relation can be used to determine the viscosity η of the network from the measured diffusion coefficient D.

$$\eta = \frac{k_B T}{D 6\pi R_s} \tag{4.14}$$

However, this relation assumes that the MSDs scale linearly with lag time and that the sample is a Newtonian fluid; assumptions which are often invalid for biopolymer networks which typically display viscoelastic properties, as shown in figure 4.3(C) and (D). In such cases, GSER can be used to determine viscoelastic moduli, as I describe below.

4.2.1 Single-particle tracking microrheology (SPTM)

For viscoelastic materials, particle MSDs measured via particle-tracking can be used to determine elastic and viscous moduli of the surrounding biopolymer network using GSER, as I describe in chapter 3, sections 3.2.1.4 and 3.2.4 (figures 4.3(C) and (D)). Briefly, GSER replaces the viscosity η in the Stokes–Einstein relation (equation (4.11)) with the frequency-dependent complex viscosity $\eta^*(\omega)$, which can be written as

$$\eta^*(\omega) = \eta'(\omega) - i\eta''(\omega) \tag{4.15}$$

where the real and imaginary parts relate to $G'(\omega)$ and $G''(\omega)$, via the relations

$$G^*(\omega) = -i\omega\eta^*(\omega) = G'(\omega) + iG''(\omega) \tag{4.16}$$

The Einstein relation (equation (4.1)) is then used to relate the diffusion coefficient in equation (4.11) to the measured MSD of the probes (Mason and Weitz 1995, Mason *et al* 1997, Squires and Mason 2010, Zia 2018).

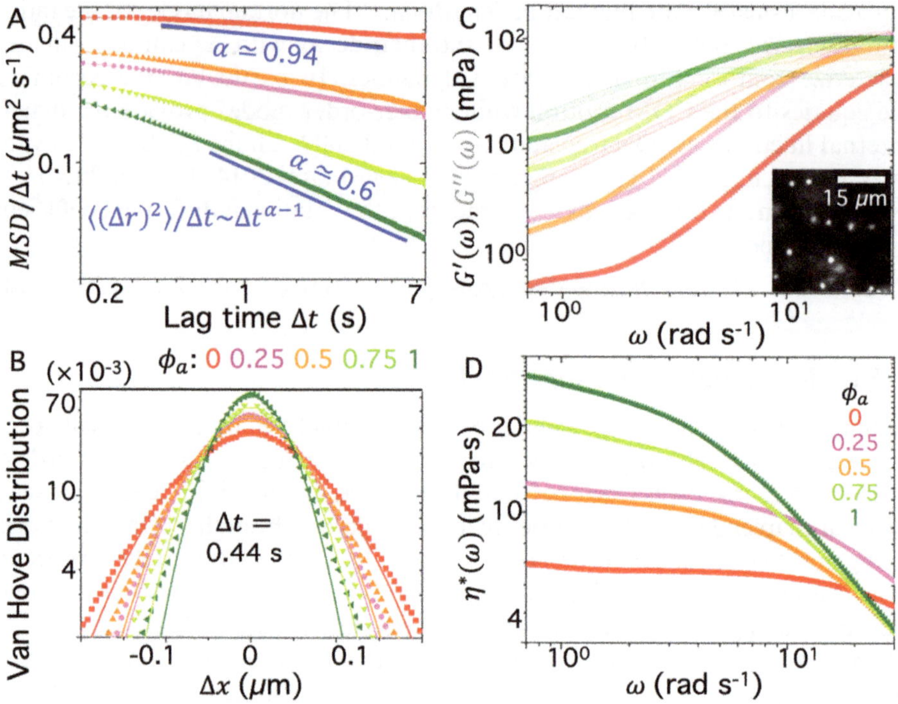

Figure 4.3. Single-particle tracking (SPT) measures displacements of diffusing probes to provide particle transport properties and viscoelastic moduli of the surrounding medium. Tracking single embedded 1 μm probes (see inset in C) in composite networks of actin and microtubules with varying molar fractions of actin ϕ_a reveal (A) subdiffusion, (B) non-Gaussian van Hove distributions; and ϕ_a-dependent (C) viscoelastic moduli $G'(\omega)$ and $G''(\omega)$ and (D) complex viscosity $\eta^*(\omega)$. (A) Log–log plot of MSDs scaled by lag time Δt highlights the extent to which particle motion deviates from normal diffusion, in which $\frac{\text{MSD}}{\Delta t} \sim \Delta t^0$ (i.e., $\alpha - 1 = 0$) manifesting as a Δt-independent horizontal line. Composites exhibit an increasing degree of subdiffusion with increasing ϕ_a, as seen by progressively steeper negative slopes, ranging from $\alpha - 1 \simeq -0.4$ for $\phi_a = 1$ to $\alpha - 1 \simeq -0.06$ for $\phi_a = 0$, corresponding to $\alpha \simeq 0.6$ and 0.94. (B) van Hove distributions of particle displacements Δx (squares, triangles) for $\Delta t = 0.44$, and corresponding fits to Gaussian functions (solid lines), show that particles exhibit non-Gaussian features including exponential large-displacement tails that extend beyond the Gaussian profile. The deviation from Gaussianity increases with increasing ϕ_a. (C) $G'(\omega)$ (filled symbols) and $G''(\omega)$ (open symbols) computed from the MSDs shown in (A) using GSER. The magnitude of $G'(\omega)$ increases and the frequency dependence decreases with increasing ϕ_a, indicating increased elasticity. (D) The complex viscosity $\eta^*(\omega)$ determined from $G'(\omega)$ and $G''(\omega)$ shows that the zero-shear viscosity η_0, approximated as the low frequency $\eta^*(\omega)$ value, increases with increasing ϕ_a. The degree of shear-thinning, $\eta^*(\omega) \sim \omega^{-x}$, shown as a power-law decrease of $\eta^*(\omega)$ with increasing ω, likewise increases with increasing ϕ_a. Adapted with permission from Anderson *et al* (2019). Copyright (2019) American Chemical Society.

Implementing the GSER approach relies on accurately computing the Fourier transform of the particle MSD, denoted as $\langle(\Delta\tilde{r})^2(\omega)\rangle$, which transforms to the complex modulus via the relation

$$G^*(\omega) = G'(\omega) + iG''(\omega) = \frac{k_B T}{i\omega\ \langle(\Delta\tilde{r})^2(\omega)\rangle \pi R_s} \tag{4.17}$$

$\langle(\Delta\tilde{r})^2(\omega)\rangle$ can be approximated via the expansion:

$$-\omega^2\langle(\Delta\tilde{r})^2(\omega)\rangle = (1 - e^{-i\omega\,\Delta t_1})\frac{\langle\Delta r^2(\Delta t_1)\rangle}{\Delta t_1} +$$

$$2De^{-i\omega\,\Delta t_N} + \sum_{k=2}^{N}\left(\frac{\langle\Delta r^2(\Delta t_k)\rangle - \langle\Delta r^2(\Delta t_{k-1})\rangle}{\Delta t_k - \Delta t_{k-1}}\right)(e^{-i\omega\,\Delta t_{k-1}} - e^{-i\omega\,\Delta t_k}) \tag{4.18}$$

where subscripts 1 and N represent the first and last point from the oversampled $\langle(\Delta r)^2(\Delta t)\rangle$.

The elastic and viscous moduli can then be computed from $G^*(\omega)$ via the relations

$$G'(\omega) = \mid G^*(\omega) \mid \cos(\pi\upsilon(\omega)/2) \tag{4.19}$$

$$G''(\omega) = \mid G^*(\omega) \mid \sin(\pi\upsilon(\omega)/2) \tag{4.20}$$

where $\upsilon(\omega)$ is the local logarithmic slope of $\langle(\Delta r)^2(\Delta t)\rangle$ at the frequency of interest:

$$\upsilon(\omega) = \left.\frac{d\ln\langle(\Delta r)^2(\Delta t)\rangle}{d\ln\Delta t}\right|_{\omega^{-1}=\Delta t} \tag{4.21}$$

As I describe in section 3.4.1, there are several alternative paths for going from $\langle(\Delta r)^2(\Delta t)\rangle$ to $G^*(\omega)$, including evaluating the Laplace transform of $\langle(\Delta r)^2(\Delta t)\rangle$, and estimating the amplitude of the complex modulus via

$$\mid G^*(\omega) \mid = \frac{k_BT}{\pi R_s\langle(\Delta r)^2(1/\omega)\rangle\Gamma[1 + \upsilon(\omega)]} \tag{4.22}$$

where Γ is the gamma function (Mason 2000, Zia 2018).

4.2.2 Two-point microrheology

Because biopolymer networks can have hierarchical, heterogeneous, and/or non-continuum rheological properties, the viscoelastic signatures measured using particle-tracking microrheology often do not match those measured using bulk rheology techniques described in chapter 3 (figures 4.4(D) and (E)) (Buchanan *et al* 2005, Liu *et al* 2006, DePuit and Squires 2012, Falzone *et al* 2015, Weigand *et al* 2017).

While this mismatch is fortuitous in many cases, as it sheds light on the scale-dependent rheology (Gardel *et al* 2004, Buchanan *et al* 2005, DePuit and Squires 2012, Falzone *et al* 2015, Weigand *et al* 2017), it is often difficult to perform both types of measurements on biopolymer networks due to the large sample volumes needed for bulk rheology. While microrheology measurements can be performed on $\sim$10 μL samples, bulk rheometers typically require >100 μL for soft and liquid-like materials that do not exert substantial stresses. The cost and preparation time required for many biopolymer systems thus renders them suboptimal for bulk rheology measurements.

An alternative approach to circumvent the small spatiotemporal scales that bound SPTM measurements, is to perform two-point microrheology (TPM). TPM analyzes the same videos of diffusing particles that are used for SPTM, also referred to as one-point microrheology. However, rather than analyzing the MSDs of individual particles,

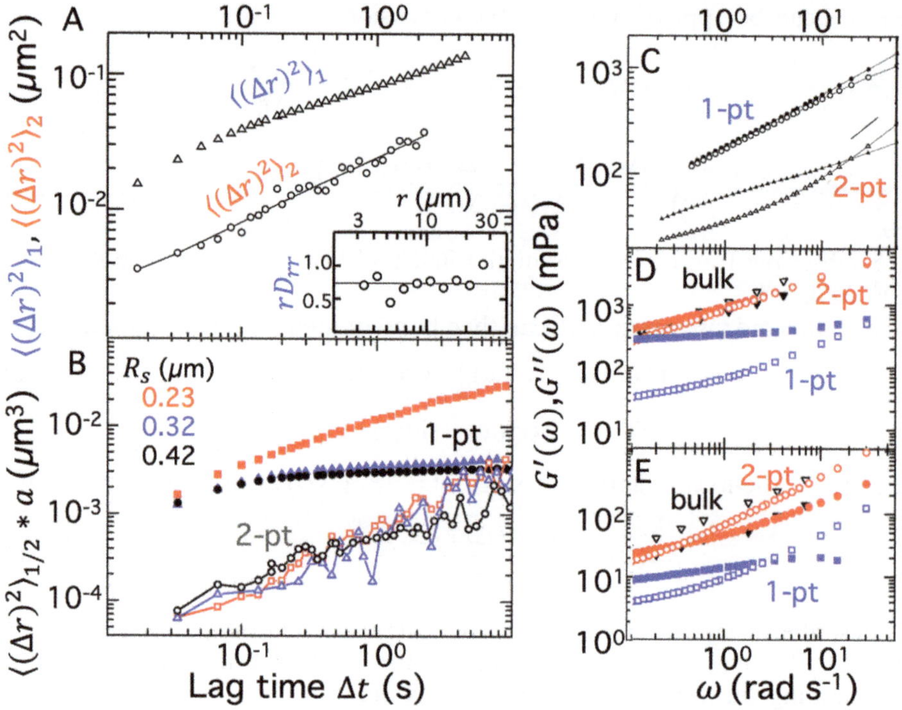

Figure 4.4. Comparison of one-point (SPTM) and two-point (TPM) microrheology of entangled actin networks at varying concentrations c_a using probes of varying sizes R_s. (A) Single-particle (1-pt, triangles) and cross-correlated (2-pt, circles) mean-squared displacements, $\langle(\Delta r)^2(\Delta t)\rangle_1$ and $\langle(\Delta r)^2(\Delta t)\rangle_2$, show that single-particle (1-pt) tracking measures faster dynamics than two-point microrheology ($\langle(\Delta r)^2(\Delta t)\rangle_1 > \langle(\Delta r)^2(\Delta t)\rangle_2$) that becomes increasingly subdiffusive (shallower slope) at larger Δt. Conversely, $\langle(\Delta r)^2(\Delta t)\rangle_2$ exhibits constant subdiffusive scaling with $\alpha \simeq 0.5$ (solid line). These differences suggest that 1-pt microrheology is measuring the dynamics of the particles diffusing within network cages, while 2-pt measures the dynamics resulting from the larger-scale network. The inset shows that the cross-correlated diffusion coefficient D_{rr} scaled by probe separation ρ is independent of ρ, as expected for measurements that detect the bulk network properties. (B) MSDs scaled by the probe size for 1-pt and 2-pt tracking using probes with radii (μm) of $R_s = 0.23$ (red), 0.32 (blue), and 0.42 (black) show that 2-pt results are independent of probe size, as needed for unequivocal determination of network properties, while 1-pt measurements show stronger caging for larger probes. (C–E) $G'(\omega)$ (filled symbols) and $G''(\omega)$ (open symbols) determined via 1-pt (black triangles in C, blue squares in D and E), 2-pt (black circles in C and red circles in D–E), and bulk rheology (black inverted triangles in D and E) show that 1-pt microrheology underestimates the magnitudes of $G'(\omega)$ and $G''(\omega)$ and overestimates the elastic contribution to the stress response, shown as a higher G'/G'' ratio and weaker frequency dependence of G' as compared to 2-pt and bulk measurements. (D, E) 2-pt measurements for different actin concentrations and probe sizes consistently show agreement with bulk measurements that differ from 1-pt. (A, C) Adapted with permission from Crocker *et al* (2000). Copyright (2000) by the American Physical Society. (B, D, E) Adapted with permission from Gardel *et al* (2003). Copyright (2003) by the American Physical Society.

as in one-point microrheology, TPM evaluates the cross-correlation D_{rr} of the motion of pairs of particles separated by a radial distance ρ at a lag time Δt, defined as

$$D_{rr}(\rho, \Delta t) = \langle \Delta r_1(\Delta t) \Delta r_2(\Delta t) \rangle \tag{4.23}$$

where $\Delta r_1(\Delta t)$ and $\Delta r_2(\Delta t)$ are the displacements of the two particles (Crocker *et al* 2000, Levine and Lubensky 2001, Tseng and Wirtz 2001, Starrs and Bartlett 2002, Buchanan *et al* 2005, Crocker and Hoffman 2007, Rowlands and So 2013, Shechtman *et al* 2015).

To relate D_{rr} to rheological properties, an effective two-point MSD can be defined:

$$\langle(\Delta r)^2(\Delta t)\rangle_2 = \frac{2\rho}{R_s}D_{rr} \tag{4.24}$$

and $\langle(\Delta r)^2(\Delta t)\rangle_2$ can be used instead of the single-particle MSD $\langle(\Delta r)^2(\Delta t)\rangle_1$ (figure 4.4(A), (B)), in the GSER framework to determine $G'(\omega)$ and $G''(\omega)$ (figure 4.4C–E).

Because $\langle(\Delta r)^2(\Delta t)\rangle_2$ depends not only on lag time but also on the distance ρ between the two particles, lengthscale-dependent viscoelastic moduli can be resolved to determine the extent to which the rheological properties are hierarchical or otherwise scale-dependent. In the simple case, in which there is limited dependence on ρ, as in a uniform continuum material, the moduli determined for each ρ can be averaged over to give a measure of the 'bulk' rheological properties, as shown in figure 4.4. Specifically, figure 4.4 shows that $G'(\omega)$ and $G''(\omega)$ measured via two-point microrheology match those measured using bulk rheology, while one-point microrheology underestimates the moduli. Moreover, figures 4.4(A) and (B) show that two-point microrheology is able to overcome the bead size dependence and caging that often arises with one-point measurements (Gardel *et al* 2003, Squires and Mason 2010, Chapman *et al* 2014, Weigand *et al* 2017).

It is important to note that two-point microrheology has much higher statistical noise compared to one-point microrheology because the cross-correlated displacements between particles is much smaller than the corresponding displacements of the individual particles. Further, because the measurement relies on pairs of particles instead of single particles, it is highly sensitive to the number of probes in a field of view. For example, for videos with $\sim$100 particles in the FOV, accurate two-point microrheology typically requires at least 10× more videos than its one-point counterpart (Crocker *et al* 2000).

4.3 Particle-image velocimetry (PIV)

Particle-image velocimetry is similar to particle-tracking in that it connects positions of features in a given image at time t_1 to those in an image at time t_2, which are separated by a lag time $\Delta t = t_2 - t_1$ (Bastiaans 1993, Kadem n.d.). However, unlike single-particle tracking, which locates and tracks the positions of individual particles in the images, PIV algorithms divide each image of $p_x \times p_y$ pixels into a grid of $n_x \times n_y$ user-specified interrogation windows of size $p_x/n_x \times p_y/n_y$, and computes an average displacement $\Delta\vec{x}$ of features within each window by spatially cross-correlating the two images (Keane and Adrian 1992, Bastiaans 1993, Kadem n.d.). The corresponding average velocity is computed as $\vec{v} = \Delta\vec{x}/\Delta t$, such that a $p_x \times p_y$ image of $n_x \times n_y$ vector arrows can be reconstructed that represents the velocity flow field of the system at $t_1 + \frac{1}{2}\Delta t$ with spatial resolution p/n (figure 4.5(A.ii–C.ii)). Dividing $\Delta\vec{x}$ by the chosen Δt provides the spatially resolved velocities $\vec{v}$.

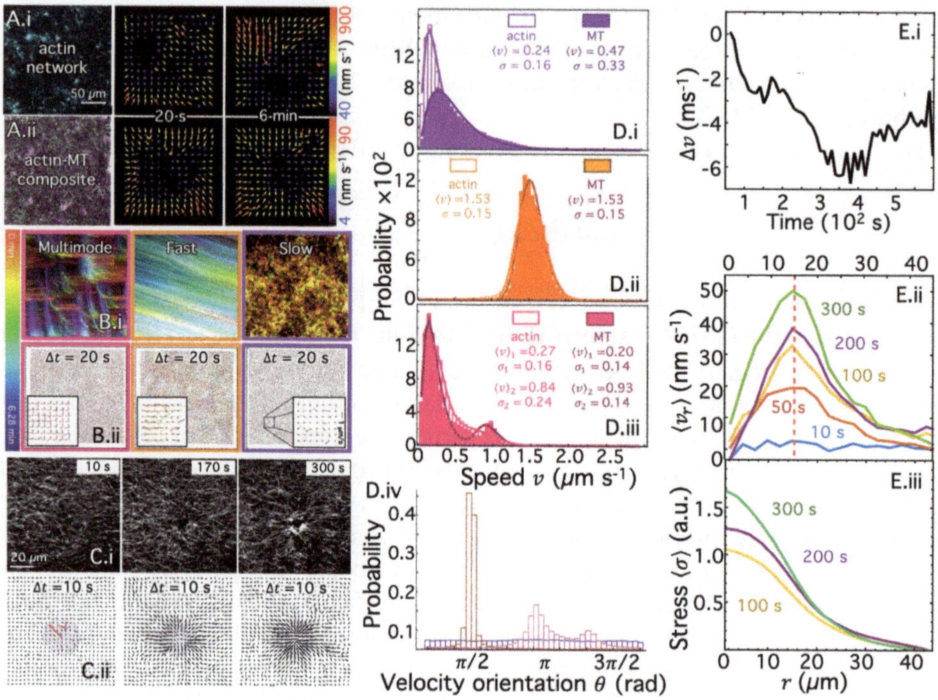

Figure 4.5. Particle Image Velocimetry (PIV) characterizes velocity flow fields of time-evolving heterogeneous systems. PIV analysis is performed on (A) myosin-driven actin networks (left) and equimolar actin-microtubule composites (right), (B, D) crosslinked and entangled actin-microtubule composites driven by kinesin, and (C and E) actomyosin networks selectively activated by blebbistatin deactivation in a central circular region. (A) Images (i) and vector fields for $\Delta t = 20$ s (ii) for an actin network (left) and actin-microtubule composite (right), with the different vector field rows corresponding to different measurement times, as listed, and the different colors corresponding to different speeds, as indicated by the color scales at the bottom. Images show (left) actin (cyan) and (right) actin (green) and microtubules (magenta). (B) Temporal color maps (i) and PIV vector fields (ii) computed from sample videos of kinesin-driven composites displaying three classes of motion: multimodal restructuring (magenta, left), fast flow (middle, orange), and slow athermal fluctuations (right, purple). The different colors in (i) correspond to different times during the video, as indicated by the color scale to the left. (C) Images (i) and PIV vector fields (ii) of actomyosin networks at different times (listed) after blebbistatin deactivation (myosin activation) in a central circular region depicted in (ii). Over time, actin contracts more strongly towards the activation zone, as shown by the larger vector arrows all pointing towards the center. (D) Probability distributions of speeds (i–iii) and velocity orientations (iv) determined from the vector fields shown in (B) for slow (purple), fast (orange), and multimode (magenta) videos. Solid lines in (i–iii) are fits of the distributions to one (i) or two (iii) Schulz distributions with corresponding average speed $\langle v \rangle$ and standard deviation σ_v listed for actin (open) and microtubules (filled) separately. (E) Analysis of PIV fields of networks shown in (C) that show the (i) divergence of the velocity $\nabla \vec{v}$ versus post-activation time, the average radially directed (ii) speed $\langle v_r \rangle$ and (iii) stress $\langle \sigma \rangle$ as functions of radial distance r from the activation center, with different colors corresponding to different post-activation times, as listed. Contractile motion is observed for all times (i, $\nabla \vec{v} < 0$), reaching a peak at ~300 s. This increasing contractility correlates with increasing speeds (ii) and stresses (iii). Modified from Lee *et al* (2021b). © The Authors, some rights reserved; exclusive licensee AAAS. (B, D) Adapted from McGorty *et al* (2023). CC BY 4.0. (C, E) Adapted from Linsmeier *et al* (2016). CC BY 4.0.

The window size $p_x/n_x \times p_y/n_y$ requires careful optimization to enable statistically significant signal-to-noise ratios, which improve with larger windows, while allowing for fine enough spatial resolution, which improves with smaller windows, to accurately capture heterogeneities in the velocity field across the image. Because PIV typically requires interrogation windows of at least several pixels, it has inherently lower spatial resolution compared to SPT, which can locate positions with subpixel accuracy (Rogers *et al* 2007, Parthasarathy 2012, Manzo and Garcia-Parajo 2015). The advantage of PIV is its versatility as it does not require tracking separate non-interacting particles or fiducial markers, but can instead work on images of dense biopolymer networks or other amorphous or structurally complex systems and/or images (figure 4.5(A.i–C.i)) (Linsmeier *et al* 2016, Seara *et al* 2018, Lee *et al* 2021b, McGorty *et al* 2023).

PIV may also be more useful and appropriate than SPT for aging or active systems that have dynamics and/or structure that is changing significantly on the timescale of the acquired videos (Bate *et al* 2022, McGorty *et al* 2023). SPT algorithms rely on averaging together all particle squared displacements separated by a given lag time Δt, regardless of the values of t_1 and t_2, such that any temporal variations in the MSDs are hidden in the averaging. In contrast, PIV produces a unique vector field for each pair of images, which can be evaluated to determine how the flow field changes in time over the course of the video (figure 4.5(E)) (Linsmeier *et al* 2016, Lee *et al* 2021b, Bate *et al* 2022). However, the temporal resolution of PIV, set by the minimum lag time Δt at which there is sufficient signal-to-noise, is almost always larger than the time between two consecutive frames, unlike particle-tracking that typically has frame rate resolution. For this reason, the appropriate method will depend on how quickly the system is moving relative to the frame rate of the video and how the system is evolving over longer timescales (tens of frames).

Another important consideration when deciding if PIV or particle-tracking is more appropriate is the expected type of motion in a given video. For isotropic Brownian motion, the PIV output will be a grid of randomly oriented velocity vectors with limited information from which to determine dynamic metrics such as MSDs, diffusion coefficients, and/or anomalous scaling exponents. However, if there is directional flow and/or spatially heterogenous dynamics, PIV is better equipped to characterize the motion.

From the vector fields that PIV produces, the distribution of speeds v or velocity components (e.g., v_x, v_y, v_r, v_θ) across a single image or stack of images can be evaluated (figure 4.5(D)), as well as the distribution of vector orientations θ (figure 4.5(D.iv)). From the distributions, the mean $\langle v \rangle$, mode $v_{\max}$, and standard deviation σ_v of speeds can be computed. Moreover, the functional form of the distribution, i.e., Gaussian, Schulz, gamma, as well as possible multimode behavior, exhibited as multiple peaks (see figure 4.5(D.iii)), can also provide valuable information regarding the dynamics of the system.

PIV is also well equipped to determine characteristics of a flow field that indicate whether motion is contractile, i.e., moving to a sink (figure 4.5(C)); extensile or expandable, i.e. moving outward from a source; or unidirectional, with no sources or sinks.

The divergence of the two-dimensional velocity vector $\vec{v} = (v_x, v_y)$:

$$\nabla\vec{v} = \frac{\partial v_x}{\partial x} + \frac{\partial v_y}{\partial y} \tag{4.25}$$

is the most widely used measure of contractility versus expansion based on the following relations:

$\nabla\vec{v} > 0$ contractile, moving towards a sink;
$\nabla\vec{v} < 0$ extensile/expandable, moving from a source;
$\nabla\vec{v} = 0$ unidirectional motion, no net change in the velocity flux across any boundary.

The greater $|\nabla\vec{v}\,|$ is, the stronger the contraction or extension. By averaging over the entire vector field, or a particular region of interest, a global rate of, i.e., contraction, can be determined, as shown in figure 4.5(E.i). Conversely, in cases in which the motion is not uniform across the field of view, PIV can generate heat maps or position-dependent distributions that spatially resolve regions of contractility, extension, flow, and/or stress in a given image (figure 4.5(E.ii)) (Muresan *et al* 2022).

The divergence can also be used to quantify network strain ε and strain rate $d\varepsilon/dt$ to connect dynamics to mechanical properties. Specifically, the strain is computed by integrating the velocity fields over time to determine a local displacement field $\vec{u}(T)$:

$$\vec{u}(T) = \sum\nolimits_{t=0}^{t=T} \vec{v}\Delta t \tag{4.26}$$

then taking the divergence of this displacement field:

$$\varepsilon_{xy}(T) = \frac{1}{2}\nabla\vec{u}(T) = \frac{1}{2}\left(\frac{\partial u_x}{\partial x} + \frac{\partial u_y}{\partial y}\right) \tag{4.27}$$

to arrive at an accumulated strain ε_{xy} in the x,y plane as a function of elapsed time T.

The strain rate can be determined from the divergence of the velocity field (equation (4.19)):

$$\frac{d\varepsilon}{dt} = \nabla\vec{v} \tag{4.28}$$

Another useful quantity that PIV can determine is the shear T, which we can understand as the extent to which the displacements at the boundaries of an interrogation window move antiparallel to one another. For a system undergoing flow, the shear is zero as all displacement vectors point in the same direction. A contracting or expanding network may also have limited shear as there are very few near neighbor regions of the network that are being displaced in opposite directions.

In practice, the shear can be computed by performing principal component analysis on the strain tensor ε_{12} (equation (4.27)), to determine the two eigenvalues ε_1

and ε_2 that represent the major and minor axis of the local strain ellipse that indicates the strain shape (Keane and Adrian 1992, Hayes *et al* 2008, Linsmeier *et al* 2016, Kadem n.d.). The shear strain T can then be computed by evaluating the difference between the principal strains:

$$\mathrm{T} = |\ \varepsilon_1 - \varepsilon_2\ |/2 \tag{4.29}$$

Zero shear cases include unidirectional flow, in which $\varepsilon_1 = \varepsilon_2 = 0$, because there is no divergence of $\vec{u}$, and isotropic motion, with $\varepsilon_1 = \varepsilon_2 \neq 0$ because there is no difference between the principal strains (Hayes *et al* 2008).

In cases in which the network can be approximated as an elastic gel, with no dissipative component, and the motion can be assumed to be radially symmetric, as in, e.g., a contracting actomyosin network, then the stress can be computed from the strain via the relation:

$$\sigma_r(r) = -\frac{\zeta_r}{h_\perp}\int_r^R dr' v_r(r') \tag{4.30}$$

where ζ_r and $h_\perp$ are the radial friction coefficient and the perpendicular height of the gel, both of which can be treated as constant, such that they can be neglected when evaluating the dependence of (unitless) stress σ_r on radial distance r and time t (figure 4.5(E.iii)).

Finally, PIV vector fields can be analyzed to determine the extent to which the motion is 'swirling' or circulating, and quantify the corresponding directionality and rate of this circulation by computing the curl of the 2D velocity:

$$\nabla \times \vec{v} = \left(\frac{\partial v_y}{\partial x} - \frac{\partial v_x}{\partial y}\right)\hat{z} \tag{4.31}$$

where $\hat{z}$ indicates the curl direction, with $\hat{z} > 0$ and $\hat{z} < 0$ indicating counter-clockwise and clockwise motion, respectively (Wu *et al* 2017, Ayegba and Edomwonyi-Otu 2020).

4.4 Differential dynamic microscopy (DDM)

The methods discussed above all rely on real-space analysis of images, which can suffer from image noise and difficulty in resolving and characterizing spatiotemporal patterns (e.g., fluctuations, mesh sizes). Fourier analysis methods instead perform calculations in reciprocal space, by transforming an image, $I(\vec{x})$, which is simply a real-space intensity function $I(\vec{x})$, into a function of reciprocal space $I(\vec{q})$, where $\vec{q} = 2\pi/\vec{x}$ is the spatial frequency or wave vector (Giavazzi and Cerbino 2014). Differential Dynamic Microscopy (DDM) is one such Fourier analysis method that can extract dynamics from videos by evaluating the difference between image pairs in reciprocal space, as introduced and described in Cerbino and Trappe (2008) and Cerbino and Cicuta (2017).

DDM is particularly useful for microscopy data in which the biopolymers are too small, fast, and/or dim to accurately track, or in which the network is too dense to resolve the positions of individual polymers and stitch them together in time (requirements for particle-tracking and PIV). Similar to dynamic light scattering, which I describe in chapter 3, DDM evaluates the temporal decay of signal correlations in reciprocal space to extract the dynamics of the system, e.g., diffusion coefficients. The power of DDM, as compared to DLS, lies in the fact that the correlation analysis can be performed on videos acquired using a wide range of optical microscopy modalities, such as epifluorescence, LSCM, TIRF, bright-field, dark-field, light-sheet, etc), making it applicable to diverse systems and compatible with other image analysis methods such as PIV and particle-tracking.

4.4.1 DDM basics

As introduced and detailed in Cerbino and Trappe (2008), Giavazzi *et al* (2009), Lu *et al* (2012), Bayles *et al* (2017), Cerbino and Cicuta (2017), Cerbino *et al* (2022), and Verwei *et al* (2022), DDM analyzes correlations in the Fourier transform of image differences as a function of lag time between the differences to determine the decay rate of density fluctuations in a system as a function of wave vector $\vec{q}$. This decay rate can be analyzed to determine the type of dynamics, e.g., ballistic, diffusive, subdiffusive, etc.

In practice, DDM is performed on a stack of images $I(x, t)$, where t runs from the first frame t_1 to the last frame t_N and x signifies the pixel position (figure 4.6(A.i)), by first subtracting all pairs of images separated by a given Δt to provide a stack of image differences $\Delta I(\vec{x}, \Delta t)$ for each lag time Δt:

$$\Delta I_n(\vec{x}, \Delta t) = I(\vec{x}, t_n) - I(\vec{x}, t_n + \Delta t) \tag{4.32}$$

Taking the Fourier transform of $\Delta I_n(\vec{x}, \Delta t)$ converts each 2D real-space image $\Delta I(\vec{x}, \Delta t)$ to a 2D Fourier-space image $\Delta \tilde{I}(\vec{q}, \Delta t)$ that represents the density correlations that occur at varying $\vec{q}$ values (figure 4.6(A.ii)). If the system is spatially isotropic and the dynamics are not changing appreciably over the course of the image stack, each $\Delta \tilde{I}_n(\vec{q}, \Delta t)$ can be azimuthally averaged over $\vec{q}$. Then all resulting one-dimensional $\Delta \tilde{I}_n(q, \Delta t)$ functions for a given Δt can be averaged over all times t_n, resulting in a single value for each magnitude of q and Δt. The 1D image structure function $D(q, \Delta t)$ that results from this computation:

$$D(q, \Delta t) = \langle \Delta \tilde{I}^2(q, \Delta t) \rangle_{t_n} \tag{4.33}$$

is typically plotted as a function of Δt for each magnitude of q (figures 4.6(A.iii) and (C.i)).

$D(q, \Delta t)$ can be interpreted as the decorrelation of density fluctuations in a system, which typically increases exponentially to a maximum plateau value at sufficiently large Δt values, indicating complete decorrelation. The magnitude of $D(q, \Delta t)$ increases with decreasing q values as the system dynamics become more decorrelated at larger lengthscales (smaller q values), as shown in figure 4.6(A.iii).

The decay rate of density fluctuations can be determined by fitting $D(q, \Delta t)$ to an exponential function of the form

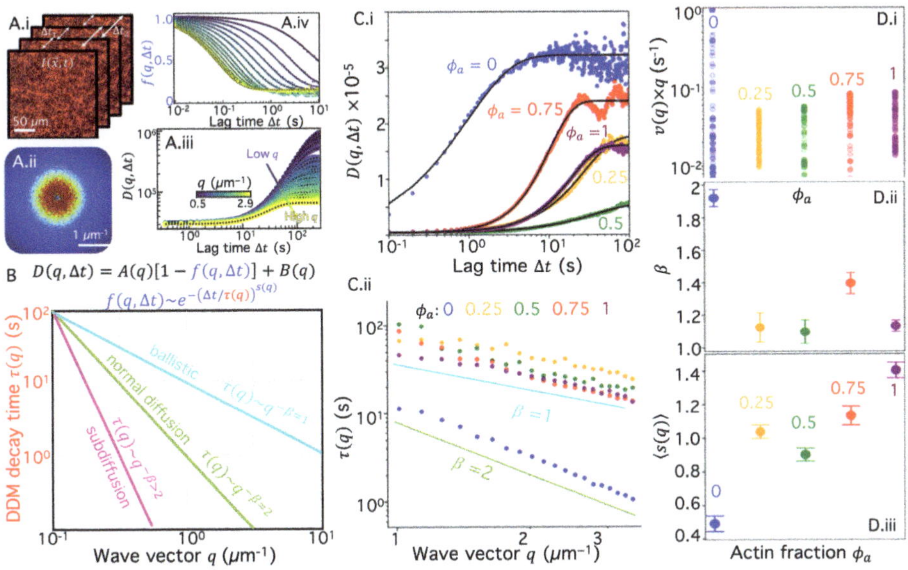

Figure 4.6. Differential Dynamic Microscopy (DDM) characterizes dynamics of biopolymer networks over a range of spatiotemporal scales. (A) DDM analysis converts a stack of images (i) to a stack of image differences that are transformed into Fourier space, resulting in a 2D image structure function $D(\vec{q}, \Delta t)$ for each lag time Δt (ii). If $D(\vec{q}, \Delta t)$ is radially symmetric (as shown in (ii), it can be azimuthally-averaged over every $|\vec{q}| = q$, resulting in a one-dimensional image structure function $D(q, \Delta t)$ as a function of Δt for each wave vector of magnitude q (iii). Fitting $D(q, \Delta t)$ to the equation shown provides $f(q, \Delta t)$ as function of Δt (iv). Different curves in (iii) and (iv) correspond to different q values as indicated by the color scale in (ii). (B) The decay time $\tau(q)$ determined from $f(q, \Delta t)$ displays power-law scaling with q, $\tau(q) \sim q^{-\beta}$ with the exponent β reporting the type of dynamics: diffusive ($\beta = 2$, olive), subdiffusive ($\beta > 2$, magenta), superdiffusive ($1 < \beta < 2$), and ballistic ($\beta = 1$, cyan). (C) Image structure functions (i) and decay times (ii) measured for microspheres embedded in myosin-driven actin-microtubule composites with fixed overall concentration $c_A + c_T = 5.8\ \mu$M and [myosin]:[actin] ratio $R_m = 0.08$, and varying molar fractions of actin ϕ_a: 0 (blue), 0.25 (gold), 0.5 (green), 0.75 (red), and 1 (purple). In the absence of actin ($\phi_a = 0$), dynamics are diffusive ($\beta = 2$), while all $\phi_a > 0$ composites exhibit ballistic scaling ($\beta = 1$). (D) Mobility metrics for each ϕ_a determined from $f(q, \Delta t)$ and $\tau(q)$ include: (i) mobility rate $\tau^{-1}(q) = \langle v \rangle \times q$ for all q values plotted in (C.ii) with the gradient going from low (dark) to high (light) q values, (ii) scaling exponents β determined from power-law fits to $\tau(q)$, and (iii) average stretching exponent $\langle s(q) \rangle$. Data show that transport in the $\phi_a = 0$ network is (i) faster than $\phi_a > 1$ composites, (ii) diffusive as compared to ballistic for $\phi_a > 1$ composites, and (iii) exhibits stretched exponential scaling ($s < 1$) suggestive of crowding or confinement, compared to compressed exponential scaling ($s < 1$ for $\phi_a > 1$ composites, indicative of active transport. (C, D) Adapted from Sheung *et al* (2022). CC BY 4.0.

$$D(q, \Delta t) = A(q)[1 - f(q, \Delta t)] + B(q) \tag{4.34}$$

where $f(q, \Delta t)$ is the intermediate scattering function (ISF), similar to that measured in DLS, $B(q)$ accounts for the background noise, and $A(q)$ is the static amplitude that encodes information about the network structure and contrast (figure 4.6(A.iv)).

The ISF encodes the dynamics of the system and can often be described by an exponential decay function

$$f(q, \Delta t) = e^{-\Delta t/\tau(q)} \tag{4.35}$$

that provides the q-dependent characteristic decay time of dynamic correlations $\tau(q)$, which typically displays power-law scaling of the form

$$\tau(q) = 1/Kq^{\beta} \tag{4.36}$$

As shown in figures 4.6(B), (C.ii), and (D.ii) the scaling exponent β describes the type of motion, as follows:

$\beta = 2$ Brownian diffusion
$\beta = 1$ ballistic motion
$1 < \beta < 2$ anomalous superdiffusion
$\beta > 2$ anomalous subdiffusion

K is the generalized transport coefficient that equates to the diffusion coefficient D when $\beta = 2$ and speed v when $\beta = 1$ (figure 4.6(D.i)).

4.4.2 Microrheology considerations

For systems in which the particles analyzed by DDM are non-interacting, and where the dynamics can be treated as spatially homogeneous and steady-state over the ROI and timescales probed, $f(q, \Delta t)$ can be transformed into the real-space MSD of the particles in the system (Bayles *et al* 2017, Gu *et al* 2021, Cerbino *et al* 2022). From the transformed MSDs, the same GSER computations used in single-particle tracking microrheology can be performed to determine G^*. See section 4.2.1 for further details.

Importantly, determining G^* from MSDs is only valid when considering spherical probes of a known size. However, one of the advantages of DDM over real-space tracking methods is that it can be performed directly on the images of the biopolymers themselves to unequivocally characterize dynamics without the need to embed tracers to infer dynamics (Regan *et al* 2019, Wulstein *et al* 2019, Lee *et al* 2021b, Verwei *et al* 2022, McGorty *et al* 2023).

4.4.3 DDM analysis for complex dynamics

For certain systems with anomalous transport characteristics such as caging or coarsening, the ISF cannot be well-fit with a simple exponential but instead is better described by a stretched or compressed exponential of the form

$$f(q, \Delta t) = e^{-(\Delta t/\tau(q))^{s(q)}} \tag{4.37}$$

with a stretching exponent $s(q) \neq 1$.

ISFs with $s(q) < 1$ or $s(q) > 1$ are often seen for systems that exhibit subdiffusion and caging or active contractility, respectively (figure 4.6(D.iii)) (Lee *et al* 2021b, Sheung *et al* 2022, Verwei *et al* 2022).

Similar to particle-tracking, DDM can also discern the extent to which a system displays non-ergodic behavior. Specifically, the ISF of a non-ergodic system cannot be well-fit to the stretched exponential shown in equation (4.30), but instead exhibits a non-zero offset captured in the following function:

$$f(q, \Delta t) = (1 - C(q))\left[e^{-\left(\frac{\Delta t}{\tau(q)}\right)^{s(q)}}\right] + C(q) \tag{4.38}$$

where $C(q)$ is the ergodicity-breaking parameter (Cho *et al* 2020). For ergodic systems, $C(q) = 0$ and equation (4.37) is recovered, while the greater the magnitude of $C(q)$, the more non-ergodic the system (Cho *et al* 2020, Anderson *et al* 2021).

Equations (4.34)–(4.38) are specifically considering 1D image structure functions (equation (4.34)), determined by azimuthal averaging over the two-dimensional image structure function

$$D(q_1, q_2, \Delta t) \tag{4.39}$$

where q_1 and q_2 are the components of the wave vector in two orthogonal directions, such as $\hat{r}$ and $\hat{\theta}$, $\hat{x}$ and $\hat{y}$, or the two principal eigenvalue components.

Also implicit in the construction above is an average over measurement time t of the full instantaneous image structure function:

$$D(q_1, q_2, \Delta t) = \frac{1}{T}\sum\int_0^T D_i(q_1, q_2, \Delta t, t)dt \tag{4.40}$$

where D_i differentiates the instantaneous time-dependent image structure function from the time-averaged $D(\vec{q}, \Delta t)$, and where $t = 0$ and $t = T$ refer to the times of the initial and final frame of the video. This process reduces the time-dependent image structure function to one in which the only temporal dependence is on lag time Δt.

These two spatiotemporal reductions average out any spatial anisotropies and time-dependence to reduce the dimensionality of the dataset and simplify analysis. However, many biopolymer networks may exhibit dynamics that are aligned along a particular axis, or have distinct dynamics along their two principal axes, such as nematically aligned networks or those undergoing directed flow (e.g., figures 4.6(B) and (D)) (Lu *et al* 2012, Fürthauer *et al* 2019, Opathalage *et al* 2019, McGorty *et al* 2023). Moreover, many biopolymer networks exhibit time-varying dynamics due to active stresses, aging, gelation, or other non-equilibrium processes (e.g., figures 4.5(A), (C), and (E)) (Aarts *et al* 2005, Bertrand *et al* 2012, Linsmeier *et al* 2016, Harmon *et al* 2017, Nguyen and Saleh 2017, Gurmessa *et al* 2018, Seara *et al* 2018, Lee *et al* 2021a, Meleties *et al* 2022, Michieletto *et al* 2022, Marfai *et al* 2023). In these cases, azimuthal and time-averaged quantities may not accurately or fully capture or characterize dynamics, and instead the spatial and temporal dependence of the dynamics need to be evaluated.

To determine the extent to which dynamics are aligned along a particular axis, the 2D image structure function can be expressed in polar coordinates:

$$D(|\vec{q}|, \theta, \Delta t) \tag{4.41}$$

and an alignment factor $A_F(q, \Delta t)$ can be determined by evaluating

$$A_F(q, \Delta t) = \frac{\int_0^{2\pi} D(|\vec{q}|, \theta, \Delta t)\cos(2\theta)d\theta}{\int_0^{2\pi} D(|\vec{q}|, \theta, \Delta t)d\theta} \tag{4.42}$$

where θ is defined relative to the positive y-axis such that a positive $A_F > 0$ corresponds to dynamics along $\hat{y}$ and $A_F < 0$ corresponds to dynamics along $\hat{x}$ (Walker and Wagner 1996, Varga and Swan 2018). $A_F = 0$ is the trivial case of isotropic dynamics. This chosen orientation of θ is arbitrary, and can instead be aligned along any pair of orthogonal axes, to assess alignment along a direction of interest, such as the director of a nematic or the direction of an imposed strain (Peddireddy *et al* 2022).

To elucidate potential temporal heterogeneities or evolution in the dynamics, the distribution of values of the instantaneous image structure function $D_i(\vec{q}, \Delta t, t)$, can be evaluated for a given Δt and q. For steady-state homogeneous dynamics, this distribution $G(D_i)$ should be a Gaussian function

$$G(D_i) \sim e^{-D_i^2/2\sigma_D^2} \tag{4.43}$$

where σ_D is the standard deviation, for all values of Δt and q.

Deviations from Gaussianity suggest sporadic events that cause larger than typical decorrelations of the structure (Gao *et al* 2015), as often seen near transition points of non-equilibrium systems or in systems with heterogeneous or time-evolving dynamics (Chan and Mohraz 2014, Gao *et al* 2015, Cherstvy *et al* 2018, McGorty *et al* 2023, Weirich *et al* 2019). While there are several metrics to quantify deviation from Gaussianity, one example is the skewness S_K, defined as

$$S_K = (\langle D_i - D \rangle)^3 / (\langle (D_i - D)^2 \rangle)^{\frac{3}{2}} \tag{4.44}$$

where D and D_i are the time-averaged and instantaneous image structure functions and the average is over time. Skewness is a measure of how asymmetric the distribution is, and $S_K > 0$ and $S_K < 0$ describe distributions with the mode shifted to the left or right of the mean, respectively. The kurtosis κ of the $D_i(t)$ distribution can also be evaluated to determine the extent to which it exhibits heavy tails that extend beyond Gaussian (e.g., figures 4.1(F), 4.6(B)) or fewer than expected large values.

4.4.4 And more…

There are several alternatives and extensions to this exact implementation of DDM for systems with, e.g., more complex dynamics, extensive photobleaching, spatio-temporal heterogeneities, etc (Garamella *et al* 2020, Khanal *et al* 2022, Verwei *et al* 2022). Some of these alternatives include: determining $\tau(q)$ directly from the image structure function $D(q, \Delta t)$ rather than from $f(q, \Delta t)$ (Lee *et al* 2021a, 2021b, Verwei *et al* 2022) and fitting the image structure function to models that account for a distribution of speeds v_i (McGorty *et al* 2023).

4.5 Spatial image autocorrelation

The techniques described above focus on extracting dynamics and rheology of biopolymer networks, which are often more complex than their structure. For example, solutions of entangled flexible biopolymers such as DNA adopt no visible structure above the optical resolution limit. However, crosslinked and bundled polymer networks, composite systems that de-mix, and networks of rigid and extended biopolymers often exhibit structural properties and features of order $\sim 10^0$–10^2 μm (figures 4.7(A) and (D)) (Alvarado *et al* 2013, Stam *et al* 2017, Bashirzadeh and Liu 2019, Edozie *et al* 2019, Gurmessa *et al* 2019, Weirich *et al* 2019, Peddireddy *et al* 2021, Bate *et al* 2022, McGorty *et al* 2023). Characterizing the network structure of these systems, and connecting structure to dynamics, sheds important light on the interactions and physics dictating the network properties.

One of the most important and universal parameters used to characterize structure is the structural correlation length ξ, which is a measure of the average size of features in a network. For entangled and crosslinked polymer networks, ξ can be understood as the mesh size or pore size, which are measures of the average spacing between polymer segments within the network. Conversely, for systems comprising large aggregates, bundles, droplets, foci, or phase-separated domains, ξ is often related to the size of these larger-scale features (figures 4.7(C) and (F)) (Lee *et al* 2021a, Peddireddy *et al* 2021, Sheung *et al* 2021). In practice, this correlation length can be determined from a microscope image of a network by evaluating spatial correlations in pixel intensities. Specifically, ξ can be defined as the separation distance r between two pixels at which their intensities become decorrelated.

Spatial Image Autocorrelation (SIA) is a Fourier analysis technique that computes this pixel correlation function and the corresponding correlation lengthscale (Robertson and Robertson 2012, Sheung *et al* 2021).

SIA acts on single images, $I(\vec{x})$, rather than the image differences, $\Delta I(\vec{x}, \Delta t)$, that DDM uses, such that SIA characterizes the static structure of the network at a given snapshot in time, while DDM characterizes dynamics. SIA computes the autocorrelation of intensities of pixels separated by a displacement $\Delta\vec{x}$, and averages over all such pairs to arrive at an autocorrelation function $g(\Delta\vec{x})$.

For isotropic systems, it is standard to azimuthally average over $\Delta\vec{x}$ to compute $g(r)$, where r is the radial separation between two pixels. In practice, this computation is performed by:

1. taking the fast Fourier transform of the 2D image $F(I(\Delta\vec{x}))$;
2. azimuthally averaging over all directions to give the one-dimensional transform $F(I(r))$;
3. multiplying by its complex conjugate $F^*(I(r))$;
4. applying an inverse Fourier transform F^{-1} to convert from reciprocal space back to real-space;
5. normalizing by the squared intensity $[I(r)]^2$ at each r.

This process results in an r-dependent correlation function:

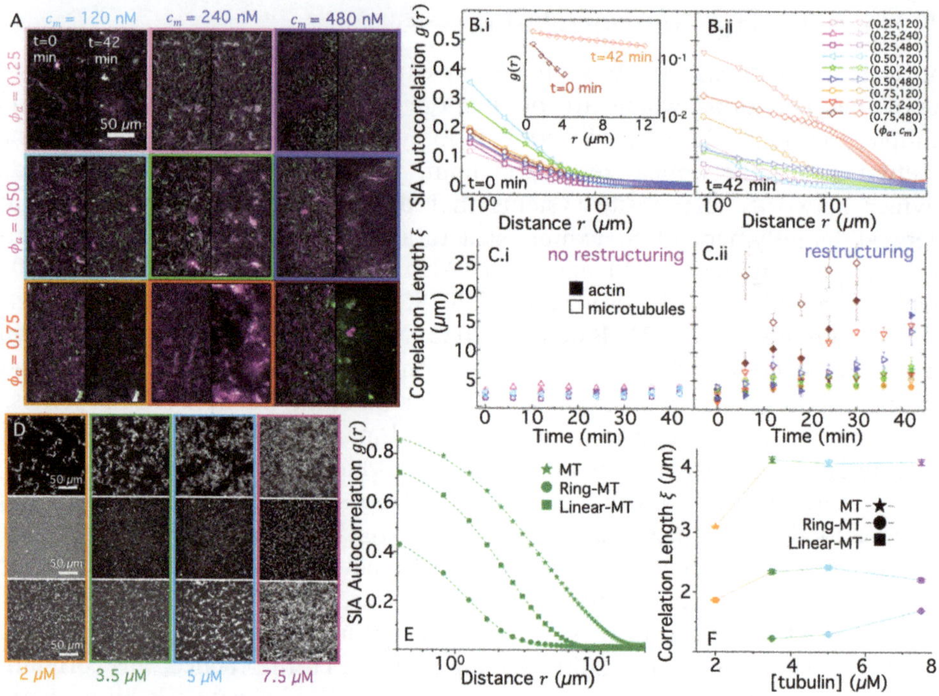

Figure 4.7. Spatial Image Autocorrelation (SIA) analysis characterizes structural features and lengthscales of biopolymer networks. Spatial image autocorrelation analysis characterizes the structural correlation length ξ as a function of time and network composition for (A–C) myosin-driven actin-microtubule composites of varying molar actin fractions ϕ_a and myosin concentrations c_m. (D–F) Networks of microtubules polymerized from varying concentrations of tubulin within solutions of ring or linear DNA. (A) Images of actin (green) and microtubules (magenta) in composites of varying ϕ_a (rows) and c_m (columns) before myosin activation ($t = 0$, left) and after $t = 42$ mins of actomyosin activity (right) show varying degrees of composite restructuring and clustering that depend on ϕ_A and c_m. (B) Azimuthally-averaged SIA autocorrelation functions $g(r)$ for microtubules in the composites shown in A at (i) $t = 0$ and (ii) $t = 42$ min, with color-coding matching the image boundary colors in A. As shown, myosin activity leads to longer-range structural correlations for actin-rich composites, seen as weaker decay of $g(r)$ with distance r. Fitting the decaying region of each curve to an exponential $g(r) = e^{-r/\xi}$ (equation (4.46)), as shown by the solid lines in the inset, provides a structural correlation length ξ which is plotted in (C) as a function of time and composition (ϕ_A, c_m). (C) Time-dependent correlation lengths $\xi(t)$ for actin (solid symbols) and microtubules (open symbols) are used to classify composites into those that undergo (i) minimal myosin-driven restructuring, evidenced as a correlation length that does not change significantly over time, or (ii) substantial restructuring, as evidenced by increasing ξ over time. Note that for most composites, the structure of actin and microtubule networks are similar, indicating strong steric interactions and co-entanglement, except in actin-rich composites with high motor concentration (maroon, red) where they separate, and the microtubules undergo more substantial restructuring and clustering. (D) Images of microtubules polymerized from tubulin in buffer (top row) or in a $\rho = 0.65$ mg mL^{-1} solution of ring (middle) or linear (bottom) DNA of $L \simeq 38$ μm (115 kbp). Increasing molarities of tubulin are shown from left to right: c_T (μM) = 2 (orange), 3.5 (green), 5 (cyan), and 7.5 (purple). (E) $g(r)$ curves computed from the images for the $c_T = 3.5$ μM case with no DNA (MT, stars), ring DNA (circles), and linear DNA (squares) show that rings suppress microtubule network formation while linear chains promote network formation. The larger $g(r)$ for the microtubules without DNA correspond to larger clusters and reduced connectivity as compared to the linear DNA case, as seen in D. (F) Correlation lengths are computed from fits of $g(r)$ for the different composite compositions showing non-monotonic dependence of ξ with c_T for

the composite with linear DNA, small ξ values that increase modestly with c_T for ring DNA, and large ξ values in the absence of DNA which are consistent with the size of larger clusters seen in D. (A–C) Adapted from Lee *et al* (2021a), with permission from the Royal Society of Chemistry. (D–F) Adapted with permission from Peddireddy *et al* (2021). Copyright (2021) American Chemical Society.

$$g(r) = \frac{F^{-1}(|F(I(r))|^2)}{[I(r)]^2} \tag{4.45}$$

that spans values of $g(r = 0) = 1$ to $g(r \to \infty) = 0$ (figures 4.7(B) and (E)).

The autocorrelation function can often be described by a simple exponential decay function

$$g(r) = e^{-r/\xi} \tag{4.46}$$

where ξ is the structural correlation length (figures 4.6(C) and (F)).

Multi-component or otherwise more structurally complex systems may exhibit more complex functional forms that cannot be well-fit by equation (4.46). For example, $g(r)$ may be better fit to a sum of exponentials, indicating multiple distinct correlation lengthscales ξ_i:

$$g(r) = \sum_i e^{-r/\xi_i} + g_\infty \tag{4.47}$$

where I have included a long-range residual correlation term g_∞ to account for potential structural lengthscales that extend beyond the image FOV.

Alternatively, networks that display fractal-like structure or a broad spectrum of correlation lengthscales that are not spatially well-separated may exhibit power-law decay of $g(r)$

$$g(r) \sim r^{-\chi} \tag{4.48}$$

with a scaling exponent χ that characterizes the structure.

Finally, for anisotropic networks that are not radially symmetric, such as those that display nematic ordering or preferential alignment in a certain direction (Hitt *et al* 1990, Kas *et al* 1996, Wu *et al* 2017), the 1D correlation function $g(r)$ computed by azimuthal averaging of $g(\Delta\vec{x})$ is likely not an accurate measure of the structure.

In these systems, $g(\Delta\vec{x})$ can be evaluated along two orthogonal directions, parallel and perpendicular to the director. Principal component analysis can also be performed on $g(\Delta\vec{x})$ to find the major and minor axes directions of the $g(\Delta\vec{x})$ ellipse, $\hat{r}_1$ and $\hat{r}_2$. Then $g(r_1)$ and $g(r_2)$ can be computed following the steps outlined above but omitting the azimuthal average step (step 2). Specifically, from the 2D Fourier transform $F(I(\Delta\vec{x}))$, the 2D correlation function can be computed as

$$g(\Delta\vec{x}) = \frac{F^{-1}(|F(I(\Delta\vec{x}))|^2)}{[I(\Delta\vec{x})]^2} \tag{4.49}$$

after which principal component analysis can determine $\hat{r}_1$ and $\hat{r}_2$ (Ringnér 2008, Shlens 2014), and the corresponding 1D correlation functions along each direction:

$$g(r_1) = \quad g(\Delta\vec{x}) \cdot \hat{r}_1 \tag{4.50a}$$

$$g(r_2) = \quad g(\Delta\vec{x}) \cdot \hat{r}_2 \tag{4.50b}$$

$g(r_1)$ and $g(r_2)$ can be fit to the appropriate function, e.g., equations (4.46)–(4.48), to determine the correlation lengthscale(s) along each direction, ξ_1 and ξ_2, as well as potential higher-order structural characteristics, such as power-law decay, quantified by χ, or long-range order, quantified by g_∞.

4.6 Advanced techniques and further reading

The set of analysis techniques described above are certainly not intended to be exhaustive but rather to provide a foundation to help beginners get started and experts to build upon. There have been many advances to this set of analyses developed in recent years, as well complementary approaches to extracting dynamics, rheology, and mechanics (Tychinskii 2007, Brangwynne *et al* 2008, Lu *et al* 2012, 2012, Stuhrmann *et al* 2012, Colin *et al* 2014, Plotnikov *et al* 2014, Bayles *et al* 2016, Hsiao *et al* 2017, Aime and Cipelletti 2019, Arko and Petelin 2019, Cho *et al* 2020, Nishi *et al* 2021, 2021, Peddireddy *et al* 2022, Leech *et al* 2023).

For example, Optical-Tweezers-integrating-Differential-Dynamic-Microscopy (OpTiDDM) couples DDM with nonlinear optical tweezers microheology to map the spatiotemporal propagation of nonlinear strains in polymer networks (Peddireddy *et al* 2022). OpTiDDM characterizes the deformation field and dynamics of biopolymer networks subject to local straining, and directly couples the measured force response and relaxation to the polymer deformations and dynamics. This technique builds on other methods that couple single-molecule tracking to OTM (Falzone and Robertson-Anderson 2015, Gurmessa *et al* 2017). Several other methods have also been introduced that combine rheological measurements (e.g., bulk rheology, OTM, microfluidics) with image analysis methods (e.g., DDM, single-molecule tracking, multiple-particle-tracking, PIV) to characterize polymer dynamics. A few of these advanced techniques are described in Liu *et al* (2007), De Vlaminck and Dekker (2012), Chan and Mohraz (2014), Falzone and Robertson-Anderson (2015), Cerbino and Cicuta (2017), Gurmessa *et al* (2017), Aime and Cipelletti (2019), A. Richards *et al* (2021), Edera *et al* (2021), Richards *et al* (2021).

Methods to more accurately characterize time-varying dynamics of active, aging, and otherwise non-equilibrium systems, have also been introduced (MacKintosh and Levine 2008, Toyota *et al* 2011, Lu *et al* 2012, 2012, Seara *et al* 2018, Garamella *et al* 2020, Meleties *et al* 2022, Verwei *et al* 2022, McGorty *et al* 2023).

Finally, to characterize structure, many real-space methods have been introduced that complement spatial image autocorrelation. Some of these techniques include skeletonization, thresholding, domain-boundary identification, and cluster size analysis (Brangwynne *et al* 2008, DiMarzio 2008, Zheng *et al* 2011, Schindelin *et al* 2012, Gao and Helgeson 2014, Cash *et al* 2018, Glover *et al* 2019, Leech *et al* 2023).

I will describe these and other advanced methods in more detail in subsequent chapters as the need arises.

References

Aarts D G A L, Lekkerkerker H N W, Guo H, Wegdam G H and Bonn D 2005 Hydrodynamics of droplet coalescence *Phys. Rev. Lett.* **95** 164503

Aime S and Cipelletti L 2019 Probing shear-induced rearrangements in Fourier space. II. differential dynamic microscopy *Soft Matter* **15** 213–26

Alvarado J, Sheinman M, Sharma A, MacKintosh F C and Koenderink G H 2013 Molecular motors robustly drive active gels to a critically connected state *Nat. Phys.* **9** 591–7

Amblard F, Maggs A C, Yurke B, Pargellis A N and Leibler S 1996 Subdiffusion and anomalous local viscoelasticity in actin networks *Phys. Rev. Lett.* **77** 4470–3

Anderson S J, Garamella J, Adalbert S, McGorty R J and Robertson-Anderson R M 2021 Subtle changes in crosslinking drive diverse anomalous transport characteristics in actin-microtubule networks *Soft Matter* **17** 4375–85

Anderson S J, Matsuda C, Garamella J, Peddireddy K R, Robertson-Anderson R M and McGorty R 2019 Filament rigidity vies with mesh size in determining anomalous diffusion in cytoskeleton *Biomacromolecules* **20** 4380–8

Aporvari M S, Dang S, Marfai J, Coursey K, McGorty R and Robertson-Anderson R M 2022 Crowding and confinement act in concert to slow DNA diffusion within cell-sized droplets *iScience* **25** 105122

Arko M and Petelin A 2019 Cross-differential dynamic microscopy *Soft Matter* **15** 2791–7

Ayegba P O and Edomwonyi-Otu L C 2020 Turbulence statistics and flow structure in fluid flow using particle image velocimetry technique: a review *Eng. Rep.* **2** e12138

Bashirzadeh Y and Liu A P 2019 Encapsulation of the cytoskeleton: towards mimicking the mechanics of a cell *Soft Matter* **15** 8425–36

Bastiaans R J M 1993 Cross-correlation PIV; theory, implementation and accuracy *EUT reports* Vol. 99-W-001 (Technische Universiteit Eindhoven)

Bate T E, Varney M E, Taylor E H, Dickie J H, Chueh C-C, Norton M M and Wu K-T 2022 Self-mixing in microtubule-kinesin active fluid from nonuniform to uniform distribution of activity *Nat. Commun.* **13** 6573

Bayles A V, Squires T M and Helgeson M E 2016 Dark-field differential dynamic microscopy *Soft Matter* **12** 2440–52

Bayles A V, Squires T M and Helgeson M E 2017 Probe microrheology without particle tracking by differential dynamic microscopy *Rheol. Acta* **56** 1–7

Bertrand O J N, Fygenson D K and Saleh O A 2012 Active, motor-driven mechanics in a DNA gel *Proc. Natl. Acad. Sci.* **109** 17342–7

Betzig E, Patterson G H, Sougrat R, Lindwasser O W, Olenych S, Bonifacino J S, Davidson M W, Lippincott-Schwartz J and Hess H F 2006 Imaging intracellular fluorescent proteins at nanometer resolution *Science* **313** 1642–5

Brangwynne C P, Koenderink G H, MacKintosh F C and Weitz D A 2008 Nonequilibrium microtubule fluctuations in a model cytoskeleton *Phys. Rev. Lett.* **100** 118104

Buchanan M, Atakhorrami M, Palierne J F and Schmidt C F 2005 Comparing macrorheology and one- and two-point microrheology in wormlike micelle solutions *Macromolecules* **38** 8840–4

Burla F, Sentjabrskaja T, Pletikapic G, van Beugen J and Koenderink G H 2020 Particle diffusion in extracellular hydrogels *Soft Matter* **16** 1366–76

Cash C E, Wang J, Martirossyan M M, Ludlow B K, Baptista A E, Brown N M, Weissler E J, Abacousnac J and Gerbode S J 2018 Local melting attracts grain boundaries in colloidal polycrystals *Phys. Rev. Lett.* **120** 018002

Cerbino R and Cicuta P 2017 Perspective: differential dynamic microscopy extracts multi-scale activity in complex fluids and biological systems *J. Chem. Phys.* **147** 110901

Cerbino R, Giavazzi F and Helgeson M E 2022 Differential dynamic microscopy for the characterization of polymer systems *J. Polym. Sci.* **60** 1079–89

Cerbino R and Trappe V 2008 Differential dynamic microscopy: probing wave vector dependent dynamics with a microscope *Phys. Rev. Lett.* **100** 188102

Chan H K and Mohraz A 2014 Microdynamics of dense colloidal suspensions and gels under constant-stress deformation *J. Rheol.* **58** 1419–39

Chapman C D, Gorczyca S and Robertson-Anderson R M 2015 Crowding induces complex ergodic diffusion and dynamic elongation of large DNA molecules *Biophys. J.* **108** 1220–8

Chapman C D, Lee K, Henze D, Smith D E and Robertson-Anderson R M 2014 Onset of non-continuum effects in microrheology of entangled polymer solutions *Macromolecules* **47** 1181–6

Chapman C D, Shanbhag S, Smith D E and Robertson-Anderson R M 2012 Complex effects of molecular topology on diffusion in entangled biopolymer blends *Soft Matter* **8** 9177–82

Chechkin A V, Seno F, Metzler R and Sokolov I M 2017 Brownian yet non-Gaussian diffusion: from superstatistics to subordination of diffusing diffusivities *Phys. Rev.* X **7** 021002

Cherstvy A G, Nagel O, Beta C and Metzler R 2018 Non-Gaussianity, population heterogeneity, and transient superdiffusion in the spreading dynamics of amoeboid cells *Phys. Chem. Chem. Phys.* **20** 23034–54

Cho J H, Cerbino R and Bischofberger I 2020 Emergence of multiscale dynamics in colloidal gels *Phys. Rev. Lett.* **124** 088005

Chun M-S, Kim C and Lee D E 2009 Conformation and translational diffusion of a xanthan polyelectrolyte chain: Brownian dynamics simulation and single molecule tracking *Phys. Rev.* E **79** 051919

Colin R, Zhang R and Wilson L G 2014 Fast, high-throughput measurement of collective behaviour in a bacterial population *J. R. Soc. Interface* **11** 20140486

Crocker J C and Hoffman B D 2007 Multiple-particle tracking and two-point microrheology in cells *Methods in Cell Biology.* (Amsterdam: Elsevier) pp 141–78

Crocker J C, Valentine M T, Weeks E R, Gisler T, Kaplan P D, Yodh A G and Weitz D A 2000 Two-point microrheology of inhomogeneous soft materials *Phys. Rev. Lett.* **85** 888–91

De Vlaminck I and Dekker C 2012 Recent advances in magnetic tweezers *Annu. Rev. Biophys.* **41** 453–72

Delarue M and Sanejouand Y-H 2002 Simplified normal mode analysis of conformational transitions in DNA-dependent polymerases: the elastic network model *J. Mol. Biol.* **320** 1011–24

DePuit R J and Squires T M 2012 Micro–macro-discrepancies in nonlinear microrheology: I. Quantifying mechanisms in a suspension of Brownian ellipsoids *J. Phys. Condens. Matter* **24** 464106

DiMarzio C A 2008 Full-field quantitative phase imaging *Three-Dimensional and Multidimensional Microscopy: Image Acquisition and Processing XV. Presented at the Three-Dimensional and Multidimensional Microscopy: Image Acquisition and Processing XV* (International Society for Optics and Photonics) p 686107

Edera P, Brizioli M, Zanchetta G, Petekidis G, Giavazzi F and Cerbino R 2021 Deformation profiles and microscopic dynamics of complex fluids during oscillatory shear experiments *Soft Matter* **17** 8553–66

Edozie B, Sahu S, Pitta M, Englert A, do Rosario C F and Ross J L 2019 Self-organization of spindle-like microtubule structures *Soft Matter* **15** 4797–807

Falzone T T, Blair S and Robertson-Anderson R M 2015 Entangled F-actin displays a unique crossover to microscale nonlinearity dominated by entanglement segment dynamics *Soft Matter* **11** 4418–23

Falzone T T and Robertson-Anderson R M 2015 Active entanglement-tracking microrheology directly couples macromolecular deformations to nonlinear microscale force response of entangled actin *ACS Macro Lett.* **4** 1194–9

Fürthauer S, Lemma B, Foster P J, Ems-McClung S C, Yu C-H, Walczak C E, Dogic Z, Needleman D J and Shelley M J 2019 Self-straining of actively crosslinked microtubule networks *Nat. Phys.* **15** 1295–300

Gao Y and Helgeson M E 2014 Texture analysis microscopy: quantifying structure in low-fidelity images of dense fluids *Opt. Express* **22** 10046

Gao Y, Kim J and Helgeson M E 2015 Microdynamics and arrest of coarsening during spinodal decomposition in thermoreversible colloidal gels *Soft Matter* **11** 6360–70

Garamella J, Regan K, Aguirre G, McGorty R J and Robertson-Anderson R M 2020 Anomalous and heterogeneous DNA transport in biomimetic cytoskeleton networks *Soft Matter* **16** 6344–53

Gardel M L, Shin J H, MacKintosh F C, Mahadevan L, Matsudaira P A and Weitz D A 2004 Scaling of F-actin network rheology to probe single filament elasticity and dynamics *Phys. Rev. Lett.* **93** 188102

Gardel M L, Valentine M T, Crocker J C, Bausch A R and Weitz D A 2003 Microrheology of entangled F-actin solutions *Phys. Rev. Lett.* **91** 158302

Giavazzi F, Brogioli D, Trappe V, Bellini T and Cerbino R 2009 Scattering information obtained by optical microscopy: differential dynamic microscopy and beyond *Phys. Rev.* E **80** 031403

Giavazzi F and Cerbino R 2014 Digital Fourier microscopy for soft matter dynamics *J. Opt.* **16** 083001

Glover Z J, Ersch C, Andersen U, Holmes M J, Povey M J, Brewer J R and Simonsen A C 2019 Super-resolution microscopy and empirically validated autocorrelation image analysis discriminates microstructures of dairy derived gels *Food Hydrocoll.* **90** 62–71

Gong Z and van der Maarel J R C 2014 Translational and reorientational dynamics of entangled DNA *Macromolecules* **47** 7230–7

Gorczyca S M, Chapman C D and Robertson-Anderson R M 2015 Universal scaling of crowding-induced DNA mobility is coupled with topology-dependent molecular compaction and elongation *Soft Matter* **11** 7762–8

Gu M, Luo Y, He Y, Helgeson M E and Valentine M T 2021 Uncertainty quantification and estimation in differential dynamic microscopy *Phys. Rev.* E **104** 034610

Gurmessa B, Francis M, Rust M J, Das M, Ross J L and Robertson-Anderson R M 2019 Counterion crossbridges enable robust multiscale elasticity in actin networks *Phys. Rev. Res.* **1** 013016

Gurmessa B, Ricketts S and Robertson-Anderson R M 2017 Nonlinear actin deformations lead to network stiffening, yielding, and nonuniform stress propagation *Biophys. J.* **113** 1540–50

Gurmessa B J, Bitten N, Nguyen D T, Saleh O A, Ross J L, Das M and Robertson-Anderson R M 2019 Triggered disassembly and reassembly of actin networks induces rigidity phase transitions *Soft Matter* **15** 1355–44

Harmon T S, Holehouse A S, Rosen M K and Pappu R V 2017 Intrinsically disordered linkers determine the interplay between phase separation and gelation in multivalent proteins *eLife* **6** e30294

Hayes K A, Buckley M R, Cohen I and Archer L A 2008 High resolution shear profile measurements in entangled polymers *Phys. Rev. Lett.* **101** 218301

Hitt A L, Cross A R and Williams R C 1990 Microtubule solutions display nematic liquid crystalline structure *J. Biol. Chem.* **265** 1639–47

Hsiao K-W, Dinic J, Ren Y, Sharma V and Schroeder C M 2017 Passive non-linear micro-rheology for determining extensional viscosity *Phys. Fluids* **29** 121603

Hu Y S, Zimmerley M, Li Y, Watters R and Cang H 2014 Single-molecule super-resolution light-sheet microscopy *ChemPhysChem.* **15** 577–86

Huang B, Babcock H and Zhuang X 2010 Breaking the diffraction barrier: super-resolution imaging of cells *Cell* **143** 1047–58

Introduction to trackpy n.d. http://soft-matter.github.io/trackpy/v0.3.0/introduction.html

Jaques C, Jaques C, Pignat E, Pignat E, Calinon S, Calinon S, Liebling M and Liebling M 2019 Temporal super-resolution microscopy using a hue-encoded shutter *Biomed. Opt. Express* **10** 4727–41

Kadem L n.d. Particle image velocimetry for fluid dynamics measurements (Laboratory for Cardiovascular Fluid Dynamics MIE – Concordia University)

Kas J, Strey H, Tang J X, Finger D, Ezzell R, Sackmann E and Janmey P A 1996 F-actin, a model polymer for semiflexible chains in dilute, semidilute, and liquid crystalline solutions *Biophys. J.* **70** 609–25

Keane R D and Adrian R J 1992 Theory of cross-correlation analysis of PIV images *Appl. Sci. Res.* **49** 191–215

Khanal P, Peddireddy K R, Marfai J, McGorty R and Robertson-Anderson R M 2022 DNA topology dictates emergent bulk elasticity and hindered macromolecular diffusion in DNA-dextran composites *J. Rheol.* **66** 699–715

Lee G, Leech G, Lwin P, Michel J, Currie C, Rust M J, Ross J L, McGorty R J, Das M and Robertson-Anderson R M 2021a Active cytoskeletal composites display emergent tunable contractility and restructuring *Soft Matter* **17** 10765–76

Lee G, Leech G, Rust M J, Das M, McGorty R J, Ross J L and Robertson-Anderson R M 2021b Myosin-driven actin-microtubule networks exhibit self-organized contractile dynamics *Sci. Adv.* **7** eabe4334

Leech G *et al* 2023 Timed material self-assembly controlled by circadian clock proteins arXiv:2303.00779v2

Levine A J and Lubensky T C 2001 Two-point microrheology and the electrostatic analogy *Phys. Rev.* E **65** 011501

Li Y, Kröger M and Liu W K 2014 Dynamic structure of unentangled polymer chains in the vicinity of non-attractive nanoparticles *Soft Matter* **10** 1723

Linsmeier I, Banerjee S, Oakes P W, Jung W, Kim T and Murrell M P 2016 Disordered actomyosin networks are sufficient to produce cooperative and telescopic contractility *Nat. Commun.* **7** 12615

Liu J, Gardel M L, Kroy K, Frey E, Hoffman B D, Crocker J C, Bausch A R and Weitz D A 2006 Microrheology probes length scale dependent rheology *Phys. Rev. Lett.* **96** 118104

Liu J, Koenderink G H, Kasza K E, MacKintosh F C and Weitz D A 2007 Visualizing the strain field in semiflexible polymer networks: strain fluctuations and nonlinear rheology of *F*-actin gels *Phys. Rev. Lett.* **98** 198304

Liu S-L, Li J, Zhang Z-L, Wang Z-G, Tian Z-Q, Wang G-P and Pang D-W 2013 Fast and high-accuracy localization for three-dimensional single-particle tracking *Sci. Rep.* **3** 2462

Lu P J, Giavazzi F, Angelini T E, Zaccarelli E, Jargstorff F, Schofield A B, Wilking J N, Romanowsky M B, Weitz D A and Cerbino R 2012 Characterizing concentrated, multiply scattering, and actively driven fluorescent systems with confocal differential dynamic microscopy *Phys. Rev. Lett.* **108** 218103

MacKintosh F C and Levine A J 2008 Nonequilibrium mechanics and dynamics of motor-activated gels *Phys. Rev. Lett.* **100** 018104

Manzo C and Garcia-Parajo M F 2015 A review of progress in single particle tracking: from methods to biophysical insights *Rep. Prog. Phys.* **78** 124601

Mardoum W M, Gorczyca S M, Regan K E, Wu T-C and Robertson-Anderson R M 2018 Crowding induces entropically-driven changes to DNA dynamics that depend on crowder structure and ionic conditions *Front. Phys.* **6** 53

Marfai J, McGorty R J and Robertson-Anderson R M 2023 Cooperative rheological state-switching of enzymatically-driven composites of circular DNA and dextran *Adv. Mater.* **35** 2305824

Mason T G 2000 Estimating the viscoelastic moduli of complex fluids using the generalized Stokes–Einstein equation springerlink *Rheol. Acta* **39** 371–8

Mason T G, Ganesan K, van Zanten J H, Wirtz D and Kuo S C 1997 Particle tracking microrheology of complex fluids *Phys. Rev. Lett.* **79** 3282–5

Mason T G and Weitz D A 1995 Optical measurements of frequency-dependent linear viscoelastic moduli of complex fluids *Phys. Rev. Lett.* **74** 1250–3

Matlab Particle Tracking n.d. https://site.physics.georgetown.edu/matlab/ (accessed 9 September 2023)

McGorty R J *et al* 2023 Kinesin and myosin motors compete to drive rich multiphase dynamics in programmable cytoskeletal composites *PNAS Nexus* **2** pgad245

Meleties M, Britton D, Katyal P, Lin B, Martineau R L, Gupta M K and Montclare J K 2022 High-throughput microrheology for the assessment of protein gelation kinetics *Macromolecules* **55** 1239–47

Memmolo P, Miccio L, Paturzo M, Caprio G D, Coppola G, Netti P A and Ferraro P 2015 Recent advances in holographic 3D particle tracking *Adv. Opt. Photonics* **7** 713–55

Metzler R, Klafter J and Sokolov I M 1998 Anomalous transport in external fields: continuous time random walks and fractional diffusion equations extended *Phys. Rev.* E **58** 1621–33

Michieletto D, Nahali N and Rosa A 2017 Glassiness and heterogeneous dynamics in dense solutions of ring polymers *Phys. Rev. Lett.* **119** 197801

Michieletto D, Neill P, Weir S, Evans D, Crist N, Martinez V A and Robertson-Anderson R M 2022 Topological digestion drives time-varying rheology of entangled DNA fluids *Nat. Commun.* **13** 4389

Muresan C G, Sun Z G, Yadav V, Tabatabai A P, Lanier L, Kim J H, Kim T and Murrell M P 2022 F-actin architecture determines constraints on myosin thick filament motion *Nat. Commun.* **13** 7008

Nguyen D T and Saleh O A 2017 Tuning phase and aging of DNA hydrogels through molecular design *Soft Matter* **13** 5421–7

Nishi K, MacKintosh F C and Schmidt C F 2021 Multiscale microrheology using fluctuating filaments as stealth probes *Phys. Rev. Lett.* **127** 158001

Opathalage A, Norton M M, Juniper M P N, Langeslay B, Aghvami S A, Fraden S and Dogic Z 2019 Self-organized dynamics and the transition to turbulence of confined active nematics *Proc. Natl. Acad. Sci.* **116** 4788–97

Parthasarathy R 2012 Rapid, accurate particle tracking by calculation of radial symmetry centers *Nat. Methods* **9** 724–6

Peddireddy K R, Clairmont R, Neill P, McGorty R and Robertson-Anderson R M 2022 OpTiDDM (Optical Tweezers integrating Differential Dynamic Microscopy) maps the spatiotemporal propagation of nonlinear stresses in polymer blends and composites *Nat. Commun.* **13** 5180

Peddireddy K R, Michieletto D, Aguirre G, Garamella J, Khanal P and Robertson-Anderson R M 2021 DNA conformation dictates strength and flocculation in DNA–microtubule composites *ACS Macro Lett.* **10** 1540–8

Plotnikov S V, Sabass B, Schwarz U S and Waterman C M 2014 High-resolution traction force microscopy ed J C Waters and T Wittman *Methods in Cell Biology, Quantitative Imaging in Cell Biology* (New York: Academic) ch 20 pp 367–94

Quirin S, Pavani S R P and Piestun R 2012 Optimal 3D single-molecule localization for superresolution microscopy with aberrations and engineered point spread functions *Proc. Natl. Acad. Sci.* **109** 675–9

Rawat N and Biswas P 2009 Size, shape, and flexibility of proteins and DNA *J. Chem. Phys.* **131** 165104

Regan K, Wulstein D, Rasmussen H, McGorty R and Robertson-Anderson R M 2019 Bridging the spatiotemporal scales of macromolecular transport in crowded biomimetic systems *Soft Matter* **15** 1200–9

Reverey J F, Jeon J-H, Bao H, Leippe M, Metzler R and Selhuber-Unkel C 2015 Superdiffusion dominates intracellular particle motion in the supercrowded cytoplasm of pathogenic acanthamoeba castellanii *Sci. Rep.* **5** 11690

Richards J A, Martinez V A and Arlt J 2021 Characterising shear-induced dynamics in flowing complex fluids using differential dynamic microscopy *Soft Matter* **17** 8838–49

Richards J A, Martinez V A and Arlt J 2021 Exploring particle dynamics in flowing complex fluids using differential dynamic microscopy ArXiv: 210712946 Cond-Mat

Ringnér M 2008 What is principal component analysis? *Nat. Biotechnol.* **26** 303–4

Robertson C and Robertson S C 2012 Theory and practical recommendations for autocorrelation-based image correlation spectroscopy *J. Biomed. Opt.* **17** 080801

Rogers S S, Waigh T A, Zhao X and Lu J R 2007 Precise particle tracking against a complicated background: polynomial fitting with Gaussian weight *Phys. Biol.* **4** 220

Rose K A, Molaei M, Boyle M J, Lee D, Crocker J C and Composto R J 2020 Particle tracking of nanoparticles in soft matter *J. Appl. Phys.* **PGNP** 191101

Rowlands C J and So P T C 2013 On the correction of errors in some multiple particle tracking experiments *Appl. Phys. Lett.* **102** 021913

Rust M J, Bates M and Zhuang X 2006 Sub-diffraction-limit imaging by stochastic optical reconstruction microscopy (STORM) *Nat. Methods* **3** 793–6

Schindelin J *et al* 2012 Fiji: an open-source platform for biological-image analysis *Nat. Methods* **9** 676–82

Schröder A and Schanz D 2023 3D lagrangian particle tracking in fluid mechanics *Annu. Rev. Fluid Mech.* **55** 511–40

Seara D S, Yadav V, Linsmeier I, Tabatabai A P, Oakes P W, Tabei S M A, Banerjee S and Murrell M P 2018 Entropy production rate is maximized in non-contractile actomyosin *Nat. Commun.* **9** 4948

Sentjabrskaja T, Zaccarelli E, De Michele C, Sciortino F, Tartaglia P, Voigtmann T, Egelhaaf S U and Laurati M 2016 Anomalous dynamics of intruders in a crowded environment of mobile obstacles *Nat. Commun.* **7** 11133

Sharonov A and Hochstrasser R M 2006 Wide-field subdiffraction imaging by accumulated binding of diffusing probes *Proc. Natl. Acad. Sci.* **103** 18911–6

Shechtman Y, Weiss L E, Backer A S, Sahl S J and Moerner W E 2015 Precise three-dimensional scan-free multiple-particle tracking over large axial ranges with tetrapod point spread functions *Nano Lett.* **15** 4194–9

Sheung J Y *et al* 2021 Motor-driven restructuring of cytoskeleton composites leads to tunable time-varying elasticity *ACS Macro Lett.* **10** 1151–8

Sheung J Y, Garamella J, Kahl S K, Lee B Y, McGorty R J and Robertson-Anderson R M 2022 Motor-driven advection competes with crowding to drive spatiotemporally heterogeneous transport in cytoskeleton composites *Front. Phys.* **10** 1055441

Shin S, Dorfman K D and Cheng X 2017 Shear-banding and superdiffusivity in entangled polymer solutions *Phys. Rev.* E **96** 062503

Shlens J 2014 A tutorial on principal component *Analysis*

Singh R K, Mahato J, Chowdhury A, Sain A and Nandi A 2020 Non-Gaussian subdiffusion of single-molecule tracers in a hydrated polymer network *J. Chem. Phys.* **152** 024903

Sokolov I M 2012 Models of anomalous diffusion in crowded environments *Soft Matter* **8** 9043–52

Squires T M and Mason T G 2010 Fluid mechanics of microrheology *Annu. Rev. Fluid Mech.* **42** 413–38

Stam S, Freedman S L, Banerjee S, Weirich K L, Dinner A R and Gardel M L 2017 Filament rigidity and connectivity tune the deformation modes of active biopolymer networks *Proc. Natl. Acad. Sci.* **114** E10037–45

Starrs L and Bartlett P 2002 One- and two-point micro-rheology of viscoelastic media *J. Phys. Condens. Matter* **15** S251

Stuhrmann B, Soares e Silva M, Depken M, MacKintosh F C and Koenderink G H 2012 Nonequilibrium fluctuations of a remodeling *in vitro* cytoskeleton *Phys. Rev.* E **86** 020901

Toprak E, Balci H, Blehm B H and Selvin P R 2007 Three-dimensional particle tracking via bifocal imaging *Nano Lett.* **7** 2043–5

Toyota T, Head D A, Schmidt C F and Mizuno D 2011 Non-Gaussian athermal fluctuations in active gels *Soft Matter* **7** 3234–9

Tseng Y and Wirtz D 2001 Mechanics and multiple-particle tracking microheterogeneity of α-actinin-cross-linked actin filament networks *Biophys. J.* **81** 1643–56

Tychinskii V P 2007 Dynamic phase microscopy: is a 'dialogue' with the cell possible? *Phys.-Uspekhi* **50** 513

Vallotton P, van Oijen A M, Whitchurch C B, Gelfand V, Yeo L, Tsiavaliaris G, Heinrich S, Dultz E, Weis K and Grünwald D 2017 Diatrack particle tracking software: review of applications and performance evaluation *Traffic* **18** 840–52

Varga Z and Swan J W 2018 Large scale anisotropies in sheared colloidal gels *J. Rheol.* **62** 405–18

Verwei H N, Lee G, Leech G, Petitjean I I, Koenderink G H, Robertson-Anderson R M and McGorty R J 2022 Quantifying cytoskeleton dynamics using differential dynamic microscopy *J. Vis. Exp.* **15** e63931

Walker L M and Wagner N J 1996 SANS analysis of the molecular order in poly(γ-benzyl l-glutamate)/deuterated dimethylformamide (PBLG/d-DMF) under shear and during relaxation *Macromolecules* **29** 2298–301

Wang B, Anthony S M, Bae S C and Granick S 2009 Anomalous yet Brownian *Proc. Natl. Acad. Sci.* **106** 15160–4

Wang B, Kuo J, Bae S C and Granick S 2012 When Brownian diffusion is not Gaussian *Nat. Mater.* **11** 481–5

Weeks E and Crocker J M n.d. *Particle tracking using IDL* https://physics.emory.edu/faculty/weeks/idl/

Weigand W J, Messmore A, Tu J, Morales-Sanz A, Blair D L, Deheyn D D, Urbach J S and Robertson-Anderson R M 2017 Active microrheology determines scale-dependent material properties of chaetopterus mucus *PLoS One* **12** e0176732

Weirich K L, Dasbiswas K, Witten T A, Vaikuntanathan S and Gardel M L 2019 Self-organizing motors divide active liquid droplets *Proc. Natl. Acad. Sci.* **116** 11125–30

Wu K-T, Hishamunda J B, Chen D T N, DeCamp S J, Chang Y-W, Fernández-Nieves A, Fraden S and Dogic Z 2017 Transition from turbulent to coherent flows in confined three-dimensional active fluids *Science* **355** eaal1979

Wulstein D M, Regan K E, Garamella J, McGorty R J and Robertson-Anderson R M 2019 Topology-dependent anomalous dynamics of ring and linear DNA are sensitive to cytoskeleton crosslinking *Sci. Adv.* **5** eaay5912

Zheng G, Kolner C and Yang C 2011 Microscopy refocusing and dark-field imaging by using a simple LED array *Opt. Lett.* **36** 3987–9

Zia R N 2018 Active and passive microrheology: theory and simulation *Annu. Rev. Fluid Mech.* **50** 371–405

IOP Publishing

Biopolymer Networks
Design, dynamics and discovery
Rae M Robertson-Anderson

Chapter 5

Biopolymer network design, dynamics, and mechanics

In this chapter, I review the design and properties of several widely-studied biopolymer networks, classified by the properties of the biopolymers, their interactions, and overall network morphology. I focus on networks of flexible DNA, semiflexible actin filaments, rigid microtubules, and heterogenous intermediate filaments. However, many of the general design principles and properties are broadly transferrable to other biopolymer networks. I cover mechanical and structural properties as well as design considerations. Some of the details I provide may be redundant with those from chapters 1 and 2. This redundancy is purposeful and intended to provide reinforcement of important points.

5.1 DNA solutions: from dilute to highly entangled

5.1.1 DNA as a model polymer—visualizing the reptation model

Pierre Gilles de Gennes won the 1991 Nobel Prize in Physics for the reptation model and blob theory that he pioneered in the 1970s (figure 5.1(A)) (de Gennes 1979, de Gennes 2003), which I discuss in chapters 1 and 2. However, at that time no one had actually witnessed the proposed reptation of an entangled polymer or de Gennes' proposed tube. Researchers instead relied on bulk rheology and dynamic light scattering measurements to validate the theory based on predicted relations between the properties of the individual polymers and the bulk rheology (Doi and Edwards 1988, Rubinstein and Colby 2003). In 1994, this feat was accomplished by researchers using optical tweezers to drag a fluorescent-labeled DNA molecule through an entangled DNA solution in the shape of an R (for reptation), stretching it beyond its native primitive path length L_0 in the process (Perkins *et al* 1994a). After pulling the DNA into the R shape, they allowed the DNA to relax from its entropically-stretched state, with an extended length $L > L_0$, back to its native state with length L_0. What they found was that the DNA relaxed in a direction nearly

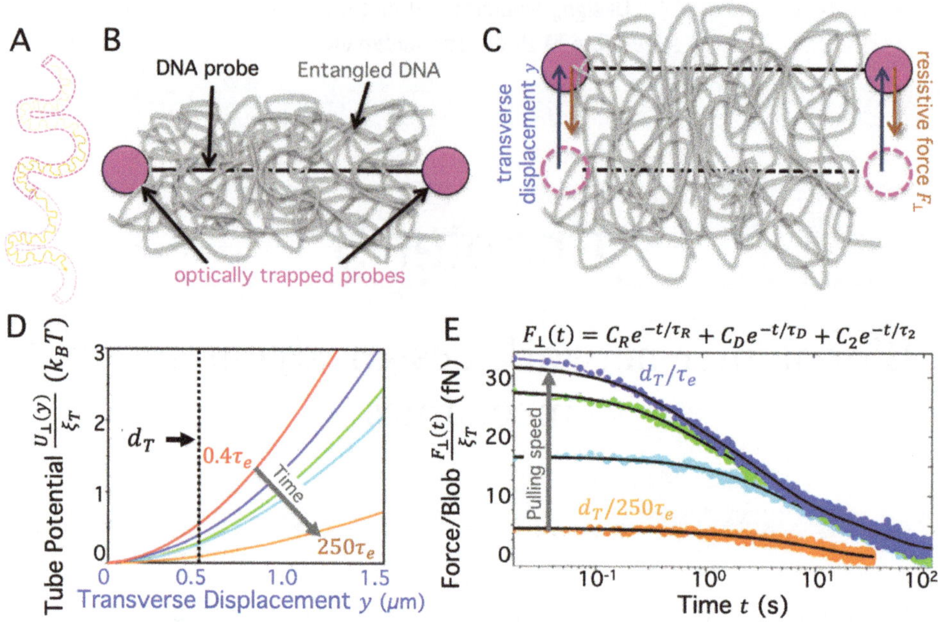

Figure 5.1. Direct evidence and measurement of reptation and tube confinement using entangled DNA. (A) Cartoon of an entangled polymer undergoing reptation within a tube (magenta) formed by the surrounding entangling polymers. (B–E) In Robertson and Smith (2007a), a 25 kbp DNA polymer was (B) attached at either end to optically trapped probes and (C) pulled transverse to its x-aligned contour through a displacement y (blue) while the force $F_\perp(y)$ resisting the displacement (orange) was measured. (D) The confining potential $U_\perp(y)$ associated with the theoretical entanglement tube, computed via equation (5.1), was shown to be quadratic with an effective tube diameter d_T (dashed vertical line) defined in equation (5.2). Counter to the traditional tube model, but in line with more recent predictions, the potential was shown to widen or 'dilate' over time from $0.4\tau_e$ (red) to $250\tau_e$ (orange) (Zhou and Larson 2006). (E) The relaxation of the confining force per blob $F_\perp(t)/\xi_T$ over time t following the transverse strain was measured for varying pulling speeds ranging from $\sim\frac{d_T}{250\tau_e}$ (orange) to $\frac{d_T}{\tau_e}$ (blue) indicated by the grey arrow. All relaxation curves were well described by a sum of three exponentials with well-separated time constants τ_R, τ_2, τ_D as displayed above the plot. The measured timescales correlate with predicted timescales for elastic Rouse relaxation with $\tau_1 \simeq 0.45$ s $\simeq \tau_R$, tube disengagement via reptation with $\tau_3 \simeq 34$ s $\simeq \tau_D$, and a non-classical process of initial tube stretching and lateral shrinking followed by recoil and re-expansion with $\tau_2 \simeq 5.4$ s. (D, E) Adapted with permission from Robertson and Smith (2007a). Copyright (2007) by the American Physical Society.

entirely along its backbone, as if recoiling within a tube aligned parallel with its contour—exactly as predicted by de Gennes.

Since that seminal work, DNA has been extensively investigated as a model system to probe open questions in polymer physics, as I describe in chapter 1 (Pecora 1991, Schroeder *et al* 2004, Robertson and Smith 2007a, 2007b, Teixeira *et al* 2007, Pan *et al* 2014, Chapman and Robertson-Anderson 2014, Pan *et al* 2014, Regan *et al* 2016, Hsiao *et al* 2017, Khan *et al* 2019, Zhou *et al* 2019, Soh and Doyle 2020, Banik *et al* 2021, Kong *et al* 2022).

For example, in 2007, the transverse confining potential $U_\perp(y)$ associated with the theoretical tube was directly measured by using dual optical tweezers to pull an entangled strand of DNA in a direction transverse to its contour and measure the force $F_{\perp}(y)$ resisting the displacement (Robertson and Smith 2007a) (figures 5.1(B) and (C)). Integrating $F(y)$, which scaled linearly with y

$$F_{\perp}(y) \sim y \tag{5.1}$$

as expected for an elastic (Hookean) restoring force, provided a confinement tube potential $U(y)$ that the surrounding entanglements imposed on the DNA (figure 5.1(D)):

$$U_{\perp}(y) = \int F_{\perp}(y)dy \tag{5.2}$$

This transverse potential was quadratic, as expected for an elastic potential

$$U_{\perp}(y) \sim y^2 \tag{5.3}$$

From the potential, the tube diameter d_T can be defined as the displacement y at which the potential per unit polymer segment, i.e., thermal blob of size ξ_T, is comparable to the thermal energy k_BT

$$U_{\perp}(d_T)/\xi_T = k_BT \tag{5.4}$$

It follows that the probability distribution of transverse displacements $P_{\perp}(y)$ of an entangled polymer from its primitive path (Zhou and Larson 2006, Wang *et al* 2010)

$$P_{\perp}(y) = P_0 e^{-U_{\perp}(y)/k_BT} \tag{5.5}$$

combined with the definition

$$P_{\perp}(d_T) = e^{-1} \tag{5.6}$$

(see equation (5.2)), yields the expression

$$P_{\perp}(y) = P_0 e^{-y^2/d_T^2} \tag{5.7}$$

as also predicted in Zhou and Larson (2006) and Wang *et al* (2010).

Importantly, not captured in equations (5.1)–(5.7), is the finding that the tube potential weakens over time (figure 5.1(D)) (Zhou and Larson 2006, Robertson and Smith 2007a, Wang *et al* 2010), indicative of the predicted dilation of the confinement tube, but at odds with classical reptation theory, as I discuss in chapter 2.

The same study described above (Robertson and Smith 2007a), demonstrated that a single entangled DNA strand relaxes stress over three distinct timescales that align with the classically-predicted Rouse time τ_R and disengagement time τ_D (Doi and Edwards 1988), as well as an intermediate non-classical timescale τ_2 (Mhetar and Archer 1999). Specifically, the force relaxation data was well described by a sum of three exponential decays

$$F_{\perp}(t) = C_1 e^{-t/\tau_1} + C_2 e^{-t/\tau_2} + C_3 e^{-t/\tau_3} \tag{5.8}$$

where τ_i is the characteristic relaxation timescale associated with each term, $\tau_1 \simeq 0.45$ s, $\tau_2 \simeq 5.4$ s $\tau_3 \simeq 34$ s, and τ_1 and τ_3 align with predicted values for, respectively, the Rouse time and disengagement time, $\tau_R \simeq 0.6$ s and $\tau_D \simeq 40$ s (figure 5.1(E)) (Robertson and Smith 2007a). The intermediate timescale τ_2 is in line with predictions of a non-classical process of initial tube stretching and lateral shrinking followed by recoil and re-expansion, which occur over a timescale $\tau_R < \tau_2 < \tau_D$ (Mhetar and Archer 1999).

The prefactors C_i for each term provide a measure of the relative contribution c_i of each process to the overall relaxation

$$c_i = C_i/\sum C_i \tag{5.9}$$

where $\sum c_i = 1$. For the data in figure 5.1(E), each term contributes equally to the relaxation, such that $c_1 \approx c_2 \approx c_3 \approx \frac{1}{3}$ (Robertson and Smith 2007a).

5.1.2 Advantages to using DNA

Beyond the facile ability to fluorescent-label and visualize DNA, another advantageous feature compared to synthetic polymers for investigating questions in polymer physics is its 'thinness'. DNA has a diameter $d \simeq 2$ nm and Kuhn length $l_k \simeq 100$ nm, allowing DNA chains to form substantial entanglements while still comprising very modest volume fractions (e.g., <1%) in solution (Chapman and Robertson-Anderson 2014). In contrast, the smaller aspect ratio of synthetic polymers often requires that they be in melt phase (no solvent) to achieve sufficient entanglement densities. This requirement limits the ability of synthetic polymer studies to test predicted scaling relations between polymer concentration and experimentally measured properties such as diffusion coefficients, relaxation timescales, and the elastic plateau modulus G^0, as I describe in chapter 2 (Doi and Edwards 1988).

DNA is able to overcome this challenge to directly test predictions and reveal new scaling relations between dynamic properties and network concentration (Hur *et al* 2001, Heo and Larson 2005, Robertson and Smith 2007b, Teixeira *et al* 2007, Bravo-Anaya *et al* 2016, Hsiao *et al* 2017, Pan *et al* 2018, Peddireddy *et al* 2020b). This feature also allows researchers to conduct measurements at concentrations that span the poorly-understood crossover regimes between dilute ($c \ll c^*$), semidilute unentangled ($c^* < c < c_e$), and entangled dynamics ($c > c_e$) (Schroeder *et al* 2004, Robertson and Smith 2007b, Pan *et al* 2014, Peddireddy *et al* 2020b).

The lengths of DNA molecules can also be precisely controlled down to the basepair ($l_{bp} \simeq 0.34$ nm), and the replication process to extract and purify specified DNA constructs from cells results in highly monodisperse samples with all of the DNA polymers being the exact same length, programmed by their sequence (Laib *et al* 2006). Conversely, all samples of synthetic polymers have a polydispersity index above 1 that results from the synthesis process (Kumar *et al* 2014, Bellone *et al* 2015, Li *et al* 2019).

5.1.3 Design considerations

As I discuss in chapter 1, an important consideration when working with DNA is its negative charge density of $\frac{Q}{L} = -2e$ bp^{-1} in solution. To avoid complications of charge interactions, it is common practice to include NaCl to screen the negative charge, such that DNA can be treated as a neutral flexible polymer with an effective diameter d^* that depends on the salt concentration [NaCl]. Predictions for d^*[NaCl] (Toan and Micheletti 2006), that align with experimental observations (Robertson *et al* 2006), are shown in figure 5.2.

The concentration and valency of the salts included in the solvent also affect the persistence length, as shown in figures 2.1(A) and 5.2, and demonstrated in Marko and Siggia (1995), Toan and Micheletti (2006), Manning (2006), and Guilbaud *et al* (2019), as well as the degree of swelling and self-avoidance of the random coil (Maarel 2008, Pan *et al* 2014). At [NaCl] $\approx$ 10 mM, DNA is considered to be in good solvent conditions with appreciable exclude volume effects and self-avoidance (Robertson *et al* 2006, Pan *et al* 2014, Banik *et al* 2021). At higher salt concentrations, [NaCl] $>$ 50 mM, DNA has a smaller effective diameter, due to stronger charge screening (figure 5.2) so is more accurately modeled as a non-swollen ideal coil in theta solvent conditions (Pecora 1991, Pan *et al* 2014, 2018). In the limit of very low salt concentrations, the polyelectrolyte nature of the DNA must be taken into account, as in Maarel (2008), Stevens *et al* (2012) and Pan *et al* (2014).

DNA of sufficient length, $L \gtrsim 5$ kbp, $N \gtrsim 50$, have been shown to behave as flexible rather than semiflexible polymers (Pecora 1991, Robertson *et al* 2006, Robertson and Smith 2007b, Banik *et al* 2021). However, the length at which DNA can be considered flexible is still debated (Tree *et al* 2013). In the long-chain limit, DNA can be reasonably modeled as a freely-jointed or bead-spring chain. However, for shorter DNA chains, $L \lesssim 2$ kbp, $N \lesssim 20$, the semiflexible nature of DNA manifests and the worm-like chain model is necessary to accurately model dynamics (Aragon and Pecora 1985, Marko and Siggia 1995, Kroy and Frey 1996, Tree *et al* 2013).

Most of the commercially available DNA constructs are supercoiled plasmids with lengths $L < 10$ kbp ($N < 30$), which are prohibitively small to form appreciable entanglements in soluble conditions (Mason *et al* 1998, Robertson and Smith 2007b, Bravo-Anaya *et al* 2016). They are also too small to easily visualize using fluorescence microscopy as their coil sizes are below the optical resolution limit

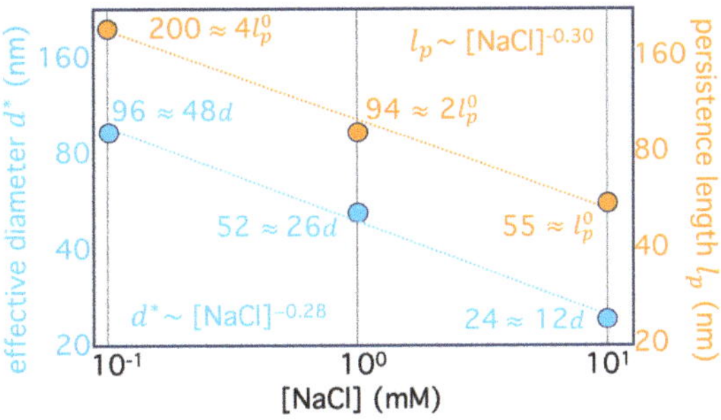

Figure 5.2. Effect of counterions on the width and stiffness of DNA. Predicted values from Toan and Micheletti (2006) for the effective diameter d^* (cyan) and persistence length l_p (orange) of dsDNA as a function of molar concentration of NaCl. The values corresponding to each data point are listed in units of nm as well as units of the native DNA diameter $d \simeq 2$ nm (cyan) or standard assumed DNA persistence length $l_p^0 \simeq 50$ nm in experimental conditions (orange). The power-law scalings of the two lengthscales with salt concentration, as listed, are remarkably close to one another.

(though super-resolution microscopy can detect these molecules (Huang *et al* 2010)), and cannot be treated as model polymers due to their stiffness, as described above (Tree *et al* 2013). Finally, because most purified DNA constructs are plasmids that are supercoiled or relaxed circular, they must be treated with a site-specific restriction endonuclease to convert them to linear chains (if desired). This process requires knowing the DNA sequence so the proper restriction endonuclease can be chosen (Laib *et al* 2006) using digestion map software such as the New England BioLabs NEBCutter ('NEBcutter 3.0,' n.d.).

The most widely-used commercially available DNA construct that meets the required length and topology requirements to investigate biopolymer dynamics is λ-DNA (Pecora 1991, Perkins *et al* 1994a, 1994b, Schroeder *et al* 2003, Boukany *et al* 2010, Regan *et al* 2016, Hsiao *et al* 2017, Banik *et al* 2021, Kong *et al* 2022), which is a 48.5 kbp ($L \simeq 16\ \mu$m, $N \simeq 162$) linear chain, typically supplied at 50 ng μL^{-1}. Calf thymus DNA is another viable commercial construct (Bravo-Anaya *et al* 2016, Mason *et al* 1998), which is supplied as a polydisperse solution of linear chains of lengths ~10–13 kbp ($L \simeq 3.3$–$4.3\ \mu$m, $N \simeq 33$–43).

To expand the available options of DNA amenable to polymer dynamics investigations, researchers developed a library of DNA constructs with lengths ranging from 6 kbp to 115 kbp that can be replicated in *Escherichia coli* and purified via scaled-up lysis and purification protocols, as described in Laib *et al* (2006). This 'home-grown' DNA, available freely to any researcher upon request, affords the opportunity to measure bulk rheological properties and examine length dependence without the prohibitive costs of purchasing large quantities of commercially available DNA. The DNA sequences were also carefully screened to allow for linearization of the circular constructs with cost-effective and widely-available restriction endonucleases, including BamHI, ApaI, and MluI (Laib *et al* 2006).

To visualize DNA molecules, researchers typically use high-quantum-yield intercalating dyes such as YOYO-I, TOTO-3, and others in this trademarked family from Molecular Probes (see table 3.1), to uniformly label the DNA backbone at dye: basepair ratios of ~1:3–1:10 (Robertson *et al* 2006, Chapman *et al* 2015, Garamella *et al* 2020). This labeling density does not alter the DNA conformation or flexibility, but does increase L and l_p by ~35%, which needs to be considered in measurements (Smith *et al* 1996).

An alternative labeling method is to use covalent dyes, such as Mirus Label IT linkers, that covalently and non-specifically attach fluorophores such as MFP488, Cy3, Cy5, rhodamine, and fluorescein to nucleic acids along the DNA backbone ('Label IT nucleic acid labeling reagents—research reagent products,' n.d.). The photostability during measurements, as well as the stability of the labeled DNA, is greatly improved over intercalating dyes; and lower labeling ratios (~1:20–1:50) as compared to intercalating dyes, can achieve the same signal-to-noise (Aporvari *et al* 2022). To resolve single DNA molecules within entangled and dense networks, researchers typically include only a trace amount of labeled DNA, <1% of the overall DNA concentration, such that each labeled molecule is separated by several $\sim R_G$. However, this concentration depends on the desired microscopy modality and analysis methods, as I describe in chapters 3 and 4. For example, sparse labeling is necessary for accurate single-molecule tracking, while DDM measurements benefit from more signal and do not require single labeled molecules to be isolated from one another (Regan *et al* 2019).

5.1.4 Network dynamics

Many papers have been published over the past few decades on the polymer physics of DNA, including several exhaustive review articles, such as Pecora (1991), Maarel (2008), Tree *et al* (2013), Regan *et al* (2016), Banik *et al* (2021). For the purposes of this text, I will not discuss studies examining single-chain dynamics or dilute solution dynamics, but will instead focus on the current understanding of the physics of networks of overlapping and entangled DNA.

The critical entanglement concentration for DNA, i.e., the concentration at which entanglement dynamics manifest, has been measured to be $c_e \simeq 4\text{–}9c^*$ depending on the solvent conditions (figures 5.3(A)–(C)) (Banik *et al* 2021, Robertson *et al* 2006). Below this critical concentration, but still above the overlap concentration c^*, solutions of linear DNA of lengths 11–115 kbp have been reported to exhibit concentration-dependent diffusion coefficients with scaling $D \sim c^{-1/2}$ (figure 5.3(A)), and modest shear thinning of $\eta^* \sim \omega^{-1/2}$ (figure 5.2(B)), both in line with Rouse model predictions (Rouse 1953, Doi and Edwards 1988, Robertson *et al* 2006, Chapman *et al* 2014). Linear viscoelastic moduli also largely exhibit terminal regime behavior with $G'' \sim \omega^1 > G' \sim \omega^2$ scaling for most of the frequency range, with scaling weakening and G' approaching G'' at higher frequencies (figures 5.3(C) and (D)) (Chapman *et al* 2014, Banik *et al* 2021).

For $c > c_e$, solutions of linear DNA exhibit key predicted signatures of entanglements, such as diffusion coefficient scaling $D \sim c^{-7/4}$ (figure 5.3(A)) and shear thinning $\eta^* \sim \omega^{-x}$ with exponents of $x \simeq 0.6\text{–}1$ (figures 5.3(B) and (E)) (Doi and Edwards 1988, Rubinstein and Colby 2003, Chapman *et al* 2014, Chapman and Robertson-Anderson 2014). Both bulk rheology and OTM measurements display entanglement regime rheology in the linear regime, in which the viscoelastic moduli crossover at $\omega_c = 2\pi/\tau_D$ from the terminal regime to an extended rubbery plateau regime where $G' \simeq G^0 \sim \omega^0$ (figures 5.3(C) and (D)). Plateau modulus values of $G^0 \simeq 0.1\text{–}20$ Pa have been reported, following empirical scaling relations $G^0 \sim c^y$ with $y \simeq 2\text{–}2.3$ (Banik *et al* 2021, Khanal *et al* 2022) and $G^0 \sim L^0$ (figure 5.3(D)) (Chapman *et al* 2014). From measured ω_c values, disengagement times of $\tau_D \simeq 10^0\text{–}10^4$ s have been reported, which strongly depend on the entanglement density $Z = L/l_e$ and may be impacted by non-classical mechanisms described in chapter 2, such as contour length fluctuations (CLF), tube dilation, and constraint release. For example, for modestly entangled DNA solutions ($Z \lesssim 10$), bulk rheology measurements have shown that contour length fluctuations can reduce τ_D by nearly three orders of magnitude (Khanal *et al* 2022).

Constant-rate straining and relaxation measurements using optical tweezers microrheology (OTM), described in chapter 3, can also be used to directly measure the disengagement time τ_D, as well as faster relaxation timescales such as the

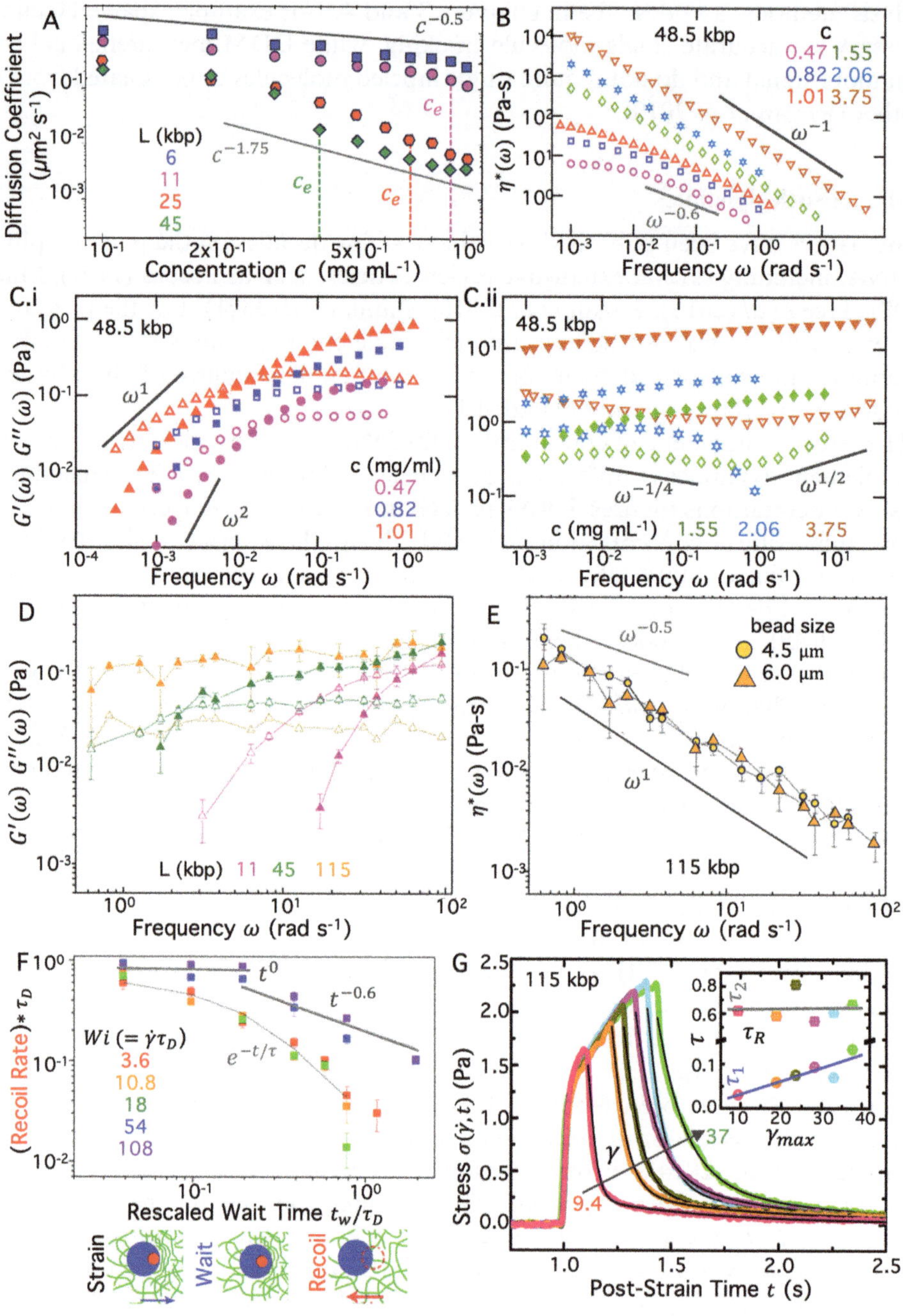

Figure 5.3. Dynamics and rheology of semidilute and entangled DNA solutions. (A) Diffusion coefficients of linear DNA of varying lengths L (kbp) follow power-law scaling with DNA concentration in line with predictions from the Rouse model ($D \sim c^{-0.5}$) or reptation model ($D \sim c^{-1.75}$) with a crossover between the two scalings indicating the critical entanglement concentration $c_e \approx 6c^*$. Adapted with permission from Robertson and Smith (2007b). Copyright (2007) American Chemical Society. (B and C) Bulk rheology measurements for 48.5 kbp λ DNA at varying concentrations exhibit (B) complex viscosities that display shear thinning $\eta^* \sim \omega^{-x}$ with exponents x that increase from $x \simeq 0.6$ to $x \simeq 1$ with increasing concentration.

Adapted with permission from Banik *et al* (2021). Copyright (2021) American Chemical Society. (C) Linear viscoelastic moduli, $G'(\omega)$ and $G''(\omega)$ that follow (C.i) terminal regime scaling ($G' \sim \omega^2$; $G'' \sim \omega^1$) at low frequencies and concentrations and (C.ii) reptation model scaling ($G' \sim \omega^0$; $G'' \sim \omega^{-1/4}$, $G'' \sim \omega^{1/2}$) at high frequencies and concentrations. Adapted with permission from Banik *et al* (2021). Copyright (2021) American Chemical Society. (D–G) Optical tweezers microrheology measurements for 1 mg mL^{-1} solutions of DNA of varying lengths (listed in each plot). (D) $G'(\omega)$ and $G''(\omega)$ cross over from terminal regime to entanglement regime scaling, reaching a length-independent plateau modulus of $G^0 \approx 0.2$ Pa at high frequencies. (E) Complex viscosities exhibit shear thinning $\eta^* \sim \omega^{-1}$ in line with tube model predictions and independent of bead probe size. (F) Non-classical relaxation dynamics of 45 kbp linear DNA following fast (nonlinear) strains (Weissenberg number $Wi > 20$; purple, blue), measured from the elastic recoil of a bead released from an optical trap (depicted in the cartoon), follows two-phase power-law decay with time, scaling as t^0 and $t^{-0.6}$. Recoil dynamics following slower (linear) strains ($Wi < 20$; red, orange, green) exhibit classical exponential decay $e^{-t/\tau}$ with time. (G) The stress relaxation profiles following nonlinear (large, fast) oscillatory strains ($\gamma = 9.4$–37; red to green) are well described by a sum of two exponentials with time constants (see inset) that correlate with a strain-independent Rouse time $\tau_2 \simeq \tau_R \sim \gamma_{\max}^0$ and a faster time $\tau_1 \sim \gamma_{\max}^1$ associated with the trapping force. (D, E) Adapted with permission from Chapman *et al* (2014). Copyright (2014) American Chemical Society. (F) Adapted with permission from Chapman and Robertson-Anderson (2014). Copyright (2014) by the American Physical Society. (G) Adapted with permission from Khan *et al* (2019). Copyright (2019) by the American Physical Society.

entanglement time τ_e and Rouse time τ_R. OTM measurements performed on DNA solutions with concentrations $c_e < c < 5c_e$ have reported relaxation times of $\tau_D \simeq 2$–40 s, $\tau_R \simeq 0.1$–0.6 s, and $\tau_e \simeq 10$–60 ms, depending on the DNA length and concentration (Chapman *et al* 2014, Chapman and Robertson-Anderson 2014, Khan *et al* 2019, Peddireddy *et al* 2020a, 2022). In response to nonlinear OTM strains, i.e., when the strain is fast enough and large enough to push the system far from steady-state, DNA solutions have been reported to relax imposed stress on faster timescales than the linear steady-state regime disengagement time τ_D due to non-classical mechanisms including tube dilation and convective constraint release (CCR) (Viovy *et al* 1991, Chapman and Robertson-Anderson 2014, Khan *et al* 2019, Peddireddy *et al* 2020a, Khanal *et al* 2022). As I describe in chapter 2, tube dilation arises from alignment of the polymers with the strain-induced flow, which decreases the local entanglement density Z and thus dilates or expands the tube diameter d_T (Viovy *et al* 1991). CCR, which also locally decreases Z, describes the strain-induced disentanglement or 'constraint release' of polymers surrounding the chain of interest, which facilitates disengagement and thus decreases τ_D in a manner that depends on the strain rate $\dot{\gamma}$ (Ianniruberto and Marrucci 2014).

Moreover, in the experiments described in figures 5.1(B)–(E), another non-classical relaxation mode, intermediate between τ_R and τ_D, was measured and attributed to the relaxation of the entanglement tube from a longitudinally stretched (and laterally shrunken) state back to its equilibrium length L_0 and diameter d_T, before the polymer can effectively relax stress via reptation (disengagement) (Mhetar and Archer 1999, Sussman and Schweizer 2013a).

The concept of a dynamic, time-dependent tube, that stretches, dilates, shrinks, and re-equilibrates over time, has also been suggested to give rise to two-phase power-law force relaxation measured for entangled 45 kbp linear DNA via non-linear OTM (figure 5.3(F)) (Chapman and Robertson-Anderson, 2014). In these studies, the probe was released from the optical trap following a wait time t_w after the strain and the rate of recoil of the probe was measured. Force relaxation profiles were determined by examining the dependence of the recoil rate—which should scale inversely with the disengagement time, (recoil rate $\sim \tau_D^{-1}$)—on the wait time. This analysis (figure 5.3(F)) revealed that entangled DNA solutions exhibited an initial period of minimal relaxation, recoil rate $\sim t^0$, followed by a power-law slowing of the relaxation with time, recoil rate $\sim \tau_D^{-1} \sim t^{-0.6}$.

Power-law relaxation indicates a spectrum of relaxation timescales that are not well-separated in time, in contrast to exponential decay in which the time constants report discrete, static relaxation times, as described above. In the measurements shown in figure 5.3(F), power-law decay is indicative of a spectrum of disengagement times $\tau_D(t)$ that arise from strain-induced tube dilation and subsequent healing. Specifically, $\tau_D(t)$ is initially shorter than that classically predicted, but steadily increases as the dilated tube shrinks back to its steady-state tube diameter d_T (Sussman and Schweizer 2013b, 2013a). The initial time-independent plateau is a result of competing effects of retraction of the stretched tube, which increases d_T, and shrinking of the dilated tube, which decreases d_T (Mhetar and Archer 1999, Sussman and Schweizer 2013a).

Finally, for certain nonlinear strain profiles, such as microscale large-amplitude oscillatory strains (MLAOS), the effect of CCR and tube dilation is substantial enough to effectively eliminate the need for disengagement to contribute to relaxation, such that the entangled DNA can completely relax its stress via Rouse relaxation modes (figure 5.3(G)) (Khan *et al* 2019).

5.2 Entangled and crosslinked actin networks

5.2.1 Actin as a model semiflexible polymer—visualizing the reptation model

Beyond their obvious biological relevance, networks of entangled actin filaments have been extensively studied for decades as a model system for probing questions in polymer physics (Isambert and Maggs 1996, Käs *et al* 1996, Everaers *et al* 1999, Hiraiwa and Ohta 2009, Broedersz and MacKintosh 2014), such as the nature of the tube confinement restricting the motion of entangled polymers (figure 5.4(A)) (Morse 1998, Hinsch *et al* 2007, Wang *et al* 2010), and the extent to which theoretical models, such as the Zimm model, Rouse model, and reptation model developed for flexible polymers need to be altered to describe semiflexible polymers with $l_p \approx L$ (Isambert and Maggs 1996, Sussman and Schweizer 2011, 2012).

In 1996, researchers used actin filaments to show the first direct evidence of tube confinement and reptation of a quiescent entangled polymer (Kas *et al* 1996) (figure 5.4(A)). The tube diameter and diffusion coefficient D_R associated with reptation was determined by visualizing fluorescent-labeled actin filaments embedded within entangled networks of unlabeled filaments, and analyzing their thermal fluctuations in directions perpendicular and parallel to the filament contour. Specifically, the tube diameter was quantified by measuring the transverse width of the distribution of filament contours from 64 successive images separated by $\Delta t = 0.1$ s. By performing this analysis for varying actin concentrations, researchers

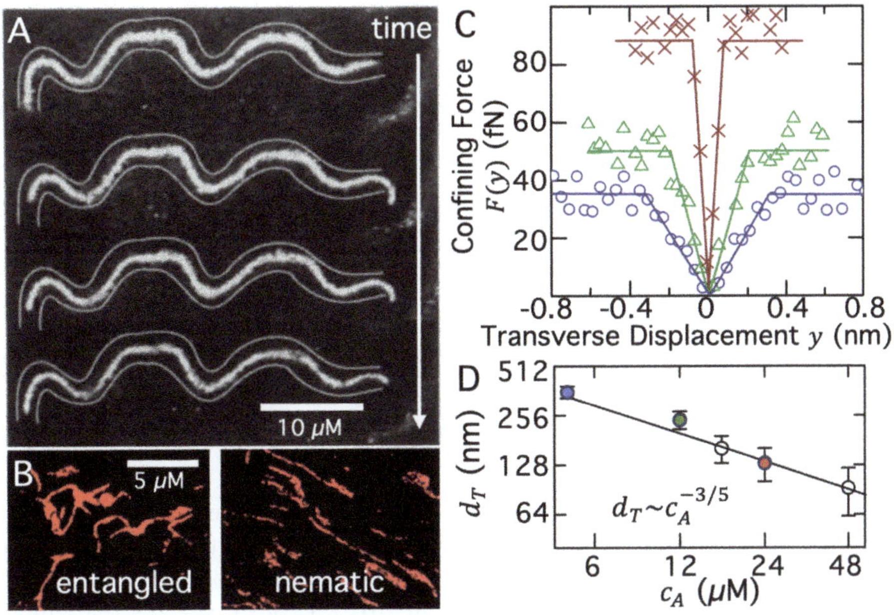

Figure 5.4. Actin as a model semiflexible polymer system to characterize tube-like confinement of entangled polymers. (A) A single fluorescent-labeled actin filament with $L \approx 40$ μm, entangled with unlabeled filaments at a concentration $c_A \simeq 48$ μM, is visualized using epifluorescence microscopy. From top to bottom are successive snapshots of the thermally fluctuating filament separated by $\Delta t = 8$ s. The images show the filament move to the right, partially leaving the initial tube, then moving back to the left. This slow diffusive process of reptation leads to a disengagement time of $\tau_D \simeq 61$ min measured for this filament. The outline is a guide to the eye to depict the theoretical confinement tube. (B) The same seminal study in (A) showed that actin filaments (red) can form isotropic entanglement networks (left) at concentrations of $c_A \simeq 2.4$–48 μM, and transition to nematic alignment (right) for $c_A > 48$ μM. In the images shown, a sparse number of filaments are labeled and embedded among networks of unlabeled filaments with $c_A \simeq 33$ μM (left) and $c_A \simeq 95$ μM (right). (C) The confining force $F_\perp(y)$ associated with the entanglement tube potential, computed from the distribution of transverse fluctuations of entangled actin filaments, following eqs. (5.14) and (5.15), for $c_A \simeq 4.8$ μM (blue), 12 μM (green), and 24 μM (red). The solid lines through the data show linear scaling $F_\perp(y) \sim y$ at small displacements and $F_\perp(y) \sim y^0$ at large displacements, indicative of a Hookean tube potential that softens at large displacements. (D) Entanglement tube diameter, determined from the same probability distribution $P_\perp(y)$ from which the data in (C) are computed, as a function of actin concentration c_A shows power-law scaling $d_T \sim c_A^{-3/5}$. The colored data points are computed from the corresponding data shown in C. (A, B) Adapted from Kas *et al* (1996). © 1996 by the Biophysical Society. (C, D) Adapted with permission from Wang *et al* (2010). Copyright (2010) by the American Physical Society.

revealed a power-law scaling relation $d_T \sim c^{-3/5}$, which has been verified in several subsequent works (Isambert and Maggs 1996, Wang *et al* 2010, Gurmessa *et al* 2016a).

The curvilinear diffusion coefficient D_R associated with reptation was determined by analyzing the correlated motion of the chain ends, which revealed a universal scaling relation with filament contour length $D_R \sim L^{-1}$. This scaling differs from the reptation model scaling $D_R \sim L^{-2}$ for flexible chains (Doi and Edwards 1988), and is a consequence of the different lengthscales over which chains of different flexibilities are assumed to reptate over the disengagement time τ_D.

Specifically, if we start with the universal relations:

$$D_R \sim L_0^2/\tau_D \tag{5.10}$$

$$\tau_D \sim L^3 \tag{5.11}$$

and consider the l_p-dependent relations

$$L_0 \sim R_G \sim L^{1/2} \quad (l_p \ll L) \tag{5.12a}$$

$$L_0 \sim L \quad (l_p \sim L) \tag{5.12b}$$

it follows that

$$D_R \sim L^{-2} \quad (l_p \ll L) \tag{5.13a}$$

$$D_R \sim L^{-1} \quad (l_p \sim L) \tag{5.13b}$$

as shown in Isambert and Maggs (1996).

Building on this seminal work (Kas *et al* 1996), researchers used similar image analysis methods to measure the probability distribution of transverse fluctuations $P_\perp(y)$ of entangled actin filaments from their primitive paths for varying actin concentrations ($c_A \simeq 4.8$–$48\ \mu$M) (Wang *et al* 2010). From $P_\perp(y)$, the confining tube potential was computed via equation (5.3):

$$U_\perp(y) = -k_BT \ln(P_\perp(y)/P_0) \tag{5.14}$$

and the corresponding restoring force computed from the derivative

$$F_\perp(y) = dU_\perp(y)/dy \tag{5.15}$$

As shown in figure 5.4(C), this restoring force is of similar magnitude as values reported for entangled DNA (figure 5.1(D)) and follows similar linear scaling, $F_\perp \sim y$ (Robertson and Smith 2007a). Moreover, the effective spring constant increased with increasing c_A, indicating a smaller tube diameter, as expected due to the increasing entanglement density. The corresponding concentration-dependent tube diameters, computed using equation (5.7), which establishes d_T as the characteristic lengthscale associated with a Gaussian probability distribution of displacements, exhibited comparable magnitudes and the same scaling relation $d_T \sim c^{-3/5}$ as previously reported (figure 5.4(D)) (Isambert and Maggs 1996, Kas *et al* 1996).

Importantly, researchers also reported non-classical softening of the tube potential at larger transverse displacements, similar to that reported in Robertson and Smith (2007a) and Li *et al* (2019) and manifested as a nearly y-independent force at larger y values (figure 5.4(C)). This phenomenon is consistent with tube dilation and spatiotemporal heterogeneities of the confining potential (Wang *et al* 2010).

5.2.2 Advantages to using actin

The unique semiflexibility of actin filaments, with $l_p \simeq 10\ \mu$m and $L \approx 1$–$40\ \mu$m, and the ability to uniformly fluorescent-label their backbone, similar to DNA, allows for direct visualization of a single extended polymer (figures 5.4(A) and (B)). In contrast, the backbone of an individual DNA molecule, which adopts a random coil conformation in solution, cannot be resolved using fluorescence microscopy, unless stretched under tension (Perkins *et al* 1994b, Laib *et al* 2006, Gorczyca *et al* 2015). This increased rigidity of actin filaments also significantly lengthens their relaxation timescales, as compared to DNA and other flexible polymers, such that their thermal fluctuations can be captured on experimentally accessible timescales, as demonstrated in the studies discussed above (figure 5.4) (Kas *et al* 1996, Wang *et al* 2010).

Another advantage to working with actin is its commercial availability from trusted companies such as Cytoskeleton, Inc., along with well-vetted preparation and handling protocols ('Pure actin, pyrene actin, fluorescent actin, rhodamine actin, pre-formed actin filaments,' n.d.). Commercially purified non-muscle actin is typically supplied as globular actin monomers, purified from rabbit skeletal tissue, that have been lyophilized with necessary salts and buffer reagents, rendering them stable at 4°C for several months and nearly indefinitely at −80°C. Reconstitution of lyophilized powders also allows for versatility in the actin concentration in solution and buffer conditions, as needed for different studies. Nevertheless, many researchers also purify actin 'in-house' from rabbit or chicken skeletal tissue, if they are equipped and expert in protein purification (Pardee and Aspudich 1982, Schafer *et al* 1998, Hansen *et al* 2013). In-house purification provides more versatility and control over the purity and allows researchers to use 'fresh' actin (i.e., not lyophilized or previously frozen) which may improve its viability and ability to polymerize.

Finally, because of its extended conformation, actin filaments can form entangled networks at much lower concentrations than their flexible counterparts, providing a wide range of concentrations over which entanglement dynamics and corresponding scalings of network properties with concentration can be investigated. Specifically, actin filaments form isotropic entangled networks for over an order of magnitude of concentrations, $c_A \approx 2.4$–$60\ \mu\text{M}$ ($\rho_A \approx 0.1$–$2.5\ \text{mg mL}^{-1}$) (Kas *et al* 1996, Gardel *et al* 2003, 2008, Wang *et al* 2010, Gurmessa *et al* 2016a), with corresponding mesh sizes

$$\xi \simeq 0.3\rho_A^{-1/2} \tag{5.16}$$

where ρ_A has units of mg mL^{-1} and ξ is in μm.

Moreover, for concentrations $c_A \gtrsim 95\ \mu\text{M}$ ($\rho_A \gtrsim 4\ \text{mg mL}^{-1}$), actin filaments nematically align and form liquid crystal-like structures with a preferred 'director' direction that runs parallel with the filament contours (figure 5.4(B)) (Isambert and Maggs 1996, Kas *et al* 1996, Popp *et al* 2006, Viamontes *et al* 2006 Gardel *et al* 2008, Lai *et al* 2008). A co-existence regime with both entangled and nematic phases also emerges for $c_A \approx 60$–$95\ \mu\text{M}$ ($\rho_A \approx 2.5$–$4\ \text{mg mL}^{-1}$). This feature allows researchers to investigate the dynamics of polymeric nematics, the phase transition between isotropic and nematic regimes, and the effect of anisotropic organization on the dynamics (Popp *et al* 2006, Viamontes *et al* 2006, Gentry *et al* 2009, Zhang *et al* 2018).

5.2.3 Design considerations

Unlike DNA, in which the replication process to prepare concentrated solutions results in monodisperse solutions of polymers of exactly the same length, the polymerization of actin filaments from monomers results in a distribution of filament lengths (Kas *et al* 1996, Sept *et al* 1999, Gurmessa *et al* 2018). The length distribution is typically exponential or gamma distributed and can be quite broad, with an average filament length $\langle L \rangle$ that is expected to increase with actin concentration, based on the nucleation-elongation polymerization process I describe in chapter 1 (Pollard 1986, Fujiwara *et al* 2002). However, several studies have shown that the average filament length is unexpectedly robust to varying actin concentrations, attributed to the important contributions of filament annealing and fragmentation to the steady-state length distribution (Sept *et al* 1999, Gurmessa *et al* 2016a).

The filament length can be more precisely controlled using actin binding proteins (ABP), such as the capping and severing ABP gelsolin (Ermentrout and Edelstein-Keshet 1998, Ditsch and Wegner 1994). As I describe in chapter 1, gelsolin controls the filament length by capping actin nuclei and promoting polymerization from the capped nuclei, such that elongation proceeds nearly entirely from gelsolin-capped nuclei (Khaitlina and Hinssen 1997, Kasza *et al* 2010). As such, the number of filaments formed from a pool of monomers of concentration c_A equates to the number of gelsolin molecules, rendering the resulting filament length inversely related to the molar concentration of gelsolin c_G according to the relation

$$L_A \simeq (2.7 \text{ nm}) c_A / c_G \tag{5.17}$$

(Khaitlina and Hinssen 1997, Kasza *et al* 2010). This process also results in a much narrower distribution of filament lengths compared to polymerization without ABPs. The capping ABP CapZ, has also been shown to act in a similar fashion as gelsolin to control and shorten filament lengths (Xu *et al* 1999).

Moreover, as I describe in chapter 1, while actin filaments maintain steady-state lengths following polymerization, they undergo continuous ATP-fueled treadmilling, whereby monomers at the pointed and barbed ends continuously dissociate and bind, respectively, via ATP hydrolysis (see figure 1.2(F)). Because this process requires a constant supply of ATP, experiments on concentrated actin solutions should be performed with saturating ATP concentrations, typically >1 mM, to ensure steady-state filament lengths are maintained.

An alternative to ensure stable lengths of actin filaments and reduce the need to maintain a supply of ATP and optimized buffer conditions, is to stabilize actin filaments with phalloidin, a peptide that is toxic to cells due to its ability to stabilize actin filaments against depolymerization (Cooper 1987, Wendel and Dancker 1987). Phalloidin selectively binds to actin in filamentous form by binding at the interface between neighboring actin monomers comprising a filament, which prevents depolymerization and blocks ATP hydrolysis (Barden *et al* 1987, Wendel and Dancker 1987). Experiments that demonstrate successful actin stabilization via phalloidin typically use saturating phalloidin:actin ratios of 1:2 or 1:1 (Gittes *et al* 1993, Adami *et al* 1999, Gardel *et al* 2008, Kasza *et al* 2010).

Phalloidin also lowers the critical concentration for polymerization, $c_p \approx 0.05\text{–}1\ \mu\text{M}$, up to ~10-fold by suppressing depolymerization at the pointed end (Wendel and Dancker 1987, Sampath and Pollard 1991, Weber 1999, 1999).

The reduction in c_p allows actin to polymerize into long filaments at low concentrations and facilitates the introduction of trace amounts of labeled filaments into unlabeled actin networks, various buffers, or other media without the filaments depolymerizing upon dilution. This stabilization is critical to experiments that rely on imaging single isolated filaments such as those in figure 5.4.

Another important consideration when working with phalloidin is that it stiffens actin filaments beyond their native rigidity, resulting in a nearly 2-fold increase in the persistence length from $l_p \simeq 10$ μm to $\sim$17 μm (Gittes *et al* 1993), which needs to be considered when comparing measured dynamics with theoretical predictions that rely on l_p, such as those I describe in section 2.7.3 of chapter 2.

There are numerous other ABPs that alter the polymerization kinetics, treadmilling rates, steady-state lengths, and critical polymerization concentrations by nucleating, capping, and severing proteins (Pollard and Cooper 1986, Weber 1999). For example, profilin, formin, and tropomodulin/tropomyosin nucleate actin filaments to lower c_p and increase the rate of polymerization (Blanchoin *et al* 2000, Adami *et al* 2003), while severing and sequestering proteins such as cofilin and thymosin can increase c_p and depolymerize filaments (Nachmias, 1993, Bamburg 1999, Blanchoin *et al* 2000, 2000, Goldstein *et al* 2005, Andrianantoandro and Pollard 2006,). These and other ABPs, some of which I will discuss in later chapters as needed, have been used in numerous studies to alter actin network dynamics and architecture (Pollard and Cooper 1986, Xu *et al* 2000, Adami *et al* 2003, Gardel *et al* 2008, Kim *et al* 2014), and offer a wide parameter space of tuning knobs to control network structure and dynamics.

Perhaps the mostly widely-used method for investigating actin networks is to image actin filaments and their networks using various forms of fluorescence microscopy (as I discuss in chapter 2). This approach is facilitated by a range of commercially available phalloidins and actin monomers conjugated with fluorescent moieties ('Alexa Fluor™ 594 Phalloidin,' n.d., 'Pure actin, pyrene actin, fluorescent actin, rhodamine actin, pre-formed actin filaments,' n.d.).

Conjugated phalloidins are available with a wide range of excitation/emission wavelengths from the Alexa Fluor (ThermoFisher), Atto (Sigma Aldrich), and Acti-Stain (Cytoskeleton, Inc.) fluorophore families ('Acti-stain 488 phalloidin,' n. d.,'Alexa Fluor™ 594 Phalloidin,' n.d., 'Phalloidin–Atto 532 suitable for fluorescence, $\geqslant$90.0% (HPLC) Sigma Aldrich,' n.d.), as well non-trademarked moieties such as rhodamine and fluorescein. The use of phalloidins enables labeling filaments after polymerization, varying their intensity via the phalloidin:actin monomer ratio, and stabilizing filaments against depolymerization. Moreover, because phalloidins only bind to filamentous actin, free actin monomers in solution (which are unavoidable) will not be labeled so will not contribute to background fluorescence signal.

A few considerations when using phalloidin to label actin filaments is that it suppresses treadmilling and increases the filament stiffness, as I discussed above. As such, phalloidin should not be used in studies that require dynamic depolymerization, treadmilling, or turnover; and the increased persistence length of phalloidin-stabilized filaments needs to be taken into account when designing experiments and interpreting data.

An alternative to phalloidin-labeling is to use actin monomers that are conjugated directly with fluorophores. There are a few commercially available options, such as rhodamine actin from Cytoskeleton, Inc. ('Pure actin, pyrene actin, fluorescent actin, rhodamine actin, pre-formed actin filaments,'). Researchers can also label actin monomers in-house by conjugating the NHS ester form of commercially available fluorophores (e.g., Alexa Fluor, Atto, etc) to the amine group of actin monomer cysteines following standard protocols (Gittes *et al* 1993, Andrianantoandro and Pollard 2006, Viamontes *et al* 2006, Murrell and Gardel 2012).

To resolve single filaments within dense networks, it is standard practice to add a trace amount of pre-polymerized labeled filaments to networks of unlabeled ('dark') filaments. For these applications, high labeling ratios are optimal to ensure high signal-to-noise and combat photobleaching. For phalloidin-labeling, a 1:1 phalloidin:actin ratio typically provides the best signal. When using labeled actin monomers, they should be incorporated into the pool of dark monomers at a 1:1 ratio of labeled:unlabeled monomers. Importantly, labeled actin monomers will not bind to each other so at least half of actin monomers must be unlabeled to form labeled filaments.

While adding pre-formed labeled filaments to networks of dark filaments is excellent for resolving single filaments within the network and measuring single-polymer dynamics and structure, the downside to this approach is that, because the filaments are polymerized separately from the rest of the network, they may not accurately report the true network properties. For example, if the labeled filaments are polymerized at a different concentration than the rest of the network, their lengths may not be representative of the lengths of the dark filaments in the network. Moreover, mixing labeled and unlabeled filaments can introduce heterogeneities, and flowing pre-formed filaments into a sample chamber can cause artificially imposed filament alignment.

An alternative approach that alleviates the aforementioned issues, and enables resolving the structure and dynamics of dense networks, is to sparsely label the entire network of filaments, by incorporating a low ratio of labeled:unlabeled monomers or a low concentration of phalloidin into the sample prior to polymerization and assembly (Gurmessa *et al* 2018, 2019, Lee *et al* 2021, Ricketts *et al* 2019, Regan *et al* 2019). Typical ratios used in this approach are ~1:10–1:50 but need to be optimized for different network concentrations and fluorophores (Regan *et al* 2019, Gurmessa *et al* 2021, Dwyer *et al* 2022, McGorty *et al* 2023). Importantly, while this method prevents high-resolution imaging of single filaments, it transparently displays the native characteristics of the network.

Finally, it is important to keep in mind that actin, like DNA, is negatively charged in solution ($\frac{Q}{L} = -4e\ \mathrm{nm}^{-1}$), so the exact properties of the filaments and network depend on the ionic conditions (Tang and Janmey 1996, Henle and Pincus 2005, Viamontes *et al* 2006, Huber *et al* 2012, 2015b, Schnauß *et al* 2016, Gurmessa *et al* 2018, 2019, Ricketts *et al* 2020). For example, in the absence of other co-factors, $MgCl_2$ is required to promote polymerization of actin filaments and network assembly, so it is included in most network buffers at a concentration of $[MgCl_2] \approx 2$ mM (Frieden 1983, Tang and Janmey 1996, Gurmessa *et al* 2018, Fujiwara *et al* 2002). However, at higher $MgCl_2$ concentrations, $[MgCl_2] \gtrsim 12$ mM, or with the inclusion of other salts such as KCl, actin filaments can crosslink and nematically bundle via counterion-crossbridging (Lai *et al* 2007, Huber *et al* 2012, 2015b, Schnauß *et al* 2016, Gurmessa *et al* 2019), which can have dramatic effects on the dynamics and rheology of the networks, as shown in figure 5.5(A), (B) (Henle and Pincus 2005, Lai *et al* 2007, Schnauß *et al* 2016, Gurmessa *et al* 2019, 2021, Ricketts *et al* 2020).

5.2.4 Network dynamics

The dynamical and rheological properties of entangled actin networks have been intensely investigated for decades, perhaps more so than any other biopolymer (Kas *et al* 1996, Isambert and Maggs 1996, Hinner *et al* 1998, Xu *et al* 1998, Gisler and Weitz 1999, Mason *et al* 2000, Schmidt *et al* 2000, Dichtl and Sackmann 2002, Gardel *et al* 2003, 2008, Pollard 2003, Wong *et al* 2004, Buchanan *et al* 2005, Uhde *et al* 2005b, 2005a, Koenderink *et al* 2006, Liu *et al* 2006, Andrianantoandro and Pollard 2006, Semmrich *et al* 2008, Romanowska *et al* 2009, Kasza *et al* 2010, Hansen *et al* 2013, Broedersz and MacKintosh 2014, Kirchenbuechler *et al* 2014, Falzone and Robertson-Anderson 2015, Jensen *et al* 2015, Gurmessa *et al* 2016b, 2018, Pegoraro *et al* 2017, Hohmann and Dehghani 2019, Ricketts *et al* 2020).

The wealth of literature on the topic is due, in part, to its understood role in dictating the viscoelastic properties of cells (Janmey *et al* 2007, Pegoraro *et al* 2017, Rigato *et al* 2017, Simon *et al* 2018, Hohmann and Dehghani 2019), its unique semiflexibility (Gittes *et al* 1993, Isambert and Maggs 1996, Dichtl and Sackmann 2002, Broedersz and MacKintosh 2014), and ease of fluorescence visualization (Kas *et al* 1996, Brau *et al* 2006, Wang *et al* 2010, Kirchenbuechler *et al* 2014, Ricketts *et al* 2020). Below, I attempt to summarize this body of literature, focusing on key results and properties that play important roles in understanding more complex systems such as those I describe in chapters 6–9. This summary is certainly not exhaustive but, instead, intended to orient you to what to expect when performing experiments with entangled actin, and how the properties of simple entangled actin solutions may impact the rheology and dynamics of more complex systems or synthetic analogs with similar properties.

5.2.4.1 Linear viscoelasticity

Entangled actin networks are viscoelastic with frequency-dependent moduli $G'(\omega)$ and $G''(\omega)$ that depend on the concentration of actin monomers c_A and lengths L of the filaments (figure 5.5) (Xu *et al* 1998, Gisler and Weitz 1999, Gardel *et al* 2003, Liu *et al* 2006). Because of their very long disengagement time, $\tau_D \approx 10^4$ s (Isambert and Maggs 1996, Wang *et al* 2010), entangled actin solutions do not display the low-frequency terminal flow regime that their flexible polymer counterparts exhibit (figures 5.3(C) and (E) and 2.4(A)). Rather, entangled actin networks exhibit rubbery plateau behavior that extends to the lowest end of experimentally accessible

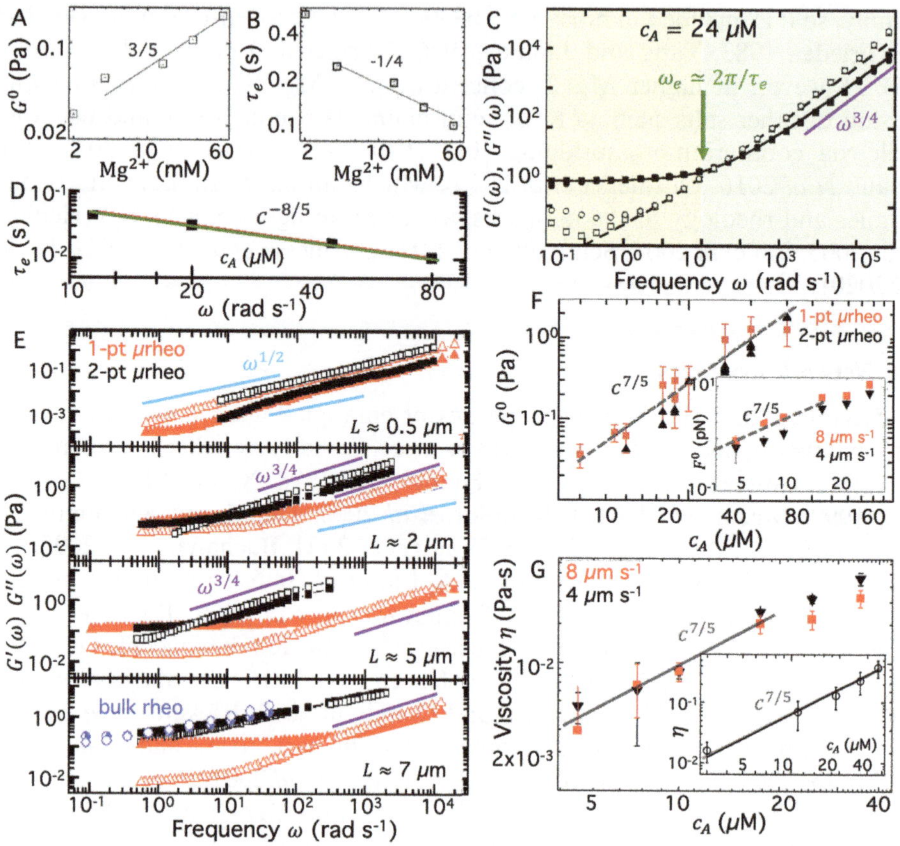

Figure 5.5. Linear viscoelasticity of entangled actin. (A and B) Due to the polyelectrolyte nature of actin, the rheological properties and dynamics of entangled actin networks are dependent on ionic conditions. Increasing concentrations of the divalent ion Mg^{2+} promote bundling and crosslinking which manifests as a power-law (A) increase in the plateau modulus $G^0 \sim [Mg^{2+}]^{3/5}$ and (B) decrease in the entanglement time $\tau_e \sim [Mg^{2+}]^{-1/4}$ for entangled actin networks with $c_A = 12\ \mu M$. (C) $G'(\omega)$ (filled symbols) and $G''(\omega)$ (open symbols) as a function of frequency ω for entangled actin networks with $c_A = 24\ \mu M$ show the low-frequency entanglement regime (yellow) in which G' exhibits a frequency-independent plateau G^0 with a value greater than G'', and the high-frequency regime (green) dominated by single-chain dynamics and exhibiting scaling $G'(\omega) \sim G''(\omega) \sim \omega^{3/4}$ (equation 5.14). The entanglement frequency $\omega_e = 2\pi/\tau_e$ separates the two regimes and is marked by a crossover point in which $G' = G''$ (green arrow). Squares and circles correspond to data collected from two different samples using diffusing wave spectroscopy. Solid and dashed lines are theoretical predictions that account for the high-frequency scaling $G^* \sim \omega^{3/4}$ as well as an additional term that scales as $G^* \sim \omega^{1/3}$ to account for the broad crossover regime that connects the high- and low-frequency regimes. (D) The entanglement time τ_e determined from the crossover frequency $\omega_e = 2\pi/\tau_e$ as a function of actin concentration c_A with the line showing the expected scaling $\tau_e \sim c_A^{-8/5}$. (E) Viscoelastic moduli $G'(\omega)$ (filled symbols) and $G''(\omega)$ measured using 1-point (red) and 2-point (black) microrheology as well as bulk rheology (blue) for entangled actin solutions with $c_A = 24\ \mu M$. The stacked panel corresponds to networks with increasing filament lengths L from top ($L \approx 0.5\ \mu m$) to bottom ($L \approx 7\ \mu m$), controlled by gelsolin. The expected high-frequency scaling for entangled semiflexible polymers $\omega^{3/4}$ (purple) and Rouse scaling $\omega^{1/2}$ (cyan) are shown. (F) Low-frequency plateau modulus G^0 measured for actin networks with varying concentrations c_A, measured using 1-pt (black) and 2-pt (red) microrheology. (Inset) Plateau force F_0, which scales linearly with G^0, as a function c_A, measured using

optical tweezers microrheology performed at 4 μm s^{-1} (red) and 8 μm s^{-1} (black). Grey dashed lines correspond to expected scaling $G^0 \sim c_A^{7/5}$. (G) Viscosity η versus actin concentration c_A, determined from the same OTM measurements shown in (F), and as well as magnetic tweezers microrheology measurements (inset), follow predicted scaling $\eta \sim c_A^{7/5}$ (solid grey lines). (A, B) Adapted from Gurmessa *et al* (2019). CC BY 4.0. (C) Adapted from Mason *et al* (2000), with the permission of AIP Publishing. (D, E) Adapted with permission from Liu *et al* (2006). Copyright (2006) by the American Physical Society. (F) Adapted with permission from Gardel *et al* (2003). Copyright (2003) by the American Physical Society. (F inset) Adapted with permission from Gurmessa *et al* (2016a). Copyright (2016) American Chemical Society. (G) Adapted with permission from Gurmessa *et al* (2016a). Copyright (2016) American Chemical Society. (G inset) Adapted with permission from Uhde *et al* (2005b). Copyright (2005) by the American Physical Society.

frequencies ($\omega \gtrsim 10^{-3}$ rad s^{-1}), as seen in figures 5.5(C) and (E). This low-ω regime is characterized by a frequency-independent plateau modulus $G^0 \sim \omega^0$ with a magnitude of order $G^0 \approx 0.1$ Pa, depending on the actin length and concentration (Liu *et al* 2006), which is larger than $G''(\omega)$ and scales with concentration as

$$G^0 \sim c_A^{7/5} \tag{5.18}$$

(Figure 5.5(F)) (Frey *et al* 1999, Gardel *et al* 2003, Gurmessa *et al* 2016b).

Tube confinement dominates the network response in this low-frequency range, which is bounded from above by the concentration-dependent entanglement rate $\omega_e \simeq 2\pi/\tau_e$, defined as the frequency at which $G'(\omega) = G''(\omega)$ before $G''(\omega) > G'(\omega)$. The dependence of ω_e on actin concentration has been shown to follow power-law scaling

$$\omega_e \sim c_A^{8/5}, \tag{5.19}$$

as seen in figure 5.5(D) in which

$$\tau_e \sim \omega_e^{-1} \sim c_A^{-8/5} \tag{5.20}$$

is observed (Liu *et al* 2006).

The reported range of values, $\omega_e \approx 10^0$–10^2 rad s^{-1} (Koenderink *et al* 2006, Liu *et al* 2006), correspond to entanglement times of order $\tau_e \approx 10^{-2}$–10^0 s (figures 5.5(A)–(C)) (Isambert and Maggs, 1996, Falzone *et al* 2015a, Falzone and Robertson-Anderson, 2015).

For $\omega > \omega_e$, the rheology is dominated by single-chain dynamics rather than entanglements, which manifests as a crossover to $G'' > G'$ and power-law scaling

$$G'(\omega) \sim G''(\omega) \sim \omega^{3/4} \tag{5.21}$$

(figures 5.5(E) and (F)) (Gittes *et al* 1997, Gittes and MacKintosh 1998, 1998, Gisler and Weitz 1999, Mason *et al* 2000, Koenderink *et al* 2006, Liu *et al* 2006).

However, the crossover regime connecting the entanglement scaling and single-chain scaling has been shown to be broad due to additional relaxation mechanisms, such as filament bending and axial chain end retraction, that enhance relaxation at intermediate timescales (Gittes *et al* 1997, Morse 1998, Xu *et al* 1998, Gisler and Weitz 1999, Mason *et al* 2000, Koenderink *et al* 2006). Specifically, this enhanced intermediate relaxation can be captured by an additional broadening term in the complex modulus that scales as $\omega^{1/3}$ (Gittes *et al* 1997, Gisler and Weitz 1999).

Moreover, unlike flexible polymers, actin filaments do not exhibit shear thinning in the linear regime. Rather the viscosity is independent of frequency ($\eta^* \sim \omega^0$), and scales with concentration as

$$\eta \sim c_A^{7/5} \tag{5.22}$$

(figure 5.5(G)) (Uhde *et al* 2005b, Gurmessa *et al* 2016b).

Importantly, the rheological properties described above have been measured using various methods including one-point (SPTM) and two-point (MPT) tracking microrheology (figures 5.5(D)–(F)), magnetic tweezers microrheology (figures 5.5(D)–(F)), optical tweezers microrheology (figures 5.5(A), (F), and (G)), diffusing wave spectroscopy (figure 5.5(C)), and bulk rheology (figures 5.5(D) and (E)). While results are generally consistent across the different methods, one-point microrheology does underestimate $G'(\omega)$ and $G''(\omega)$ and overestimate ω_e, as compared to two-point and bulk rheology for highly entangled networks (figure 5.5(E)), for reasons I explain in chapter 4.

5.2.4.2 Nonlinear mechanical response

The behavior summarized above describes the linear viscoelastic response of actin networks, in which G' and G'' are independent of the strain amplitude γ, i.e., $G'(\gamma) \sim G''(\gamma) \sim \gamma^0$, and the stress scales linearly with strain ($\sigma \sim \gamma, \frac{d^2\sigma}{d\gamma^2} = 0$), such that the differential modulus, $K = \frac{d\sigma}{d\gamma}$, is constant. This linear viscoelasticity manifests for actin networks in response to strains that are small enough to maintain the network in steady-state (see chapter 2 for further details). For larger strains, that push the filaments far from steady-state, actin networks exhibit nonlinear viscoelasticity, whereby the stress displays a nonlinear dependence on strain, which can be classified as either softening or stiffening, in which the slope of $\sigma(\gamma)$ either decreases, i.e., $\frac{K}{K_0} < 0\ \frac{d^2\sigma}{d\gamma^2} < 0$, or increases, i.e., $\frac{K}{K_0} > 0, \frac{d^2\sigma}{d\gamma^2} > 0$.

Entangled actin networks can display both stiffening and softening, depending on the scale of the strain as well as the concentration and lengths of the filaments (Semmrich *et al* 2008, Broedersz and MacKintosh 2014, Falzone *et al* 2015a, Falzone and Robertson-Anderson 2015, Chen *et al* 2023). For example, macrorheology measurements have largely shown that entangled actin networks stress-soften, explained by theoretical models to be a result of non-affine bending and disentanglements (Isambert and Maggs 1996, Frey *et al* 1999, Head *et al* 2005, Das *et al* 2007, Liu *et al* 2007, Broedersz and MacKintosh 2014, Chen *et al* 2023). However, a few studies have reported stress-stiffening at the macroscale (figures 5.6(A) and (B)) (Xu *et al* 1998, Semmrich *et al* 2008).

At the microscale, stress-stiffening, rather than softening, is observed in response to strain rates $\dot{\gamma} \gtrsim \tau_e^{-1}$ (figures 5.6(C) and (D)) due to local entanglements being 'frozen' on the timescale of the strain, such that they cannot move relative to another to facilitate non-affine deformations (Falzone *et al* 2015a, Falzone and Robertson-Anderson 2015, Gurmessa *et al* 2016a). Instead, filaments deform primarily via affine entropic stretching, akin to reported behavior of crosslinked actin networks,

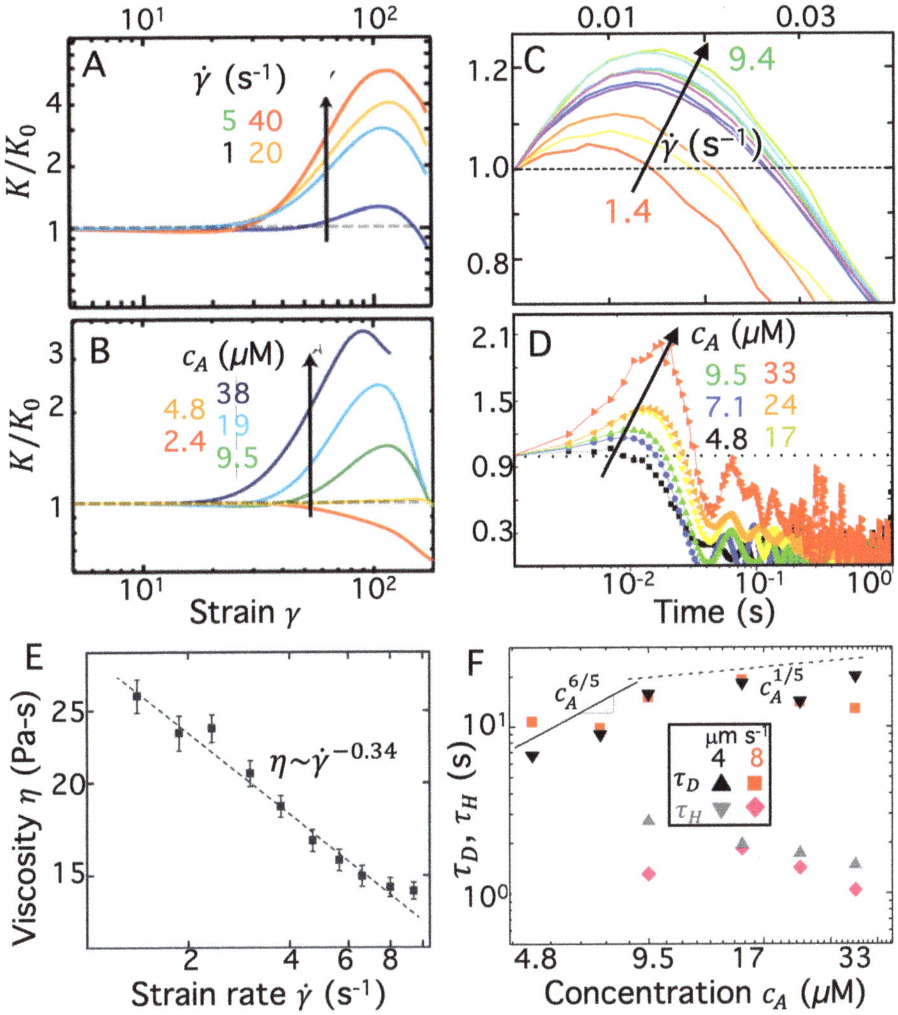

Figure 5.6. Nonlinear stiffening, thinning, and tube dilation of entangled actin. (A and B) Differential modulus K, scaled by the linear (low-γ limit) value K_0, versus strain γ, measured via nonlinear bulk rheology measurements of varying strain rates $\dot{\gamma} = 1$–$40\ \mathrm{s}^{-1}$ (as listed by color) (A) for entangled actin networks of varying concentrations c_A (as listed by color) (B) show stress-stiffening for $\dot{\gamma} \gtrsim 5\ \mathrm{s}^{-1}$ (A) and $c_A \gtrsim 9.5\ \mu\mathrm{M}$ (B). (C and D) K/K_0 versus time (from the start of the strain), measured via constant-rate OTM strains of varying rates $\dot{\gamma} = 1$–$9.4\ \mathrm{s}^{-1}$ (increasing from red to purple) (C) for entangled actin networks of varying concentrations c_A (as listed by color) (D) show stress-stiffening for $\dot{\gamma} \gtrsim 3\ \mathrm{s}^{-1}$ (C) and $c_A \gtrsim 9.5\ \mu\mathrm{M}$ (D). (E) Steady-state viscosity η versus strain rate $\dot{\gamma}$, measured via OTM, shows shear thinning with scaling exponent $x \simeq 0.34$ (dashed line). (F) The force relaxation curves following nonlinear OTM strains with speeds of $4\ \mu\mathrm{m\ s}^{-1}$ (black/grey) and $8\ \mu\mathrm{m\ s}^{-1}$ (red/magenta) are well fit to a sum of two exponentials with characteristic timescales, τ_H (grey, magenta) and τ_D (black, red). The scaling of the relaxation timescales with concentration c_A align with predictions for τ_D that incorporate tube dilation in the nonlinear regime, and the ~10× faster non-classical relaxation mechanism of entanglement hopping that occurs on a timescale τ_H. (A, B) Adapted from Semmrich *et al* (2008) with permission from the Royal Society of Chemistry. (C, E) Adapted from Falzone *et al* (2015a) with permission from the Royal Society of Chemistry. (D, F) Adapted with permission from Gurmessa *et al* (2016a). Copyright (2016) American Chemical Society.

rather than bending and disentanglement (Das *et al* 2007, Broedersz and MacKintosh 2014), as discussed further below. Importantly, these nonlinear features only emerge for entangled networks above a critical concentration $c_{A,nl} \approx 9.5\ \mu$M, ~4-fold higher than the critical entanglement concentration $c_e \approx 2.4\ \mu$M (figures 5.6(B) and (D)) (Semmrich *et al* 2008, Gurmessa *et al* 2016a). This effect demonstrates the need for ample entanglement density to suppress the filament bending that underlies stress-softening.

The microscale stiffening observed for $(\dot{\gamma}, c_A) \gtrsim (\tau_e^{-1}, c_{A,nl})$ transitions to softening at timescales comparable to the mesh time τ_ξ (figure 5.6(D)) (Falzone *et al* 2015a), which is the fastest predicted relaxation timescale for entangled semiflexible polymers (Isambert and Maggs 1996), and is a measure of the time it takes an entangled filament to feel the hydrodynamic effects of its neighbors (see chapter 2 for more details). Following this softening phase, the network yields to a linear viscoelastic regime at timescales comparable to the entanglement time τ_e (which is greater than τ_ξ) as shown in figure 5.6(D) (Falzone and Robertson-Anderson 2015, Gurmessa *et al* 2016a).

Entangled actin networks have also been shown to exhibit shear thinning, $\eta \sim \dot{\gamma}^{-x}$, in response to OTM nonlinear straining, albeit with a weaker scaling of $x \simeq 0.34$ (figure 5.6(E)) (Falzone *et al* 2015a) compared to $x \simeq 0.6$–1 reported for flexible polymers such as DNA (Chapman *et al* 2014, Chapman and Robertson-Anderson 2014, Peddireddy *et al* 2020a). This unique thinning was reported to arise from strain-induced dilation of the confining tube as entangling polymers are stretched in the direction of the strain (Gurmessa *et al* 2017, Sussman and Schweizer 2012, 2013b). Corresponding OTM force relaxation measurements also showed evidence of strain-induced tube dilation in the nonlinear regime, manifested as reduced scaling of the disengagement time τ_D with actin concentration (Gurmessa *et al* 2016a). Namely, τ_D transitioned from $\tau_D \sim c_A^{6/5}$ scaling in the linear regime to $\tau'_D \sim c_A^{1/5}$ in the nonlinear regime (figure 5.6(F)), in line with predicted tube dilation scaling

$$d'_T/d_T \sim c_A^{1/2} \tag{5.23}$$

where d'_T and τ'_D are the dilated tube diameter and correspondingly faster disengagement time (Sussman and Schweizer 2012, 2013b). Recognizing the relation $\tau_D \sim d_T^{-2}$ then provides

$$(d'_T/d_T)^2 \sim c_A^1 \sim \frac{c_A^{6/5}}{c_A^{1/5}} \sim \frac{\tau_D}{\tau'_D} \tag{5.24}$$

Another relaxation mechanism, not predicted by traditional reptation theory for semiflexible polymers, has also been reported to emerge at the microscale in the nonlinear regime due to lateral hopping of entangled segments between entanglement 'cages' (Gurmessa *et al* 2016a, 2017, Ricketts *et al* 2018). This lateral hopping can also be understood as convective constraint release (CCR) whereby the strain temporarily disrupts an entanglement comprising the confining tube of an entangled polymer, allowing the polymer to laterally 'hop', via thermal fluctuations, into a new tube (Sussman and Schweizer, 2012, 2013a). This hopping process, therefore, allows the entangled polymer to relax its constraints from the entanglement tube on a much faster timescale, $\tau_H \approx \frac{\tau_D}{10}$, than that associated with reptating out of a deformed tube and into a new tube (figure 5.6(F)).

Caging and hopping can also be readily observed in the thermal transport characteristics of microspheres embedded in actin networks (Gardel *et al* 2003, Wong *et al* 2004, Wang *et al* 2012, Anderson *et al* 2019). Specifically, deviations from canonical Brownian motion, such as subdiffusive scaling of the mean-squared displacement, $MSD \sim \Delta t^{\alpha}$ with $\alpha < 1$, and van Hove distributions of particle displacements that deviate from Gaussianity (see chapter 4 for further discussion), are often indicative of caging and hopping (Bouchaud and Georges 1990, Wong *et al* 2004, Wang *et al* 2009, Chechkin *et al* 2017, Regan *et al* 2019, Garamella *et al* 2020).

5.2.4.3 Crosslinked actin networks

In the cytoskeleton, actin filaments are often crosslinked to one another by ABPs such as α-actinin, scruin, fascin, and filamin (Pollard and Cooper 1986, Pollard 2003, Gardel *et al* 2008, Jensen *et al* 2015), which can dramatically alter their structural and rheological properties, as compared to networks with only steric interactions (entanglements) between filaments (figure 5.7) (Gardel *et al* 2004, 2008, Janmey *et al* 2007, Liu *et al* 2007, Broedersz and MacKintosh 2014, Kim *et al* 2014, Dwyer *et al* 2022). Their combined physiological relevance and rheological impact have made crosslinked actin networks the topic of intense research over the past several decades (Xu *et al* 2000, Gardel *et al* 2004, 2008, Claessens *et al* 2006, Wagner *et al* 2006, Liu *et al* 2007, Tharmann *et al* 2007, Lieleg *et al* 2008, Kasza *et al* 2010, Stricker *et al* 2010, Yao *et al* 2011, Gurmessa *et al* 2017, Ricketts *et al* 2020, Dwyer *et al* 2022). They have also served as a model system for testing more general theoretical predictions for semiflexible polymer networks and gels, such as those based on rigidity percolation theory (MacKintosh *et al* 1995, Gittes and MacKintosh 1998, Head *et al* 2005, Das *et al* 2007, Lieleg *et al* 2007, Broedersz *et al* 2010, Broedersz and MacKintosh 2014, Punter *et al* 2020, Chen *et al* 2023).

Physiological crosslinking ABPs, such as widely-studied α-actinin, are transient, with varying binding and dissociation rates, duty ratios, and binding affinities that impact the dynamics of the network (Xu *et al* 2000, Gardel *et al* 2008, Yao *et al* 2011). For example, crosslinking suppresses relaxation mechanisms such as reptation and bending by restricting center-of-mass motion of the filaments (Janmey *et al* 1994, Gardel *et al* 2004, 2008, Luan *et al* 2008, Lee *et al* 2010, Broedersz and MacKintosh 2014, Chen *et al* 2023). At the same time, the transient nature of ABPs introduces additional relaxation mechanisms with distinct characteristic timescales such as ABP unbinding (figure 5.7(B)) and slippage, filament buckling and rupture, and turnover (Janmey *et al* 1994, Lieleg *et al* 2008, Yao *et al* 2011, Kim *et al* 2011, 2014, De La Cruz and Gardel 2015).

To suppress the relaxation mechanisms associated with dynamic crosslinkers, researchers also employ the strong, permanent avidin-biotin bond to statically crosslink actin networks (figures 5.7(D)–(F), (L), and (M)) (Koenderink *et al* 2006, Gurmessa *et al* 2017, 2018, Ricketts *et al* 2020). Specifically, commercially available biotinylated actin monomers (b-actin), can be included in the pool of actin monomers

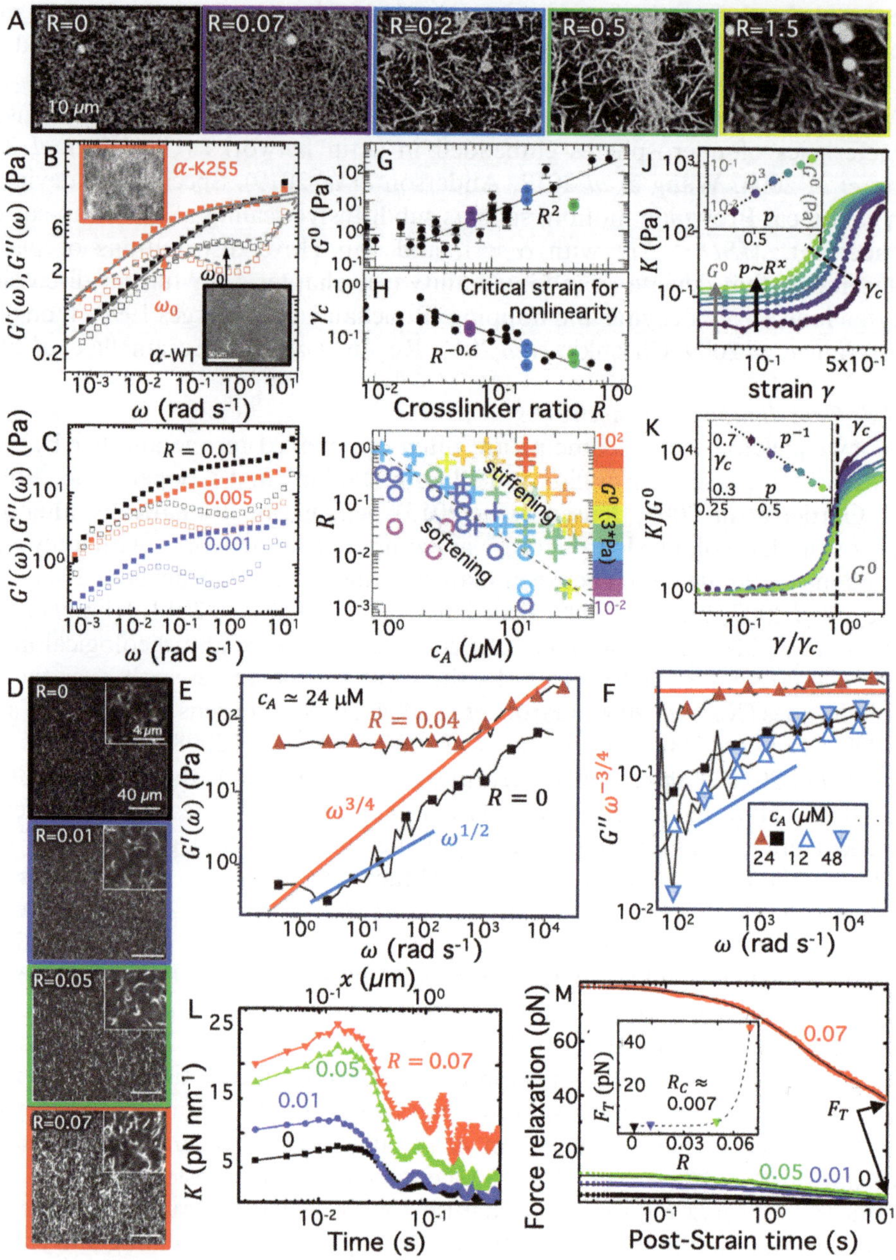

Figure 5.7. Crosslinked actin network rheology. (A, B, and D) Confocal micrographs showing actin networks crosslinked by (A) scruin, (B insets) wild-type (α-wt, black border) and strongly binding K255 mutant (α-K255, red border) α-actinin, and (D) biotin-NeutrAvidin of varying ABP:actin ratios (A) $R = 0$–1.5, (B) $R = 0.005$, (D) $R = 0$–0.07. (B) Bulk linear rheology measurements of actin networks with $c_A = 24\ \mu$M and crosslinked by α-wt (black) and α-K255 (red) show that the dissociation rate ω_0, signified by the local maximum in G'', governs the onset of the low-frequency relaxation regime and is ~20-fold slower for α-K255 versus α-wt. Crosslinker unbinding and rebinding renders the network more fluid-like in this regime, so the

$\sim$20-fold longer binding time ω_0^{-1} for α-K255 is consistent with its $\sim$6-fold higher dissociation constant (Yao *et al* 2011). Dashed and solid lines are fits of the data to a mean-field crosslink-governed dynamics model (Broedersz *et al* 2010). (C) Networks crosslinked with varying ratios of α-K255 ($R = 0.001$, black; $R = 0.005$, red; $R = 0.01$, blue) show similar ω_0 values and frequency-dependence of $G'(\omega)$ and $G''(\omega)$, but the magnitudes of G', G'' and G^0 increase with R. (E and F) $G'(\omega)$ (E) and $G''(\omega)$ (F), measured using two-point microrheology, for actin networks crosslinked with biotin-NA at $R = 0.04$ (red triangles), show that (E) crosslinking extends the frequency range over which a plateau in G' is apparent by over three decades in ω, increases G^0 nearly $\sim 10^2$-fold beyond that of the $R = 0$ network (black squares), and (F) suppresses the intermediate scaling regime $G'(\omega) \sim G''(\omega) \sim \omega^{1/2}$ (blue lines) that connects the low- and high-frequency scaling behavior, $G'(\omega) \sim \omega^0$ and $G'(\omega) \sim G''(\omega) \sim \omega^{3/4}$ (red lines), respectively. (F) The intermediate $\omega^{1/2}$ scaling of G'' is apparent for entangled networks with $c_A \simeq 12$ μM (open triangles), 24 μM (black squares), and 48 μM (blue triangles), which only asymptotically approach the $\omega^{3/4}$ scaling that the crosslinked network exhibits. (G–I) Bulk rheology measurements of actin networks with $c_A \simeq 12$ μM and crosslinked by scruin show that the (G) plateau modulus increases with crosslinker ratio as $G^0 \sim R^2$; (H) the critical strain γ_c at which the networks transition from linear response to nonlinear stiffening decreases with increasing R, according to $\gamma_c \sim R^{-0.6}$; and (I) the nonlinear response of crosslinked networks transitions from stress-softening (circles) to stiffening (crosses) at sufficiently large R and c_A values, which correlate with larger G^0 values (color coded according to scale on the right). (J and K) Simulations of crosslinked semiflexible filament networks of varying crosslinker coverage p (increasing from purple to green), which is expected to scale with R^x, show the transition from linear elasticity, in which $K = G^0 \sim \gamma^0$, to nonlinear stiffening, with $K > G^0$, $\frac{dK}{d\gamma} > 0$, at a critical strain γ_c. $G^0 (=K_0)$ increases and γ_c decreases with increasing p according to power-law scaling relations (J inset) $G^0 \sim p^3$ and (K inset) $\gamma_c \sim p^{-1}$. All data shown in J collapses to a single universal curve when K and γ are scaled by G^0 and γ_c, respectively. (L and M) Nonlinear OTM measurements of actin networks with $c_A \simeq 12$ μM and crosslinked by biotin-NA at $R = 0$ (black), 0.01 (blue), 0.05 (green), and 0.07 (red) show (L) the initial stiffness K_0, the degree of stress-stiffening (increase in K), the final stiffness K_f at the end of the strain, and (M) the terminal force F_T retained at the end of the relaxation period following the strain all increase with increasing R. (M) The terminal post-strain force F_T, a measure of the retained elastic memory of the network, increases exponentially with R, $F_T \sim e^{-R/R_c}$, with a critical value $R_c \simeq 0.007$ for ample elasticity. (A, G, H) Adapted from Shin *et al* (2004) with permission of PNAS. Copyright (2004) National Academy of Sciences, U.S.A. (B, C) Adapted from Yao *et al* (2011), Copyright (2011), with permission from Elsevier. (D, L, M) Adapted from Gurmessa *et al* (2017), Copyright (2017), with permission from Elsevier. (E, F) Adapted with permission from Koenderink *et al* (2006). Copyright (2006) by the American Physical Society. (J and K) Adapted with permission from Syed *et al* (2022). Copyright (2022) American Chemical Society. (I) Adapted from Gardel *et al* (2004). © American Association for the Advancement of Science.

to be polymerized into filaments, with the ratio of b-actin to unlabeled actin controlling the crosslinking density. A crosslinked network can then be formed by including a protein from the avidin family, the most widely used being NeutrAvidin (NA) due to its reduced non-specific binding compared to other avidins, to crosslink b-actin monomers from different filaments. Because avidins have four biotin binding sites, to reduce clustering and bundling of filaments, free biotin can be included at a 1:1 b-actin:biotin ratio (Gurmessa *et al* 2017, Ricketts *et al* 2020).

For crosslinked networks, the crosslinker:actin molar ratio R is the principal determinant of the network rheology, dynamics, and morphology, with actin concentration and crosslinker type also contributing (figure 5.7) (Gardel *et al* 2004, Broedersz *et al* 2010, Broedersz and MacKintosh 2014, Gurmessa *et al* 2017). For physiological ABPs,

$$R = [ABP]/[actin] \tag{5.25}$$

where [] denotes molarity, while for biotin-NeutrAvidin crosslinking

$$R = \frac{[b \cdot actin]}{2([b \cdot actin] + [actin])} \tag{5.26}$$

$$[b \cdot actin] = [free\ \ biotin] = 2[NA] \tag{5.27}$$

Molar ratios of $R \simeq 0.005$–0.1 are typically used in experiments to form isotropic crosslinked filament networks, while higher R values often cause nematic filament bundling (figures 5.7(A), (B), and (D)) (Xu *et al* 2000, Shin *et al* 2004, Gardel *et al* 2004, Lieleg *et al* 2007, Schmoller *et al* 2010, Falzone *et al* 2012, Gurmessa *et al* 2017). However, for certain crosslinkers, such as scruin and fascin, bundles can form at lower R values, as discussed below (Shin *et al* 2004, Lieleg *et al* 2007).

Crosslinking with any ABP increases the elastic plateau modulus G^0 of actin networks above that of their entangled counterparts, and generally scales with the crosslinker ratio R as

$$G^0 \sim R^\chi \tag{5.28}$$

figure 5.7(C), (G), (J), and (L). Studies using scruin as crosslinkers report a scaling exponent of $\chi \approx 2$ for $R = 0.01$–1 (figure 5.7(C)) (Gardel *et al* 2004). However, experiments using heavy meromyosin (HMM) and fascin observe distinct scaling regimes for ratios below and above a crossover at $R \approx R_c$ (Lieleg *et al* 2007, Luan *et al* 2008), and experiments with biotin-NA crosslinking observe exponential dependence $G^0 \sim e^{R/R_c}$ (Gurmessa *et al* 2017). For HMM, $\chi_{R<R_c} \approx 0.1$, $\chi_{R>R_c} \approx 1.2$ and $R_c \approx 5e^{-4}$ (Luan *et al* 2008); for fascin, $\chi_{R<R_c} \approx 0.1$, $\chi_{R>R_c} \approx 1.5$ and $R_c \approx 0.01$ (Lieleg *et al* 2007); and for biotin-NA $R_c \approx 0.015$ (Gurmessa *et al* 2017). The different scaling exponents and functional dependence for the different crosslinkers can be explained, in part, by the propensity for the different crosslinkers to form bundles versus maintaining isotropic crosslinks. HMM and biotin-NA have limited bundling (figure 5.7(D)) (Luan *et al* 2008, Gurmessa *et al* 2017), while scruin and fascin are more prone to forming bundles (figure 5.7(A)) (Shin *et al* 2004, Lieleg *et al* 2007).

For permanent crosslinkers such as biotin-NA, the elastic plateau modulus $G^0 \sim \omega^0$ extends to the lowest measurable frequencies (figure 5.7(E)) as there is no mechanism to relax the stress stored in the crosslinks (ignoring filament fragmentation, bond-breakage, and other mechanisms that may arise in the nonlinear regime). Conversely, for transient ABPs such as α-actinin and HMM, the ABP binding/dissociation rate ω_o dominates the viscoelastic response at low frequencies, with networks displaying a crossover from elastic-like dynamics, i.e.,

$$G'(\omega) \sim \omega^0, \ \text{for}\ \omega > \omega_o, \tag{5.29}$$

to a power-law regime

$$G'(\omega) \sim G''(\omega) \sim \omega^{1/2}\ \text{for}\ \omega < \omega_o, \tag{5.30}$$

(see figures 5.7(B) and (C)) indicative of network rearrangement via transient ABP bond release and reformation (Broedersz *et al* 2010, Yao *et al* 2011).

The high-frequency behavior that follows the entanglement plateau regime ($\omega > \omega_e$), dominated by single-chain dynamics, is independent of the bond lifetime, with crosslinked networks generally displaying

$$G'(\omega) \sim G''(\omega) \sim \omega^{3/4} \text{ for } \omega > \omega_e \tag{5.31}$$

similar to entangled actin networks. Recall that entangled actin networks display a broad crossover from the plateau regime to this high-frequency scaling regime (as described above), with the approximate scaling $G'(\omega) \sim G''(\omega) \sim \omega^{1/2}$ (Gisler and Weitz 1999, Koenderink *et al* 2006). However, while crosslinking essentially eliminates this crossover regime and instead a sharp transition from $G'(\omega) \sim \omega^0$ to $G'(\omega) \sim G''(\omega) \sim \omega^{3/4}$ is observed (figures 5.7(E) and (F)).

Finally, for the uniquely large and flexible ABP, filamin, the network rheology has been shown to be dictated by the dynamics and flexibility of the filamin linkers rather than the actin filaments, resulting in an increased dependence of the rheological properties on the lengths of actin filaments as compared to the smaller, rigid ABPs discussed above (Tseng *et al* 2004, Esue *et al* 2009, Schmoller *et al* 2009, Kasza *et al* 2010, Wang *et al* 2020, 2023).

In the nonlinear regime, both microrheology and bulk rheology measurements show that crosslinking leads to stress-stiffening, due to the filaments extending and stretching affinely (i.e., in the direction of the strain) (figures 5.7(I)–(L)) (Gardel *et al* 2004, Liu *et al* 2007, Gurmessa *et al* 2017, Syed *et al* 2022). The degree of stiffening increases with increasing R (figures 5.7(J)–(L)), while the critical strain γ_c at which nonlinear stiffening ensues decreases (figures 5.7(H), (J), and (K)). The subsequent stress-softening observed for entangled actin is also greatly suppressed (figures 5.7(J)–(L)). For example, in response to nonlinear OTM strains, entangled actin networks soften and yield to a largely viscous regime with negligible stiffness or elasticity, i.e., $K_f \approx 0$ (figure 5.6(D)). Conversely, biotin-NA crosslinked networks maintain non-zero stiffness at the end the strain ($K_f > 0$) with the value of K_f increasing exponentially with increasing R (figure 5.7(L)). Similarly, simulations (figures 5.7(J) and (K)) show that, following an initial period of strong stiffening ($\frac{dK}{d\gamma} \gg 0$), the stiffening weakens and K approaches a new steady-state plateau value that is greater than K_0 (figures 5.7(J) and (K)).

This sustained elasticity is also seen in the force relaxation curves which maintain a residual terminal force F_T at the end of the relaxation phase, unlike entangled actin solutions in which the force completely relaxes ($F_T \sim 0$) as the system returns to equilibrium (figure 5.7(M)). This suppressed energy dissipation is a direct result of permanent crosslinkers preventing bending and reptation. The relaxation and softening that does remain in the presence of crosslinkers has been shown to arise from filament recoil and strain-induced crosslink rupturing and rebinding (Yang *et al* 2012a, Gurmessa *et al* 2017). Moreover, experiments and simulations have shown that the long-lived stress following strain is likely maintained by only a small fraction of highly-strained filaments that form percolating stress fibers throughout the network, while the majority of the filaments can relax and recoil (Onck *et al* 2005, Abhilash *et al* 2012, Kim *et al* 2014, Žagar *et al* 2015, Gurmessa *et al* 2017).

An alternative to crosslinking and bundling actin with ABPs is to use high concentrations of multivalent counterions such as Mg^{2+} to form counterion cross-bridges, as I describe in section 5.2.3 (Henle and Pincus 2005, Huber *et al* 2012, Schnauß *et al* 2016, Gurmessa *et al* 2019). For example, $MgCl_2$ concentrations above ~10 mM, have been reported to produce actin bundles with ~4× larger persistence length compared to that of individual filaments, i.e.,

$$l_p^{\mathrm{Mg}^{2+}} \simeq 4l_p^0 \simeq 40\ \mu\mathrm{m} \tag{5.32}$$

(Schnauß *et al* 2016, Gurmessa *et al* 2019), with the increased stiffness arising from both the bundle density and the crosslinks formed between bundles.

Microrheology experiments have shown that it is the crosslinking between fibers, rather than increased stiffness from bundling, that dictates the linear regime rheology, with reported scaling relations $G^0 \sim [\mathrm{Mg}^{2+}]^{3/5}$ and $\tau_e \sim [\mathrm{Mg}^{2+}]^{-1/4}$ (figures 5.5(A) and (B)). Conversely, the nonlinear response was shown to be dominated by the increased stiffness from nematic bundling rather than crosslinking, as nonlinear straining was sufficient to disrupt crosslinks (Gurmessa *et al* 2019). Bundling also strongly suppressed nonlinear force relaxation, with networks retaining nearly 98% of the induced stress. Moreover, the relaxation timescales associated with the small degree of observed relaxation were longer than those for entangled actin networks, which was shown to be due to the ~4-fold larger persistence length of the counterion-bundled fibers. Specifically, the relaxation times aligned with predicted values for the mesh time τ_ξ and entanglement time τ_e (see chapter 2 for details) when taking into account equation (5.28) and recognizing the following predicted scaling relations

$$\tau_\xi \sim l_p^{1/5} \tag{5.33}$$

$$\tau_e \sim l_p \tag{5.34}$$

such that

$$\tau_\xi^{\mathrm{Mg}^{2+}} \simeq 4^{1/5}\tau_\xi^0 \simeq 1.32\tau_\xi^0 \tag{5.35}$$

$$\tau_e^{\mathrm{Mg}^{2+}} \simeq 4\tau_e^0 \tag{5.36}$$

(Gurmessa *et al* 2019).

5.3 Entangled and crosslinked networks of microtubules

5.3.1 Microtubules as an advantageous model rigid rod polymer

Similar to DNA and actin serving as model systems for understanding the physics of flexible and semiflexible polymers, respectively, networks of microtubules (MTs) have been employed for decades as model rigid rod polymer systems (Lin *et al* 2007, Maarel 2008, Hawkins *et al* 2010, Wen and Janmey 2011, Yang *et al* 2012b, Lopez and Valentine 2015, Peddireddy *et al* 2021).

As I describe in chapter 1, microtubules are essentially rigid rods, with a persistence length $l_p \approx 1$ mm far larger than typical contour lengths of $L \simeq 1$–$40\ \mu$m (Hawkins *et al* 2010). This rigidity renders microtubule networks of a given tubulin concentration

c_T substantially more elastic than networks of actin or DNA with comparable molar concentrations c_A and c_{DNA} (Ricketts *et al* 2018, Wen and Janmey 2011, Peddireddy *et al* 2021). Moreover, due to their reduced thermal fluctuations and slower relaxation modes, microtubules are easier to visualize and resolve with high signal-to-noise as compared to actin and DNA (figures 5.8(A.i) and (B.i)), making them model systems for directly measuring the reptative dynamics of entangled rigid rod polymers and testing corresponding theoretical predictions (Odijk 1983, Doi and Edwards, 1988, Höfling *et al* 2008, Sussman and Schweizer 2011, Glaser and Kroy 2010, 2011, Schweizer and Sussman 2016).

5.3.2 Design considerations

Despite the reported increased bulk rigidity of entangled microtubules as compared to networks of entangled actin or DNA, it is important to consider that the mesh size of a microtubule network ξ_{MT} with a given tubulin molarity c_T is larger than that of an actin network of the same concentration ($c_T = c_A$) due to the larger molar mass of tubulin compared to actin subunits ($M_{w,T} \simeq 110$ kDa versus $M_{w,A} \simeq 42$ kDa) as well as the smaller length that each subunit adds to the polymer, $l_T \simeq \frac{8}{13}$ nm versus $l_A \simeq 2.7$ nm. Specifically, the mesh size, which depends on the subunit size a and subunits per volume c_N, via equation (2.80)

$$\xi \approx 1/\sqrt{c_N a} \tag{2.80}$$

(Schmidt *et al* 1989, Lin *et al* 2007) can be expressed as

$$\xi_{MT} \simeq 0.89\rho_T^{-1/2} \tag{5.37}$$

$$\xi_{MT} \simeq 890\left[M_w c_T\right]^{-\frac{1}{2}} \simeq 2.68 c_T^{-1/2} \tag{5.38}$$

where ξ_{MT} is in μm, ρ_T is the mass concentration of tubulin in mg mL^{-1}, and c_T is the molar concentration.

In comparison, the equivalent expressions for actin (see equation (5.16)) yield:

$$\xi_A \simeq 0.3\rho_A^{-1/2} \simeq 300\left[M_w c_A\right]^{-\frac{1}{2}} \simeq 1.46 c_A^{-1/2} \tag{5.39}$$

From these relations, we can see that for actin and microtubule networks with equal molar concentrations c or mass concentrations ρ, the mesh size for microtubules is larger than for actin according to:

$$\frac{\xi_{MT}}{\xi_A}(c) \simeq 1.84 \tag{5.40}$$

$$\frac{\xi_{MT}}{\xi_A}(\rho) = 2.97 \tag{5.41}$$

The tubulin concentration required to induce polymerization into microtubules in standard buffer conditions has been shown to be $c_p \approx 22$ μM (Hawkins *et al* 2010,

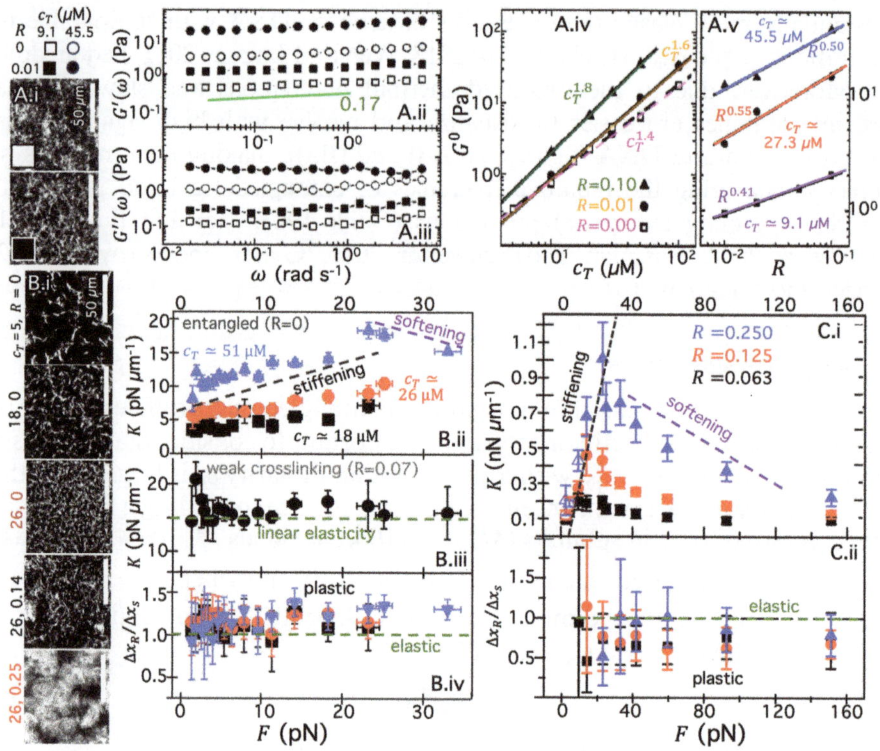

Figure 5.8. Microtubule network dynamics. (A) Bulk rheology measurements of entangled (white symbols, $R = 0$) and crosslinked ($R = 0.01$, black symbols) microtubule networks with $c_T \simeq 9.1$ μM (A.i, squares) and $c_T \simeq 45.5$ μM (circles) show that the viscoelastic moduli $G'(\omega)$ (ii) and $G''(\omega)$ (iii) for the higher concentration networks (circles) are substantially larger than those for the lower concentration network. Crosslinking (black symbols) also increases the magnitudes of $G'(\omega)$ and $G''(\omega)$ as compared to the entangled networks (white symbols), but to a lesser degree than the effect of c_T. The elastic modulus exhibits weak scaling of $G'(\omega) \sim \omega^{0.17}$ with frequency for all networks, while $G''(\omega)$ is independent of frequency across the entire frequency range. The elastic plateau modulus scales with concentration as $G^0 \sim c_T^b$ (A.iv) with the scaling exponent weakly increasing from $b \approx 1.4$ for $R = 0$ (magenta) to $b \approx 1.8$ for $R = 0.1$ (green). In a similar manner, G^0 follows power-law scaling $G^0 \sim R^y$ (A.v) with scaling exponents $y \approx 0.41$ (purple), 0.55 (red), and 0.50 (blue) for networks with $c_T \simeq 9.1$ μM, 27.3 μM, and 45.5 μM, respectively. (B and C) Magnetic tweezers microrheology measurements of entangled (B.ii,iv) and crosslinked (B.iii,C) microtubule networks with varying combinations of concentrations c_T (μM) (B) and crosslinker ratios R (C) as listed next to the corresponding confocal images in B.i. show that increasing c_T decreases the mesh size (top three images) while increasing R increases network heterogeneity (bottom three images). (B.i) The stiffness K measured as a function of force F applied on a magnetically trapped bead to move it through entangled microtubule networks with $c_T = 18$ μM (black), 26 μM (red), and 51 μM (blue) shows that the initial stiffness K_0 and degree of stiffening (black dashed line) increase with c_T, and, for the highest concentration, stiffening is followed by softening (purple dashed). (B.iii) Introducing a low-level of crosslinking ($R = 0.07$) increases K_0 by ~2-fold as compared to entangled networks at the same c_T (red data in B.ii), but eliminates the nonlinear stiffening and softening that entangled networks display (B.ii), as seen by the limited deviation of data points from the horizontal dashed line. (B.iv) The distance the bead recoils towards its starting position Δx_R following force cessation, scaled by its force-induced displacement Δx_F through the network as a function of applied force F. $\frac{\Delta x_R}{\Delta x_F} = 1$ signifies complete elastic recovery, as indicated by the green dashed line and observed for all networks in the low-force limit. Conversely, $\frac{\Delta x_R}{\Delta x_F} > 1$ suggests polymer buildup and depletion at the respective leading and lagging edges of the probe, enabling the probe to travel beyond its

starting point, as seen for higher forces ($F \gtrsim 10$ pN) and network concentrations. $\frac{\Delta x_R}{\Delta x_F} < 1$, only observed for crosslinked networks (C.ii), indicates stress dissipation via network rearrangement. The two $\frac{\Delta x_R}{\Delta x_F} \neq 1$ behaviors are types of plastic deformations, i.e., irreversible stress-induced network restructuring that prevents elastic recovery. (C) The same metrics shown in B.ii and B.iii for crosslinked microtubule networks with $R = 0.063$ (black), 0.125 (red), and 0.250 (blue). C.i shows that crosslinking increases the low-force stiffness K_0 of entangled networks ~20-fold and likewise substantially increases the degree of stiffening (black dashed line) in an R-dependent manner, with K increasing ~5-fold for the highest R value. Following stiffening, all networks transition to a pronounced softening regime (purple dashed line) at a crossover force F_c (black dashed line) which scales linearly with R. C.ii shows that crosslinked networks undergo dissipative plastic deformation ($\frac{\Delta x_R}{\Delta x_F} < 1$) opposite to that seen for entangled networks. (A) Adapted with permission from Lin *et al* (2007). Copyright (2007) American Chemical Society. (B) Adapted from Yang *et al* (2012a) with permission from the Royal Society of Chemistry. (C) Adapted from Yang *et al* (2012b) with permission from the Royal Society of Chemistry.

Wen and Janmey 2011, Hohmann and Dehghani 2019), which is quite high compared to that of actin and compared to the critical concentration to form entanglements. Moreover, as I describe in chapter 1, microtubules continuously undergo catastrophe and rescue events that abruptly change the length of the microtubules in a stochastic manner, making *in vitro* experiments difficult to perform and the interpretation of results equally complicated.

However, the presence of the cancer drug, paclitaxel (Taxol), during or after polymerization stabilizes microtubules against catastrophe and lowers the critical polymerization concentration to $c_p \approx 0.1$–$4\ \mu$M, thereby suppressing the dynamic instability that MTs often exhibit *in vitro* (O'Brien *et al* 1990, Hawkins *et al* 2010, Wen and Janmey 2011, Mirigian *et al* 2013, Huber *et al* 2015a). An alternative stabilization method often used is to replace GTP with its nonhydrolyzable analog GMPCPP during polymerization to halt depolymerization caused by GTP hydrolysis (Hawkins *et al* 2010, Chandrakar *et al* 2022). GMPCPP also lowers the critical polymerization concentration to $c_p \approx 150$ nM.

When choosing the stabilization method, it is important to consider that the polymerization kinetics, stiffness, and contour lengths are highly dependent on the stabilization method (Gittes *et al* 1993, Mickey and Howard 1995, Desai and Mitchison 1997, Hawkins *et al* 2010, Wen and Janmey 2011). Moreover, there is not clear consensus on the effect of Taxol stabilization on microtubule stiffness (Hawkins *et al* 2010). For example, Taxol has typically been observed to result in longer and more flexible microtubules that can form branched networks, while GMPCPP typically produces very short microtubules with an increased persistence length as compared to unstabilized microtubules (Wilson *et al* 1985, Mickey and Howard 1995, Hawkins *et al* 2010, Ricketts *et al* 2020, Chandrakar *et al* 2022). Various microtubule associated proteins (MAPs) and tau protein have also been shown to impact the stability, rigidity, and polymerization kinetics of microtubules, and may be incorporated into assays as desired. For example, tau protein and MAP2 have been shown to increase the rigidity of microtubules by ~3–4-fold without greatly impacting c_p (Felgner *et al* 1997).

Most previous studies investigating microtubule networks have used tubulin dimers purified from bovine or porcine brain tissue. Porcine brain tubulin is commercially available from, Cytoskeleton, Inc. ('Tubulin protein (>99% pure),' n.d.), while most in-house purification methods use bovine brain tissue (Miller and Wilson 2010 p. 1). Tubulin dimers labeled with fluorophores such as rhodamine, x-rhodamine, HiLyte Fluor 488, HiLyte Fluor 647, and AMCA are also commercially available from Cytoskeleton, Inc., allowing for fluorescence imaging of microtubules over a broad spectral range. In-house covalent labeling of tubulin dimers is also possible following standard carboxyl chemistry protocols as described in Yang *et al* (2012b).

Similar to incorporating labeled actin into actin networks (as I describe in section 5.2.3), microtubules can be visualized within networks by either doping in a small fraction of pre-formed microtubules, labeled at a high labeled:unlabeled dimer ratio (~1:1–1:4); or incorporating labeled dimers into the solution, at a lower ratio (~1:10–1:50), prior to network formation. Moreover, like actin, commercially available biotinylated tubulin dimers can be incorporated into networks to enable crosslinking of microtubules via NeutrAvidin, using equations (5.25–5.27) to determine the concentrations of tubulin, b-tubulin, NeutrAvidin, and biotin needed to reach a desired crosslinking ratio R.

The critical concentration for microtubules to form an entangled network has been reported as $c_e \approx 0.9\ \mu\text{M}$ ($\rho_T \approx 0.1\ \text{mg mL}^{-1}$), with networks remaining isotropically entangled up to $c_T \approx 45\ \mu\text{M}$ ($\rho_T \approx 5\ \text{mg mL}^{-1}$) (Lin *et al* 2007, Yang *et al* 2012b, Ricketts *et al* 2018). For higher concentrations, $c_T \gtrsim 50\ \mu\text{M}$, nematic crystal structures emerge in which large regions of microtubules are bundled together and oriented along a similar director (Hitt *et al* 1990, Lin *et al* 2007).

5.3.3 Network dynamics

5.3.3.1 Entangled microtubules

In the entangled regime, microtubule networks are predominantly elastic, with $G'(\omega) > G''(\omega)$ across the entire measurable frequency range, and $G'(\omega)$ weakly scaling as $\omega^{0.17}$ (figures 5.8(A.ii, iii)). The corresponding plateau moduli are of order $G^0 \approx 1$–10 Pa (figures 5.8(A.iv, v)) significantly larger than G^0 for entangled actin networks (figures 5.5(E) and (F)). However, the reported scaling with concentration, $G^0 \sim c_T^{7/5}$ (figure 5.8(A.iv)), aligns remarkably well with $G^0 \sim c_A^{7/5}$ observed for actin networks (figures 5.5(F) and (G)).

Magnetic tweezers microrheology (MTM) experiments probing the microscale response of entangled microtubule networks with $c_T \simeq 18$–$51\ \mu\text{M}$, showed that microtubule networks exhibit largely linear elastic response characteristics, similar to bulk rheology results (figure 5.8(A)), for applied forces up to $F \approx 15$ pN (figure 5.8(B.ii)). This linear elasticity was demonstrated by the stiffness K being independent of the force F such that its value remains near the low-force linear-limit value K_0

$$K \simeq K_0 \sim F^0 \tag{5.42}$$

(Yang *et al* 2012b). To understand how K is measured and quantified in MTM, recall that a set force F is applied to the probe in MTM and the distance Δx_F that the probe moves in response to that force is measured (as I describe in chapter 3), providing a measure of stiffness

$$K = F/\Delta x_F \tag{5.43}$$

similar to that measured with OTM (Lin and Valentine 2012). However, in OTM the distance that the probe moves is controlled and the resulting force is measured (Robertson-Anderson 2018).

In the linear elastic regime (eq. 5.37), the MTM-measured stiffness was reported to scale linearly with tubulin concentration,

$$K_0 \sim c_T^b \tag{5.44}$$

where $b \simeq 1$, in contrast to the $b \simeq 7/5$ scaling observed in bulk rheology measurements of microtubule networks (figure 5.8(A.iv)) as well as semiflexible actin networks (figure 5.5(F)). These different scaling exponents suggest that the micro-scale elasticity of microtubule networks is mechanical in origin as opposed to the entropic elasticity that dictates the response of semiflexible polymers and may play an more important role in the response of microtubule networks at macroscopic scales in which entropic bending and stretching may be more accessible (Gardel *et al* 2003, Yang *et al* 2012b, Gurmessa *et al* 2016a).

Beyond the linear elastic limit, $F > 15$ pN, entangled microtubule networks exhibit stress-stiffening in response to MTM strains (figure 5.8(Bii)), followed by modest softening for the highest concentration network. Unlike flexible and semi-flexible polymers, in which stiffening is expected to arise from entropic affine stretching of the polymers in the direction of the strain (Gurmessa *et al* 2017, Fitzpatrick *et al* 2018), at odds with the linear regime MTM scaling, these studies showed that stiffening resulted from the buildup of microtubules at the leading edge of the probe, increasing the local entanglement density and providing a higher restoring force (Yang *et al* 2012b).

Modest crosslinking of entangled microtubule networks was shown to increase the stiffness by ~3-fold while at the same time eliminating nonlinear stiffening and softening (figure 5.8(B.iii)), further supporting the physical picture of stiffening resulting from polymer buildup at the leading edge of the probe, as crosslinking would restrict this structural rearrangement. To conserve density, polymer buildup at the leading edge of the probe, which increases the local entanglement density, should result in a reduced entanglement density wake or void behind the moving probe. This density mismatch should be reflected as a difference in the distance that the bead travels in response to the applied force Δx_F compared to the distance that it recoils back towards its starting position following the cessation of force Δx_R. Namely, $\frac{\Delta x_R}{\Delta x_F} = 1$ would indicate uniform density throughout and a linear elastic response, while $\frac{\Delta x_R}{\Delta x_F} > 1$ would indicate that the probe experiences less steric hindrances in the recoil as compared to the force-induced displacement. As shown in figure 5.8(B.iv), $\frac{\Delta x_R}{\Delta x_F}$ becomes increasingly greater than unity for higher forces and network concentrations, consistent with the physical picture of polymer accumulation and depletion at the leading and lagging edges of the probe (Yang *et al* 2012b).

OTM experiments have also measured the nonlinear response of entangled microtubules at $c_T \simeq 11.6\ \mu$M (Ricketts *et al* 2018), showing that microtubules are more susceptible to buckling and breaking in response to large strains as compared to actin due to their inability to entropically stretch or appreciably bend in response to strain (Brangwynne *et al* 2006, Yang *et al* 2012b, Ricketts *et al* 2018). This property manifests in entangled microtubule networks as heterogeneous force responses with large peaks and valleys corresponding to buckling events (Yang *et al* 2012a, Ricketts *et al* 2018).

For strains smaller than those required to buckle filaments, OTM measurements showed that entangled microtubules behave as poroelastic solids (Kalcioglu *et al* 2012, Moeendarbary *et al* 2013, Punter *et al* 2020) with fast poroelastic draining rates of $\upsilon_p \approx 25$ kHz, ~40× faster than υ_p of actin networks with the same molar concentration (Ricketts *et al* 2018), and orders of magnitude faster than the <10 Hz strain rates used in the OTM experiments. This poroelastic response resulted in lower force resistance at small strains as compared to actin networks of the same concentration. However, at larger strains, microtubules exhibit stress-stiffening similar to that seen in MTM experiments (figure 5.8(Bii)), likely due to the rigid microtubules accumulating at the leading edge of the probe.

Following the nonlinear OTM straining described above, entangled microtubules were shown to relax the imposed force via power-law decay $F_R \sim t^{-0.35}$, similar to that measured for entangled actin networks (Falzone *et al* 2015b), following an initial period $\Delta t_0 \approx 20$ ms of minimal relaxation. The initial 'stalling' period for microtubules is consistent with poroelastic models (Moeendarbary *et al* 2013, Punter *et al* 2020), and indicates the lack of available network relaxation mechanisms for these short times $t < \Delta t_0$. Notably, similar two-phase power-law relaxation was also measured for entangled linear DNA subject to nonlinear straining (figure 5.3(F)) as well as composites of entangled DNA and actin (Chapman and Robertson-Anderson 2014, Fitzpatrick *et al* 2018), with the second power-law phase indicative of dynamic tube dilation and re-equilibration (Sussman and Schweizer 2012, Chapman and Robertson-Anderson 2014). This universal relaxation profile suggests that strain-induced variations to the equilibrium entanglement tube may be relatively insensitive to polymer stiffness.

Particle-tracking experiments have also been performed on entangled microtubule networks at the same concentration as in the OTM measurements described above ($c_T \simeq 11.6\ \mu$M), to characterize particle transport within the networks as well as their linear microrheological properties (Anderson *et al* 2019). These studies revealed that particles diffusing in entangled microtubule networks exhibited very weak subdiffusion, with a scaling exponent of $\alpha \simeq 0.94$, in contrast to $\alpha \simeq 0.58$ measured for actin networks at the same molar concentration. Corresponding van Hove distributions of particle displacements were also distinctly more Gaussian in microtubule networks compared to actin networks and the corresponding transport coefficients, $\vartheta = MSD/\Delta t^{\alpha}$, were ~4× larger (Anderson *et al* 2019).

These effects were reported to arise from the ~1.8× larger mesh size of microtubule networks compared to their actin counterparts (see equation 5.40), as well as their enhanced rigidity, which allows for greater separation between dynamic timescales of the particles and mesh (Regan *et al* 2019). Entangled microtubules also exhibited $\sim$4-fold lower viscosity ($\eta_{o,MT} \simeq 7$ mPa s versus $\eta_{o,A} \simeq 30$ mPa s) and $\sim$6-fold lower average shear modulus ($\langle G'_{MT}\rangle \simeq 10$ mPa versus $\langle G'_{MT}\rangle \simeq 60$ mPa), as compared to actin networks, as well as a greater frequency dependence of $G'(\omega)$, and weaker shear thinning—all indicators of reduced elasticity (Anderson *et al* 2019). These findings are in contrast to bulk rheological measurements that show that entangled microtubules have a higher shear modulus and weaker scaling of G' and G'' with frequency than actin (Lin *et al* 2007), suggesting a scale-dependent hierarchy of mechanical responses and the need for measurements to be performed across several scales.

5.3.3.2 Crosslinked microtubules

In vitro microtubule networks can be crosslinked via an array of physiological crosslinking MAPs (microtubule associated proteins). One such MAP that has been used broadly in studies on *in vitro* networks, is MAP65, which crosslinks antiparallel microtubules (Edozie *et al* 2019, Farhadi *et al* 2020, Hawkins *et al* 2010, Hess and Ross, 2017, Pringle *et al* 2013). MAP65 crosslinking sorts isotropic microtubule networks into arrays of nematic bundles (Edozie *et al* 2019), enhancing the network rigidity, while at the same time allowing for relative sliding between linked filaments due to the compliant nature of MAP65 linkers (Subramanian *et al* 2010).

Microtubules can also be crosslinked via biotin-Neutravidin bonding by incorporating biotinylated tubulin dimers into microtubules, similar to the method described above to crosslink actin filaments. Confocal imaging, MTM, and bulk rheology measurements have been performed on crosslinked microtubule networks with tubulin concentrations $c_T \simeq 2.9$–$45.5\ \mu$M and ratios $R = 0.01$–0.25 (Lin *et al* 2007, Yang *et al* 2012a). These studies demonstrated that increasing crosslinking ratios increase the degree of structural heterogeneity of microtubule networks (figures 5.8(A.i) and (B.i)). Moreover, bulk rheology measurements showed that a modest crosslinking density of $R = 0.01$ led to a $\sim$3-fold and $\sim$6-fold increase in the plateau modulus G^0 from the entangled network value for respective network concentrations of $c_T \simeq 9.1\ \mu$M and $c_T \simeq 45.5\ \mu$M (figures 5.8(A.ii, iii)) (Lin *et al* 2007, Yang *et al* 2012a). However, the scaling relations $G^0 \sim c_T^b$ (figure 5.8(A.iv)) and $G^0 \sim R^y$ (figure 5.8(A.v)) were not universal, but instead scaling exponents of $b \approx 1.4$–1.8 and $y \approx 0.41$–0.55 were measured for varying R and c_T values, respectively (figures 5.8(A.iv,v)).

MTM measurements on highly crosslinked microtubule networks, similar to those performed for entangled microtubule networks (figure 5.8(B)), showed that crosslinking substantially increases the low-force stiffness K_0 and the degree of stress-stiffening above that of entangled networks. Specifically, K_0 was measured to be $\sim$20-fold higher, and stiffening led to a peak value of $K/K_0 \approx 5$ for the highest R value (figure 5.8(C.i)). After reaching a crossover force F_c, which scales linearly with R, crosslinked networks transitioned from stiffening to softening, displaying a more pronounced softening regime as compared to entangled networks, in opposition to results for entangled and crosslinked actin networks (Gardel *et al* 2004, Shin *et al* 2004). Notably, for all crosslinking ratios, K nearly returned to the initial linear-limit K_0 value in the high-force limit (figure 5.8(C.i)), suggestive of dissipative dynamics and plastic restructuring (Yang *et al* 2012a). This physical picture is supported by the reduced recoil of the probe following force cessation, i.e., $\frac{\Delta x_R}{\Delta x_F} < 1$, which was suggested to arise from forced crosslinker unbinding, allowing for larger displacements Δx_F, and rebinding, leading to reduced recoil Δx_R as filaments behind the moving probe reform connections that hinder its reverse motion. Notably, these dynamics are in direct opposition to those observed for entangled microtubule networks in which $\frac{\Delta x_R}{\Delta x_F} > 1$ due to polymer buildup and depletion (figures 5.8(B.iv) and (C.ii)). Moreover, despite this plastic deformation and dissipation, the networks maintain substantial elasticity following strain (figure 5.8(C.i)), indicating that the stress is sustained by a small fraction of stably crosslinked stress-bearing microtubules, while the majority of the network can relax via unlinking and re-linking. A similar phenomenon has been shown to play an important role in the nonlinear response of crosslinked actin networks (Kim *et al* 2014, Gurmessa *et al* 2017). An additional contribution to the sustained elasticity is suggested to arise from the balanced formation and breakage of bonds (Yang *et al* 2012a).

5.4 Intermediate filament (IF) networks

5.4.1 Intermediate filaments as diverse and tunable flexible polymers

Unlike their cytoskeletal partners, actin and microtubules, intermediate filaments constitute an entire class of polymers, including, e.g., vimentin, keratin, neurofilaments, lamins, and desmins, each with distinct properties and functions (Herrmann *et al* 2007, Wen and Janmey 2011, Block *et al* 2015, Charrier and Janmey 2016). As I describe in chapter 1, intermediate filaments assemble via annealing of ULFs at high ionic strength, forming flexible filaments with $d \simeq 9$–13 nm, $l_p \approx 0.3$–1 μm, and $L \approx 5$–20 μm. Similar to other flexible polymers, intermediate filaments typically assume random coil conformations in solution, and form entangled networks at $\rho_e \approx 0.2$–10 mg mL^{-1} (Herrmann *et al* 2007, Block *et al* 2015, Charrier and Janmey 2016).

In response to stresses, intermediate filaments can also undergo substantial entropic stretching, from random coil to extended conformations ($R_0 \rightarrow L$), as well as mechanical stretching to lengths beyond their unstressed contour lengths ($L \rightarrow L + \Delta L$) (Wen and Janmey 2011, Köster *et al* 2010, 2015, Pegoraro *et al* 2017, Aufderhorst-Roberts and Koenderink 2019). This unique extensibility, inaccessible to actin and microtubules, allows intermediate filaments to withstand much higher stresses than actin and microtubules without rupturing or buckling. Similar to actin, intermediate filaments can also form crosslinks and bundles in the presence of counterions such as Mg^{2+} at millimolar concentrations (figures 5.5(A) and (B) and 5.9) (Schopferer *et al* 2009, Lin *et al* 2010a, Köster *et al* 2015). The extent of bundling versus crosslinking via counterion-crossbridging differs among different types of intermediate filaments, which, in turn, has been shown to play a dominant role in the structure and mechanics of their networks (figure 5.9(A)) (Schopferer *et al* 2009, Lin *et al* 2010a, 2010b, Pawelzyk *et al* 2014, Köster *et al* 2015, Aufderhorst-Roberts and Koenderink 2019, Elbalasy *et al* 2021).

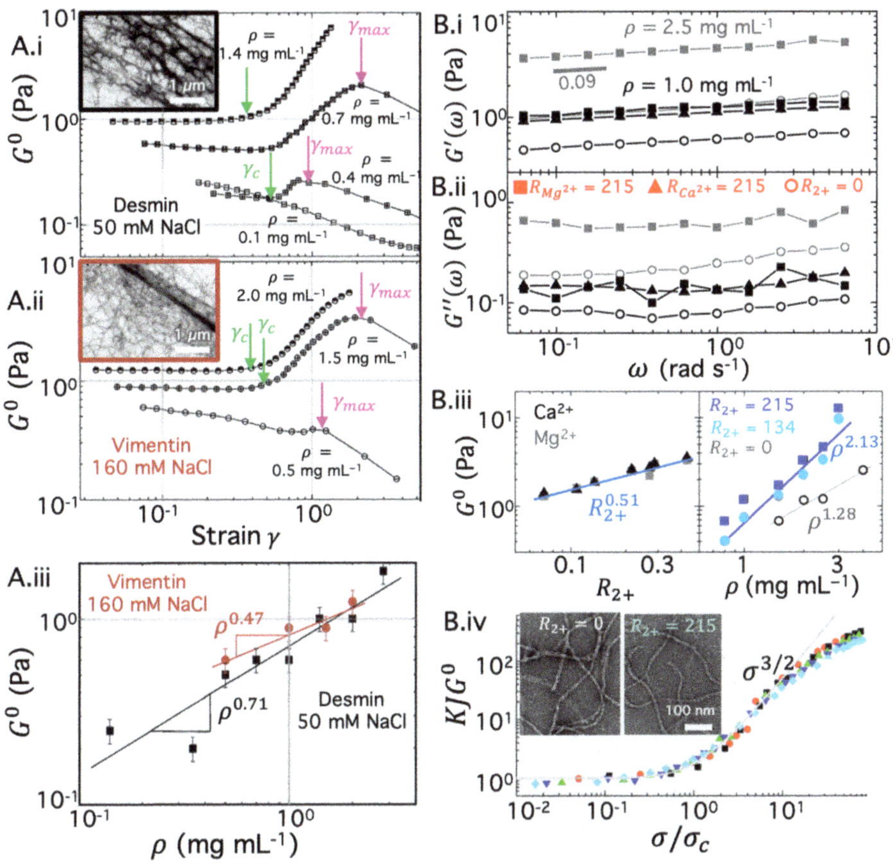

Figure 5.9. Dynamics and structure of networks of intermediate filaments. (A) The distinct structure (insets) and rheological properties of (i) desmin in low salt conditions ([NaCl] = 50 mM) and (ii) vimentin in high salt conditions ([NaCl] = 160 mM) at mass concentrations ρ of (i) ρ_d = 0.1–1.4 mg mL^{-1} and (ii) ρ_v = 0.5–2.0 mg mL^{-1}; and (iii) their different scalings of the shear modulus with concentration $G^0 \sim \rho^b$. Insets show that desmin (i, black border) undergoes substantial bundling and crosslinking at much lower salt (50 mM NaCl) than is required to crosslink vimentin (ii, red border). (iii) G^0 for desmin also exhibits steeper scaling with concentration compared to vimentin, with exponents of $b_d \simeq 0.71$ (black) and $b_v \simeq 0.47$ (red). (i, ii) Despite these distinct linear regime rheological properties, both intermediate filaments at concentrations $\rho \geqslant 0.4$ mg mL^{-1} crossover to nonlinear stiffening at the same critical strain $\gamma_c \approx 0.5$ (i, ii). However, the degree of stiffening, $G_{\max}/G^0$, as well as the strain at which stiffening yields to softening γ_y (blue arrows), does increase with ρ and differs between desmin and vimentin. (B) Dependence of linear (i–iii) and nonlinear (iv) rheological properties of vimentin networks on the concentrations of vimentin ρ_v and the molar ratio R_{2+} of divalent counterions (Mg^{2+} or Ca^{2+}) to vimentin. (i) $G'(\omega)$ and (ii) $G''(\omega)$ for vimentin networks at ρ_v = 1 mg mL^{-1} (black symbols) and ρ_v = 2.5 mg mL^{-1} (grey symbols) with $R_{2+} = 0$ (open circles), $R_{Mg^{2+}} = 215$ (filled squares), and $R_{Ca^{2+}} = 215$ (filled triangles), reveal elastic-like properties across all compositions and frequencies, including $G'(\omega) > G''(\omega)$ and very minimal dependence of G' with frequency. Both moduli increase with increasing ρ_v and R_{2+} as further quantified by (iii) the scaling of G^0 with R_{2+} (left) and ρ_v (right). The scaling relation $G^0 \sim R_{2+}^{0.51}$ is measured for vimentin networks with ρ_v = 2 mg mL^{-1} in the presence of either Mg^{2+} (grey) or Ca^{2+} (black). The scaling exponent relating G^0 to ρ_v is $b_v \simeq 2.13$ for both $R_{Mg^{2+}} = 215$ (blue) and $R_{Mg^{2+}} = 134$ (cyan), but drops to $b_v \simeq 1.28$ in the no salt condition ($R_{2+} = 0$, open circles). (iv) In response to nonlinear straining, vimentin networks with varying concentrations of vimentin and salt collapse onto a single master curve that exhibits stress-stiffening $K/G^0 \sim \sigma^{3/2}$ for stresses above the critical stress σ_c that follows the prediction for affine deformation of crosslinked polymer networks (grey line). The different colors correspond to

networks with different crosslinker lengths l_c in μm [0.69 (red circles), 0.65 (black squares), 0.54 (green triangles), 0.45 (purple inverted triangles), 0.39 (cyan diamonds)] computed for each (ρ_v, R_{2+}) combination via equations (5.45) and (5.46). Insets show transmission electron micrographs of vimentin networks assembled without divalent counterions ($R_{2+} = 0$) or in presence of Mg^{2+} at $R_{2+} = 215$. (A) Adapted from Schopferer *et al* (2009), Copyright (2009), with permission from Elsevier. (B) Adapted from Lin *et al* (2010a), Copyright (2010), with permission from Elsevier.

5.4.2 Design considerations

The diversity of intermediate filaments demands many approaches to purification and preparation (Köster *et al* 2015), with very few commercially available options. Moreover, a common property among most intermediate filaments is their surprising insolubility *in vitro* under physiological conditions. For this reason, intermediate filaments are typically purified in denaturing conditions, using buffers that contain high concentrations of urea or guanidine HCl. A common approach to refolding purified intermediate filaments into their native conformations, is to perform step-wise dialysis to incrementally remove the urea. During this process, the buffer remains at low ionic strength (typically 5 mM Tris-HCl, pH 8.5), to prevent assembly of dimers and tetramers into filaments (Köster *et al* 2015, Patteson *et al* 2020). To initiate polymerization, the ionic strength of the buffer is increased by adding 160 mM NaCl and 20 mM Tris-HCl. During this assembly step, intermediate filaments often form bundles or crosslinks, which can be tuned by the concentrations and types of intermediate filaments and counterions (figure 5.9) (Schopferer *et al* 2009, Lin *et al* 2010b, 2010a, Köster *et al* 2010, 2015, Charrier and Janmey 2016, Aufderhorst-Roberts and Koenderink, 2019). Given the tendency of intermediate filaments to aggregate and 'crash out' of solution, polymerized intermediate filaments solutions are typically only considered viable for 1–3 days when stored at 4°C.

5.4.3 Network dynamics

5.4.3.1 Linear viscoelasticity

The linear rheological response of networks of intermediate filaments has been shown to be largely elastic, with $G'(\omega) > G''(\omega)$ and minimal frequency-dependence across measurable frequency ranges (figures 5.9(B.i, ii)). The mechanism for this linear elasticity is understood to be the entropic stretching of thermally coiled filaments, similar to other flexible polymers (MacKintosh *et al* 1995, Lin *et al* 2010b). Plateau modulus values of $G^0 \approx 0.2$–50 Pa and scaling relations $G^0 \sim \rho^b$, with $b \simeq 0.5$–2.5 have been reported, with G^0 and b values dependent on the type of intermediate filament and ionic conditions (figure 5.9(A.iii)) (Schopferer *et al* 2009, Broedersz *et al* 2010, Köster *et al* 2010, Lin *et al* 2010a, 2010b, Pawelzyk *et al* 2014, Charrier and Janmey 2016). For example, $G^0 \approx 10$ Pa was measured for networks of neurofilaments at $\rho = 2$ mg mL^{-1} and $[Mg^{2+}] = 5$ mM, which is ~5× higher than $G^0 \approx 2$ Pa reported for vimentin networks at the same mass concentration and ionic conditions (Lin *et al* 2010b). For many more comparisons like this one, see Charrier and Janmey (2016) for a comprehensive table of properties and references organized by intermediate filament type and concentration.

Counterion-crosslinking has also been shown to play an important role in the mechanical response of intermediate filament networks, with the impact of salt concentration and valency on the viscoelastic and structural network properties being highly dependent on the type of intermediate filament (Schopferer *et al* 2009, Lin *et al* 2010a, 2010b, Yao *et al* 2010, Leitner *et al* 2012, Charrier and Janmey 2016). For example, G^0 for vimentin networks at $\rho = 2$ mg mL^{-1} was reported to scale with the ratio R_{2+} of divalent crosslinkers to vimentin according to the power-law relation $G^0 \sim R_{2+}^{\mho}$ with $\mho \simeq 0.51$ (Lin *et al* 2010a), for both Mg^{2+} and Ca^{2+}, while $G^0 \sim [Mg^{2+}]^{3/5}$ was reported for neurofilaments (Lin *et al* 2010b), similar to the reported scaling for actin networks (Gurmessa *et al* 2019). This dependence is directly linked to the extent of crosslinking of filaments by the counterions which increases the elastic modulus according to

$$G^0 = 6c_N k_B T \frac{l_p^2}{l_c^3} \tag{5.45}$$

where $c_N \sim \rho$ is the filament number density and $l_c \sim R_{2+}^{-\mho/3}$ is the length between counterion crosslinks, such that

$$G^0 \sim \rho R_{2+}^{\mho} \tag{5.46}$$

for intermediate filaments that primarily form crosslinks rather than bundles in the presence of salt.

5.4.3.2 Nonlinear rheology

In response to nonlinear straining, networks of intermediate filaments have been shown to stress-stiffen in response to strains that induce softening in networks of actin and microtubules (Schopferer *et al* 2009, Yao *et al* 2010, Lin *et al* 2010b, Pawelzyk *et al* 2014, Block *et al* 2015, Žagar *et al* 2015, Charrier and Janmey 2016, Aufderhorst-Roberts and Koenderink 2019). The origin of this robust stiffening behavior has been shown to be mechanical (enthalpic) stretching and crosslink-governed affine deformation (Broedersz *et al* 2010, Lin *et al* 2010b, 2010a, Aufderhorst-Roberts and Koenderink, 2019), the latter of which relies heavily on counterions to crosslink filaments.

In this nonlinear stiffening regime, which occurs at stresses above a critical stress σ_c, the differential modulus has been reported to increase by over two orders of magnitude, depending on the type and concentration of intermediate filaments and ionic conditions (figures 5.9(A.i, ii) and (B.iv)) (Leitner *et al* 2012, Žagar *et al* 2015, Charrier and Janmey 2016, Aufderhorst-Roberts and Koenderink 2019), and scale universally with stress according to

$$K \sim \sigma^{3/2} \tag{5.47}$$

This scaling aligns with theoretical predictions for crosslinked networks of semiflexible filaments (MacKintosh *et al* 1995, Kasza *et al* 2009) and experimental results for crosslinked actin networks (Gardel *et al* 2004).

Like the value of K, the critical nonlinear stress σ_c also depends on the network composition according to the predicted relation

$$\sigma_c = c_N k_B T \frac{l_p}{l_c^2} \tag{5.48}$$

which provides the experimentally accessible scaling relation

$$\sigma_c \sim \rho R_{2+}^{\mho/2} \tag{5.49}$$

Using equations (5.46) and (5.49) to scale K and σ by their respective G^0 and σ_c values, data for a range of concentrations of intermediate filaments and counterions can be plotted together to demonstrate universal data collapse in the stiffening regime that aligns with equation 5.47 (figure 5.9(B.iv)).

Another important feature of intermediate filament networks in the nonlinear regime, which varies among different network compositions, is the critical stress $\sigma_{\max}$ at which stiffening transitions to softening, yielding, or rupture. For example, counterion-crosslinking has been shown to play a key role in sustaining vimentin networks against rupture and softening, thereby increasing $\sigma_{\max}$ (Aufderhorst-Roberts and Koenderink 2019). In contrast, $\sigma_{\max}$ for desmin networks has been reported to be relatively insensitive to ionic strength, which has been rationalized as arising from the increased propensity for counterions to bundle desmin filaments rather than form isotropic crosslinks (Schopferer *et al* 2009).

5.5 Canonical building blocks for complex biopolymer networks

The systems described in this chapter are model systems for probing open questions in polymer physics and design challenges in materials engineering. They also serve as well-characterized foundational building blocks from which to engineer a vast array of more complex biopolymer networks that I discuss in the remaining chapters. The four canonical systems discussed in this chapter span orders of magnitude in stiffness, from flexible (DNA, intermediate filaments) to semiflexible (actin filaments), to rigid (microtubules). They are all linear chains, and form entangled networks over a range of polymer concentrations in solution, facilitating comparison with other linear polymer systems, including synthetic polymers, and testing well-established theoretical predictions for linear polymers.

The persistence lengths, contour lengths, and monomeric subunits of these canonical biopolymers are also well-defined and characterized to enable broad use with established protocols. While the phase space of dynamics and rheological properties of DNA and actin networks have been exhaustively explored, there are comparatively fewer studies for microtubules and intermediate filaments, which are also more complex in terms of their length distributions, polymerization conditions, and interactions with counterions.

Armed with the design tips, descriptions and rheological characterizations of these four canonical biopolymer networks, I encourage you to mix and match these building blocks to design and interrogate novel material platforms, biomimetic networks, and other experimental systems that you can dream up to advance our current understanding of polymer physics, soft matter, biophysics, and beyond.

The following chapters will provide examples of such biopolymer networks with layered complexity, focusing on the effects of polymer topology (chapter 6), mixing polymers of different species (chapter 7), non-equilibrium active processes (chapter 8), and heterogeneous structures (chapter 9), on the dynamics, structure, and rheological properties of a diverse range of biopolymer networks.

References

Abhilash A S, Purohit P K and Joshi S P 2012 Stochastic rate-dependent elasticity and failure of soft fibrous networks *Soft Matter* **8** 7004–16

Acti-stain 488 phalloidin [WWW Document] n.d. https://cytoskeleton.com/phdg1 (accessed 21 September 2023)

Adami R, Choquet D and Grazi E 1999 Rhodamine phalloidin F-actin: critical concentration versus tensile strength *Eur. J. Biochem.* **263** 270–5

Adami R, Cintio O, Trombetta G, Choquet D and Grazi E 2003 On the stiffness of the natural actin filament decorated with alexa fluor tropomyosin *Biophys. Chem.* **104** 469–76

Alexa FluorTM 594 Phalloidin [WWW Document] n.d. https://thermofisher.com/order/catalog/product/A12381 (accessed 21 September 2023)

Anderson S J, Matsuda C, Garamella J, Peddireddy K R, Robertson-Anderson R M and McGorty R 2019 Filament rigidity vies with mesh size in determining anomalous diffusion in cytoskeleton *Biomacromolecules* **20** 4380–8

Andrianantoandro E and Pollard T D 2006 Mechanism of actin filament turnover by severing and nucleation at different concentrations of ADF/Cofilin *Mol. Cell* **24** 13–23

Aporvari M S, Dang S, Marfai J, Coursey K, McGorty R and Robertson-Anderson R M 2022 Crowding and confinement act in concert to slow DNA diffusion within cell-sized droplets *iScience* **25** 105122

Aragon S R and Pecora R 1985 Dynamics of wormlike chains *Macromolecules* **18** 1868–75

Aufderhorst-Roberts A and Koenderink G H 2019 Stiffening and inelastic fluidization in vimentin intermediate filament networks **15** 7127–36

Bamburg J R 1999 Proteins of the ADF/Cofilin Family: essential regulators of actin dynamics *Annu. Rev. Cell Dev. Biol.* **15** 185–230

Banik S, Kong D, San Francisco M J and McKenna G B 2021 Monodisperse lambda DNA as a model to conventional polymers: a concentration-dependent scaling of the rheological properties *Macromolecules* **54** 8632–54

Barden J A, Miki M, Hambly B D and G. Dos Remedios C 1987 Localization of the phalloidin and nucleotide-binding sites on actin *Eur. J. Biochem.* **162** 583–8

Bellone D E, Bours J, Menke E H and Fischer F R 2015 Highly selective molybdenum ONO pincer complex initiates the living ring-opening metathesis polymerization of strained alkynes with exceptionally low polydispersity indices *J. Am. Chem. Soc.* **137** 850–6

Blanchoin L, Pollard T D and Mullins R D 2000 Interactions of ADF/cofilin, Arp2/3 complex, capping protein and profilin in remodeling of branched actin filament networks *Curr. Biol.* **10** 1273–82

Block J, Schroeder V, Pawelzyk P, Willenbacher N and Köster S 2015 Physical properties of cytoplasmic intermediate filaments *Biochim. Biophys. Acta (BBA)—Mol. Cell Res., Mechanobiol.* **1853** 3053–64

Bouchaud J-P and Georges A 1990 Anomalous diffusion in disordered media: statistical mechanisms, models and physical applications *Phys. Rep.* **195** 127–293

Boukany P E, Hemminger O, Wang S-Q and Lee L J 2010 Molecular imaging of slip in entangled DNA solution *Phys. Rev. Lett.* **105** 027802

Brangwynne C P, MacKintosh F C, Kumar S, Geisse N A, Talbot J, Mahadevan L, Parker K K, Ingber D E and Weitz D A 2006 Microtubules can bear enhanced compressive loads in living cells because of lateral reinforcement *J. Cell Biol.* **173** 733–41

Brau R R, Tarsa P B, Ferrer J M, Lee P and Lang M J 2006 Interlaced optical force-fluorescence measurements for single molecule biophysics *Biophys. J.* **91** 1069–77

Bravo-Anaya L M, Rinaudo M and Martínez F A S 2016 Conformation and rheological properties of calf-thymus DNA in solution *Polymers* **8** 51

Broedersz C P, Depken M, Yao N Y, Pollak M R, Weitz D A and MacKintosh F C 2010 Cross-link-governed dynamics of biopolymer networks *Phys. Rev. Lett.* **105** 238101

Broedersz C P and MacKintosh F C 2014 Modeling semiflexible polymer networks *Rev. Mod. Phys.* **86** 995–1036

Buchanan M, Atakhorrami M, Palierne J F and Schmidt c f 2005 Comparing macrorheology and one- and two-point microrheology in wormlike micelle solutions *Macromolecules* **38** 8840–4

Chandrakar P *et al* 2022 Engineering stability, longevity, and miscibility of microtubule-based active fluids *Soft Matter* **18** 1825–35

Chapman C D, Gorczyca S and Robertson-Anderson R M 2015 Crowding induces complex ergodic diffusion and dynamic elongation of large DNA molecules *Biophys. J.* **108** 1220–8

Chapman C D, Lee K, Henze D, Smith D E and Robertson-Anderson R M 2014 Onset of non-continuum effects in microrheology of entangled polymer solutions *Macromolecules* **47** 1181–6

Chapman C D and Robertson-Anderson R M 2014 Nonlinear microrheology reveals entanglement-driven molecular-level viscoelasticity of concentrated DNA *Phys. Rev. Lett.* **113** 098303

Charrier E E and Janmey P A 2016 Chapter Two—Mechanical properties of intermediate filament proteins ed M B Omary and R K H Liem *Methods in Enzymology, Intermediate Filament Proteins* (New York: Academic) pp 35–57

Chechkin A V, Seno F, Metzler R and Sokolov I M 2017 Brownian yet non-Gaussian diffusion: from superstatistics to subordination of diffusing diffusivities *Phys. Rev.* X **7** 021002

Chen S, Markovich T and MacKintosh F C 2023 Nonaffine deformation of semiflexible polymer and fiber networks *Phys. Rev. Lett.* **130** 088101

Claessens M M a E, Tharmann R, Kroy K and Bausch A R 2006 Microstructure and viscoelasticity of confined semiflexible polymer networks *Nat. Phys.* **2** 186–9

Cooper J A 1987 Effects of cytochalasin and phalloidin on actin *J. Cell Biol.* **105** 1473–8

Das M, MacKintosh F C and Levine A J 2007 Effective medium theory of semiflexible filamentous networks *Phys. Rev. Lett.* **99** 038101

de Gennes P-G 1979 *Scaling Concepts in Polymer Physics* (Ithaca, NY: Cornell University Press)

de Gennes P G 2003 Reptation of a polymer chain in the presence of fixed obstacles *J. Chem. Phys.* **55** 572–9

De La Cruz E M and Gardel M L 2015 Actin mechanics and fragmentation *J. Biol. Chem.* **290** 17137–44

Desai A and Mitchison T J 1997 Microtubule polymerization dynamics *Annu. Rev. Cell Dev. Biol.* **13** 83–117

Dichtl M A and Sackmann E 2002 Microrheometry of semiflexible actin networks through enforced single-filament reptation: frictional coupling and heterogeneities in entangled networks *Proc. Natl Acad. Sci. USA* **99** 6533–8

Ditsch A and Wegner A 1994 Nucleation of actin polymerization by gelsolin *Europ. J. Biochem.* **224** 223–7

Doi M and Edwards S F 1988 *The Theory of Polymer Dynamics* (Oxford: Clarendon)

Dwyer M E, Robertson-Anderson R M and Gurmessa B J 2022 Nonlinear microscale mechanics of actin networks governed by coupling of filament crosslinking and stabilization *Polymers* **14** 4980

Edozie B, Sahu S, Pitta M, Englert A, do Rosario c f and Ross J L 2019 Self-organization of spindle-like microtubule structures *Soft Matter* **15** 4797–807

Elbalasy I, Mollenkopf P, Tutmarc C, Herrmann H and Schnauß J 2021 Keratins determine network stress responsiveness in reconstituted actin–keratin filament systems *Soft Matter* **17** 3954–62

Ermentrout G B and Edelstein-Keshet L 1998 Models for the length distributions of actin filaments: II. Polymerization and fragmentation by gelsolin acting together *Bull. Math. Biol.* **60** 477–503

Esue O, Tseng Y and Wirtz D 2009 α-Actinin and filamin cooperatively enhance the stiffness of actin filament networks *PLoS One* **4** e4411

Everaers R, Jülicher F, Ajdari A and Maggs A C 1999 Dynamic fluctuations of semiflexible filaments *Phys. Rev. Lett.* **82** 3717–20

Falzone T T, Blair S and Robertson-Anderson R M 2015a Entangled F-actin displays a unique crossover to microscale nonlinearity dominated by entanglement segment dynamics *Soft Matter* **11** 4418–23

Falzone T T, Blair S and Robertson-Anderson R M 2015b Entangled F-actin displays a unique crossover to microscale nonlinearity dominated by entanglement segment dynamics *Soft Matter* **11** 4418–23

Falzone T T, Lenz M, Kovar D R and Gardel M L 2012 Assembly kinetics determine the architecture of α-actinin crosslinked F-actin networks *Nat. Commun.* **3** 861

Falzone T T and Robertson-Anderson R M 2015 Active entanglement-tracking microrheology directly couples macromolecular deformations to nonlinear microscale force response of entangled actin *ACS Macro Letters* **4** 1194–9

Farhadi L, Ricketts S N, Rust M J, Das M, Robertson-Anderson R M and Ross J L 2020 Actin and microtubule crosslinkers tune mobility and control co-localization in a composite cytoskeletal network *Soft Matter*

Felgner H, Frank R, Biernat J, Mandelkow E-M, Mandelkow E, Ludin B, Matus A and Schliwa M 1997 Domains of neuronal microtubule-associated proteins and flexural rigidity of microtubules *J. Cell Biol.* **138** 1067–75

Fitzpatrick R, Michieletto D, Peddireddy K R, Hauer C, Kyrillos C, Gurmessa B J and Robertson-Anderson R M 2018 Synergistic interactions between DNA and actin trigger emergent viscoelastic behavior *Phys. Rev. Lett.* **121** 257801

Frey E, Kroy K and Wilhelm J 1999 Viscoelasticity of biopolymer networks and statistical mechanics of semiflexible polymers *Advances in Structural Biology* (Amsterdam: Elsevier) pp 135–68

Frieden C 1983 Polymerization of actin: mechanism of the Mg^{2+}-induced process at pH 8 and 20 degrees C *Proc. Natl Acad. Sci. USA* **80** 6513–7

Fujiwara I, Takahashi S, Tadakuma H, Funatsu T and Ishiwata S 2002 Microscopic analysis of polymerization dynamics with individual actin filaments *Nat. Cell Biol.* **4** 666–73

Garamella J, Regan K, Aguirre G, McGorty R J and Robertson-Anderson R M 2020 Anomalous and heterogeneous DNA transport in biomimetic cytoskeleton networks *Soft Matter* **16** 6344–53

Gardel M L, Kasza K E, Brangwynne C P, Liu J and Weitz D A 2008 Mechanical response of cytoskeletal networks *Methods Cell Biol.* **89** 487–519

Gardel M L, Shin J H, MacKintosh F C, Mahadevan L, Matsudaira P and Weitz D A 2004 Elastic behavior of cross-linked and bundled actin networks *Science* **304** 1301

Gardel M L, Valentine M T, Crocker J C, Bausch A R and Weitz D A 2003 Microrheology of entangled F-actin solutions *Phys. Rev. Lett.* **91** 1 58302

Gentry B, Smith D and Käs J 2009 Buckling-induced zebra stripe patterns in nematic F-actin *Phys. Rev.* E **79** 031916

Gisler T and Weitz D A 1999 Scaling of the microrheology of semidilute F-actin solutions *Phys. Rev. Lett.* **82** 1606–9

Gittes F and MacKintosh F C 1998 Dynamic shear modulus of a semiflexible polymer network *Phys. Rev.* E **58** R1241–4

Gittes F, Mickey B, Nettleton J and Howard J 1993 Flexural rigidity of microtubules and actin filaments measured from thermal fluctuations in shape *J. Cell Biol.* **120** 923–34

Gittes F, Schnurr B, Olmsted P D, MacKintosh F C and Schmidt c f 1997 Microscopic viscoelasticity: shear moduli of soft materials determined from thermal fluctuations *Phys. Rev. Lett.* **79** 3286–9

Glaser J and Kroy K 2011 Tube-width fluctuations of entangled stiff polymers *Phys. Rev.* E **84** 051801

Glaser J and Kroy K 2010 Fluctuations of stiff polymers and cell mechanics *Biopolymers* ed M Elnashar (IntechOpen)

Goldstein A L, Hannappel E and Kleinman H K 2005 Thymosin β4: actin-sequestering protein moonlights to repair injured tissues *Trends Mol. Med.* **11** 421–9

Gorczyca S M, Chapman C D and Robertson-Anderson R M 2015 Universal scaling of crowding-induced DNA mobility is coupled with topology-dependent molecular compaction and elongation *Soft Matter* **11** 7762–8

Guilbaud S, Salomé L, Destainville N, Manghi M and Tardin C 2019 Dependence of DNA persistence length on ionic strength and ion type *Phys. Rev. Lett.* **122** 028102

Gurmessa B, Fitzpatrick R, Falzone T T and Robertson-Anderson R M 2016a Entanglement density tunes microscale nonlinear response of entangled actin *Macromolecules* **49** 3948–55

Gurmessa B, Fitzpatrick R, Falzone T T and Robertson-Anderson R M 2016b Entanglement density tunes microscale nonlinear response of entangled actin *Macromolecules* **49** 3948–55

Gurmessa B, Francis M, Rust M J, Das M, Ross J L and Robertson-Anderson R M 2019 Counterion crossbridges enable robust multiscale elasticity in actin networks *Phys. Rev. Res.* **1** 013016

Gurmessa B, Ricketts S and Robertson-Anderson R M 2017 Nonlinear actin deformations lead to network stiffening, yielding, and nonuniform stress propagation *Biophys. J.* **113** 1540–50

Gurmessa B J, Bitten N, Nguyen D T, Saleh O A, Ross J L, Das M and Robertson-Anderson R M 2018 Triggered disassembly and reassembly of actin networks induces rigidity phase transitions *Soft Matter* **15** 1335–44

Gurmessa B J, Rust M J, Das M, Ross J L and Robertson-Anderson R M 2021 Salt-mediated stiffening, destruction, and resculpting of actomyosin network *Front. Phys.* **9** 760340

Hansen S D, Zuchero J B and Mullins R D 2013 Cytoplasmic actin: purification and single molecule assembly assays ed A S Coutts *Adhesion Protein Protocols, Methods Mol. Biol.* (Totowa, NJ: Humana Press) pp 145–70

Hawkins T, Mirigian M, Selcuk Yasar M and Ross J L 2010 Mechanics of microtubules *J. Biomech.* **43** 23–30

Head D A, Levine A J and MacKintosh F C 2005 The mechanical response of semiflexible networks to localized perturbations *Phys. Rev.* E **72** 061914

Henle M and Pincus P 2005 Equilibrium bundle size of rodlike polyelectrolytes with counterion-induced attractive interactions *Phys. Rev.* E **71** 060801

Heo Y and Larson R G 2005 The scaling of zero-shear viscosities of semidilute polymer solutions with concentration *J. Rheol.* **49** 1117–28

Herrmann H, Bär H, Kreplak L, Strelkov S V and Aebi U 2007 Intermediate filaments: from cell architecture to nanomechanics *Nat. Rev. Mol. Cell Biol.* **8** 562–73

Hess H and Ross J L 2017 Non-equilibrium assembly of microtubules: from molecules to autonomous chemical robots *Chem. Soc. Rev.* **46** 5570–87

Hinner B, Tempel M, Sackmann E, Kroy K and Frey E 1998 Entanglement, elasticity, and viscous relaxation of actin solutions *Phys. Rev. Lett.* **81** 2614–7

Hinsch H, Wilhelm J and Frey E 2007 Quantitative tube model for semiflexible polymer solutions *Eur. Phys. J. E. Soft Matter.* **24** 35–46

Hiraiwa T and Ohta T 2009 Viscoelasticity of a single semiflexible polymer chain *Macromolecules* **42** 7553–62

Hitt A L, Cross A R and Williams R C 1990 Microtubule solutions display nematic liquid crystalline structure *J. Biol. Chem.* **265** 1639–47

Höfling F, Munk T, Frey E and Franosch T 2008 Entangled dynamics of a stiff polymer *Phys. Rev.* E **77** 060904

Hohmann T and Dehghani F 2019 The cytoskeleton—a complex interacting meshwork *Cells* **8** 362

Hsiao K-W, Samsal C, Prakash J R and Schroeder C M 2017 Direct observation of DNA dynamics in semi-dilute solutions in extensional flow *J. Rheol.* **61** 151–67

Huang B, Babcock H and Zhuang X 2010 Breaking the diffraction barrier: super-resolution imaging of cells *Cell* **143** 1047–58

Huber F, Boire A, López M P and Koenderink G H 2015a Cytoskeletal crosstalk: when three different personalities team up *Curr. Opin. Cell Biol., Cell Archit.* **32** 39–47

Huber F, Strehle D and Käs J 2012 Counterion-induced formation of regular actin bundle networks *Soft Matter* **8** 931–6

Huber F, Strehle D, Schnauß J and Käs J 2015b Formation of regularly spaced networks as a general feature of actin bundle condensation by entropic forces *New J. Phys.* **17** 043029

Hur J S, Shaqfeh E S G, Babcock H P, Smith D E and Chu S 2001 Dynamics of dilute and semidilute DNA solutions in the start-up of shear flow *J. Rheol.* **45** 421–50

Ianniruberto G and Marrucci G 2014 Convective constraint release (CCR) revisited *J. Rheol.* **58** 89–102

Isambert H and Maggs A C 1996 Dynamics and rheology of actin solutions *Macromolecules* **29** 1036–40

Janmey P A, Georges P C and Hvidt S 2007 Basic rheology for biologists *Methods Cell. Biol.* Cell Mech. **83** 1–27

Janmey P A, Hvidt S, Käs J, Lerche D, Maggs A, Sackmann E, Schliwa M and Stossel T P 1994 The mechanical properties of actin gels. Elastic modulus and filament motions *J. Biol. Chem.* **269** 32503–13

Jensen M H, Morris E J and Weitz D A 2015 Mechanics and dynamics of reconstituted cytoskeletal systems *Biochim. Biophys. Acta (BBA)—Mol. Cell Res., Mechanobiol.* **1853** 3038–42

Kalcioglu Z I, Mahmoodian R, Hu Y, Suo Z and Van Vliet K J 2012 From macro- to microscale poroelastic characterization of polymeric hydrogels via indentation *Soft Matter* **8** 3393

Käs J, Strey H, Tang J X, Finger D, Ezzell R, Sackmann E and Janmey P A 1996 F-actin, a model polymer for semiflexible chains in dilute, semidilute, and liquid crystalline solutions *Biophys. J.* **70** 609–25

Kas J, Strey H, Tang J X, Finger D, Ezzell R, Sackmann E and Janmey P A 1996 F-actin, a model polymer for semiflexible chains in dilute, semidilute, and liquid crystalline solutions *Biophys. J.* **70** 609–25

Kasza K E, Broedersz C P, Koenderink G H, Lin Y C, Messner W, Millman E A, Nakamura F, Stossel T P, MacKintosh F C and Weitz D A 2010 Actin filament length tunes elasticity of flexibly cross-linked actin networks *Biophys. J.* **99** 1091–100

Kasza K E, Koenderink G H, Lin Y C, Broedersz C P, Messner W, Nakamura F, Stossel T P, MacKintosh F C and Weitz D A 2009 Nonlinear elasticity of stiff biopolymers connected by flexible linkers *Phys. Rev.* E **79** 041928

Khaitlina S and Hinssen H 1997 Conformational changes in actin induced by its interaction with gelsolin *Biophys. J.* **73** 929–37

Khan M, Regan K and Robertson-Anderson R M 2019 Optical tweezers microrheology maps the dynamics of strain-induced local inhomogeneities in entangled polymers *Phys. Rev. Lett.* **123** 038001

Khanal P, Peddireddy K R, Marfai J, McGorty R and Robertson-Anderson R M 2022 DNA topology dictates emergent bulk elasticity and hindered macromolecular diffusion in DNA-dextran composites *J. Rheol.* **66** 699–715

Kim T, Gardel M L and Munro E 2014 Determinants of fluidlike behavior and effective viscosity in cross-linked actin networks *Biophys. J.* **106** 526–34

Kim T, Hwang W and Kamm R D 2011 Dynamic role of cross-linking proteins in actin rheology *Biophys. J.* **101** 1597–603

Kirchenbuechler I, Guu D, Kurniawan N A, Koenderink G H and Lettinga M P 2014 Direct visualization of flow-induced conformational transitions of single actin filaments in entangled solutions *Nat. Commun.* **5** 5060

Koenderink G H, Atakhorrami M, MacKintosh F C and Schmidt c f 2006 High-frequency stress relaxation in semiflexible polymer solutions and networks *Phys. Rev. Lett.* **96** 138307

Kong D, Banik S, San Francisco M J, Lee M, Robertson Anderson R M, Schroeder C M and McKenna G B 2022 Rheology of entangled solutions of ring–linear DNA blends *Macromolecules* **55** 1205–17

Köster S, Lin Y-C, Herrmann H and Weitz D A 2010 Nanomechanics of vimentin intermediate filament networks *Soft Matter* **6** 1910–4

Köster S, Weitz D A, Goldman R D, Aebi U and Herrmann H 2015 Intermediate filament mechanics *in vitro* and in the cell: from coiled coils to filaments, fibers and networks *Curr. Opin. Cell Biol., Cell Archit.* **32** 82–91

Kroy K and Frey E 1996 Force-extension relation and plateau modulus for wormlike chains *Phys. Rev. Lett.* **77** 306–9

Kumar A, Hasan J, Majji A, Avhale A, Gopinathan S, Sharma P, Tarange D, Bajpai R and Kumar A 2014 Continuous-flow synthesis of regioregular poly(3-hexylthiophene): ultrafast polymerization with high throughput and low polydispersity index *J. Flow Chem.* **4** 206–10

Label It Nucleic Acid Labeling Reagents—Research Reagent Products [WWW Document] n.d. https://mirusbio.com/products/labeling/label-it-nucleic-acid-labeling-reagents (accessed 19 September 2023)

Lai G H, Butler J C, Zribi O V, Smalyukh I I, Angelini T E, Purdy K R, Golestanian R and Wong G C L 2008 Self-organized gels in DNA/F-actin mixtures without crosslinkers: networks of induced nematic domains with tunable density *Phys. Rev. Lett.* **101** 218303

Lai G H, Coridan R, Zribi O V, Golestanian R and Wong G C L 2007 Evolution of growth modes for polyelectrolyte bundles *Phys. Rev. Lett.* **98** 187802

Laib S, Robertson R M and Smith D E 2006 Preparation and characterization of a set of linear DNA molecules for polymer physics and rheology studies *Macromolecules* **39** 4115–9

Lee G, Leech G, Rust M J, Das M, McGorty R J, Ross J L and Robertson-Anderson R M 2021 Myosin-driven actin-microtubule networks exhibit self-organized contractile dynamics *Sci. Adv.* **7** eabe4334

Lee H, Ferrer J M, Nakamura F, Lang M J and Kamm R D 2010 Passive and active microrheology for cross-linked F-actin networks *in vitro Acta Biomater.* **6** 1207–18

Leitner A, Paust T, Marti O, Walther P, Herrmann H and Beil M 2012 Properties of intermediate filament networks assembled from keratin 8 and 18 in the presence of Mg2+ *Biophys. J.* **103** 195–201

Li S, Wang Y, Ma L, Zhang X, Dong S, Liu L, Zhou X, Wang C and Shi Z 2019 Synthesis of PAN with adjustable molecular weight and low polydispersity index (PDI) value via reverse atom transfer radical polymerization *Des. Monomers Polym.* **22** 180–6

Lieleg O, Claessens M M A E, Heussinger C, Frey E and Bausch A R 2007 Mechanics of bundled semiflexible polymer networks *Phys. Rev. Lett.* **99** 088102

Lieleg O, Claessens M M A E, Luan Y and Bausch A R 2008 Transient binding and dissipation in cross-linked actin networks *Phys. Rev. Lett.* **101** 108101

Lin J and Valentine M T 2012 High-force NdFeB-based magnetic tweezers device optimized for microrheology experiments *Rev. Sci. Instrum.* **83** 053905

Lin Y-C, Broedersz C P, Rowat A C, Wedig T, Herrmann H, MacKintosh F C and Weitz D A 2010a Divalent cations crosslink vimentin intermediate filament tail domains to regulate network mechanics *J. Mol. Biol.* **399** 637–44

Lin Y-C, Koenderink G H, MacKintosh F C and Weitz D A 2007 Viscoelastic properties of microtubule networks *Macromolecules* **40** 7714–20

Lin Y-C, Yao N Y, Broedersz C P, Herrmann H, MacKintosh F C and Weitz D A 2010b Origins of elasticity in intermediate filament networks *Phys. Rev. Lett.* **104** 058101

Liu J, Gardel M L, Kroy K, Frey E, Hoffman B D, Crocker J C, Bausch A R and Weitz D A 2006 Microrheology probes length scale dependent rheology *Phys. Rev. Lett.* **96** 118104

Liu J, Koenderink G H, Kasza K E, MacKintosh F C and Weitz D A 2007 Visualizing the strain field in semiflexible polymer networks: strain fluctuations and nonlinear rheology of *F*-actin gels *Phys. Rev. Lett.* **98** 198304

Lopez B J and Valentine M T 2015 Molecular control of stress transmission in the microtubule cytoskeleton *Biochim. Biophys. Acta (BBA)—Mol. Cell Res.* **1853** 3015–24

Luan Y, Lieleg O, Wagner B and Bausch A R 2008 Micro- and macrorheological properties of isotropically cross-linked actin networks *Biophys. J.* **94** 688–93

MacKintosh F C, Kas J and Janmey P A 1995 Elasticity of semiflexible biopolymer networks *Phys. Rev. Lett.* **75** 4425–8

Manning G S 2006 The persistence length of DNA is reached from the persistence length of its null isomer through an internal electrostatic stretching force *Biophys. J.* **91** 3607–16

Marko J F and Siggia E D 1995 Stretching DNA *Macromolecules* **28** 8759–70

Mason T G, Dhople A and Wirtz D 1998 Linear viscoelastic moduli of concentrated DNA solutions *Macromolecules* **31** 3600–3

Mason T G, Gisler T, Kroy K, Frey E and Weitz D A 2000 Rheology of F-actin solutions determined from thermally driven tracer motion *J. Rheol.* **44** 917–28

McGorty R J *et al* 2023 Kinesin and myosin motors compete to drive rich multiphase dynamics in programmable cytoskeletal composites *PNAS Nexus* **2** pgad245

Mhetar V and Archer L A 1999 Nonlinear viscoelasticity of entangled polymeric liquids *J. Non-Newton Fluid* **81** 71–81

Mickey B and Howard J 1995 Rigidity of microtubules is increased by stabilizing agents *J. Cell Biol.* **130** 909–17

Microscale mechanics of plug-and-play *in vitro* cytoskeleton networks IntechOpen [WWW Document] n.d. https://intechopen.com/books/parasitology-and-microbiology-research/micro-scale-mechanics-of-plug-and-play-in-vitro-cytoskeleton-networks (accessed 21 June 2020)

Miller H P and Wilson L 2010 Chapter 1—Preparation of microtubule protein and purified tubulin from bovine brain by cycles of assembly and disassembly and phosphocellulose chromatography ed L Wilson and J J Correia *Methods in Cell Biology, Microtubules, In Vitro* (New York: Academic) pp 2–15

Mirigian M, Mukherjee K, Bane S and Sackett D 2013 Measurement of *in vitro* microtubule polymerization by turbidity and fluorescence *Methods Cell. Biol.* **115** 215–29

Moeendarbary E, Valon L, Fritzsche M, Harris A R, Moulding D A, Thrasher A J, Stride E, Mahadevan L and Charras G T 2013 The cytoplasm of living cells behaves as a poroelastic material *Nat. Mater.* **12** 253–61

Morse D C 1998 Viscoelasticity of tightly entangled solutions of semiflexible polymers *Phys. Rev.* E **58** R1237–40

Murrell M P and Gardel M L 2012 F-actin buckling coordinates contractility and severing in a biomimetic actomyosin cortex *PNAS* **109** 20820–5

Nachmias V T 1993 Small actin-binding proteins: the β-thymosin family *Curr. Opin. Cell Biol.* **5** 56–62

NEBcutter 3.0 [WWW Document] n.d. https://nc3.neb.com/NEBcutter/ (accessed 19 September 2023)

O'Brien E T, Salmon E D, Walker R A and Erickson H P 1990 Effects of magnesium on the dynamic instability of individual microtubules *Biochemistry* **29** 6648–56

Odijk T 1983 The statistics and dynamics of confined or entangled stiff polymers *Macromolecules* **16** 1340–4

Onck P R, Koeman T, van Dillen T and van der Giessen E 2005 Alternative explanation of stiffening in cross-linked semiflexible networks *Phys. Rev. Lett.* **95** 178102

Pan S, At Nguyen D, Sridhar T, Sunthar P and Ravi Prakash J 2014 Universal solvent quality crossover of the zero shear rate viscosity of semidilute DNA solutions *J. Rheol.* **58** 339–68

Pan S, Nguyen D A, Dünweg B, Sunthar P, Sridhar T and Ravi Prakash J 2018 Shear thinning in dilute and semidilute solutions of polystyrene and DNA *J. Rheol.* **62** 845–67

Pardee J D and Aspudich J 1982 Purification of muscle actin *Methods in Enzymology, Structural and Contractile Proteins Part B: The Contractile Apparatus and the Cytoskeleton* (New York: Academic) pp 164–81

Patteson A E, Vahabikashi A, Goldman R D and Janmey P A 2020 Mechanical and non-mechanical functions of filamentous and non-filamentous vimentin *BioEssays* **42** 2000078

Pawelzyk P, Mücke N, Herrmann H and Willenbacher N 2014 Attractive interactions among intermediate filaments determine network mechanics *in vitro PLoS One* **9** e93194

Pecora R 1991 DNA: a model compound for solution studies of macromolecules *Science* **251** 893–8

Peddireddy K R, Clairmont R, Neill P, McGorty R and Robertson-Anderson R M 2022 OpTiDDM (Optical Tweezers integrating Differential Dynamic Microscopy) maps the spatiotemporal propagation of nonlinear stresses in polymer blends and composites *Nat. Commun.* **13** 5180

Peddireddy K R, Lee M, Schroeder C M and Robertson-Anderson R M 2020a Viscoelastic properties of ring-linear DNA blends exhibit nonmonotonic dependence on blend composition *Phys. Rev. Res.* **2** 023213

Peddireddy K R, Lee M, Zhou Y, Adalbert S, Anderson S, Schroeder C M and Robertson-Anderson R M 2020b Unexpected entanglement dynamics in semidilute blends of supercoiled and ring DNA *Soft Matter* **16** 152–61

Peddireddy K R, Michieletto D, Aguirre G, Garamella J, Khanal P and Robertson-Anderson R M 2021 DNA conformation dictates strength and flocculation in DNA–microtubule composites *ACS Macro Lett.* **10** 1540–8

Pegoraro A F, Janmey P and Weitz D A 2017 Mechanical properties of the cytoskeleton and cells *Cold Spring Harb. Perspect. Biol.* **9** a022038

Perkins T T, Quake S R, Smith D E and Chu S 1994a Relaxation of a single DNA molecule observed by optical microscopy *Science* **264** 822–6

Perkins T T, Smith D E and Chu S 1994b Direct observation of tube-like motion of a single polymer chain *Science* **264** 819–22

Phalloidin–Atto 532 suitable for fluorescence, ⩾90.0% (HPLC) Sigma-Aldrich [WWW Document] n.d. http://sigmaaldrich.com/ (accessed 21 September 2023)

Pollard T D 2003 The cytoskeleton, cellular motility and the reductionist agenda *Nature* **422** 741–5

Pollard T D 1986 Rate constants for the reactions of ATP- and ADP-actin with the ends of actin filaments *J. Cell Biol.* **103** 2747–54

Pollard T D and Cooper J A 1986 Actin and actin-binding proteins. a critical evaluation of mechanisms and functions *Annu. Rev. Biochem.* **55** 987–1035

Popp D, Yamamoto A, Iwasa M and Maéda Y 2006 Direct visualization of actin nematic network formation and dynamics *Biochem. Biophys. Res. Commun.* **351** 348–53

Pringle J, Muthukumar A, Tan A, Crankshaw L, Conway L and Ross J L 2013 Microtubule organization by kinesin motors and microtubule crosslinking protein MAP65 *J. Phys. Condens. Matter* **25** 374103

Punter M T J J M, Vos B E, Mulder B M and Koenderink G H 2020 Poroelasticity of (bio) polymer networks during compression: theory and experiment *Soft Matter* **16** 1298–305

Pure actin, pyrene actin, fluorescent actin, rhodamine actin, pre-formed actin filaments, [WWW Document] n.d. https://cytoskeleton.com/actin/proteins (accessed 21 September 2023)

Regan K, Ricketts S and Robertson-Anderson R 2016 DNA as a model for probing polymer entanglements: circular polymers and non-classical dynamics *Polymers* **8** 336

Regan K, Wulstein D, Rasmussen H, McGorty R and Robertson-Anderson R M 2019 Bridging the spatiotemporal scales of macromolecular transport in crowded biomimetic systems *Soft Matter* **15** 1200–9

Ricketts S N, Khanal P, Rust M J, Das M, Ross J L and Robertson-Anderson R M 2020 Triggering cation-induced contraction of cytoskeleton networks via microfluidics *Front. Phys.* **8** 596699

Ricketts S N, Gurmessa B and Robertson-Anderson R M 2019 *Microscale Mechanics of Plug-and-Play In Vitro Cytoskeleton Networks* (IntechOpen)

Ricketts S N, Ross J L and Robertson-Anderson R M 2018 Co-entangled actin-microtubule composites exhibit tunable stiffening and power-law stress relaxation

Rigato A, Miyagi A, Scheuring S and Rico F 2017 High-frequency microrheology reveals cytoskeleton dynamics in living cells *Nat. Phys.* **13** 771–5

Robertson R M, Laib S and Smith D E 2006 Diffusion of isolated DNA molecules: dependence on length and topology *PNAS* **103** 7310–4

Robertson R M and Smith D E 2007a Direct measurement of the intermolecular forces confining a single molecule in an entangled polymer solution *Phys. Rev. Lett.* **99** 126001

Robertson R M and Smith D E 2007b Self-diffusion of entangled linear and circular DNA molecules: dependence on length and concentration *Macromolecules* **40** 3373–7

Robertson-Anderson R M 2018 Optical tweezers microrheology: from the basics to advanced techniques and applications *ACS Macro Lett.* **7** 968–75

Romanowska M, Hinsch H, Kirchgeßner N, Giesen M, Degawa M, Hoffmann B, Frey E and Merkel R 2009 Direct observation of the tube model in F-actin solutions: tube dimensions and curvatures *EPL* **86** 26003

Rouse P E 1953 A theory of the linear viscoelastic properties of dilute solutions of coiling polymers *J. Chem. Phys.* **21** 1272–80

Rubinstein M and Colby R H 2003 *Polymer Physics* (Oxford: Oxford University Press)

Sampath P and Pollard T D 1991 Effects of cytochalasin, phalloidin and pH on the elongation of actin filaments *Biochemistry* **30** 1973–80

Schafer D A, Jennings P B and Cooper J A 1998 Rapid and efficient purification of actin from nonmuscle sources *Cell Motil.* **39** 166–71

Schmidt c f, Baermann M, Isenberg G and Sackmann E 1989 Chain dynamics, mesh size, and diffusive transport in networks of polymerized actin: a quasielastic light scattering and microfluorescence study *Macromolecules* **22** 3638–49

Schmidt F G, Hinner B and Sackmann E 2000 Microrheometry underestimates the values of the viscoelastic moduli in measurements on F-actin solutions compared to macrorheometry *Phys. Rev.* E **61** 5646–53

Schmoller K M, Fernández P, Arevalo R C, Blair D L and Bausch A R 2010 Cyclic hardening in bundled actin networks *Nat. Commun.* **1** 134

Schmoller K M, Lieleg O and Bausch A R 2009 Structural and viscoelastic properties of actin/filamin networks: cross-linked versus bundled networks *Biophys. J.* **97** 83–9

Schnauß J, Händler T and Käs J A 2016 Semiflexible biopolymers in bundled arrangements *Polymers* **8** 274

Schopferer M, Bär H, Hochstein B, Sharma S, Mücke N, Herrmann H and Willenbacher N 2009 Desmin and vimentin intermediate filament networks: their viscoelastic properties investigated by mechanical rheometry *J. Mol. Biol.* **388** 133–43

Schroeder C M, Babcock H P, Shaqfeh E S and Chu S 2003 Observation of polymer conformation hysteresis in extensional flow *Science* **301** 1515–9

Schroeder C M, Shaqfeh E S G and Chu S 2004 Effect of hydrodynamic interactions on DNA dynamics in extensional flow: simulation and single molecule experiment *Macromolecules* **37** 9242–56

Schweizer K S and Sussman D M 2016 A force-level theory of the rheology of entangled rod and chain polymer liquids. I. Tube deformation, microscopic yielding, and the nonlinear elastic limit *J. Chem. Phys.* **145** 214903

Semmrich C, Larsen R J and Bausch A R 2008 Nonlinear mechanics of entangled F-actin solutions *Soft Matter* **4** 1675

Sept D, Xu J, Pollard T D and Andrew McCammon J 1999 Annealing accounts for the length of actin filaments formed by spontaneous polymerization *Biophys. J.* **77** 2911–9

Shin J H, Gardel M L, Mahadevan L, Matsudaira P and Weitz D A 2004 Relating microstructure to rheology of a bundled and cross-linked F-actin network *in vitro Proc. Natl Acad. Sci.* **101** 9636–41

Simon C, Caorsi V, Campillo C and Sykes C 2018 Interplay between membrane tension and the actin cytoskeleton determines shape changes *Phys. Biol.* **15** 065004

Smith D E, Perkins T T and Chu S 1996 Dynamical scaling of DNA diffusion coefficients *Macromolecules* **29** 1372–3

Stevens M J, McIntosh D B and Saleh O A 2012 Simulations of stretching a strong, flexible polyelectrolyte *Macromolecules* **45** 5757–65

Stricker J, Falzone T and Gardel M L 2010 Mechanics of the F-actin cytoskeleton *J. Biomech.* **43** 9–14 (Special Issue on Cell Mechanobiology)

Subramanian R, Wilson-Kubalek E M, Arthur C P, Bick M J, Campbell E A, Darst S A, Milligan R A and Kapoor T M 2010 Insights into antiparallel microtubule crosslinking by PRC1, a conserved nonmotor microtubule binding protein *Cell* **142** 433–43

Sussman D M and Schweizer K S 2013a Entangled polymer chain melts: orientation and deformation dependent tube confinement and interchain entanglement elasticity *J. Chem. Phys.* **139** 234904

Sussman D M and Schweizer K S 2013b Entangled rigid macromolecules under continuous startup shear deformation: consequences of a microscopically anharmonic confining tube *Macromolecules* **46** 5684–93

Sussman D M and Schweizer K S 2012 Microscopic theory of quiescent and deformed topologically entangled rod solutions: general formulation and relaxation after nonlinear step strain *Macromolecules* **45** 3270–84

Sussman D M and Schweizer K S 2011 Microscopic theory of the tube confinement potential for liquids of topologically entangled rigid macromolecules *Phys. Rev. Lett.* **107** 078102

Syed S, MacKintosh F C and Shivers J L 2022 Structural features and nonlinear rheology of self-assembled networks of cross-linked semiflexible polymers *J. Phys. Chem.* B **126** 10741–9

Tang J X and Janmey P A 1996 the polyelectrolyte nature of f-actin and the mechanism of actin bundle formation *J. Biol. Chem.* **271** 8556–63

Teixeira R E, Dambal A K, Richter D H, Shaqfeh E S G and Chu S 2007 The individualistic dynamics of entangled DNA in solution *Macromolecules* **40** 2461–76

Tharmann R, Claessens M M A E and Bausch A R 2007 Viscoelasticity of isotropically cross-linked actin networks *Phys. Rev. Lett.* **98** 088103

Toan N M and Micheletti C 2006 Inferring the effective thickness of polyelectrolytes from stretching measurements at various ionic strengths: applications to DNA and RNA *J. Phys. Condens. Matter* **18** S269

Tree D R, Muralidhar A, Doyle P S and Dorfman K D 2013 Is DNA a good model polymer? *Macromolecules* **46** 8369–82

Tseng Y, An K M, Esue O and Wirtz D 2004 The bimodal role of filamin in controlling the architecture and mechanics of F-actin networks *J. Biol. Chem.* **279** 1819–26

Tubulin protein (>99% pure): porcine brain [WWW Document] n.d. https://cytoskeleton.com/t240 (accessed 27 September 2023)

Uhde J, Feneberg W, Ter-Oganessian N, Sackmann E and Boulbitch A 2005a Osmotic force-controlled microrheometry of entangled actin networks *Phys. Rev. Lett.* **94** 198102

Uhde J, Ter-Oganessian N, Pink D A, Sackmann E and Boulbitch A 2005b Viscoelasticity of entangled actin networks studied by long-pulse magnetic bead microrheometry *Phys. Rev.* E **72** 061916

van der Maarel J R C 2008 *Introduction to Biopolymer Physics* (Singapore: World Scientific)

Viamontes J, Oakes P W and Tang J X 2006 Isotropic to nematic liquid crystalline phase transition of *F*-actin varies from continuous to first order *Phys. Rev. Lett.* **97** 118103

Viovy J L, Rubinstein M and Colby R H 1991 Constraint release in polymer melts: tube reorganization versus tube dilation *Macromolecules* **24** 3587–96

Wagner B, Tharmann R, Haase I, Fischer M and Bausch A R 2006 Cytoskeletal polymer networks: the molecular structure of cross-linkers determines macroscopic properties *Proc. Natl Acad. Sci.* **103** 13974–8

Wang B, Anthony S M, Bae S C and Granick S 2009 Anomalous yet Brownian *Proc. Natl Acad. Sci.* **106** 15160–4

Wang B, Guan J, Anthony S M, Bae S C, Schweizer K S and Granick S 2010 Confining potential when a biopolymer filament reptates *Phys. Rev. Lett.* **104** 118301

Wang B, Kuo J, Bae S C and Granick S 2012 When Brownian diffusion is not Gaussian *Nat. Mater.* **11** 481–5

Wang X, Zhu H, Lu Y, Wang Z and Kennedy D 2020 The elastic properties and deformation mechanisms of actin filament networks crosslinked by filamins *J. Mech. Behav. Biomed. Mater.* **112** 104075

Wang X, Zhu H, Song B, Chen X, Kennedy D and Shi Y 2023 Nonlinear elastic behaviors and deformation mechanisms of nano-structured crosslinked biopolymer networks *Extreme Mech. Lett.* **61** 102017

Weber A 1999 Actin binding proteins that change extent and rate of actin monomer-polymer distribution by different mechanisms ed S Imai, I Ohtsuki and M Endo *Muscle Physiology and Biochemistry* (Boston, MA: Springer US) pp 67–74

Wen Q and Janmey P A 2011 Polymer physics of the cytoskeleton *Curr. Opin. Solid State Mater. Sci.* **15** 177–82

Wendel H and Dancker P 1987 Influence of phalloidin on both the nucleation and the elongation phase of actin polymerization *Biochim. Biophys. Acta (BBA)—Protein Struct. Molecul. Enzymol.* **915** 199–204

Wilson L, Miller H P, Farrell K W, Snyder K B, Thompson W C and Purich D L 1985 Taxol stabilization of microtubules *in vitro*: dynamics of tubulin addition and loss at opposite microtubule ends *Biochemistry* **24** 5254–62

Wong I Y, Gardel M L, Reichman D R, Weeks E R, Valentine M T, Bausch A R and Weitz D A 2004 Anomalous diffusion probes microstructure dynamics of entangled F-actin networks *Phys. Rev. Lett.* **92** 178101

Xu J, Casella J F and Pollard T D 1999 Effect of capping protein, CapZ, on the length of actin filaments and mechanical properties of actin filament networks *Cell Motil.* **42** 73–81

Xu J, Palmer A and Wirtz D 1998 Rheology and microrheology of semiflexible polymer solutions: actin filament networks *Macromolecules* **31** 6486–92

Xu J, Tseng Y and Wirtz D 2000 Strain hardening of actin filament networks: regulation by the dynamic cross-linking protein α-actinin *J. Biol. Chem.* **275** 35886–92

Yang Y, Bai M, Klug W S, Levine A J and Valentine M T 2012a Microrheology of highly crosslinked microtubule networks is dominated by force-induced crosslinker unbinding *Soft Matter* **9** 383–93

Yang Y, Lin J, Kaytanli B, Saleh O A and Valentine M T 2012b Direct correlation between creep compliance and deformation in entangled and sparsely crosslinked microtubule networks *Soft Matter* **8** 1776–84

Yao N Y, Becker D J, Broedersz C P, Depken M, MacKintosh F C, Pollak M R and Weitz D A 2011 Nonlinear viscoelasticity of actin transiently cross-linked with mutant α-Actinin-4 *J. Mol. Biol.* **411** 1062–71

Yao N Y, Broedersz C P, Lin Y-C, Kasza K E, MacKintosh F C and Weitz D A 2010 Elasticity in ionically cross-linked neurofilament networks *Biophys. J.* **98** 2147–53

Žagar G, Onck P R and van der Giessen E 2015 Two fundamental mechanisms govern the stiffening of cross-linked networks *Biophys. J.* **108** 1470–9

Zhang R, Kumar N, Ross J L, Gardel M L and de Pablo J J 2018 Interplay of structure, elasticity, and dynamics in actin-based nematic materials *Proc. Natl Acad. Sci.* **115** E124–33

Zhou Q and Larson R G 2006 Direct calculation of the tube potential confining entangled polymers *Macromolecules* **39** 6737–43

Part III

Beyond the basics—novel and complex networks

IOP Publishing

Biopolymer Networks
Design, dynamics and discovery
Rae M Robertson-Anderson

Chapter 6

Networks of topologically-novel biopolymers

Polymer physics theory is largely devoted to linear polymers and their networks; yet biopolymers naturally exist in multiple topologies such as circular (i.e., ring), branched, and torsionally strained and twisted (i.e., supercoiled) (figure 6.1). This chapter will discuss the effects of topology on biopolymer network dynamics, rheology, and structure; as well as the transport properties and conformations of their biopolymer constituents. The discussion will be framed primarily in the context of how the properties of topologically-novel biopolymer networks differ from those of linear chains (described in chapters 2 and 5). There is a vast body of literature investigating synthetic ring and branched polymers (e.g., Rubinstein 1986, Klein 1986, Brown and Szamel 1998, Suneel *et al* 2002, Saha *et al* 2006, Shanbhag *et al* 2006, Kapnistos *et al* 2008, McLeish 2008, Ge *et al* 2016a, Tsalikis *et al* 2016, Yan *et al* 2016, Michieletto *et al* 2017b, Parisi *et al* 2021), which I will only discuss in cases in which their findings shed light on the properties of circular and branched *bio*polymers such as DNA and mucins.

6.1 Relaxed circular (ring) biopolymers

Double-stranded DNA, such as plasmids and bacterial genomes, naturally occur in circular topology, with no free ends (Alberts 2004, Adams *et al* 2013). The double-helix twisting of the DNA causes circular DNA to become supercoiled and torsionally strained, similar to twisting a piece of string then attaching its ends (figure 6.1, left). However, if one of the two DNA strands is cut, such that the DNA is 'nicked' then the torsional stress is released and the DNA unwinds into a 'relaxed' circle or ring (figure 6.1, top path) (Heiter *et al* 2005, Kim *et al* 2012, Adams *et al* 2013). There are numerous naturally occurring and commercially available site-specific nicking enzymes that serve this purpose. There is also a class of enzymes known as topoisomerases that can twist and untwist DNA to alter the degree of supercoiling (Gellert 1981, Liu and Wang 1983, Seol and Neuman 2016, Bax *et al* 2019). For example, Topoisomerase II cuts both strands of supercoiled DNA in a

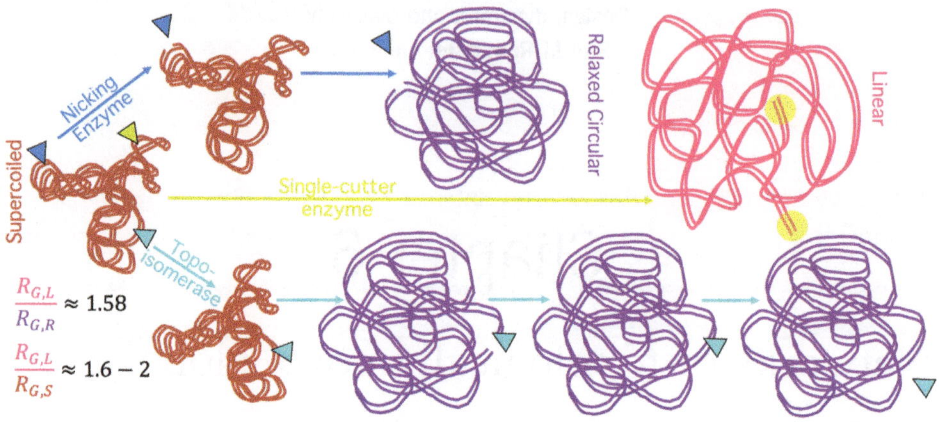

Figure 6.1. DNA naturally exists in multiple topologies with enzymes that convert from one topology to another. Prokaryotic DNA is typically replicated as double-stranded supercoiled circular constructs (red) which can be converted to relaxed rings (purple) by nicking enzymes (top path, blue triangles) that cleave one of the two strands to release the torsional stress that maintains supercoiling, or topoisomerases (bottom path, cyan triangles) that successively cleave both DNA strands, unwind the local supercoils, reseal the free ends, and repeat at another location along the backbone until all supercoils are relaxed. Supercoiled and relaxed circular DNA can also be converted to linear topology (magenta) via single-cutter enzymes (yellow triangles) that cleave both strands of the DNA at a single specific recognition site (yellow circles). The different DNA topologies differ in their size, according to the listed ratios of the radii of gyration for supercoiled ($R_{G,S}$), relaxed ring ($R_{G,R}$), and linear ($R_{G,L}$) topologies.

specific location, unwinds the local supercoils, reconnects the cleaved ends, and then repeats this process at a different location, until all supercoils are relaxed or unwound (Alberts 2004, Robertson *et al* 2006, Krajina *et al* 2018). The result is a relaxed circular (ring) polymer with both strands intact, in contrast to nicked or 'open' DNA rings that have only one intact strand.

Cytoskeletal proteins, including actin, microtubules, and vimentin, have been shown to form ring structures that typically comprise multiple filaments bundled together. Because these structures are many-polymer structures, we will not focus on their properties here, but instead refer the interested reader to, e.g., Liu *et al* (2011), Patteson *et al* (2020), and Kučera *et al* (2021).

6.1.1 Single ring dynamics

Remarkably, the simple act of connecting the ends of a linear polymer, even one that is hundreds of Kuhn lengths long, has substantial impact on its conformation and dynamics. The radius of gyration of a flexible ring polymer $R_{G,R}$ is smaller than that of its linear counterpart $R_{G,L}$ due to reduced conformational degrees of freedom, with exact values for the ratio predicted to be

$$R_{G,L}/R_{G,R} \simeq 1.33 - 1.54 \text{ (theory)} \tag{6.1}$$

(Bloomfield and Zimm 1966, Prentis 1984, Bensafi *et al* 2000). These predictions align with the value

$$R_{G,L}/R_{G,R} \simeq 1.58 \pm 0.02 \text{ (experiment)} \tag{6.2}$$

reported for DNA of lengths $L \simeq 6-289$ kbp in good solvent conditions in the dilute limit, as inferred from diffusion measurements of DNA (figure 6.2(A)) (Robertson *et al* 2006). Importantly, this L-independent relation implies that the scaling of $R_{G,R}$ with polymer length follows the same scaling as for linear chains, with both adhering to Flory scaling (Flory 1949, Robertson *et al* 2006):

$$R_{G,R} \sim R_{G,L} \sim L^{\nu} \ (\nu \simeq 0.588) \tag{6.3}$$

As I described in chapter 2, $R_{G,L}$ for a linear polymer can be determined from its experimentally measured dilute-limit diffusion coefficient $D_{0,L}$ via the relations

$$R_{H,L} = k_B T / 6\pi\eta D_{0,L} \tag{6.4}$$

and

$$R_{G,L}/R_{H,L} \simeq 1.508 \tag{6.5}$$

The same Stokes–Einstein relation holds for circular polymers, but the ratio of the radius of gyration to hydrodynamic radius is smaller, with a predicted value (Burchard and Schmidt 1980):

$$R_{G,R}/R_{H,R} \simeq (\pi/2)^{1/2} \simeq 1.253 \tag{6.6}$$

Combining equations (6.2), (6.5) and (6.6) yields the relationship between the diffusion coefficients for circular and linear polymers in good solvent conditions:

$$D_{0,R}/D_{0,L} \simeq 1.32 \pm 0.01 \tag{6.7}$$

(Figure 6.2(A)) (Robertson *et al* 2006), in agreement with predictions that rely on the Zimm model but assume less swelling (i.e., reduced excluded volume effects) for circular polymers compared to their linear counterparts in good solvent conditions (Bensafi *et al* 2000). Once again, the L-independent ratio $D_{0,R}/D_{0,L}$ relies on the assumption that the scaling relation $D_0 \sim L^{-\nu}$ is the same for rings and linear chains. Indeed, the scaling exponents measured via single-molecule tracking of ring and linear DNA were reported to be $\nu_R = 0.589 \pm 0.018$ and $\nu_L = 0.571 \pm 0.014$ (figure 6.2(A)), within error of each other and in agreement with the predicted value of $\nu \simeq 0.588$ (Flory 1949, Robertson *et al* 2006).

The relaxation times for rings in the dilute limit are faster than their linear counterparts due, primarily, to their smaller coil size. Specifically, the Zimm time, i.e., the time for a polymer coil to diffuse a distance equal to its end-to-end length R_0, scales as $\tau_Z \sim R_0^3 \sim R_G^3$ (Zimm 1956) such that

$$\tau_{Z,L}/\tau_{Z,R} \simeq (R_{G,L}/R_{G,R})^3 \simeq 3.9 \tag{6.8}$$

The Rouse time, i.e., the time associated with elastic retraction of the polymer chain, scales as $\tau_R \approx R_G^2/D_0$ (Rouse 1953), which leads to a topology dependence of the form

$$\tau_{R,L}/\tau_{R,R} \simeq (R_{G,L}/R_{G,R})^2 (D_{0,R}/D_{0,L}) \simeq (1.58)^2(1.32) \simeq 3.3 \tag{6.9}$$

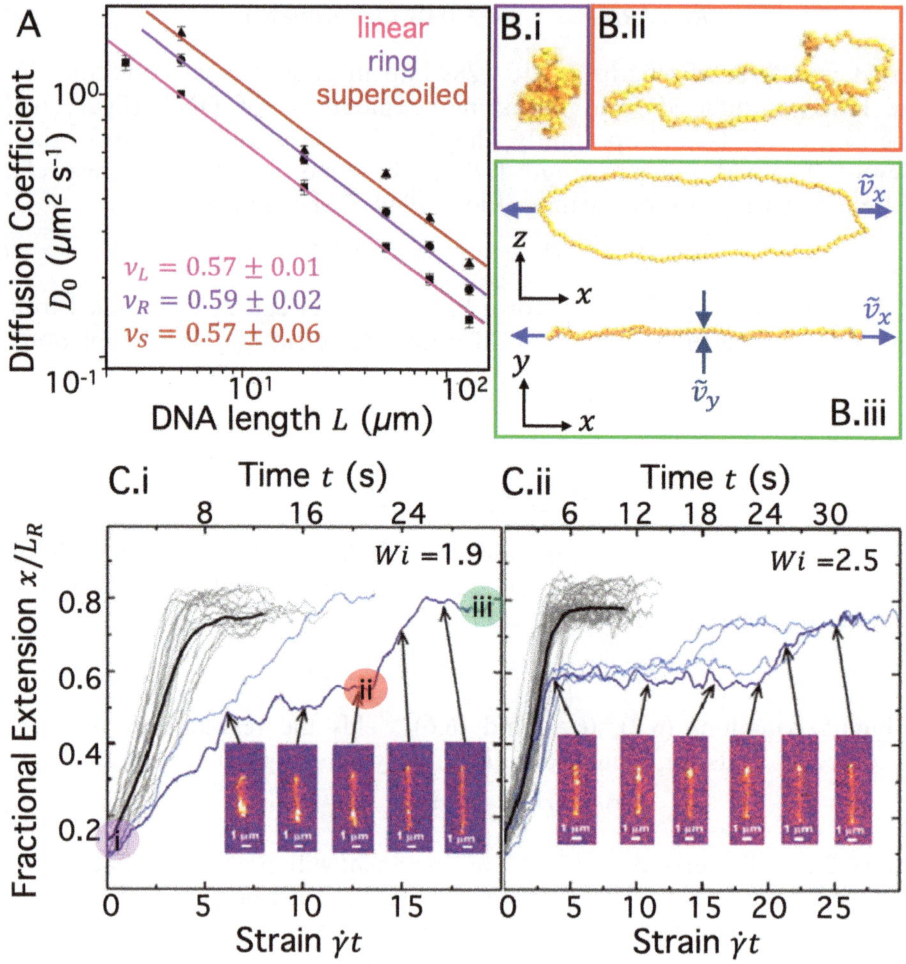

Figure 6.2. Isolated ring and linear DNA molecules exhibit distinct dynamics in steady-state and in response to elongational flow. (A) Diffusion coefficients of linear (magenta), ring (purple), and red (supercoiled) DNA of varying contour lengths L, measured via single-molecule tracking, exhibit similar scaling $D_0 \sim L^{-\nu}$, with scaling exponents (color-coded lines) $\nu_L \simeq 0.57$, $\nu_R \simeq 0.59$, and $\nu_S \simeq 0.57$. Unlike the scaling exponents, the magnitudes of D_0 do differ with $D_{0,S} > D_{0,R} > D_{0,L}$. (B) Simulated conformations of a ring in the (i) beginning coiled state (purple border), (ii) intermediate transiently knotted state (red border), and (iii) final stretched state during planar elongational flow (green border). The final ring conformation (iii) orients and opens up in $\hat{z}$, orthogonal to the $\hat{x}\hat{y}$ plane of the flow causing the maximum extension x to be less than the maximum possible extension $L_R = L/2$. (C) Fractional extension x/L_R versus time (t, top axis) and strain ($\dot{\gamma}t$, bottom axis) of 45-kbp ring DNA stretched by elongational flows with (i) $Wi = 1.9$ and (ii) $Wi = 2.5$. Besides continuous stretching trajectories (grey lines), akin to those of linear chains, rings also exhibit unique intermittent pauses and heterogeneous trajectories (blue lines). The peaks and valleys in the trajectories, which contribute to delaying the coil-stretch transition for rings compared to linear chains, arise from transient knotting events depicted in the inset fluorescence images of ring DNA at the specified points (arrows) along the trajectory. These events are more pronounced and occur more frequently at higher Wi, as seen by comparing (i) and (ii). The color-coded translucent circles correspond to the simulated ring conformations captured in B. (A) Adapted from Robertson *et al* (2006), with permission of PNAS. (B) Adapted with permission from Hsiao *et al* (2016) Copyright (2016) American Chemical Society. (C) Adapted with permission from Li *et al* (2015). Copyright (2015) American Chemical Society.

Beyond the differences in their steady-state conformations and dynamics, ring and linear DNA respond differently to stretching and shear, as demonstrated in single-molecule microfluidics experiments (figures 6.2(B) and (C)) (Li *et al* 2015, Hsiao *et al* 2016, Mai and Schroeder 2016).

Under extensional flow, both rings and linear chains exhibit a transition from coiled to stretched conformations (figures 6.2(B) and (C)) (Li *et al* 2015). However, while a fully stretched linear chain has an end-to-end extension close to its contour length L, a ring can only extend to $L_R \simeq L/2$, in which case the two halves of the fully connected polymer align with another. However, the increased hydrodynamic interactions (HI) between the two parallel strands of the stretched ring cause the ring to swell in the direction orthogonal to the flow plane, preventing complete fractional extension $x/L_R = 1$ (figure 6.2(B.iii)), and only reaching $x/L_R \approx 0.7$. The increased HI also causes the coil−stretch transition to occur at $\sim$1.25× larger Weissenberg number (Wi), or flow strength, than for linear DNA of the same length (Hsiao *et al* 2016, Mai and Schroeder 2016). Moreover, during extensional flow, rings exhibit intermittent knotting and looping that result in heterogeneous and slow stretching trajectories that are more pronounced and frequent at higher flow strength (figure 6.2(C)) and are absent for linear chains.

Following flow cessation, ring DNA polymers relax back to their random coil configurations more quickly than their linear counterparts, but both topologies follow similar scaling of the relaxation time with contour length $\tau \sim L^{3\nu}$, with measured exponents $3\nu_R \simeq 1.41 \pm 0.10$ and $3\nu_L \simeq 1.71 \pm 0.05$ (Li *et al* 2015). The exponent for the linear chains is slightly less than the good solvent Flory exponent $\nu \simeq 0.588$, which accounts for substantial excluded volume, while the exponent for rings more closely aligns with theta solvent predictions ($\nu \simeq 0.5$). The lower value of ν_R compared to ν_L aligns with previous results that indicate decreased excluded volume effects for rings compared to linear chains (Bensafi *et al* 2000, Mai and Schroeder 2016), but is at odds with steady-state diffusion measurements that report $\nu_R \approx \nu_L \approx 0.588$, in line with the good solvent Flory exponent (figure 6.2(A)) (Robertson *et al* 2006).

Under shear flow, rather than the elongational flows discussed above, single ring DNA molecules have been reported to undergo tumbling behavior similar to linear DNA, and their fractional extension as a function of Wi is likewise similar (Tu *et al* 2020). However, a notable difference between the two topologies is the more symmetric and narrow distributions of chain extensions for rings compared to linear chains, which is likely due to the reduced degrees of freedom as well as the finding that rings swell or 'open up' in the vorticity direction (perpendicular to the shear-gradient direction). We further explore the propensity for rings to open up or swell under certain conditions in chapter 7.

6.1.2 Unentangled ring DNA solutions

As I describe in chapter 2, as the concentration of linear DNA in solution approaches the overlap concentration c^*, hydrodynamic effects become screened which causes the polymer coils to 'de-swell' such that they can be modeled as ideal random walks in space without self-avoidance. The same effect holds for ring DNA;

however, their overlap concentration c_R^* is nearly 4-fold higher than for linear DNA of the same length owing to the relations $R_{G,L}/R_{G,R} \simeq 1.58$ (Robertson *et al* 2006) and $c^* \sim R_G^{-3}$, which together yield

$$c_R^* \simeq 3.94 c_L^* \tag{6.10}$$

Single-molecule tracking studies of tracer ring or linear DNA of lengths $L \simeq 6$–45 kbp, diffusing in semidilute solutions of either ring or linear DNA, showed that all four cases—ring DNA diffusing in a solution of ring DNA (R-R), rings in a solution of linear DNA (R-L), and linear DNA in the same two solutions (L-R, L-L)—followed scaling aligned with Rouse model predictions for good solvent conditions $D \sim c^{-0.5}$ for concentrations up to $\sim 6c_L^*$ (Robertson and Smith 2007). For the two shorter DNA constructs (6, 11 kbp), the diffusion coefficients were largely independent of the topology of the tracer or solution, while for the two larger lengths (25, 45 kbp) diffusion of both rings and linear chains were substantially slower in a network of overlapping linear DNA compared to ring DNA of the same concentration (Robertson and Smith 2007, 2007a).

This effect can be understood by recalling that for the same concentration, linear DNA is more strongly overlapping than rings, equation (6.10), so they can more effectively slow tracer diffusion. Likewise, networks comprising the two smaller constructs are more weakly overlapping at the same concentration, as they have comparatively higher c^* values due their smaller radius of gyration (recall $c^* \sim R_G^{-3}$), so the topology-dependent variations in overlap density and intermolecular interactions are weaker. Finally, it is important to recall that these results are for concentrations below the entanglement concentration c_e, so the primary mode of center-of-mass motion is not 'head-first' curvilinear diffusion (reptation), that requires free ends that rings lack. As such, we expect the impact of end closure to be weaker than in the entanglement regime.

Microfluidics experiments examining the stress relaxation of rings following transient stretching in semidilute solutions of linear DNA revealed that the relaxation dynamics for many of the rings exhibited two modes, with the slow and fast modes being ~2× slower and ~5× faster than the single linear chain relaxation timescale (figure 6.3(B)). Moreover, rings exhibited much larger conformational fluctuations during relaxation compared to linear chains, as seen in figure 6.3(C) and quantified by the mean fractional fluctuation of chain extensions about the mean:

$$\frac{\langle \delta \rangle}{L_R} = \frac{\sum_{n=1}^{n=N} \sqrt{\sum_{t_{0.9x}}^{t_f} | x_n(t) - \langle x \rangle_n |^2}}{N L_R} \tag{6.11}$$

where $t_{0.9x}$ and t_f are the times at which the extension reaches 90% of the steady-state stretched value and the flow ceases, respectively, and N is the total number of trials for each condition. As shown in figure 6.3(D), $\frac{\langle \delta \rangle}{L_R}$ for rings in a solution of concentration c^* is >2-fold larger than that for linear chains at the same concentration, and remains larger even when the concentration is reduced to as low as $\sim 0.025c^*$ (Zhou *et al* 2019).

These results indicate the importance of transient threading of rings under extensional strain, even at very dilute linear chain concentrations. Namely, transient

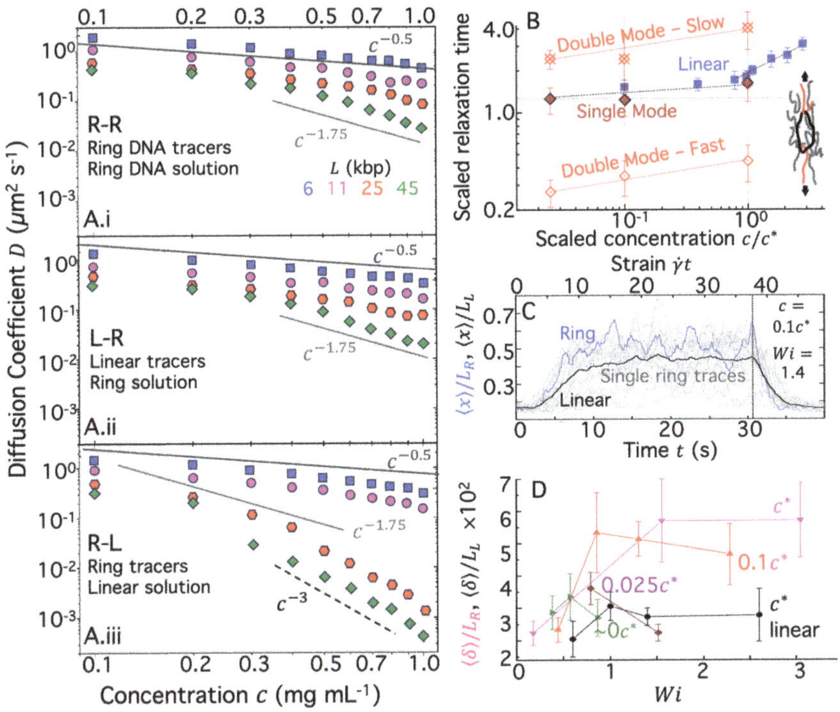

Figure 6.3. Dynamics of single ring DNA molecules in semidilute unentangled solutions are distinct from linear chains in steady-state and under flow. (A) Diffusion coefficients of ring (i, iii) and linear (ii) DNA tracers embedded in solutions of ring (i, ii) and linear (iii) DNA of varying mass concentrations *c*, measured via single-molecule tracking. Tracer and solution DNA are the same length in all cases and colors/symbols correspond to different lengths: $L = 6$ (blue squares), 11 (magenta circles), 25 (red hexagons), and 45 (green diamonds) kilobasepairs. The solid power-law scaling lines correspond to predictions from the Rouse model (dark grey, $D \sim c^{-0.5}$) and reptation model (light grey, $D \sim c^{-1.75}$); and the dashed line indicates the steeper empirical scaling for constraint release of threaded rings ($D \sim c^{-3}$). (B–D) Microfluidic elongational flow experiments with 45-kbp ring DNA embedded in semidilute solutions ($c/c^* = 0.025$, 0.1, 1) of linear 48.5-kbp λ DNA, depicted in inset in B. (B) Relaxation times τ, scaled by their tracer limit value τ_0, as a function of reduced concentration (c/c^*), determined from exponential fits to the decaying fractional extensions of the stretched rings following flow cessation. Rings exhibit either single-mode relaxation (filled red diamonds) with similar relaxation times and scaling as their linear DNA counterparts (blue squares), or double-mode relaxation with relaxation timescales that are slower (crossed open diamonds) and faster (open diamonds) than the single mode τ. Dashed lines are power-law fits of the ring data to $\tau/\tau_0 \sim (c/c^*)^w$ with scaling exponents $w \simeq 0.07$ (single mode, black dashed line), $w \simeq 0.13$ (slow mode, red dotted line), and $w \simeq 0.14$ (fast mode, red dotted line). (C) Average fractional extension versus time (t, top axis) and strain ($\dot{\gamma}t$, bottom axis) for ring ($\langle x\rangle/L_R$, blue) and linear ($\langle x\rangle/L_L$, black) DNA under elongational flow with $Wi = 1.4$ in a $0.1c^*$ solution of linear DNA. A wide range of heterogeneous stretching profiles (grey) comprise $\langle x\rangle/L_R$. (C) Average fractional fluctuations $\langle\delta\rangle/L_R$ as a function of *Wi* for rings in linear DNA solutions of $c = 0$ (green triangles), $0.025\,c^*$ (maroon diamonds), $0.1c^*$ (red triangles), and c^* (magenta inverted triangles) compared to linear chains at c^* (black circles). (A) Adapted with permission from Robertson and Smith (2007). Copyright (2007) American Chemical Society. (B–D) Adapted from Zhou *et al* (2019). CC BY 4.0.

threading and releasing of rings leads to the heterogeneous extension curves seen in figure 6.3(C) and quantified in figure 6.3(D), as well as the double-mode relaxation profiles seen in figure 6.3(B). The slow relaxation mode is due to the relaxation of threaded rings, which is slower than the retraction of linear chains, whereas the fast mode reflects the unencumbered relaxation of unthreaded rings, which is substantially faster than their linear counterparts due to their reduced conformational degrees of freedom and smaller fully-extended length (Zhou *et al* 2019).

6.1.3 Entangled ring DNA

Because a ring polymer has no free ends, i.e., no 'head' or 'tail', it cannot reptate in the traditional sense as it cannot translate its COM by diffusing 'head-first' in a direction parallel to its contour. Attempts at this process equate to a dog chasing its tail, which goes nowhere except around and around in a circle. Nevertheless, solutions of ring DNA have been shown to exhibit entanglement-like dynamics that align with theoretical models for modified reptation dynamics of rings (Iyer *et al* 2006, Robertson and Smith 2007, Robertson and Smith 2007a, 2007b, Chapman *et al* 2012, Ge *et al* 2016a, Regan *et al* 2016). However, the extent to which ring polymers can form entanglements and the nature of their dynamics, as compared to linear chains, remains a highly controversial topic in the polymer community (Rubinstein 1986, Iyer *et al* 2006, McLeish 2008, Ge *et al* 2016b, Michieletto 2016, Tsalikis *et al* 2016, Michieletto *et al* 2017b, Smrek *et al* 2019, Ubertini *et al* 2022).

In the following sections, I focus on the empirical properties of entangled ring DNA and relevant theoretical studies that shed light on the measured properties.

6.1.3.1 Experimental results

Single-molecule tracking studies of concentrated solutions of ring and linear DNA showed that, for both topologies, the scaling of the diffusion coefficient with concentration aligns with reptation model predictions for good solvent conditions

$$D_L \sim D_R \sim c^{-1.75} \tag{6.12}$$

for concentrations $c \gtrsim 6c_L^*$ (figure 6.3(A)) (Robertson and Smith 2007). For ring DNA tracers diffusing in entangled linear DNA solutions, their scaling became steeper at $\sim 10c_L^*$, more closely following a scaling of c^{-3}, indicative of threading and constraint release that slows the dynamics (figure 6.3(A)). While their scaling behavior was similar for both topologies, indicating similar mechanisms mediating the diffusion, the magnitudes of the diffusion coefficients for rings and linear chains were reported to be faster when diffusing in a solution of rings compared to linear chains, owing to the inefficiency of rings to form entanglements (figure 6.3(A)) (Robertson and Smith 2007, 2007a).

To determine the extent to which transverse motion is restricted in concentrated solutions of ring DNA (the hallmark of the reptation tube model), and characterize the nature of the tube-like confinement, optical tweezers measurements were performed to measure the force resisting polymer motion transverse to its contour in concentrated solutions of ring DNA (figures 6.4(A) and (B)) (Robertson and Smith 2007b). These studies showed the first proof of a transverse confining

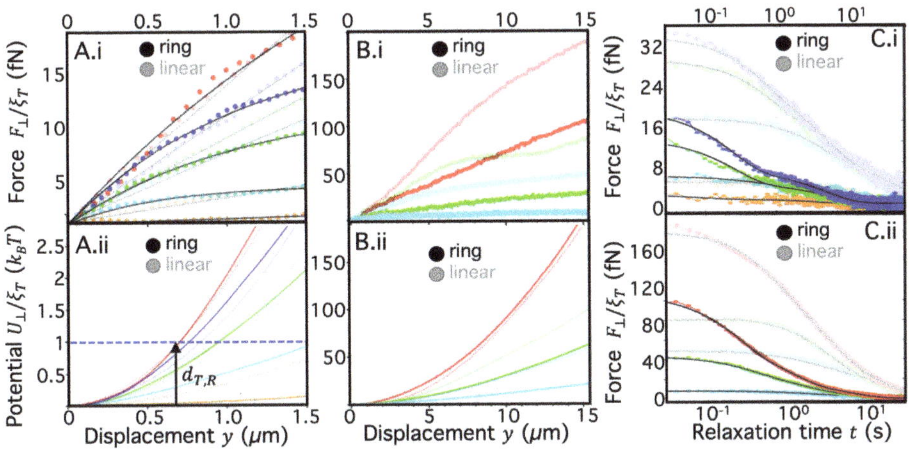

Figure 6.4. Optical tweezers measurements demonstrate that entangled ring DNA solutions exhibit tube-like confinement that is shorter range and less persistent than that of linear DNA. A 25-kbp DNA strand is pulled vertically through an entangled ($\sim 40c_L^*$) solution of 115 kbp ring DNA (solid data points and curves) or linear DNA (translucent data) and the force exerted by the surrounding entangled DNA to resist the displacement is measured during and after strains of varying pulling speeds v (μm s^{-1}): 65 (red), 25 (blue), 13 (green), 0.52 (cyan), and 0.1 (orange). These experiments are similar to those described in section 5.1.1 and shown in figure 5.1. The linear DNA data shown in A.i and C.i are the same as in figures 5.1(D) and (E). (A) The confining force per thermal blob $F_\perp(y)/\xi_T$ (i) and associated tube potential $U_\perp(y)$ (ii) computed from $F_\perp(y)$ via equation (5.1) for small displacements ($y_{\max} = 1.5\ \mu$m). The solid lines are fits to $F_\perp(y) = F_{\max}(1 - e^{-\kappa y})$ (black, ring data) and $F_\perp(y) = Ky$ (grey, linear data), and the dashed blue line indicates $U_\perp(y = d_{T,R})/\xi_T = k_BT$ from which a tube diameter of $d_{T,R} \simeq 0.6\ \mu$m $\simeq 0.75 d_{T,L}$ is determined (black arrow). (B) The same measurements shown in A, performed over 10× larger displacements ($y_{\max} = 15\ \mu$m) show substantial softening of force (i) and potential (ii) for rings compared to linear DNA. (C) The relaxation of the confining forces $F_\perp(t)/\xi_T$ shown in A following transverse displacements of $y_{\max} = 1.5\ \mu$m (i) and $y_{\max} = 15\ \mu$m (ii) are much faster for entangled rings compared to linear chains. All linear DNA data (i, ii) and the large displacement ring data (ii) are well fit to a sum of three exponential decays (black lines) with fast, intermediate, and slow time constants τ_1, τ_2 and τ_3 that align with topology-dependent Rouse relaxation τ_R, tube stretching and shrinking τ_2, and tube disengagement τ_D, respectively. For entangled rings relaxing following small displacement strains (i), the fast and intermediate decay modes are sufficient for complete relaxation, i.e., the curves are fit to a sum of two exponentials with $\tau_1 \approx \tau_{R,R}$ and τ_2. Adapted with permission from Robertson and Smith (2007b, 2007c). Copyright (2007) by the American Physical Society.

potential in entangled ring solutions, akin to the expected tube potential (figure 6.4(Aii)) (Zhou and Larson 2006, Robertson and Smith 2007c, Wang *et al*). However, the tube diameter $d_{T,R}$, measured via equation (5.4):

$$U_\perp(d_{T,R})/\xi_T = k_BT$$

is ~25% smaller than that for linear DNA of the same length and concentration ($d_{T,R} \approx 0.6\ \mu$m versus $d_{T,L} \approx 0.8\ \mu$m) (figure 6.4(A.ii)), in line with theoretical predictions based on the pom-pom ring (PPR) model described in the following section (Iyer *et al* 2006) and demonstrating stronger short-range confinement (figure 6.4(A)).

However, while for entangled linear DNA, the transverse force increases linearly with displacement

$$F_{\perp,L}(y) = Ky \tag{6.13}$$

with a spring constant of stiffness K and a quadratic potential,

$$U_{\perp}(y) \sim Ky^2 \tag{6.14}$$

as expected for a Hookean restoring force, entangled ring DNA elicit a softer exponential force response described by

$$F_{\perp}(y) = F_{\max}(1 - e^{-\kappa y}) \tag{6.15}$$

where $F_{\max}$ is the asymptotic force value (nonexistent for linear DNA) and κ is an effective stiffness (Robertson and Smith 2007b). The result is that the tube confinement formed by rings is stronger than their linear counterparts for small lengthscales $\lesssim d_T$, but becomes much weaker as y increases beyond d_T (figures 6.4(A) and (B)). Of note, this effect is only apparent for speeds $v \geqslant 13\ \mu\text{m s}^{-1}$, below which $U_{\perp}(y)$ for rings is markedly weaker than that for linear DNA at all lengthscales, indicating faster relaxation timescales for entangled rings compared to linear chains (figure 6.4(A)).

Figure 6.4(C) corroborates this interpretation by showing that the strain-induced force on entangled rings $F_{\perp}(t)$ relaxes much more quickly over time t than for linear chains, regardless of the displacement size ($y_{\max} = 1.5\ \mu\text{m}$ (i) or $y_{\max} = 15\ \mu\text{m}$ (ii)) or speed ($v = 0.1-65\ \mu\text{m s}^{-1}$). Fits of the relaxation profiles to a sum of three exponential decays (see equation (5.8)), revealed decay times of $\tau_1 \simeq 0.30$ s, $\tau_2 \simeq 4.1$ s, and $\tau_3 \simeq 11$ s, with τ_1 and τ_2 being similar to those measured for linear DNA and in line with Rouse relaxation ($\tau_1 \approx \tau_{R,R}$) and non-classical tube stretching and re-equilibration (τ_2). However, the longest relaxation time, which equates to the disengagement time for entangled linear polymers, was reported to be $\sim 3\times$ shorter for rings compared to linear chains ($\tau_{D,R} \approx 11$ s vs $\tau_{D,L} \approx 34$ s), roughly consistent with the theoretically predicted ratio of disengagement times from the PPR model

$$\tau_{D,R}/\tau_{D,L} \approx 0.2 \text{ (PPR)} \tag{6.16}$$

Moreover, this longest relaxation time was shown to only significantly contribute to the relaxation profile following large displacements (figure 6.4(C.ii)), whereas for shorter displacements (figure 6.4(C.i)) the reptation that occurs during τ_2 is sufficient to relax the modest deformations from small displacements. This much faster relaxation of rings compared to linear chains suggests that ring DNA can more readily rearrange on the timescale of the imposed strains, such that the confinement forces measured at large displacements are significantly weaker in ring DNA solutions (figure 6.4(B)).

These studies showed evidence for tube-like confinement in ring DNA solutions, albeit with key differences compared to the classical tube confinement seen for entangled linear polymers. However, several bulk rheological studies on synthetic ring polymer melts have reported dynamics that are fundamentally different than those expected for entangled polymers (Roovers 1985, 1988, McKenna *et al* 1989, Kapnistos *et al* 2008, Tsalikis *et al* 2016, Yan *et al* 2016, Parisi *et al* 2021, Chen *et al* 2023), and there remains extensive debate in the field as to whether rings can form long-lived entanglements and exhibit key entanglement features like a plateau modulus G^0 (Rubinstein 1986, Kremer *et al* 2011, Halverson *et al* 2011, 2012, Michieletto *et al* 2014, 2017b, Ge *et al* 2016b, Michieletto 2016, Smrek and Grosberg 2016, Smrek *et al* 2019, Ubertini *et al* 2022).

This controversy is enhanced by the near impossibility of synthesizing highly concentrated ring polymers devoid of linear contaminants, knots, or concatenation (Roovers and Toporowski 1988, Bielawski *et al* 2002, Endo 2008, Kapnistos *et al* 2008, Takano *et al* 2009, Chen *et al* 2023). Given this caveat, I will not discuss synthetic ring polymer studies in this chapter, but will instead reserve any discussion of this expansive body of literature for chapter 8 where I discuss blends of ring and linear polymers and their relation to studies on blended solutions of ring and linear DNA.

6.1.3.2 Theoretical frameworks and predictions

To understand the entanglement-like dynamics that concentrated ring polymers exhibit, coupled with their faster relaxation compared to linear chains, several theoretical models have been proposed that suggest that rings can adopt conformations that allow for reptation-like diffusion despite their lack of free ends (figure 6.5) (Klein 1986, Cates and Deutsch 1986, Halverson *et al* 2011, Iyer *et al* 2006, Kremer *et al* 2011, Brás *et al* 2014, Michieletto *et al* 2014, Rosa and Everaers 2014, Michieletto 2016, Ge *et al* 2016b, Tsalikis *et al* 2018, Smrek *et al* 2019, Ghobadpour *et al* 2021, Michieletto and Sakaue 2021, Ubertini *et al* 2022).

For example, rings have been predicted to adopt double-folded conformations in which rings appear similar to linear chains but with length $L/2$, in which case the primary mode of diffusion is reptation (Klein 1986, Smrek *et al* 2019, Ghobadpour *et al* 2021). Several theories predicting entangled ring dynamics suggest that rings adopt tree-like or lattice-animal conformations, reminiscent of branched polymers, in which several fingers, loops, branches, or 'pom-poms' extend in different directions from the ring center-of-mass, each undergoing amoeba-like motion (Obukhov *et al* 1994, Muller *et al* 1996, 2000, Iyer *et al* 2006, Milner and Newhall 2010, Grosberg 2013, Michieletto 2016, Smrek and Grosberg 2016, Kruteva *et al* 2023). Some key differences between these theories include the extent to which the rings are considered compact, swollen, crumpled, or ideal; the size distribution, number and conformation of loops; the relative importance of the ends of the double-folded rings versus the central trunk; and the fractal dimension of the ring polymer and its central trunk (figures 6.5(A) and (B)).

Pom-Pom Ring (PPR): The pom-pom-ring model (Iyer *et al* 2006, Michieletto 2016) is one such analytical approach that treats an entangled ring polymer as a tree-like structure with a central trunk or primitive path of length

$$L_{0,p} \simeq N^{2\upsilon} l_k^2 d_T^{-1} \tag{6.17}$$

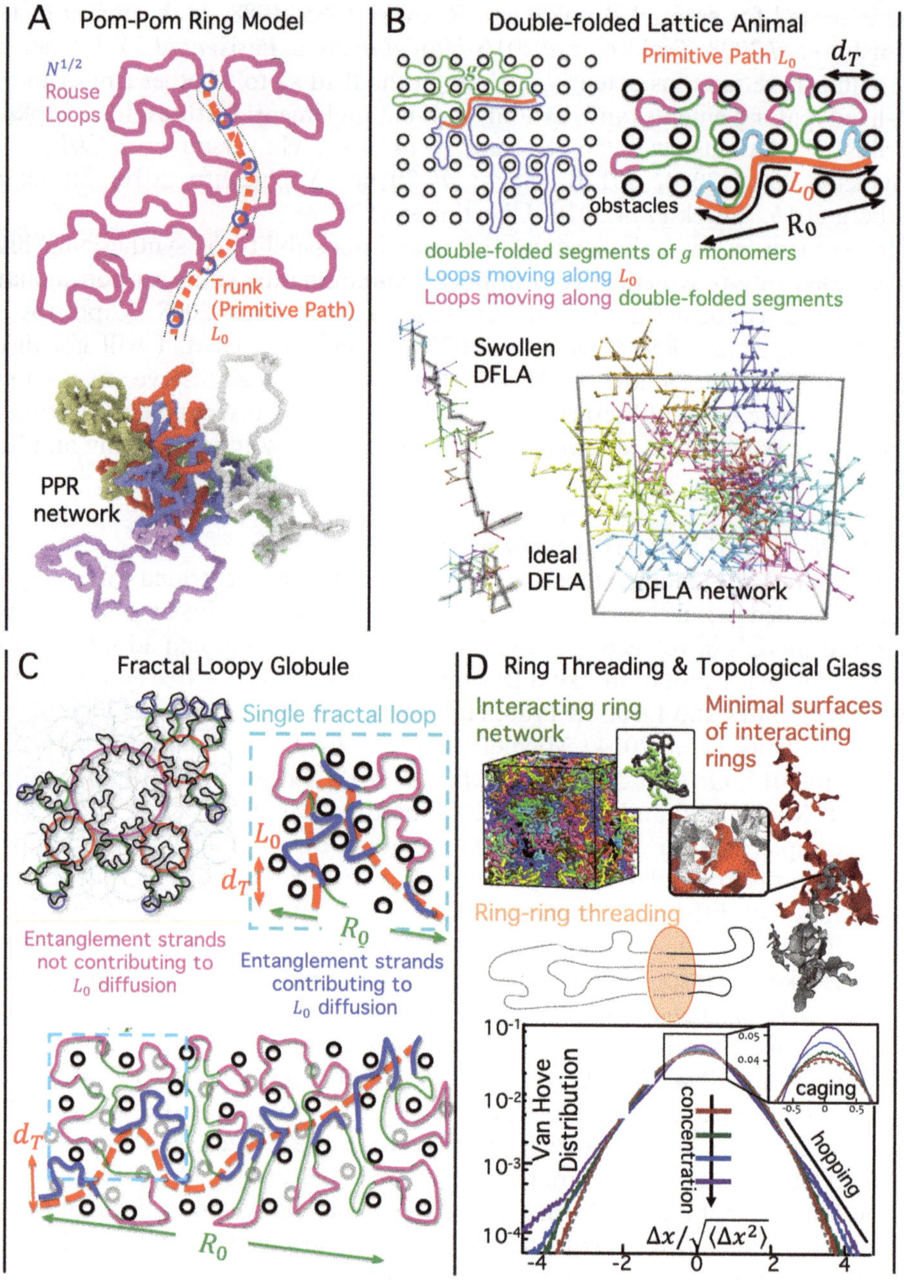

Figure 6.5. Theoretical frameworks to describe the structure and dynamics of highly overlapping ring polymers. (A) (top) The pom-pom ring (PPR) treats each ring as a central trunk (red) of length $L_{0,p} \simeq L^{2v}$ that undergoes reptation with added friction from $N_l \approx N^{1/2}$ Rouse loops (magenta) of size $n_l \approx N^{1/2}$. (bottom) The trunks of highly overlapping PPR rings entangle with one another while the loops remain collapsed and unentangled. (**B**) (top-left) Double-folded lattice animal (DFLA) models treat each ring as a chain of double-folded branches or loops (green and blue), arranged on a lattice (black circles) with spacing d_T. Each chain segment of n_p Kuhn lengths (green) is connected by a trunk or primitive path ($L_{0,p}$, red). (top-right) A small fraction of the loops (cyan) moves

curvilinearly with the primitive path, while most of the loops (magenta) move along the double-folded branches (green) so do not contribute to the tube dynamics. (bottom) Isolated DFLA rings can be modeled as either ideal or self-avoiding swollen conformations, while at high concentrations DFLA rings adopt compact conformations that entangle with one another to form a percolated overlapping network. (C) The fractal loopy globule (FLG) model describes an entangled ring as (top-left) a fractal series of loops of different sizes (indicated by circles of different colors) that can interpenetrate with one another and have the same degree of overlap at all scales. In any given loop of size R_0 (green; top-right and bottom) at any given time (e.g., t_1, t_2), only a small fraction of segments (blue) contributes to the reptation of the primitive path (dashed red line) while the majority (magenta) only provide added friction. The fraction of non-contributing segments increases with time as the relevant loop size increases, thereby increasing the entanglement spacing d_T. This effective tube dilation can be seen by comparing the grey (t_1) and black (t_2) obstacles in iii. The grey obstacles shown in the cyan bordered box are the same as those shown in black at top-right, highlighting the increase in d_T over time. Complete tube dilation over time prevents the onset of an elastic entanglement plateau. (D) Simulations of dense systems of rings (top-left) have shown that neighboring rings can interpenetrate or thread one another (inset), which halts ring diffusion and results in glassy dynamics that PPR, DFLA, and FLG models do not predict. Similarly, modeling each ring (grey) as an Interacting Branching Primitive tree (IBP) that can penetrate the minimal surface (peach) of a neighboring IBP (red) has revealed a strong propensity for ring threading that was not captured when modeling rings as DFLAs. Glassy dynamics can be seen in the non-Gaussian van Hove distributions of ring displacements that display caging and hopping dynamics, signatures of heterogeneous transport often seen near glass transitions, that are amplified with increasing concentration. (A) Adapted with permission from Iyer *et al* (2006). Copyright (2006) by the American Physical Society and from Michieletto (2016) with permission from the Royal Society of Chemistry. (B) Adapted with permission from Ge *et al* (2016a). Copyright (2016) American Chemical Society and from Ghobadpour *et al* (2021). Copyright (2021) by the American Physical Society. (C) Adapted with permission from Ge *et al* (2016b). Copyright (2016) American Chemical Society. (D) Adapted with permission from Michieletto *et al* (2017b). Copyright (2017) by the American Physical Society and from Smrek *et al* (2019). CC BY 4.0.

where $1/4 \leqslant \upsilon \leqslant 1/2$ (Muller *et al* 2000, Suzuki *et al* 2009), and, for entangled DNA in good solvent conditions, $\upsilon \simeq 0.3$ (Muller *et al* 2000, Iyer *et al* 2006, 2008).

The trunk is decorated with a series of n_l 'pom-poms' or loops of length L_l, with both quantities relating to the length of the polymer as

$$N_l \approx n_l \approx N^{1/2} \tag{6.18}$$

where, recall that $N = Ll_k^{-1}$ is the number of Kuhn lengths per polymer, such that $N_l = L_l l_k^{-1}$.

Diffusion proceeds via curvilinear reptation of the central trunk, and the longest relaxation timescale is therefore the disengagement time τ_D of the trunk. The loops, which are assumed to be unentangled due to their relatively collapsed conformation, obey Rouse dynamics and provide an added friction term to the trunk diffusion and relaxation (figure 6.5(A)) (Iyer *et al* 2006, Rosa and Everaers 2014). Because the trunk is shorter than the length of the polymer chain L (see equation (6.15)), the disengagement time for a ring $\tau_{D,R}$ is predicted to be shorter than for a linear chain of the same length, according to the expression

$$\frac{\tau_{D,R}}{\tau_{D,L}} \simeq (N_e/N)^{1-2\upsilon} \tag{6.19}$$

where, recall that $N_e = l_e l_k^{-1}$ is the entanglement length in units of l_k. PPR further predicts that N_e is the same for rings and linear chains

$$N_{e,R} \approx N_{e,L} \approx N_e \tag{6.20}$$

To determine the ability of equation (6.19) to predict $\tau_{D,R}/\tau_{D,L}$ for the $\sim 40c_L^*$ solutions of 115 kbp ($N \simeq 383$) DNA examined in figure 6.4, consider the self-avoiding random walk relationship

$$d_T \approx (l_k^2 N_e)^{\nu} \tag{6.21}$$

which can be expressed as

$$N_e \approx d_{T,L}^{1/\nu} l_k^{-2\nu} \tag{6.22}$$

where $l_k \simeq 100$ nm, $d_{T,L} \simeq 500$ nm (Doi and Edwards 1988, Robertson and Smith 2007c), and $\nu \simeq 0.588$, from which we can estimate $N_e \approx 5$.

It follows that equation (6.19) gives the relation $\tau_{D,R} \simeq 0.2\tau_{D,L}$, in reasonable agreement with the empirical ratio $\tau_{D,R} \approx 0.3\tau_{D,L}$ (figure 6.4(C)) (Robertson and Smith 2007b, 2007c).

Relaxation times measured via optical tweezers microrheology for blends of ring, supercoiled, and linear DNA of lengths 25 kbp and 45 kbp are also consistent with PPR predictions, as I discuss in chapter 7 (Peddireddy *et al* 2020a, 2020b).

PPR models that assume the equality in equation (6.20) also predict that the tube diameter for rings $d_{T,R}$ is smaller than that of equivalent linear chains $d_{T,L}$ according to the ratio

$$\frac{d_{T,R}}{d_{T,L}} = N_e^{\frac{2\upsilon - 1}{2}} = N_e^{-0.2} \tag{6.23}$$

which equates to $d_{T,R} \simeq 0.72 d_{T,L}$ for the DNA solutions in figure 6.4, in excellent agreement with the empirical relationship $d_{T,R} \simeq 0.75 d_{T,L}$ (Robertson and Smith 2007b).

Double-folded lattice animal (DFLA): The double-folded lattice animal model for entangled rings is similar to PPR; however, DFLA models treat each 'loop' as a perfectly double-folded chain segment with no penetrable space between the folds (figure 6.5(B)) (Nechaev *et al* 1987, Obukhov *et al* 1994, Kremer *et al* 2011, Grosberg 2013, Rosa and Everaers 2014, Michieletto 2016, Ghobadpour *et al* 2021). Traditional DFLA models predict that the mean end-to-end distance of the central trunk or primitive path $R_{0,p}$ can be written as

$$R_{0,p} \simeq d_T (N/N_e)^{1/d_f} \tag{6.24}$$

and its primitive path length $L_{0,p}$ as

$$L_{0,p} \simeq d_T (N/N_e)^{1/d_p} \tag{6.25}$$

where the ring is considered to have a global fractal dimension of $d_f = 4$ and its primitive path is considered an ideal random walk with fractal dimension $d_p = 2$ (Rubinstein 1986, Nechaev *et al* 1987, Obukhov *et al* 1994).

Further developments to this initial DFLA construction considered ring conformations as being fully compact or 'crumpled' on lengthscales above l_e (Grosberg 2013, Rosa and Everaers 2014, Ghobadpour *et al* 2021), and the primitive path was treated as a self-avoiding random walk rather than ideal, leading to fractal dimensions of $d_f = 3$ and $d_p = 5/3$.

This refinement provides the predicted expression for the coil size of an entangled ring

$$\langle R_G \rangle \sim R_{0,p} \sim d_T (L/l_e)^{1/3} \tag{6.26}$$

which is more compact than that of ideal entangled linear chains, $\langle R_G \rangle \sim L^{1/2}$.

The fractal nature of the loop sizes predicted by DFLA models render the corresponding relaxation dynamics of an entangled ring likewise fractal, in contrast to the relaxation dynamics of an entangled linear chain, which is dictated solely by the chain ends and is similar for all monomers. Moreover, the fractal nature of the loops leads to self-similar dynamics of an entangled ring, whereby loops of all sizes relax in a similar fashion, over timescales that scale with their size (figure 6.5(B)). At each lengthscale, the smaller loops provide added friction to the larger loops to slow their dynamics, but do not contribute to the reptation of the primitive path, similar to models for branched and polydisperse polymers (Klein 1986, Doi *et al* 1987, Leonardi *et al* 2000, Rubinstein and Colby 2003).

Fractal Loopy Globule (FLG): The fractal loopy globule model builds on the tree-like models discussed above by treating each ring as a fractal series of loops of broadly distributed sizes that have the same degree of overlap at all lengthscales (figure 6.5(C)) (Ge *et al* 2016b, Kruteva *et al* 2023). FLG models assume a fractal dimension of $d_f = 3$ for the ring conformation, and, importantly, allow loops to penetrate one another, which is prohibited by DFLA and PPR models (figure 6.5(C)) (Mirny 2011, Ge *et al* 2016b, Kruteva *et al* 2023). Like DFLA models, the relaxation dynamics are self-similar, proceeding by loops of successively larger size rearranging on successively larger timescales.

At each loop lengthscale l_l, smaller loops contribute to the friction without effecting the tube-like dynamics at that scale, which have a characteristic timescale $\tau_{D,l}$, similar to PPR. However, the large distribution of loop sizes leads to dilation of the entanglement tube over time, as can be seen by the following relations

$$l_l^2 \sim \tau_{D,l} \tag{6.27}$$

$$d_T^2 \sim \tau_D \tag{6.28}$$

FLG predicts complete dilation of the entanglement tube which eliminates the time-independent entanglement plateau ($G(t) \sim G^0$) and instead results in power-law scaling of the relaxation modulus with time

$$G(t) \sim t^{-3/7} \tag{6.29}$$

The FLG longest relaxation timescale and COM diffusion coefficient are predicted to scale with polymer length as

$$\tau_{D,R} \sim L^{7/3} \quad (6.30)$$

$$D_{R,R} \sim L^{-5/3} \quad (6.31)$$

which are weaker than the corresponding reptation model predictions for linear chains

$$\tau_{D,L} \sim L^{3} \quad (6.32)$$

$$D_{R,L} \sim L^{-2}. \quad (6.33)$$

6.1.3.3 Reconciling experiments and theory

Importantly, original implementations of PPR, DFLA, and FLG assume a background of fixed constraints, a reasonable approximation for highly entangled linear chains, but often inaccurate for describing the dynamics of more mobile tube constraints formed by rings, which can reorganize on the relaxation timescale of a confined ring (Robertson and Smith 2007b, Michieletto *et al* 2017b, Peddireddy *et al* 2020a).

One approach to incorporating the mobility of the background into these models, has been to adopt the double reptation framework (Marrucci 1985, des Cloizeaux 1988, McLeish 2002, Haley and Lodge 2005), originally developed to account for the reptation of the surrounding polymers that adds mobility to the constraints in polydisperse and blended linear polymers networks. This modification, similar to the concept of multi-ring relaxation (Rubinstein and Colby 2003, Milner and Newhall 2010, Xue *et al* 2020), leads to faster relaxation timescales with altered power-law dependence on polymer length, as well as the lack of an entanglement plateau, which has been empirically observed for synthetic ring polymers (Kapnistos *et al* 2008).

In other attempts to reconcile theoretical predictions with experimental results, the FLG model and similar frameworks (Halverson *et al* 2011, Rosa and Everaers 2014) were further developed to account for tube dilation, as discussed above, which has been evidenced in optical tweezers experiments on entangled solutions of ring and linear DNA (figures 5.3 and 6.4) (Robertson and Smith 2007b, 2007c). Importantly, the origin and nature of the tube dilation for rings is distinct from that for linear chains in which dilation is due to segments of the confined polymer 'exploring' (i.e., thermally fluctuating) larger transverse distances over time $t < \tau_D$ (Zhou and Larson 2006, Wang *et al*). Within the FLG framework, tube dilation occurs due to the successive relaxation of larger and larger loops that comprise the entangled ring (Ge *et al* 2016b). In so far as d_T can be equated to the average spacing between topological constraints (i.e., the average loop size) (figure 6.5(D)), it follows that d_T increases with time as the average size of an unrelaxed loop increases. An important distinction between the FLG model and other lattice-tree models is that it is self-consistent in its treatment of tube dilation, rather than adding it in 'by hand', by incorporating the time-varying friction component that results from the relaxation of successively larger loops (Grosberg 2013, Ge *et al* 2016b, Kruteva *et al* 2023).

A final important consideration for entangled rings, which has only more recently been appreciated, is the possible threading of rings by their neighbors, which can stall tube dilation and cause relaxation times to diverge (Michieletto *et al* 2014, 2017a, 2017b, Wang and Ge 2021, Khanal *et al* 2022, Marfai *et al* 2023). One such implementation of this idea is the Interacting Branching Primitive tree (IBP) model that builds on the DFLA model to allow branches of one ring to interpenetrate the minimal surface of a neighboring ring (Smrek and Grosberg 2016, Smrek *et al* 2019, Ubertini *et al* 2022). In the case of globally connected threadings, i.e., every ring is threaded by a neighbor, the dynamics are predicted to exhibit glassiness or 'dynamic arrest'. Notably, threadings are only predicted to occur on lengthscales below l_e while looping and branching dominate the ring conformations at lengthscales larger than l_e (Ubertini *et al* 2022). However, threadings can still alter the entanglement dynamics of rings, which occur at lengthscales $>l_e$, if their density and lengths are large enough. Above this critical threading threshold, glassy caging and hopping of rings is predicted.

These anomalous and heterogenous transport mechanisms manifest as non-Gaussian van Hove distributions (figure 6.5(D)) (Michieletto *et al* 2017b), as seen in systems near glass or jamming transitions (Bouchaud and Georges 1990, Chaudhuri *et al* 2007, Michieletto *et al* 2017b, Marfai *et al* 2023). These features are predicted to arise from populations of threaded and pinned rings with nearly halted or 'caged' displacements, and populations of unthreaded rings that can move further than expected (i.e., hop) due to mobile entanglements with surrounding rings. The populations of caged and mobile rings are predicted to be spatially segregated such that threaded and slow rings cluster together and maintain long-lived overlap with their neighbors, while more mobile, non-threaded rings maintain spatial correlations with one another but change neighbors quickly (i.e., very short-lived constraints). Importantly, this heterogeneous distribution of constraints is not seen in entangled linear polymers which exhibit largely homogeneously distributed universal constraints defined by a single lengthscale d_T and timescale τ_e.

The theoretical framework described above is strictly for ring–ring threadings in pure ring solutions, which are predicted to give rise to different dynamics than threadings of rings by linear chains, a ubiquitous feature of blends of ring and linear polymers (Helfer *et al* 2003, Halverson *et al* 2012, Peddireddy *et al* 2020a, Tsalikis and Mavrantzas 2020). Specifically, the lifetime of ring threadings are predicted to be shorter than their linear counterparts and exhibit a broader distribution of lifetimes, resulting in 'dynamic arrest' similar to glassy behavior (Michieletto *et al* 2017a, 2017b, Smrek *et al* 2019, Michieletto and Sakaue 2021). Conversely, threading of rings by linear chains results in long-lived static pinning of the ring that is only released via slow constraint release of the threading linear chain (Rubinstein and Colby 2003, Tsalikis and Mavrantzas 2020, Michieletto and Sakaue 2021). Chapter 7 will discuss in more detail the impact of ring-linear threading on the dynamics of ring-linear blends.

6.2 Supercoiled circular biopolymers

The above discussion regarding polymers without ends was restricted to relaxed ring topologies and did not consider more complex topological variations such as concatenated, knotted, or supercoiled (i.e., torsionally twisted) circular polymers. The latter is of fundamental importance in biology as the entire class of bacterial genomic and plasmid DNA is supercoiled, in part, to reduce its conformational size and protect its genetic information (Alberts 2004, Adams *et al* 2013).

In dilute conditions, supercoiling reduces the conformational size of ring polymers, as one may expect as the twists and coils inhibit swelling. One prediction for the size of a supercoiled molecule employs the WLC expression for R_G but assumes a contour length that is 40% of its actual contour length ($L_S = 0.4L$) (Latulippe and Zydney 2010):

$$R_{G,S} = l_p[(L_S/3l_p) - 1 + 2\left(\frac{l_p}{L_S}\right)^2(1 - e^{-L_S/l_p})]^{0.5} \tag{6.34}$$

In the limit of large contour lengths ($L \gg l_p$), this expression yields a reduction in the radius of gyration of a supercoiled polymer compared to its linear counterpart of

$$\frac{R_{G,L}}{R_{G,S}} \simeq 1.62 \text{ (theory)} \tag{6.35}$$

(Latulippe and Zydney 2010), which is slightly higher than the empirically inferred ratio of $R_{G,L}/R_{G,R} \simeq 1.58$ for ring versus linear DNA (Robertson *et al* 2006). Previous measurements of diffusion coefficients for supercoiled and linear DNA of lengths ~3–289 kbp reported values of

$$\frac{R_{G,L}}{R_{G,S}} \approx 1.6-2 \text{ (experiment)} \tag{6.36}$$

(Robertson *et al* 2006) (figure 6.1(A)), in line with the predicted expression, which indicates more compaction compared to relaxed rings.

However, the case of semidilute and concentrated solutions of supercoiled polymers presents a more complex story. Simulations of densely packed supercoiled polymers, with properties akin to plasmid DNA with varying degrees of supercoiling σ (figure 6.6(A)), have shown that, above a critical polymer length and concentration, the radius of gyration of supercoiled polymers $R_{G,S}$ are larger than that of their relaxed ring counterparts $R_{G,R}$ (figure 6.6(B.i)) (Smrek *et al* 2021), with this relative expansion, $R_{G,S}/R_{G,R}$, increasing with the degree of supercoiling σ and contour length L. Moreover, the increase in $R_{G,S}$ with length was shown to follow power-law scaling $R_{G,S} \sim L^{\nu}$ indicative of self-avoiding random walk statistics (i.e., $\nu \simeq 3/5$), in contrast to collapsed ($\nu \simeq 1/3$) and ideal ($\nu \simeq 1/2$) statistics for entangled and unentangled relaxed rings (figure 6.6(C.i)) (Smrek *et al* 2021). Finally, supercoiling was reported to not only increase R_G, but also significantly change the conformation of a circular polymer, leading to a more closed conformation, with reduced minimal surface area $A_{\rm ms}$ (figure 6.6(D.i)) and enhanced

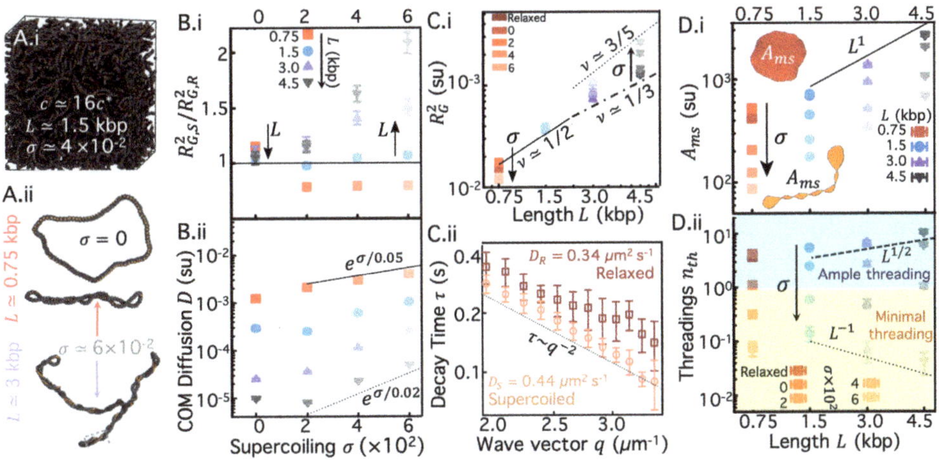

Figure 6.6. Theoretical frameworks to describe the structure and dynamics of highly overlapping rings polymers. (A) Brownian dynamics simulations of (i) highly overlapping ($c \simeq 16c^*$) supercoiled DNA polymers with (ii) varying lengths, $L \simeq 0.75$–4.5 kbp, and degree of supercoiling, $\sigma = 0$–6×10^{-2}, are used to determine (B) the effect of contour length L (color-coded according to legend) and supercoiling σ (x axis, dark to light shades) on the (i) radius of gyration R_G and (ii) COM diffusion coefficients D. The squared radius of gyration R_G^2, scaled by the value for a relaxed (i.e., nicked) ring $R_{G,R}^2$, (B.i) shows the extent to which supercoiling swells or compacts the DNA, indicated by data lying above or below the horizontal line at $R_G^2/R_{G,R}^2 = 1$. Increasing supercoiling σ causes increased swelling for all rings above $L \simeq 0.75$ kbp. Counter to the expected inverse relation between R_G and D, (B.ii) shows that increasing σ increases D in a length-dependent manner. The dashed and solid lines indicate exponential scaling $D \sim e^{a\sigma}$ with a increasing with the ring length L. (C.i) Radius of gyration values R_G^2 shown in B are plotted as a function of polymer length L and compared with theoretical scaling laws for various polymer conformations: ideal (solid line, $\nu \simeq 1/2$), compact or crumpled (dotted, $\nu \simeq 1/3$), or self-avoiding (dash-dot, $\nu \simeq 3/5$). (C.ii) DDM decay time τ versus wave vector q, experimentally measured for supercoiled (peach) and relaxed ring (maroon) DNA with $L \simeq 6$ kbp and $c \simeq 5c^*$ show diffusive scaling, $\tau \sim q^{-2}$, for both topologies, with supercoiled constructs exhibiting ~30% faster diffusion compared to relaxed rings, i.e., $D_s/D_R \simeq 1.3$. (D) Supercoiling reduces the minimal penetrable surface area of rings (i) which inhibits threading events (ii) that slow diffusion. (i) Minimal surface area, depicted in insets for $L \simeq 750$ kbp with $\sigma = 0$ (A_{ms}, top) and 0.04 (bottom) and plotted as a function of L for increasing supercoiling σ (dark to light hues), shows that increasing supercoiling universally decreases the minimal surface area (arrow). The increase in R_G (shown in B.i and C.i) is a result of the polymer conformations extending rather than swelling. The linear scaling of minimal surface area with polymer length $A_{\mathrm{ms}} \sim L^1$ is consistent with ideal random walk statistics $R_0 \sim L^{1/2}$. (ii) The number of threading events per DNA n_{th} versus L shows that only rings with $\sigma \lesssim 0.02$ have at least one threading per DNA (blue, $n_{\mathrm{th}} > 1$) while threading events are minimal for $\sigma > 0.02$ (yellow region, $n_{\mathrm{th}} < 1$). The threadings per DNA either increase or decrease with increasing L for low or high σ, following scalings of $n_{\mathrm{th}} \sim L^{1/2}$ (dashed line) or $n_{\mathrm{th}} \sim L^{-1}$ (dotted line). Modified from Smrek *et al* (2021). © The Authors, some rights reserved; exclusive licensee AAAS.

intra-chain interactions. This conformation more closely mimics a stiffer and shorter linear or branched polymer, with the degree of branching and asymmetry increasing with increasing polymer length (figures 6.6(A.ii) and (D.i)). The measured power-law relation

$$A_{\mathrm{ms}} \sim L^1 \tag{6.37}$$

(figure 6.6D.i)) is consistent with ideal random walk statistics $R_0 \sim L^{1/2}$, provided the dimensional analysis $A_{ms} \sim R_0^2$ holds.

Surprisingly, while increasing R_G increases the overlap of supercoiled polymers as compared to relaxed rings at a given concentration (recall $c/c^* \sim R_G^3$), the simulations discussed above showed that supercoiled rings with lengths $L \gtrsim 1.5$ kbp diffused faster than their relaxed ring counterparts. Moreover, D was reported to exponentially increase with σ as

$$D_s(\sigma)/D_R \approx e^{\sigma/\sigma_c} \tag{6.38}$$

where the critical degree of supercoiling σ_c decreases with increasing length L (figure 6.6(B.ii)) (Smrek *et al* 2021). Complementary DDM measurements of concentrated solutions of 6-kbp supercoiled and relaxed circular plasmid DNA at $c/c^* \simeq 5$ showed the supercoiled constructs diffused ~30% faster than their relaxed counterparts ($D_S/D_R \simeq 1.3$) (figure 6.6(C.ii)), corroborating the faster diffusion of simulated $\sim 16c^*$ supercoiled polymers as compared to relaxed rings (figure 6.6(B.ii)).

This counterintuitive coupling of enhanced mobility and larger conformational size was attributed to the lack of 'open' loops in sufficiently supercoiled rings ($\sigma > 0.02$) (figure 6.6(A.ii)), which reduces their minimal surface area compared to relaxed rings while at the same time increasing R_G by extending supercoiled constructs into asymmetric conformations (figure 6.6(D.i)). This reduced A_{ms} suppresses entanglements and threading events, which slow dynamics in a length-dependent manner (figure 6.6(Dii)). Specifically, the number of threadings per DNA n_{th} is increasingly reduced with increasing L according to the power law:

$$n_{th} \sim L^{-1} \, (\sigma > 0.02) \tag{6.39}$$

suggesting

$$n_{th} \sim A_{ms}^{-1} \, (\sigma > 0.02) \tag{6.40}$$

(figure 6.6(D.ii)). Conversely, for minimal supercoiling ($\sigma \lesssim 0.02$), the minimal surface area increases with polymer length according to

$$n_{th} \sim L^{1/2} \, (\sigma \lesssim 0.02) \tag{6.41}$$

(figure 6.6(D.ii)), suggesting that the number of threading events scales with the size of the polymer conformation R_G, which adheres to ideal random walk statistics $R_G \sim L^{1/2}$.

As I discuss in chapter 7, while supercoiled polymers cannot easily be threaded themselves, microrheology experiments on blends of supercoiled and ring DNA have shown that supercoiled constructs can be effective 'threaders' of neighboring ring DNA causing supercoiled-ring blends to exhibit entanglement dynamics at concentrations of $\sim c^*$, well below the critical entanglement concentration of $c_e \simeq 6c^*$, for linear and ring DNA (Peddireddy *et al* 2020b).

6.3 Concatenated ring biopolymers

As I discuss in chapter 1, there is a large family of endonucleases that can convert DNA from one topology to another—supercoiled to relaxed circular, circular to linear, etc (figure 6.1). An important class of these enzymes are topoisomerases that can twist and untwist circular DNA to increase or decrease the degree of supercoiling or torsional stress. For example, Topoisomerase II (T2) cuts a supercoiled DNA plasmid in a single location, locally untwists it, re-anneals the cut, moves to a new location along the DNA backbone and repeats the process until the supercoils are completely relaxed (Gellert 1981, Liu and Wang 1983). An alternative approach to untwisting supercoiled DNA is to use a nicking enzyme to cut one of the two strands of the double-stranded DNA to allow it to unwind and prevent it from storing any subsequent torsional stress (figure 6.1). As such, when T2 acts on nicked circular DNA it repeatedly cuts and reseals the DNA ring, but its unwinding action has no effect as the nicking prevents sustained twist. When this action is carried out in solutions of highly overlapping nicked DNA, the rings can become dynamically concatenated (Figure 6.7(A)) to form multi-ring structures or catenanes that resemble 'Olympic rings' or chain mail, akin to kinetoplasts (Lukeš *et al* 2002, Krajina *et al* 2018, Tubiana *et al* 2022).

Dynamic light scattering microrheology measurements (see chapter 3) of highly concentrated solutions of nicked circular DNA ($L \simeq 23$ kbp, $c \simeq 6$ mg mL$^{-1} \simeq 10c_R^*$,) showed that dynamic concatenation by T2 decreased the elastic contributions to the stress relaxation (i.e., G') and increased the relaxation rates compared to solutions without T2 (figure 6.7(B)) (Krajina *et al* 2018). Specifically, the low-frequency crossover ω_c, that demarks the onset of the terminal regime, was shown to correspond to the concatenation/de-concatenation rate $\sim \tau_{T2}^{-1}$ for solutions with active T2, rather than the slower disengagement rate $\sim \tau_D^{-1}$ expected for entangled polymer solutions (figure 6.7(B)). In the absence of T2, the relation $\omega_c \simeq \tau_D^{-1}$ was recovered with $\tau_D > \tau_{T2}$ (Krajina *et al* 2018).

Because the concatenation dynamics are faster than that of entanglements, T2 activity allows entanglements between rings to 'pass through' one another via the breakage and reannealing of entanglement segments (figure 6.7(A)), enabling rings to evade entanglement constraints and thus relax stress more quickly. This increased dissipation manifests as an extended terminal regime and lower plateau modulus for T2-active solutions compared to those without T2 (figure 6.7(B)). Conversely, by de-activating T2 via heat or chemical quenching, the concatenation dynamics can be halted, causing the rings to become 'frozen' in concatenated configurations (figure 6.7(A)).

The studies described in Krajina *et al* (2018) showed that quenching produced a nearly opposite effect to that of the active T2, eliminating the terminal regime seen without T2, and shifting the low-frequency rheological properties towards those of an elastic gel, with a rubbery plateau maintained down to the lowest measured frequency ($\omega = 0.1$ s^{-1}) (figure 6.7(C)). Conversely, in the high-frequency limit, above $\omega_e \simeq 10^3$ rad s^{-1}, solutions with active and quenched T2 exhibited similar magnitudes of $G'(\omega)$ and $G''(\omega)$, and scalings $G'(\omega) \sim \omega^{-b}$ with $b \simeq 1/2$ and

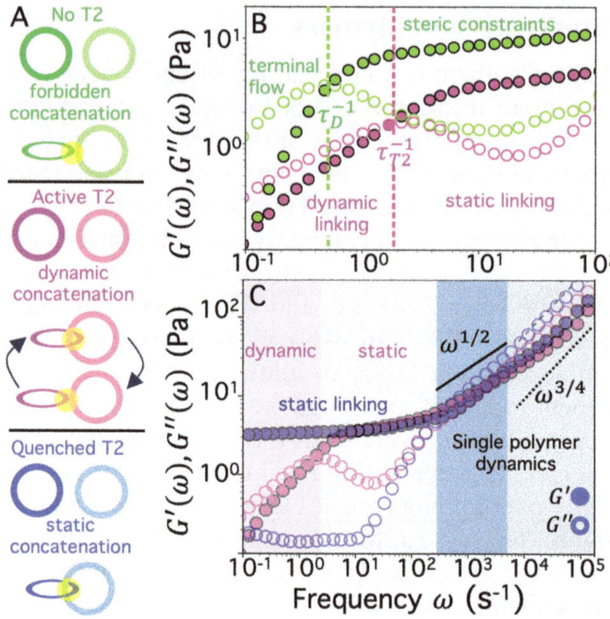

Figure 6.7. Dynamic concatenation of overlapping ring DNA via Topoisomerase II. (A) Two neighboring rings cannot become linked or concatenated (No T2, green) because their strands cannot pass through one another (yellow circle). Topoisomerase II (T2) cuts and reconnects the ends of ring DNA (Active T2, magenta), which can concatenate two neighboring rings and subsequently de-link them. Quenching of T2 activity freezes the two rings in concatenated states (Quenched T2, blue). (B and C) Linear viscoelastic moduli, $G'(\omega)$ (open symbols) and $G''(\omega)$ (filled symbols) for concentrated solutions of nicked ring DNA with length $L \simeq 23$ kbp and concentration $c \simeq 6\ \mathrm{mg\ mL^{-1}} \simeq 10c_R^*$ without T2 (green, B), with active T2 (magenta), and with quenched T2 (blue). (B) Solutions with and without T2 exhibit terminal regime scaling at low frequencies and entanglement plateaus at high frequencies, but the frequency ω_c at which the dynamics cross over to terminal regime (vertical dashed lines) is higher and the plateau modulus is lower in the presence of active T2, indicating faster relaxation dynamics and increased dissipation. This faster relaxation timescale for active T2 reflects the T2 linking/unlinking rate τ_{T2}^{-1}, which is faster than the terminal disengagement rate τ_D^{-1} of the sterically constrained rings without T2. (C) Quenching T2 (blue) prevents the terminal flow (pink shaded region) seen in the Active T2 case (magenta) by preventing rings from unlinking and disentangling, thereby eliminating τ_{T2} and τ_D. Following the entanglement regime that both solutions exhibit (light purple), both Active and Quenched T2 solutions exhibit similar properties. The dynamics at these higher frequencies, which reflect the dynamics of single polymers before they are constrained by the surrounding rings, are thus independent of any linking or lack thereof with nearest neighbors. In this regime, the scaling $G'(\omega) \sim \omega^{-b}$ for both active and quenched T2 obeys predicted scaling laws for flexible ($b \simeq 1/2$) and semiflexible ($b \simeq 3/4$) polymers at lower (dark blue) and higher (light blue) frequencies, respectively. Adapted with permission from Krajina *et al* (2018). Copyright (2018) by the American Physical Society.

$b \simeq 3/4$ for $\omega < 0.5\ \mathrm{ms^{-1}}$ and $\omega > 0.5\ \mathrm{ms^{-1}}$, respectively (figure 6.7(C)). Insofar as we can assume the predicted relation, $\omega_e \approx \tau_e^{-1}$ (figure 2.4) the similar dynamics can be attributed the fact that, at frequencies faster than the entanglement rate τ_e^{-1}, the free relaxation of single flexible chains ($b \simeq 1/2$) and semiflexible segments thereof ($b \simeq 3/4$), which are identical in both systems, dominate the rheology (figure 6.7(C)).

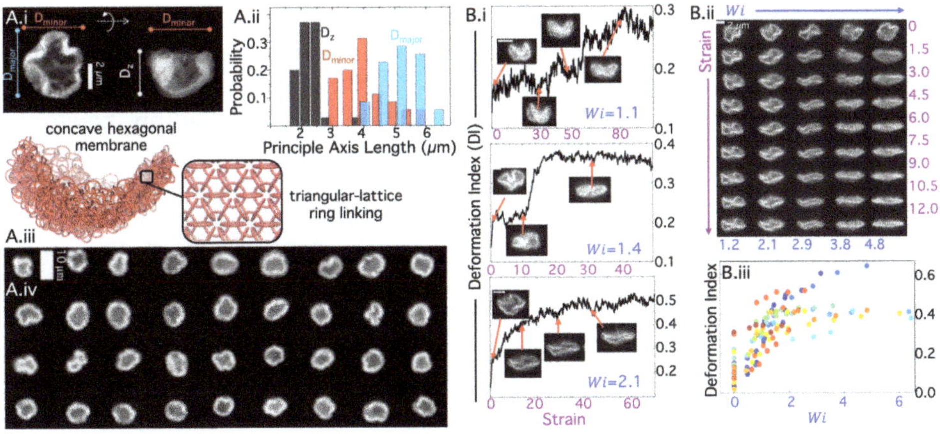

Figure 6.8. Kinetoplasts are two-dimensional membranes of interlinked DNA rings that display distinct fluctuations and deformation dynamics. (A) Kinetoplasts adopt (i) hemispherical conformations with (ii) a broad distribution of major and minor axes lengths (D_{major}, D_{minor}) and narrower distribution of heights (D_z). (iii) Simulated sheets of linked rings mimic kinetoplast structure when modeled as a hexagonal sheet of rings linked in a triangular-lattice configuration. (iv) Kinetoplasts undergo thermal fluctuations that cause a range of folding, crumpling, stretching, and swelling events. (B) Kinetoplasts undergo (i, ii) a broad range of strain-dependent deformation profiles in response to microfluidic flows of varying Weissenberg numbers Wi, quantified by the Deformation Index (DI). (i) Unlike linear DNA, kinetoplasts can exhibit periods of stalled deformation (constant DI) as well as sporadic jumps in DI as the cumulative strain (purple) increases, as seen for $Wi = 1.1$ (top) and 1.4 (middle). (ii) The degree of deformation from zero-strain conformations increases with increasing strain (top to bottom) and Wi (left to right). (iii) Steady-state DI reached at maximum strain universally increases with increasing Wi for an ensemble of 21 kinetoplasts (different colors), with no apparent coil-stretch transition. (A.i, ii, iv) Adapted from Klotz *et al* (2020) with permission of PNAS. (A.iii) Adapted from Polson *et al* (2021) with permission from the Royal Society of Chemistry. (B) Adapted with permission from Soh and Doyle (2020). Copyright (2020) American Chemical Society.

Naturally occurring kinetoplasts are another example of a concatenated ring DNA network, comprising $\sim 10^3$ very small DNA rings (minicircles, $\sim$200 nm) and $\sim 10^1$ larger rings, that adopt a 2D membrane-like geometry (Shapiro and Englund 1995, Lukeš *et al* 2002, Klotz *et al* 2020, Polson *et al* 2021, He *et al* 2023). *In vitro* fluorescence microscopy experiments have shown that kinetoplasts appear as wrinkled hemispherical sheets with a wide range of contour shapes and small-scale conformational fluctuations (figure 6.8(A)) (Klotz *et al* 2020). Simulations that model kinetoplasts as two-dimensional membranes of linked rigid rings suggest that the concavity of the kinetoplasts arises from local excluded volume interactions, which cause the membranes to swell (Polson *et al* 2021), in line with the experimental observation that kinetoplasts are swollen in good solvent conditions (Klotz *et al* 2020). These simulations further showed that concavity increased with the thickness and linking valency of rings, indicating that the most probable lattice configuration of kinetoplasts is that of triangular-lattice linking rather than lower valency square-lattice linking configuration (figure 6.8(A.iii)) (Polson *et al* 2021).

Under microfluidic confinement and deformation, kinetoplasts have been shown to elastically fold, unfold, stretch, and compress (figure 6.8(B.i)) (Klotz *et al* 2020).

Microfluidics studies have also shown that kinetoplasts stretch under extensional flow, reaching a steady-state deformation that scales with the strain rate, similar to linear polymers (figure 6.8(B)) (Soh and Doyle 2020). However, unlike single linear and ring polymers, which exhibit a cooperative coil-stretch transition, kinetoplasts were shown to steadily elongate to reach steady-state (figure 6.8(B.iii)). Moreover, when subject to nonlinear extensional flows, kinetoplasts exhibit unique stage-wise and transient elongation due to structural rearrangement (Klotz *et al* 2020).

Building on these experiments, simulation studies have examined the dynamics and conformations of ring concatenanes (Tubiana *et al* 2022) and dynamically reconnecting DNA rings (Bonato *et al* 2022). In the former study, the ends of linear chains of concatenated ring polymers were connected to form circular chains without ends, demonstrating that twist and writhe could be stored in the circular concatenanes and could be tuned by the size and stiffness of the polymer rings (Tubiana *et al* 2022). In the latter study (Bonato *et al* 2022), recombinase-like topological processes were performed on solutions of polymers that mimicked circular DNA, to show that dilute solutions of flexible rings formed isolated, unconcatenated rings while at higher concentrations and for stiffer rings, gel-like networks of large concatenanes formed. The network phase included rings with a wide range of sizes and knotting probabilities, unlike the Olympic ring gels formed via Topoisomerase II (figure 6.7), which was suggested to arise from the inherently different actions of the simulated recombinases, which randomly cut and recombine fragments of different DNA molecules, in contrast to topoisomerases which cut, untwist, and reseal single DNA strands.

6.4 Branched biopolymers

Many biopolymers, such as mucins, are best described as branched, comb, or bottlebrush polymers (Klein 1986, Beum and Cheng 2001, Suneel *et al* 2002, Rogers *et al* 2014, Hughes *et al* 2019, Fass and Thornton 2023). DNA also forms transiently branched structures during replication and recombination, and can be engineered to have stable branched junctions to form various complex architectures such as bottlebrushes, H-shapes, and multi-arm stars (Saha *et al* 2006, Adams *et al* 2013, Biffi *et al* 2013, Mai and Schroeder 2016, Dong *et al* 2020, Lee *et al* 2021, Conrad *et al* 2022, Naskar *et al* 2023). The properties of branched DNA constructs are also relevant to ring, supercoiled, and histone-bound genomic DNA (Boles *et al* 1990, Bednar *et al* 1994, Huang *et al* 2001, Fox *et al* 2014, Basbous and Constantinou 2019, Ghobadpour *et al* 2021, Smrek *et al* 2021), as well as DNA origami (Pound *et al* 2009, Shih and Lin 2010, Li *et al* 2021).

At concentrations above c^*, branched polymers are expected to exhibit a range of distinct relaxation timescales associated with interactions and entanglements between neighboring branches, trunks, and segments between branch points. These different mechanisms necessitate modifications to the reptation model to account for the distinct dynamics at different lengthscales. There is a large body of literature devoted to theoretical modeling of branched polymers (Graessley 1982, Klein 1986, Bick and McLeish 1996, McLeish and Larson 1998, Kunamaneni *et al*

2006, Read *et al* 2011, Bačová *et al* 2013, Rosa and Everaers 2016, Korolkovas 2018); and rheological measurements of entangled synthetic branched polymers (McLeish and Milner 1999, Suneel *et al* 2002, Shanbhag *et al* 2006, van Ruymbeke *et al* 2007, Hu *et al* 2011, Snijkers *et al* 2015). Here, we limit our discussion to networks of branched DNA, DNA nanostars, and mucins; and the most pertinent theories used to understand the observed properties of these systems.

6.4.1 Branched DNA

For a linear DNA chain, the only lengthscale that affects its dynamics is its contour length L, which relaxes with a single relaxation timescale. However, branched DNA constructs have multiple hardwired lengthscales including, e.g., branch lengths, the central backbone or 'trunk' length, and lengths between branches, all of which are expected to relax over different timescales (McLeish and Larson 1998, Everaers *et al* 2017).

Microfluidic extensional flow experiments have demonstrated this multi-modal relaxation using single comb DNA constructs with backbone or trunk length of $L_T = 30$ kbp and varying numbers of branches of equal length $L_B = 10$ kbp (figure 6.9(A)) (Mai *et al* 2015). Namely, the comb constructs were reported to undergo coil-stretch transitions and relax their stretch via initial fast elastic retraction, then Rouse-like conformational relaxation of both trunk segments and branches, followed, finally, by slow relaxation of the trunk (figure 6.9(A)).

The timescale of this longest relaxation mode, τ_f, associated with relaxation of the trunk, was determined from the exponentially decaying fractional extension x/L_T of the relaxing chains following stretch (figure 6.9(B)), and was reported to be slower than that of a linear chain with the same length (i.e., $L_T = L$). Moreover, τ_f increased with branch density, reporting relaxation times of $\tau_{f,1} \approx 8$ s, $\tau_{f,2} \approx 9.6$ s and $\tau_{f,3} \approx 13$ s for constructs with 1, 2, and 3 branches (figure 6.9(B)). This progressively slowing relaxation was rationalized as arising from the increased friction from more branches, in similar spirit to the lattice-animal models for rings that treat the double-folded loops along the trunk as added friction terms that slow the longest relaxation time (i.e., that of the central trunk or primitive path $L_{0,p}$) (Grosberg 2013, Ge *et al* 2016b, Michieletto 2016, Ghobadpour *et al* 2021).

A series of experiments (Heuer *et al* 2003, Saha *et al* 2004, 2006) also investigated the impact of star-like branching of DNA on its electrophoretic mobility μ, namely, the speed at which DNA moves through solution under the action of a directed electric field. These studies showed that star-like branched DNA (figure 6.9(C)), comprising varying numbers n_B of branches of equal length L_B that extend from a central core, display similar electrophoretic mobility μ_0 and random coil configurations as their linear counterparts (Saha *et al* 2006). This insensitivity to branching, seemingly at odds with the more complex and slower relaxation of branched constructs described above (figures 6.9(A) and (B)), may arise from the different lengths of the central trunk L_T and branches L_B in Mai *et al* (2015), in contrast to the star-like branched constructs that have a single defining lengthscale L_B.

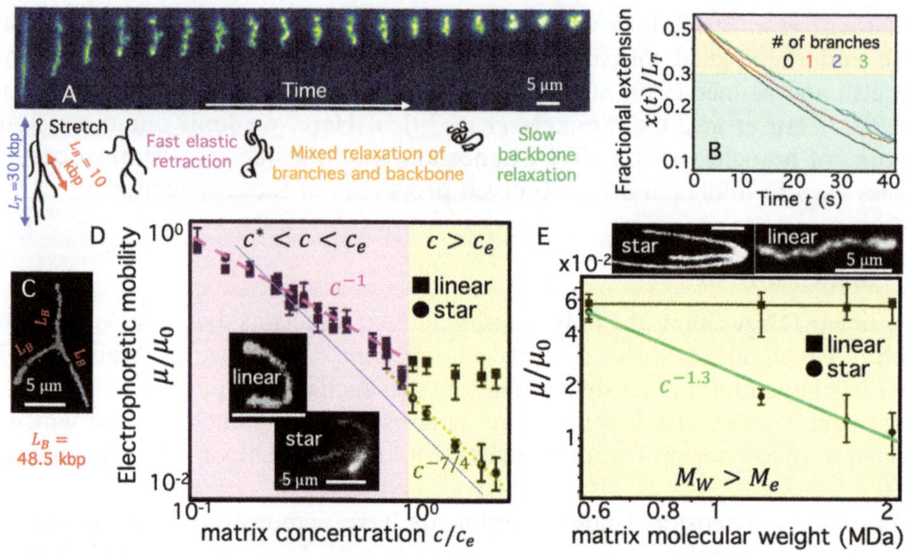

Figure 6.9. Branched DNA exhibits unique relaxation dynamics and electrophoretic mobility. (A and B) Single-molecule microfluidic stretching experiments (A) visualize the relaxation dynamics of single bottlebrush DNA molecules with trunk length $L_T = 30$ kbp and varying numbers of branches n_B of length $L_B = 10$ kbp, and (B) quantify the time-dependent fractional extension of the trunk $x(t)/L_T$ as each entropically stretched molecule relaxes back to its equilibrium random coil configuration. Data shown in (B) are for DNA with $n_B = 0$ (black, linear), 1 (red), 2 (blue), and 3 (green), and the magenta, orange, and green shaded regions show the (x, t) regions of the relaxation profile that are dominated by the color-matched modes depicted in (A), i.e., fast retraction, mixed branch/trunk relaxation, and slow trunk relaxation. (C–E) The electrophoretic behavior of star-like branched DNA with $n_B = 3$ and $L_B = 48.5$ kbp, engineered by annealing λ-DNA to each of the three branch points of a central oligo core (C), was measured for DNA moving through semidilute (pink, $c^* < c < c_e$) and entangled (yellow, $c > c_e$) solutions of linear polyacrylamide (LPA) of varying concentrations c/c_e (D) and molecular weights (E). (D and E) The electrophoretic mobility μ scaled by the dilute-limit value μ_0, for branched DNA (circles) and linear DNA (squares) of comparable total length $L \approx n_B L_B \approx 162$ kbp, with insets depicting sample configurations of linear and branched DNA subject to an electric field. For $c < c_e$ (D, pink), μ is insensitive to branching and follows approximate scaling $\mu \sim c^{-1}$ (dashed line) for both linear and branched DNA. For $c > c_e$, this concentration dependence becomes steeper for branched DNA, with approximate scaling $\mu \sim c^{-7/4}$ (dotted line), whereas μ is essentially independent of LPA concentration for linear DNA. (E) Similar trends are observed for the dependence of μ on matrix LPA molecular weight, with $\mu \sim M_W^0$ for linear chains and $\mu \sim M_W^{-1.3}$ for branched constructs. (A) Adapted with permission from Mai *et al* (2015). Copyright (2015) American Chemical Society. (B) Saha *et al* (2006). John Wiley & Sons. Copyright © 2006 WILEY-VCH Verlag GmbH & Co. KGaA, Weinheim.

However, important differences between linear and star-like DNA arise when embedded in overlapping ($c^* < c < c_e$) and entangled ($c > c_e$) polymer solutions. Specifically, in unentangled overlapping solutions ($c^* < c < c_e$), DNA stars were shown to adopt squid-like conformations, with the central core leading the electrophoretic motion, while the branches extended back in the direction of the electric field (figures 6.9(C) and (D)). Conversely, linear chains were uniformly stretched in the direction of the electric field, forming u-shaped and fully-extended conformations (figures 6.9(C) and (D)). Despite these conformational differences, the reduced electrophoretic mobility μ/μ_0 of linear and 3-branch chains (figure 6.9(C)) with similar lengths of $L = 162$ kbp and $L = 3 \times L_B = 145.5$ kbp were indistinguishable from one another. Moreover, both stars and linear chains exhibited similar scaling of μ/μ_0 with the molecular weight and concentration of the matrix linear polymers.

In entangled solutions ($c > c_e$), the topology-dependent differences in conformations were shown to be starker, with linear chains always assuming fully-extended conformations while the branches were stretched more strongly away from their leading core (figure 6.9(D)). Moreover, while the electrophoretic mobility of the linear chains was shown to be insensitive to matrix polymer length, μ/μ_0 for the DNA stars decreased strongly with increasing matrix chain length (figure 6.9(E)).

6.4.2 Self-associating DNA nanostars

DNA nanostars are a simplified version of DNA origami that are formed by the self-assembly of complementary DNA oligos to form a structure with arms that extend from a central core (figures 6.10(A) and (B)), similar in motif but much smaller than the DNA stars in figures 6.9(C)–(E) (Biffi *et al* 2013, Nguyen and Saleh 2017, Naskar *et al* 2023). By including single-strand complementary overhangs at the ends of the arms, networks of crosslinked nanostars can self-assemble into diverse structures from lattice-like percolated hydrogels to liquid-like coacervates (figures 6.10(A) and (B)) (Nguyen and Saleh 2017, Jeon *et al* 2018, Conrad *et al* 2022). Varying the length and number of arms, as well as the hybridization strength, stiffness, and lifetime of the overhangs, can tune the network architecture and aging kinetics.

For example, nanostars engineered to have four arms with flexible overhangs at their ends form liquid-like droplets, i.e., coacervates, (figure 6.10(A)) that become more spherical and coalesce over time (Jeon *et al* 2018). Conversely, when the nanostar arms are engineered to have stiff overhangs, they form fully-percolated networks (figure 6.10(B)) that contract over time (figure 6.10(C)) (Nguyen and Saleh 2017). These aging kinetics are understood to arise from the overhangs dynamically linking and unlinking to allow the network of nanostars to reconfigure into free-energy minimized states.

Studies have also shown that temperature and ionic conditions can control the structure, aging kinetics, and reversibility of the restructuring (figures 6.10(C) and (D)) (Nguyen and Saleh 2017, Naskar *et al* 2023). For example, crosslinked nanostar gels have been shown to contract and coarsen upon lowering the concentration of NaCl from 50 mM to 15 mM. Suprisingly, this contraction continues even when [NaCl] is increased back to 50 mM; and then accelerates upon subsequent lowering back to 15 mM (figure 6.10(D)). Conversely, networks formed in the presence of 10 mM $MgCl_2$ expand upon lowering [$MgCl_2$] to 1 mM and re-expand upon subsequent increase back to 10 mM (figure 6.10(D)). This process is fully reversible over several cycles of [$MgCl_2$] modulation, in stark opposition to the unidirectional contraction and rupturing mediated by monovalent salt.

Many studies have built on these seminal works on DNA nanostar networks, some of which include Spinozzi *et al* (2020), Lee *et al* (2021), Conrad *et al* (2022), Lattuada *et al* (2022), Naskar *et al* (2023) and references there within. For example, investigations of

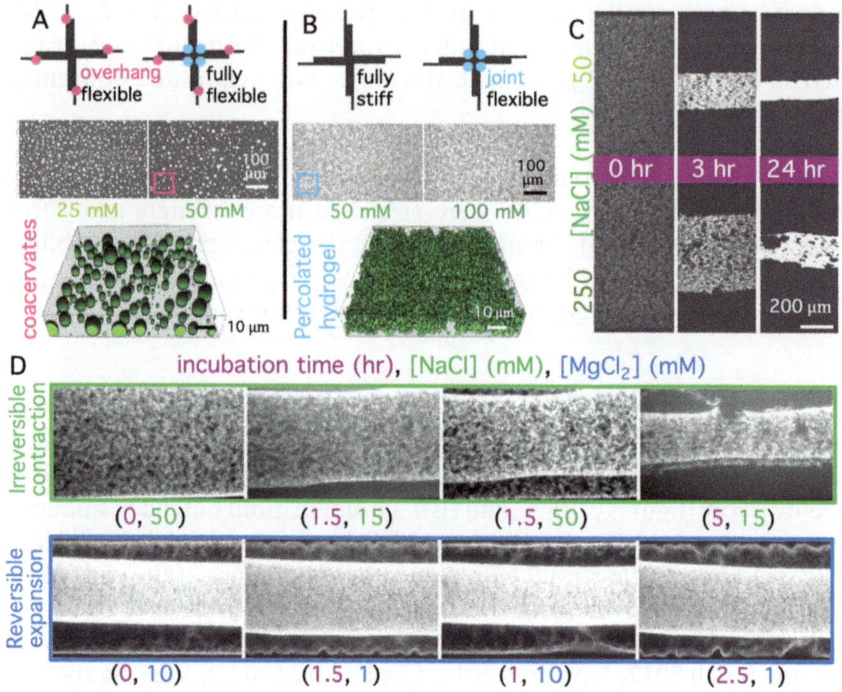

Figure 6.10. DNA nanostars crosslink to form networks that are tuned by the nanostar flexibility and ionic conditions. (A and B) (Top) DNA nanostars with four 20-bp arms, each with 6-nucleotide overhangs, are engineered by annealing four 46-nucleotide complementary single-stranded oligomers that can be made to have flexible overhangs (magenta) and/or joints (cyan) by incorporating 1 and/or 2 unmatched nucleotides into the oligos. Epiflourescence images (middle) and confocal *z*-stacks (bottom) of fluorescent-labeled nanostars in the presence of varying NaCl concentrations (green labels) show that nanostars with overhangs that are (A) flexible or (B) stiff form (A) coacervates or (B) percolated networks with properties that can be tuned by salt. The *z*-stack renderings correspond to color-coded boxed regions of the fully-flexible and fully-stiff cases. (C) Nanostar networks contract and coarsen over time, a process that is hindered at higher [NaCl]. Images show bulk nanostar networks at varying times (purple) after the addition of 50 mM (top) or 250 mM (bottom) NaCl. (D) Images of aging hydrogels with varying concentrations of monovalent NaCl (top, green) or divalent $MgCl_2$ (bottom, blue) at different points in time (purple). Images show that nanostar hydrogels undergo irreversible contraction upon cyclic decreasing and increasing of [NaCl] between 50 and 15 mM, while they reversibly expand and contract upon cyclic lowering and raising of [$MgCl_2$] between 10 and 1 mM. Adapted from Nguyen and Saleh (2017) with permission from the Royal Society of Chemistry.

nanostar coacervates have demonstrated that nanostar diffusion within the droplets is anomalous and activated by stochastic breakage of overhang bonds, a process that is hindered at the surface (Jeon *et al* 2018, Conrad *et al* 2022). The reported low surface tension, salt-mediated compaction, and anomalous transport properties suggest that the nanostar network inside the coacervate has a heterogeneous and clustered architecture due, primarily, to the nanostar flexibility (Jeon *et al* 2018).

Chapter 9 discusses coacervates and liquid–liquid phase separation of biopolymers in more detail; and chapter 8 describes in more detail the non-equilibrium aging and activity of nanostar networks.

6.4.3 Mucins

As described in chapter 1, mucins are the family of bottlebrush or comb biopolymers that give mucus its signature viscoelastic and structural properties (Bansil *et al* 1995, Celli *et al* 2005, Bansil and Turner 2006, 2018, Lai *et al* 2009, Fass and Thornton 2023). Different mucins, typically classified by their physiological function, can exhibit distinct conformations and network morphologies (Bansil *et al* 1995, Bansil and Turner 2018). For example, two distinct lung mucins, MUC5AC and MUC5B, form, respectively, isotropic crosslinked meshes with high viscoelasticity and networks of unconnected nematic bundles with low viscoelasticity (Fass and Thornton 2023). However, the majority of mucins are expected to adopt swollen random coil conformations akin to flexible polymers, and form entangled networks at high concentrations (Celli *et al* 2005, Georgiades *et al* 2014). Mucin networks also exhibit varying degrees of transient and static crosslinking and bundling via counterion crossbridges and accessory proteins; properties that are highly dependent on pH and ionic conditions (Bansil *et al* 1995, Bansil and Turner 2006, Wagner *et al* 2017, Hughes *et al* 2019).

Particle-tracking studies on networks of porcine gastrointestinal mucins, MUC5AC and MUC2 (figures 6.11(A) and (B)) (Georgiades *et al* 2014), have shown that both mucins exhibit semidilute, unentangled dynamics with viscosity scaling $\eta \sim c^{0.53}$ at neutral pH for concentrations $c^* < c < c_e$ where c_e was measured to be $\sim 20c^*$ and $\sim 30c^*$ for MUC5AC (figure 6.11(A)) and MUC2 (figure 6.11(B)), respectively. For higher concentrations $c > c_e$, the viscosities of both networks followed much steeper scalings of $\eta \sim c^{3.93}$ and $\eta \sim c^{5.1}$ for MUC5AC (figure 6.11(A)) and MUC2 (figure 6.11(B)), respectively. The MSDs for both networks, from which the viscosities were computed, generally decreased with increasing mucin concentration; and exhibited normal diffusion ($MSD \sim \Delta t^1$) at concentrations below c_e and subdiffusion with $\alpha \simeq 0.75$ above c_e (figures 6.11(A) and (B) insets).

Complementary bulk rheology measurements (Wagner *et al* 2017) showed that MUC5AC networks display largely elastic-dominated linear response, with $G' > G''$ for all pH and salt concentrations, with the viscoelastic moduli and relative elasticity of MUC5AC networks increasing upon decreasing pH (figure 6.11(C)) and increasing [NaCl] (figure 6.11(D)). This phenomenon was rationalized as resulting from, respectively, unfolding of crossbridged mucin chains and more crosslinkers with longer lifetimes (Wagner *et al* 2017).

Conversely, SPT microrheology measurements on the same samples (figures 6.11(C) and (D), solid and dashed lines) displayed largely viscous-dominated dynamics, i.e., $G'' > G'$, and generally lower values of both G' and G''. Moreover, while a similar dependence on [NaCl] was observed in both SPT and bulk rheology (figure 6.11(D)), the pH dependence measured using the two techniques were in opposition, with SPT-measured viscoelastic moduli decreasing upon decreasing pH from 4 to 2 (Wagner *et al* 2017) (figure 6.11(C)).

SPT measurements further showed that lowering the pH to 2 led to faster and less subdiffusive transport as compared to pH = 4 and pH = 7, as seen by the

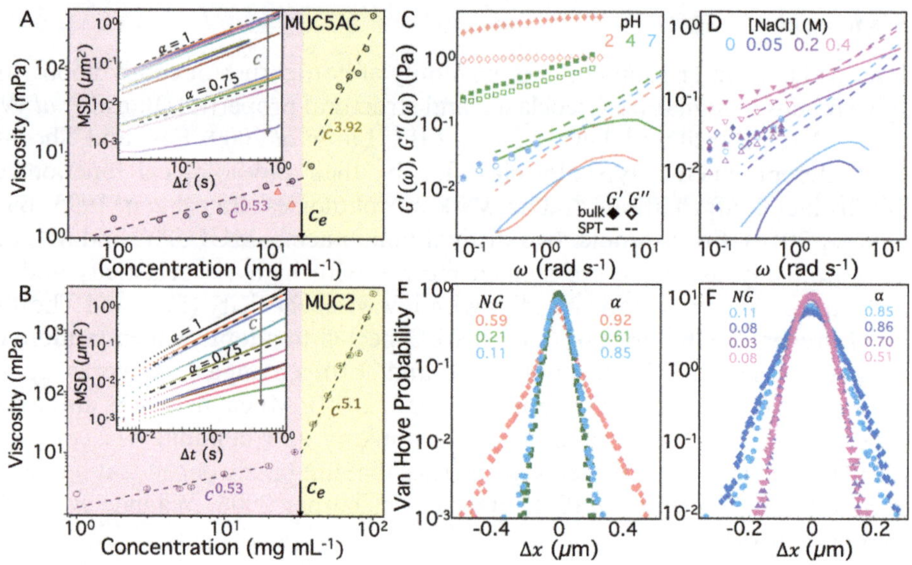

Figure 6.11. Particle-tracking microrheology and bulk rheology of *in vitro* networks of different types and concentration of mucins at varying pH and salt concentrations. (A and B) Viscosity of *in vitro* networks of porcine gastrointestinal MUC5AC (A) and MUC2 (B) as a function of mucin concentration, computed from the MSDs (insets) of embedded particles using single-particle tracking microrheology. The viscosities of both MUC5A and MUC2 increase with concentration according to power-law scaling $\eta \sim c^{0.53}$ (pink regions) for concentrations below the entanglement concentration c_e (vertical arrow), and much steeper scalings of $\eta \sim c^{3.92}$ (A) and $\eta \sim c^{5.1}$ for $c > c_e$ (yellow regions). (Insets) MSDs generally decrease with increasing concentration (vertical arrow) and transition from diffusive ($\alpha \simeq 1$) to subdiffusive ($\alpha \to 0.75$) (dashed lines). (C and D) Bulk rheology (symbols) and SPT microrheology (lines) measurements of $G'(\omega)$ and $G''(\omega)$ for MUC5AC networks in solutions with (C) pH = 2 (pink), 4 (green), and 7 (blue) with no added salt; and (D) [NaCl] = 0 M (light blue), 0.05 M (blue), 0.2 M (purple), and 0.4 M (magenta) at pH = 7. (E and F) Van Hove probability distributions of particle displacements Δx for the same networks shown in C and D at a lagtime of $\Delta t = 0.1$ *s*. The non-Gaussianity parameter *NG* and anomalous diffusion exponent α associated with particle transport in each network condition is listed in the corresponding color. Larger *NG* values indicate increased transport heterogeneity, and lower α values indicate more caging. (A, B) Adapted from Georgiades *et al* (2014). CC BY 3.0. (C–F) Adapted with permission from Wagner *et al* (2017). Copyright (2017) American Chemical Society.

broader van Hove distribution and higher anomalous exponent of $\alpha(2) \simeq 0.92$ compared to $\alpha(7) \simeq 0.85$ and $\alpha(4) \simeq 0.61$ (figure 6.11(E)). Particle transport at pH = 2 was also faster and less subdiffusive than that measured for all salt concentrations at neutral pH (figure 6.11(F)). This enhanced mobility is at odds with the increased bulk elasticity of the network seen in figure 6.11(C).

Moreover, van Hove displacement distributions revealed that particle transport at pH = 2 was markedly more heterogeneous compared to the other conditions, as seen by the larger non-Gaussianity parameter of $NG(2) \simeq 0.59$ compared to $NG(4) \simeq 0.21$ and $NG(7) \simeq 0.11$, and strongly exponential van Hove distribution (figure 6.11(D)). These results are indicative of a combination of caging, hopping, and free diffusion, suggesting that lowering the pH promotes bundling and stiffening of the mucin fibers. This bundling serves to increase bulk elasticity but also increase the structural mesh size and heterogeneity, leading particles to undergo a combination of free diffusion in large voids and caged transport in smaller pores of rigid bundles (Sokolov 2012, Wagner *et al* 2017, Anderson *et al* 2019). Conversely, increasing salt concentration increases the crosslinking density, which likewise increases the elasticity. However, salt-mediated crosslinking is suggested to be isotropic such that networks remain stable and percolated with minimal bundling and smaller mesh sizes, leading to more close matching of bulk and microscopic measurements.

Optical tweezers microrheology experiments on marine worm mucus reported similar hierarchical and heterogeneous mechanical properties (Weigand *et al* 2017). Specifically, as the radius of the microsphere probe was increased from $R_s = 1\ \mu$m to $R_s = 5\ \mu$m, the viscoelastic properties transitioned from Newtonian, to viscoelastic, to largely elastic and comparable to bulk rheological properties. These results, along with analysis of the heterogeneity of the force response, demonstrate that the mucus adopts structures akin to semidilute, unentangled networks at the microscopic scale, entangled meshworks at the mesoscopic scale, and networks of large bundles with similarly large mesh sizes at the macroscale (Weigand *et al* 2017).

6.5 Building in complexity

This chapter has provided a broad overview of our current understanding of topologically-complex biopolymers. I have focused on the most widely studied and physiologically relevant topologies: relaxed ring, supercoiled circular, and branched. There are numerous other complex topologies that biopolymers can adopt, either naturally or engineered, including the complex folded structures that most soluble proteins adopt. Protein folding constitutes an entire class of research that I will not cover here (Dill and MacCallum 2012, Flapan *et al* 2019, Wetlaufer 2019, Mirdita *et al* 2022, Tsuboyama *et al* 2023), because the resulting structures are often so compact that the polymers can be modeled as colloidal particles and the complex structure can be neglected at the scale of the network.

Other topologies and structural motifs that have been extensively investigated are hairpins and loops in RNA and ssDNA (see chapter 1) (Matthews 1992, Barr and Fearns 2010, Bikard *et al* 2010, Russell 2012, Adams *et al* 2013, Danaee *et al* 2018, Petermann *et al* 2022). Other branching geometries of DNA, including T-shaped and H-shaped constructs (Bednar *et al* 1994, Rogers *et al* 2014, Mai and Schroeder 2016, Dong *et al* 2020), as well as nanostars with varying numbers and lengths of arms (Biffi *et al* 2013, Conrad *et al* 2022, Lattuada *et al* 2022, Naskar *et al* 2023), have also been engineered and studied. Finally, theoretical investigations of tadpole constructs, in which a linear chain end is attached to a ring (Rosa *et al* 2020), and daisy chains of rings (O'Connor *et al* 2020), in which adjacent rings become knotted with one another, have been performed to shed light on the highly debated dynamics of overlapping ring polymers and blends of linear and ring chains. These different topologies will not be covered further here, but I urge the interested reader to think about how to advance our limited understanding of networks of these complex topologies.

Armed with the foundation we have established in the preceding chapters, we are now ready to turn to composite networks comprising biopolymers of varying sizes, topologies, and stiffnesses (chapter 7); non-equilibrium networks that undergo active dynamics, restructuring, or aging over time (chapter 8); and conditions in which biopolymer networks undergo liquid–liquid phase separation (chapter 9).

References

Adams R L P, Knowler J T and Leader D P 2013 *The Biochemistry of the Nucleic Acids* (Springer Science & Business Media)

Alberts B 2004 *Molecular Biology of the Cell* (Garland)

Anderson S J, Matsuda C, Garamella J, Peddireddy K R, Robertson-Anderson R M and McGorty R 2019 Filament rigidity vies with mesh size in determining anomalous diffusion in cytoskeleton *Biomacromolecules* **20** 4380–8

Bačová P, Hawke L G D, Read D J and Moreno A J 2013 Dynamics of branched polymers: a combined study by molecular dynamics simulations and tube theory *Macromolecules* **46** 4633–50

Bansil R, Stanley E and Lamont J T 1995 Mucin biophysics *Annu. Rev. Physiol.* **57** 635–57

Bansil R and Turner B S 2018 The biology of mucus: composition, synthesis and organization *Adv. Drug Deliv. Rev.* **124** 3–15

Bansil R and Turner B S 2006 Mucin structure, aggregation, physiological functions and biomedical applications *Curr. Opin. Colloid Interface Sci.* **11** 164–70

Barr J N and Fearns R 2010 How RNA viruses maintain their genome integrity *J. Gen. Virol.* **91** 1373–87

Basbous J and Constantinou A 2019 A tumor suppressive DNA translocase named FANCM *Crit. Rev. Biochem. Mol. Biol.* **54** 27–40

Bax B D, Murshudov G, Maxwell A and Germe T 2019 DNA topoisomerase inhibitors: trapping a DNA-cleaving machine in motion *J. Mol. Biol.* **431** 3427–49

Bednar J, Furrer P, Stasiak A, Dubochet J, Egelman E H and Bates A D 1994 The twist, writhe and overall shape of supercoiled DNA change during counterion-induced transition from a loosely to a tightly interwound superhelix: possible implications for DNA structure *in vivo* *J. Mol. Biol.* **235** 825–47

Bensafi A, Maschke U and Benmouna M 2000 Cyclic polymers in good solvents *Polym. Int.* **49** 175–83

Beum P V and Cheng P-W 2001 Biosynthesis and function of ß 1,6 branched mucin-type glycans ed A M Wu *The Molecular Immunology of Complex Carbohydrates—2, Advances in Experimental Medicine and Biology* (Boston, MA: Springer US) pp 279–312

Bick D K and McLeish T C B 1996 Topological contributions to nonlinear elasticity in branched polymers *Phys. Rev. Lett.* **76** 2587–90

Bielawski C W, Benitez D and Grubbs R H 2002 An 'endless' route to cyclic polymers *Science* **297** 2041–4

Biffi S, Cerbino R, Bomboi F, Paraboschi E M, Asselta R, Sciortino F and Bellini T 2013 Phase behavior and critical activated dynamics of limited-valence DNA nanostars *Proc. Natl. Acad. Sci.* **110** 15633–7

Bikard D, Loot C, Baharoglu Z and Mazel D 2010 Folded DNA in action: hairpin formation and biological functions in prokaryotes *Microbiol. Mol. Biol. Rev.* **74** 570–88

Bloomfield V and Zimm B H 1966 Viscosity, sedimentation, *et cetera*, of ring- and straight-chain polymers in dilute solution *J. Chem. Phys.* **44** 315–23

Boles T C, White J H and Cozzarelli N R 1990 Structure of plectonemically supercoiled DNA *J. Mol. Biol.* **213** 931–51

Bonato A, Marenduzzo D, Michieletto D and Orlandini E 2022 Topological gelation of reconnecting polymers *Proc. Natl. Acad. Sci.* **119** e2207728119

Bouchaud J-P and Georges A 1990 Anomalous diffusion in disordered media: statistical mechanisms, models and physical applications *Phys. Rep.* **195** 127–293

Brown S and Szamel G 1998 Structure and dynamics of ring polymers *J. Chem. Phys.* **108** 4705–8

Burchard W and Schmidt M 1980 Static and dynamic structure factors calculated for flexible ring macromolecules *Polymer* **21** 745–9

Cates M E and Deutsch J M 1986 Conjectures on the statistics of ring polymers *J. Phys. France* **47** 2121–8

Celli J, Gregor B, Turner B, Afdhal N H, Bansil R and Erramilli S 2005 Viscoelastic properties and dynamics of porcine gastric mucin *Biomacromolecules* **6** 1329–33

Chapman C D, Shanbhag S, Smith D E and Robertson-Anderson R M 2012 Complex effects of molecular topology on diffusion in entangled biopolymer blends *Soft Matter* **8** 9177–82

Chaudhuri P, Berthier L and Kob W 2007 Universal nature of particle displacements close to glass and jamming transitions *Phys. Rev. Lett.* **99** 060604

Chen D, Molnar K, Kim H, Helfer C A, Kaszas G, Puskas J E, Kornfield J A and McKenna G B 2023 Linear viscoelastic properties of putative cyclic polymers synthesized by reversible radical recombination polymerization (R3P) *Macromolecules* **56** 1013–32

Conrad N, Chang G, Fygenson D K and Saleh O A 2022 Emulsion imaging of a DNA nanostar condensate phase diagram reveals valence and electrostatic effects *J. Chem. Phys.* **157** 234203

Danaee P, Rouches M, Wiley M, Deng D, Huang L and Hendrix D 2018 bpRNA: large-scale automated annotation and analysis of RNA secondary structure *Nucleic Acids Res.* **46** 5381–94

des Cloizeaux J 1988 Double reptation vs. simple reptation in polymer melts *Europhys. Lett.* **5** 437

Dill K A and MacCallum J L 2012 The protein-folding problem, 50 years on *Science* **338** 1042–6

Doi M and Edwards S F 1988 *The Theory of Polymer Dynamics* (Oxford: Clarendon)

Doi M, Graessley W W, Helfand E and Pearson D S 1987 Dynamics of polymers in polydisperse melts *Macromolecules* **20** 1900–6

Dong Y, Yao C, Zhu Y, Yang L, Luo D and Yang D 2020 DNA functional materials assembled from branched DNA: design, synthesis, and applications *Chem. Rev.* **120** 9420–81

Endo K 2008 Synthesis and properties of cyclic polymers Synthesis and Properties of Cyclic Polymers (Advances in Polymer Science vol 217) (Springer) pp (book ref) 121–83

Everaers R, Grosberg A Y, Rubinstein M and Rosa A 2017 Flory theory of randomly branched polymers *Soft Matter* **13** 1223–34

Fass D and Thornton D J 2023 Mucin networks: dynamic structural assemblies controlling mucus function *Curr. Opin. Struct. Biol.* **79** 102524

Flapan E, He A and Wong H 2019 Topological descriptions of protein folding *Proc. Natl. Acad. Sci.* **116** 9360–9

Flory P J 1949 Statistical mechanics of dilute polymer solutions *J. Chem. Phys.* **17** 1347–8

Fox D, Yan Z, Ling C, Zhao Y, Lee D-Y, Fukagawa T, Yang W and Wang W 2014 The histone-fold complex MHF is remodeled by FANCM to recognize branched DNA and protect genome stability *Cell Res.* **24** 560–75

Ge T, Panyukov S and Rubinstein M 2016a Self-similar conformations and dynamics in entangled melts and solutions of nonconcatenated ring polymers *Macromolecules* **49** 708–22

Ge T, Panyukov S and Rubinstein M 2016b Self-similar conformations and dynamics in entangled melts and solutions of nonconcatenated ring polymers *Macromolecules* **49** 708–22

Gellert M 1981 DNA topoisomerases *Annu. Rev. Biochem.* **50** 879–910

Georgiades P, Pudney P D A, Thornton D J and Waigh T A 2014 Particle tracking microrheology of purified gastrointestinal mucins *Biopolymers* **101** 366–77

Ghobadpour E, Kolb M, Ejtehadi M R and Everaers R 2021 Monte carlo simulation of a lattice model for the dynamics of randomly branching double-folded ring polymers *Phys. Rev.* E **104** 014501

Graessley W W 1982 Entangled linear, branched and network polymer systems—molecular theories *Adv. Polym. Sci.* **47** 67–117

Grosberg A Y 2013 Annealed lattice animal model and flory theory for the melt of non-concatenated rings: towards the physics of crumpling *Soft Matter* **10** 560–5

Haley J C and Lodge T R 2005 Viscosity predictions for model miscible polymer blencils: including self-concentration, double reptation, and tube dilation *J. Rheol.* **49** 1277–302

Halverson J D, Grest G S, Grosberg A Y and Kremer K 2012 Rheology of ring polymer melts: from linear contaminants to ring-linear blends *Phys. Rev. Lett.* **108** 038301

Halverson J D, Lee W B, Grest G S, Grosberg A Y and Kremer K 2011 Molecular dynamics simulation study of nonconcatenated ring polymers in a melt. II. Dynamics *J. Chem. Phys.* **134** 204905

Halverson J D, Lee W B, Grest G S, Grosberg A Y and Kremer K 2011 Molecular dynamics simulation study of nonconcatenated ring polymers in a melt. I. Statics *J. Chem. Phys.* **134** 204904

He P, Katan A J, Tubiana L, Dekker C and Michieletto D 2023 Single-molecule structure and topology of kinetoplast DNA networks *Phys. Rev.* X **13** 021010

Heiter D F, Lunnen K D and Wilson G G 2005 Site-specific DNA-nicking mutants of the heterodimeric restriction endonuclease R.BbvCI *J. Mol. Biol.* **348** 631–40

Helfer C A, Xu G Q, Mattice W L and Pugh C 2003 Monte carlo simulations investigating the threading of cyclic poly(ethylene oxide) by linear chains in the melt *Macromolecules* **36** 10071–8

Heuer D M, Saha S and Archer L A 2003 Electrophoretic dynamics of large DNA stars in polymer solutions and gels *Electrophoresis* **24** 3314–22

Hsiao K-W, Schroeder C M and Sing C E 2016 Ring polymer dynamics are governed by a coupling between architecture and hydrodynamic interactions *Macromolecules* **49** 1961–71

Hu M, Xia Y, McKenna G B, Kornfield J A and Grubbs R H 2011 Linear rheological response of a series of densely branched brush polymers *Macromolecules* **44** 6935–43

Huang J, Schlick T and Vologodskii A 2001 Dynamics of site juxtaposition in supercoiled DNA *Proc. Natl. Acad. Sci.* **98** 968–73

Hughes G W, Ridley C, Collins R, Roseman A, Ford R and Thornton D J 2019 The MUC5B mucin polymer is dominated by repeating structural motifs and its topology is regulated by calcium and pH *Sci. Rep.* **9** 17350

Iyer B V S, Lele A K and Juvekar V A 2006 Flexible ring polymers in an obstacle environment: molecular theory of linear viscoelasticity *Phys. Rev.* E **74** 021805

Iyer B V S, Shanbhag S, Juvekar V A and Lele A K 2008 Self-diffusion coefficient of ring polymers in semidilute solution *J. Polym. Sci. Pol. Phys.* **46** 2370–9

Jeon B, Nguyen D T, Abraham G R, Conrad N, Fygenson D K and Saleh O A 2018 Salt-dependent properties of a coacervate-like, self-assembled DNA liquid *Soft Matter* **14** 7009–15

Kapnistos M, Lang M, Vlassopoulos D, Pyckhout-Hintzen W, Richter D, Cho D, Chang T and Rubinstein M 2008 Unexpected power-law stress relaxation of entangled ring polymers *Nat. Mater.* **7** 997–1002

Khanal P, Peddireddy K R, Marfai J, McGorty R and Robertson-Anderson R M 2022 DNA topology dictates emergent bulk elasticity and hindered macromolecular diffusion in DNA-dextran composites *J. Rheol.* **66** 699–715

Kim E, Kim S, Kim D H, Choi B-S, Choi I-Y and Kim J-S 2012 Precision genome engineering with programmable DNA-nicking enzymes *Genome Res.* **22** 1327–33

Klein J 1986 Dynamics of entangled linear, branched, and cyclic polymers *Macromolecules* **19** 105–18

Klotz A R, Soh B W and Doyle P S 2020 Equilibrium structure and deformation response of 2D kinetoplast sheets *PNAS* **117** 121–7

Korolkovas A 2018 5D Entanglement in star polymer dynamics *Adv. Theory Simul.* **1** 1800078

Krajina B A, Zhu A, Heilshorn S C and Spakowitz A J 2018 Active DNA olympic hydrogels driven by topoisomerase activity *Phys. Rev. Lett.* **121** 148001

Kruteva M, Allgaier J and Richter D 2023 Topology matters: conformation and microscopic dynamics of ring polymers *Macromolecules* **56** 7203–29

Kučera O, Siahaan V, Janda D, Dijkstra S H, Pilátová E, Zatecka E, Diez S, Braun M and Lansky Z 2021 Anillin propels myosin-independent constriction of actin rings *Nat. Commun.* **12** 4595

Kunamaneni S, Buzza D M A, Read D J, Parker D, Kenwright A M, Feast W J and Larsen A L 2006 Entanglement transition of randomly branched polymers in the hyperbranched class *Macromolecules* **39** 6720–36

Lai S K, Wang Y-Y, Wirtz D and Hanes J 2009 Micro- and macrorheology of mucus *Adv. Drug Deliv. Rev.* **61** 86–100

Lattuada E, Pietrangeli T and Sciortino F 2022 Interpenetrating gels in binary suspensions of DNA nanostars *J. Chem. Phys.* **157** 135101

Latulippe D R and Zydney A L 2010 Radius of gyration of plasmid DNA isoforms from static light scattering *Biotechnol. Bioeng.* **107** 134–42

Lee T, Do S, Lee J G, Kim D-N and Shin Y 2021 The flexibility-based modulation of DNA nanostar phase separation *Nanoscale* **13** 17638–47

Leonardi F, Majeste J C, Allal A and Marin G 2000 Rheological models based on the double reptation mixing rule: the effects of a polydisperse environment *J. Rheol.* **44** 675–92

Li Y, Hsiao K-W, Brockman C A, Yates D Y, Robertson-Anderson R M, Kornfield J A, Francisco M J S, Schroeder C M and McKenna G B 2015 When ends meet: circular DNA stretches differently in elongational flows *Macromolecules* **48** 5997–6001

Li Y, Pei J, Lu X, Jiao Y, Liu F, Wu X, Liu J and Ding B 2021 Hierarchical assembly of super-DNA origami based on a flexible and covalent-bound branched DNA structure *J. Am. Chem. Soc.* **143** 19893–900

Liu L, Tüzel E and Ross J L 2011 Loop formation of microtubules during gliding at high density *J. Phys. Condens. Matter* **23** 374104

Liu L F and Wang J C 1983 DNA topoisomerases-enzymes that catalyse the breaking and rejoining of DNA *Crit. Rev. Biochem.* **15** 1–24

Lukeš J, Lys Guilbride D, Votýpka J, Zíková A, Benne R and Englund P T 2002 Kinetoplast DNA network: evolution of an improbable structure *Eukaryot. Cell* **1** 495–502

Mai D J, Marciel A B, Sing C E and Schroeder C M 2015 Topology-controlled relaxation dynamics of single branched polymers *ACS Macro Lett.* **4** 446–52

Mai D J and Schroeder C M 2016 Single polymer dynamics of topologically complex DNA *Curr. Opin. Colloid Interface Sci.* **26** 28–40

Marfai J, McGorty R J and Robertson-Anderson R M 2023 Cooperative rheological state-switching of enzymatically-driven composites of circular DNA and dextran *Adv. Mater.* **35** 2305824

Marrucci G 1985 Relaxation by reptation and tube enlargement: a model for polydisperse polymers *J. Polym. Sci.: Polym. Phys. Ed.* **23** 159–77

Matthews K S 1992 DNA looping *Microbiol. Rev.* **56** 123–36

McKenna G B, Hostetter B J, Hadjichristidis N, Fetters L J and Plazek D J 1989 A study of the linear viscoelastic properties of cyclic polystyrenes using creep and recovery measurements *Macromolecules* **22** 1834–52

McLeish T 2008 Polymer dynamics floored by the rings *Nat. Mater.* **7** 933–5

McLeish T C B 2002 Tube theory of entangled polymer dynamics *Adv. Phys.* **51** 1379–527

McLeish T C B and Larson R G 1998 Molecular constitutive equations for a class of branched polymers: the pom-pom polymer *J. Rheol.* **42** 81–110

McLeish T C B and Milner S T 1999 Entangled dynamics and melt flow of branched polymers ed J Roovers *Branched Polymers II, Advances in Polymer Science* (Berlin, Heidelberg: Springer) pp 195–256

Michieletto D 2016 On the tree-like structure of rings in dense solutions *Soft Matter* **12** 9485–500

Michieletto D, Marenduzzo D, Orlandini E, Alexander G P and Turner M S 2014 Threading dynamics of ring polymers in a gel *ACS Macro Lett.* **3** 255–9

Michieletto D, Marenduzzo D, Orlandini E and Turner M S 2017a Ring polymers: threadings, knot electrophoresis and topological glasses *Polymers* **9** 349

Michieletto D, Nahali N and Rosa A 2017b Glassiness and heterogeneous dynamics in dense solutions of ring polymers *Phys. Rev. Lett.* **119** 197801

Michieletto D and Sakaue T 2021 Dynamical entanglement and cooperative dynamics in entangled solutions of ring and linear polymers *ACS Macro Lett.* **10** 129–34

Milner S T and Newhall J D 2010 Stress relaxation in entangled melts of unlinked ring polymers *Phys. Rev. Lett.* **105** 208302

Mirdita M, Schütze K, Moriwaki Y, Heo L, Ovchinnikov S and Steinegger M 2022 ColabFold: making protein folding accessible to all *Nat. Methods* **19** 679–82

Mirny L A 2011 The fractal globule as a model of chromatin architecture in the cell *Chromosome Res.* **19** 37–51

Muller M, Wittmer J P and Cates M E 2000 Topological effects in ring polymers. II. Influence of persistence length *Phys. Rev.* E **61** 4078–89

Muller M, Wittmer J P and Cates M E 1996 Topological effects in ring polymers: a computer simulation study *Phys. Rev. E Stat. Phys. Plasmas Fluids Relat. Interdiscip. Topics* **53** 5063–74

Naskar S, Bhatia D, Lin S-T and Maiti P K 2023 Mechanistic insight into the structure, thermodynamics and dynamics of equilibrium gels of multi-armed DNA nanostars *Phys. Chem. Chem. Phys.* **25** 7847–58

Nechaev S K, Semenov A N and Koleva M K 1987 Dynamics of a polymer chain in an array of obstacles *Phys.* A **140** 506–20

Nguyen D T and Saleh O A 2017 Tuning phase and aging of DNA hydrogels through molecular design *Soft Matter* **13** 5421–7

Obukhov S P, Rubinstein M and Duke T 1994 Dynamics of a ring polymer in a gel *Phys. Rev. Lett.* **73** 1263–6

O'Connor T C, Ge T, Rubinstein M and Grest G S 2020 Topological linking drives anomalous thickening of ring polymers in weak extensional flows *Phys. Rev. Lett.* **124** 027801

Parisi D *et al* 2021 Nonlinear shear rheology of entangled polymer rings *Macromolecules* **54** 2811–27

Patteson A E, Vahabikashi A, Goldman R D and Janmey P A 2020 Mechanical and non-mechanical functions of filamentous and non-filamentous vimentin *BioEssays* **42** 2000078

Peddireddy K R, Lee M, Schroeder C M and Robertson-Anderson R M 2020a Viscoelastic properties of ring-linear DNA blends exhibit nonmonotonic dependence on blend composition *Phys. Rev. Res.* **2** 023213

Peddireddy K R, Lee M, Zhou Y, Adalbert S, Anderson S, Schroeder C M and Robertson-Anderson R M 2020b Unexpected entanglement dynamics in semidilute blends of supercoiled and ring DNA *Soft Matter* **16** 152–61

Petermann E, Lan L and Zou L 2022 Sources, resolution and physiological relevance of R-loops and RNA–DNA hybrids *Nat. Rev. Mol. Cell Biol.* **23** 521–40

Polson J M, Garcia E J and Klotz A R 2021 Flatness and intrinsic curvature of linked-ring membranes *Soft Matter* **17** 10505–15

Pound E, Ashton J R, Becerril H A and Woolley A T 2009 Polymerase chain reaction based scaffold preparation for the production of thin, branched DNA origami nanostructures of arbitrary sizes *Nano Lett.* **9** 4302–5

Prentis J J 1984 Crossover between random and self-avoiding behaviour in a ring polymer *J. Phys. A: Math. Gen.* **17** 1723

Brás R, Gooßen A, Krutyeva S, Radulescu M, Farago A, Allgaier B, Pyckhout-Hintzen J, Wischnewski W, Richter A and D 2014 Compact structure and non-gaussian dynamics of ring polymer melts *Soft Matter* **10** 3649–55

Read D J, Auhl D, Das C, den Doelder J, Kapnistos M, Vittorias I and McLeish T C B 2011 Linking models of polymerization and dynamics to predict branched polymer structure and flow *Science* **333** 1871–4

Regan K, Ricketts S and Robertson-Anderson R M 2016 DNA as a model for probing polymer entanglements: circular polymers and non-classical dynamics *Polymers* **8** 336

Robertson R M, Laib S and Smith D E 2006 Diffusion of isolated DNA molecules: dependence on length and topology *PNAS* **103** 7310–4

Robertson R M and Smith D E 2007 Self-diffusion of entangled linear and circular DNA molecules: dependence on length and concentration *Macromolecules* **40** 3373–7

Robertson R M and Smith D E 2007a Strong effects of molecular topology on diffusion of entangled DNA molecules *PNAS* **104** 4824–7

Robertson R M and Smith D E 2007b Direct measurement of the confining forces imposed on a single molecule in a concentrated solution of circular polymers *Macromolecules* **40** 8737–41

Robertson R M and Smith D E 2007c Direct measurement of the intermolecular forces confining a single molecule in an entangled polymer solution *Phys. Rev. Lett.* **99** 126001

Rogers S A, Calabrese M A and Wagner N J 2014 Rheology of branched wormlike micelles *Curr. Opin. Colloid Interface Sci.* **19** 530–5

Roovers J 1988 Viscoelastic properties of polybutadiene rings *Macromolecules* **21** 1517–21

Roovers J 1985 The melt properties of ring polystyrenes *Macromolecules* **18** 1359–61

Roovers J and Toporowski P M 1988 Synthesis and characterization of ring polybutadienes *J. Polym. Sci. Part B-Polym. Phys.* **26** 1251–9

Rosa A and Everaers R 2016 Computer simulations of melts of randomly branching polymers *J. Chem. Phys.* **145** 164906

Rosa A and Everaers R 2014 Ring polymers in the melt state: the physics of crumpling *Phys. Rev. Lett.* **112** 118302

Rosa A, Smrek J, Turner M S and Michieletto D 2020 Threading-induced dynamical transition in tadpole-shaped polymers *ACS Macro Lett.* **9** 743–8

Rouse P E 1953 A theory of the linear viscoelastic properties of dilute solutions of coiling polymers *J. Chem. Phys.* **21** 1272–80

Rubinstein M 1986 Dynamics of ring polymers in the presence of fixed obstacles *Phys. Rev. Lett.* **57** 3023–6

Rubinstein M and Colby R H 2003 *Polymer Physics* (Oxford) (Oxford, New York): Oxford University Press)

Russell R 2012 *Biophysics of RNA Folding* (Springer Science & Business Media)

Saha S, Heuer D M and Archer L A 2006 Electrophoretic mobility of linear and star-branched DNA in semidilute polymer solutions *Electrophoresis* **27** 3181–94

Saha S, Heuer D M and Archer L A 2004 Effect of matrix chain length on the electrophoretic mobility of large linear and branched DNA in polymer solutions *Electrophoresis* **25** 396–404

Seol Y and Neuman K C 2016 The dynamic interplay between DNA topoisomerases and DNA topology *Biophys. Rev.* **8** 101–11

Shanbhag S, Park S J, Zhou Q and Larson R 2006 Analytical rheology: linear viscoelasticity of model and commercial long-chain-branched polymer melts *Abstr. Pap. Am. Chem. S.* 231

Shapiro T A and Englund P T 1995 The structure and replication of kinetoplast dna *Annu. Rev. Microbiol.* **49** 117–43

Shih W M and Lin C 2010 Knitting complex weaves with DNA origami *Curr. Opin. Struct. Biol. Nucleic Acids/Seq. Topol.* **20** 276–82

Smrek J, Garamella J, Robertson-Anderson R and Michieletto D 2021 Topological tuning of DNA mobility in entangled solutions of supercoiled plasmids *Sci. Adv.* **7** eabf9260

Smrek J and Grosberg A Y 2016 Minimal surfaces on unconcatenated polymer rings in melt *ACS Macro Lett.* **5** 750–4

Smrek J, Kremer K and Rosa A 2019 Threading of unconcatenated ring polymers at high concentrations: double-folded vs time-equilibrated structures *ACS Macro Lett.* **8** 155–60

Snijkers F, Pasquino R, Olmsted P D and Vlassopoulos D 2015 Perspectives on the viscoelasticity and flow behavior of entangled linear and branched polymers *J. Phys. Condens. Matter* **27** 473002

Soh B W and Doyle P S 2020 Deformation response of catenated DNA networks in a planar elongational field *ACS Macro Lett.* **9** 944–9

Sokolov I M 2012 Models of anomalous diffusion in crowded environments *Soft Matter* **8** 9043–52

Spinozzi F, Ortore M G, Nava G, Bomboi F, Carducci F, Amenitsch H, Bellini T, Sciortino F and Mariani P 2020 Gelling without structuring: a SAXS study of the interactions among DNA nanostars *Langmuir* **36** 10387–96

Suneel , Buzza D M A, Groves D J, McLeish T C B, Parker D, Keeney A J and Feast W J 2002 Rheology and molecular weight distribution of hyperbranched polymers *Macromolecules* **35** 9605–12

Suzuki J, Takano A, Deguchi T and Matsushita Y 2009 Dimension of ring polymers in bulk studied by Monte-Carlo simulation and self-consistent theory *J. Chem. Phys.* **131** 144902

Takano A, Kushida Y, Ohta Y, Masuoka K and Matsushita Y 2009 The second virial coefficients of highly-purified ring polystyrenes in cyclohexane *Polymer* **50** 1300–3

Tsalikis D G, Alatas P V, Peristeras L D and Mavrantzas V G 2018 Scaling laws for the conformation and viscosity of ring polymers in the crossover region around me from detailed molecular dynamics simulations *ACS Macro Lett.* **7** 916–20

Tsalikis D G and Mavrantzas V G 2020 Size and diffusivity of polymer rings in linear polymer matrices: the key role of threading events *Macromolecules* **53** 803–20

Tsalikis D G, Mavrantzas V G and Vlassopoulos D 2016 Analysis of slow modes in ring polymers: threading of rings controls long-time relaxation *ACS Macro Lett.* **5** 755–60

Tsuboyama K, Dauparas J, Chen J, Laine E, Mohseni Behbahani Y, Weinstein J J, Mangan N M, Ovchinnikov S and Rocklin G J 2023 Mega-scale experimental analysis of protein folding stability in biology and design *Nature* **620** 434–44

Tu M Q, Lee M, Robertson-Anderson R M and Schroeder C M 2020 Direct observation of ring polymer dynamics in the flow-gradient plane of shear flow *Macromolecules* **53** 9406–19

Tubiana L, Ferrari F and Orlandini E 2022 Circular polycatenanes: supramolecular structures with topologically tunable properties *Phys. Rev. Lett.* **129** 227801

Ubertini M A, Smrek J and Rosa A 2022 Entanglement length scale separates threading from branching of unknotted and non-concatenated ring polymers in melts *Macromolecules* **55** 10723–36

van Ruymbeke E, Orfanou K, Kapnistos M, Iatrou H, Pitsikalis M, Hadjichristidis N, Lohse D J and Vlassopoulos D 2007 Entangled dendritic polymers and beyond: rheology of symmetric cayley-tree polymers and macromolecular self-assemblies *Macromolecules* **40** 5941–52

Wagner C E, Turner B S, Rubinstein M, McKinley G H and Ribbeck K 2017 A rheological study of the association and dynamics of MUC5AC gels *Biomacromolecules* **18** 3654–64

Wang B, Guan J, Anthony S M, Bae S C, Schweizer K S and Granick S Confining potential when a biopolymer filament reptates *Phys. Rev. Lett.* **104** 118301

Wang J and Ge T 2021 Crazing reveals an entanglement network in glassy ring polymers *Macromolecules* **54** 7500–11

Weigand W J, Messmore A, Tu J, Morales-Sanz A, Blair D L, Deheyn D D, Urbach J S and Robertson-Anderson R M 2017 Active microrheology determines scale-dependent material properties of chaetopterus mucus *PLoS One* **12** e0176732

Wetlaufer D B 2019 *The Protein Folding Problem* (Routledge)

Xue K-L, Hu Y-F, Yu X-C and Hou J-X 2020 The diffusion properties of a ring polymer in a grid matrix *J. Polym. Res.* **27** 123

Yan Z-C, Costanzo S, Jeong Y, Chang T and Vlassopoulos D 2016 Linear and nonlinear shear rheology of a marginally entangled ring polymer *Macromolecules* **49** 1444–53

Zhou Q and Larson R G 2006 Direct calculation of the tube potential confining entangled polymers *Macromolecules* **39** 6737–43

Zhou Y, Hsiao K-W, Regan K E, Kong D, McKenna G B, Robertson-Anderson R M and Schroeder C M 2019 Effect of molecular architecture on ring polymer dynamics in semidilute linear polymer solutions *Nat. Commun.* **10** 10

Zimm B H 1956 Dynamics of polymer molecules in dilute solution: viscoelasticity, flow birefringence and dielectric loss *J. Chem. Phys.* **24** 269–78

Chapter 7

Biopolymer composites, blends, and crowding

While the focus of polymer physics theory and materials science has largely been on single-component polymer networks, cells take advantage of composite networks of biopolymers, such as the cytoskeleton, to enable emergent dynamical and structural properties. Composites are also of wide interest for industrial and commercial applications, as they can exhibit emergent properties such as low weight and high strength, as well as hierarchical rheological properties.

In this chapter, I will discuss composites and blends of two or more distinct biopolymers, as well as crowding of biopolymers by other macromolecules, e.g., synthetic polymers. The distinction between blends and composites in this context are that blends are fully miscible mixtures of the same polymer type (e.g., DNA) but with different sizes and/or topologies, while composites are mixtures of two or more distinct types of polymers (e.g., DNA and actin) that often exhibit varying degrees of de-mixing and phase separation.

I will focus the discussion on the dynamics, mechanical properties, and structures of key examples of these multi-constituent biopolymer networks, highlighting emergent properties and design considerations. Specific examples of networks that I will discuss include blends of linear, ring, and supercoiled DNA, as well as composites comprising different combinations of DNA, actin, microtubules, intermediate filaments, and synthetic dextran polymers.

7.1 Biopolymer blends

As I discuss in chapter 6, topology plays a key role in the dynamics of semidilute and entangled DNA networks (Schroeder *et al* 2004, Robertson and Smith 2007, 2007a, Regan *et al* 2016, Smrek *et al* 2021). Perhaps the most widely-studied and intriguing phenomenon is the threading of rings by linear chains in ring-linear blends, which is understood to dramatically slow the diffusion and relaxation of threaded rings (Robertson and Smith 2007, 2007b, McLeish 2008, Michieletto *et al* 2014, Smrek *et al* 2019, Ubertini *et al* 2022). However, the impact of this slowing on the

doi:10.1088/978-0-7503-5037-2ch7

microscopic and bulk rheological properties of ring-linear blends, the diffusion and relaxation rates of linear chains, and the conformational dynamics of threaded rings are still debated (Schroeder *et al* 2004, Iyer *et al* 2007, Halverson *et al* 2012, Michieletto *et al* 2017, Katsarou *et al* 2020, Parisi *et al* 2020, Peddireddy *et al* 2020a, Michieletto and Sakaue 2021, Zhou *et al* 2021a, McKenna *et al* 2022, O'Connor *et al* 2022). The extent to which supercoiled molecules can participate in threading, as well as the dynamics of blends comprising supercoiled biopolymers, also requires further investigation (Fathizadeh *et al* 2015, Peddireddy *et al* 2020b, Smrek *et al* 2021). As in previous chapters, I will not cover the large body of literature on synthetic polymer blends, in particular the exhaustive body of work focused on synthetic ring-linear blends, such as (Roovers, 1988; Kawaguchi *et al* 2006, Kapnistos *et al* 2008, Hur *et al* 2011, p 20222022, Halverson *et al* 2012, Tsalikis and Mavrantzas 2014, Tsalikis *et al* 2017, Kobayashi *et al* 2018, Parisi *et al* 2020, 2021) but will instead focus on topological blends of biopolymers, DNA in particular.

7.1.1 Ring-linear DNA blends

In chapter 6, I discuss the effect of topology on the diffusion of tracer DNA in an entangled DNA solution (matrix), looking at cases in which the tracer and/or matrix were rings and/or linear chains (Robertson and Smith 2007, 2007b). In brief, single-molecule tracking experiments showed that the diffusion coefficients of both ring and linear DNA tracers were lower in a matrix of linear chains compared to rings, and ring tracer diffusion in a linear matrix was markedly slower than the other three cases (Robertson and Smith 2007, 2007b).

Following on this work, similar single-molecule tracking methods were used to measure diffusion coefficients of ring and linear DNA of equal contour length $L \simeq 15\ \mu\text{m}$ (45 kbp) diffusing in blends of ring and linear DNA of the same length L with varying mass fractions of linear DNA ϕ_L (figure 7.1(A)) (Chapman *et al* 2012). At a blend concentration of $c \approx 2.5c_e$ (1 mg mL^{-1}) the diffusion coefficients for ring DNA D_R dropped sharply by ~4-fold and ~8-fold as the fraction of linear DNA in the blend increased from $\phi_L = 0$ (pure rings) to, respectively, $\phi_L = 0.2$ (20% ring, 80% linear) and $\phi_L = 0.4$ (40% ring, 60% linear), after which the decrease was much more modest, decreasing another ~2-fold as $\phi_L \to 1$ (i.e., $D_R(\phi_L = 0) \approx 16 D_R(\phi_L = 1)$) (figure 7.1(B)). This effect was attributed to threading of ring DNA by linear chains, aligning with predictions and experiments on synthetic ring-linear blends that have shown that a very small fraction of linear chains can dramatically reduce the mobility of ring-linear blends (Mills *et al* 1987, Cosgrove *et al* 1996, von Meerwall *et al* 2003, Subramanian and Shanbhag 2008, Halverson *et al* 2012, Xue *et al* 2020). A similar but more modest slowing trend was observed for more weakly entangled solutions ($c \simeq c_e$) with $D_R(\phi_L = 0) \approx 2D_R(\phi_L = 0.2) \approx 3D_R(\phi_L = 1)$ (figure 7.1(C)).

Perhaps the more surprising result of this study is the non-monotonic dependence of the linear DNA diffusion coefficient D_L on ϕ_L. Namely, D_L was highest (fastest) for pure ring solutions ($\phi_L = 0$), similar to D_R, but the linear chain diffusion coefficient actually reached a minimum $D_{L,\min}$ at $\phi_L = 0.5$, which was ~3-fold lower

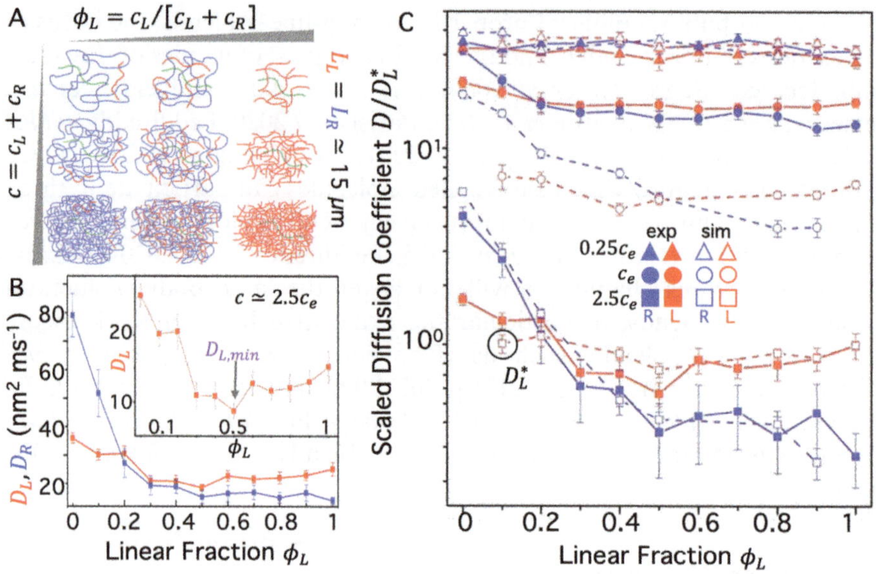

Figure 7.1. The effect of linear fraction and entanglement density on the diffusion coefficients of linear and ring tracer DNA in ring-linear DNA blends. (A) Blends of ring (blue) and linear (red) DNA of length $L \simeq 15\ \mu m$ (45 kbp) were prepared at total mass concentrations of $c = c_L + c_R \approx 0.1$, 0.5, and 1 mg mL^{-1}, equivalent to $\sim 0.25c_e$, $\sim c_e$ and $\sim 2.5c_e$, and 11 mass fractions of linear DNA spanning from $\phi_L = 0$ (pure rings) to $\phi_L = 1$ (pure linear). A trace amount of linear or ring DNA was fluorescent-labeled (green) and tracked to determine topology-dependent diffusion coefficients D_L or D_R. (B) Diffusion coefficients for ring (blue) and linear (red) DNA versus linear mass fraction ϕ_L for entangled ring-linear blends ($c \approx 2.5c_e$). The zoom-in of D_L shown in the inset highlights the non-monotonic dependence of D_L which drops by a factor of ~ 3 as ϕ_L increases from 0 to 0.5 ($D_{L,\min} \approx \frac{1}{3}D_L(\phi_L = 0)$), followed by a subsequent ~ 2-fold increase as ϕ_L increases further to $\phi_L = 1$ ($D_{L,\min} \approx \frac{1}{2}D_L(\phi_L = 1)$). (C) Brownian dynamics simulations (open symbols) showed similar diffusive behavior for both ring and linear topologies in the entangled blends examined in (B) (squares), as well as for ~ 4-fold shorter unentangled DNA chains ($L \simeq 3.7\ \mu m$, triangles). Deviations between experiment and simulations for blends with $\sim c_e$ (circles) arise from the limited ability of theoretical models to accurately capture the dynamics in the crossover region between semidilute and entangled regimes. Both simulation and experimental data are scaled by the linear chain diffusion coefficient for $\phi_L = 0.1$ and $c \approx 2.5c_e$, D_L^* (experimental value circled). Adapted from Chapman *et al* (2012) with permission from the Royal Society of Chemistry.

than D_L in pure rings, after which it increased again ~ 2-fold as $\phi_L \to 1$ (figure 7.1(B) inset). Supported by simulations (figure 7.1(C)), this non-monotonicity was attributed to a second order effect of the threaded rings in the matrix exhibiting nearly halted motion, much slower than entangled linear chains or rings. Consequently, for blends with equal fractions of rings and linear chains ($\phi_L = 0.5$), every ring may be threaded by a linear chain and every linear chain may thread a ring; so the matrix is composed almost entirely of threaded rings that have nearly halted motion. This maximally rigid matrix gives rise to the most suppressed linear chain diffusion.

Similar measurements performed with the same length DNA but at a 10-fold lower concentration of $c \approx 0.25c_e$ (0.1 mg mL^{-1}), as well with $\sim 4\times$ shorter DNA ($L \simeq 3.7\ \mu m$, 11 kbp) at the same concentration $c \simeq 1$ mg mL^{-1}, showed minimal effects of topology on diffusion coefficients (Chapman *et al* 2012) (figure 7.1(C)). This insensitivity indicates that it is the changing nature of the steric interactions between overlapping chains, rather than the topology of the individual molecules, that drive the impact of topology on diffusion.

Optical tweezers microrheology experiments on the same ring-linear DNA blends ($L \simeq 15\ \mu$m, $c = 1$ mg mL^{-1}) showed that the scaling of $G'(\omega)$ for the two ϕ_L extremes, $\phi_L = 1$ and $\phi_L = 0.14$, followed predictions from the Doi–Edwards model (D-E) for linear polymers (Doi and Edwards 1986) and the lattice animal model (DFLA) for rings (Kapnistos *et al* 2008), respectively. Conversely, intermediate ϕ_L blends exhibited weaker scaling with ω and higher $G'(\omega)$ values over the entire frequency range, indicative of enhanced elasticity (figure 7.2(A)). Moreover, all blends exhibited shear-thinning scaling $\eta^*(\omega) \sim \omega^{-x}$, with the maximum scaling exponent reached for $\phi_L \simeq 0.68$ (figure 7.2(B)).

This emergent non-monotonicity is further highlighted by the dependence of the plateau modulus G^0 and initial stress relaxation modulus G_N on ϕ_L, with both G^0 and G_N reaching maxima at $\phi_L \simeq 0.68$, which are ~3× and ~6× larger than for, respectively, the highest ($\phi_L = 1$) and lowest ($\phi_L = 0.14$) linear fractions examined (figure 7.2(C)) (Peddireddy *et al* 2020a). Moreover, the maximum shear-thinning exponent, observed for $\phi_L \simeq 0.68$ was measured to have a value of $x \approx 0.75$, in line with expected exponents of $x \approx 0.7 - 1$ for entangled linear polymers (Chapman *et al* 2014, Chapman and Robertson-Anderson 2014, Pan *et al* 2018) and ~25% and ~2-fold higher than that measured for the $\phi_L = 1$ and $\phi_L = 0.14$ blends (figure 7.2(C)). These results collectively demonstrate that ring-linear DNA blends with comparable fractions of rings and linear chains, in which threading events are maximized, display the most elastic-like and constrained dynamics which, in turn, promote chain stretching and flow alignment.

Complementary nonlinear OTM measurements exhibited similar, albeit more modest, non-monotonic dependence of the maximum force $F_{\max}$ (figure 7.2(D)) and nonlinear viscosity η_{nl} (figure 7.2(E)) on ϕ_L, indicating that ring-linear threading can withstand nonlinear straining. However, for sufficiently fast strain rates, above the predicted entanglement rate of $\tau_{e,L}^{-1} \simeq 35$ s^{-1} for the pure linear DNA networks ($\phi_L = 1$), the largely elastic force response yields, or softens, to a viscous-dominated regime at much faster timescales than for slower strains. Moreover, this softening time in the high strain rate limit is nearly independent of ϕ_L and aligns with the predicted Rouse time for the linear chains $\tau_{R,L} \simeq 0.1$ s. This agreement suggests that steric constraints (e.g., entanglements, threadings) are disrupted at these high rates, and the force response is dominated by linear chains rather than rings.

One mechanism which may lead to this rate-dependent phenomenon is forced de-threading of the linear chains by the moving probe. Namely, the moving probe forces linear chains to de-thread from rings as they deform in the direction of the strain and gather at the leading edge of the probe. The de-threaded rings, which can less easily align with the strain (evidenced by weaker shear thinning), then gather in the wake and thus do not contribute to the measured force relaxation following straining.

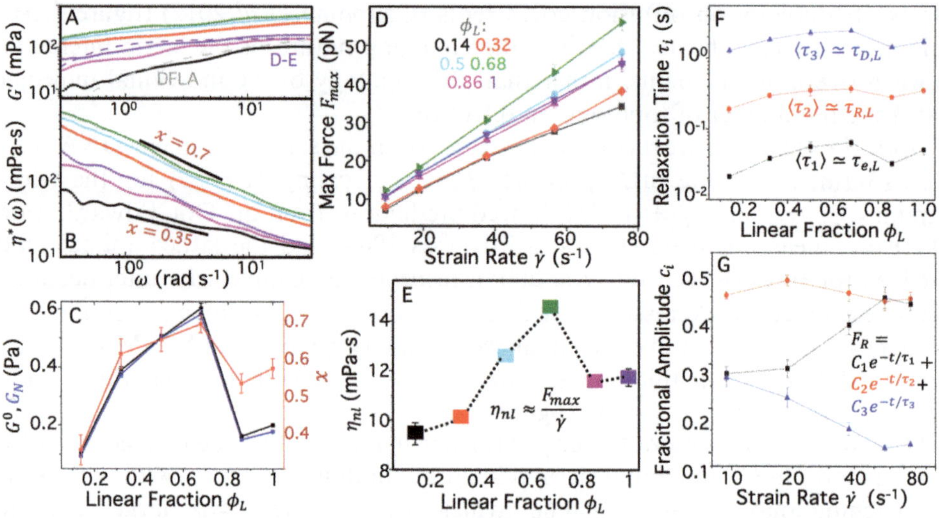

Figure 7.2. Optical tweezers microrheology of ring-linear DNA blends reveal non-monotonic dependence on linear DNA fraction ϕ_L. (A–C) Linear OTM measurements for entangled blends of ring and linear DNA of length $L \simeq 15\ \mu$m (45 kbp) and $c = c_L + c_R = 1$ mg mL^{-1}, with varying linear DNA fractions ϕ_L: 0.14 (black), 0.32 (red), 0.5 (cyan), 0.68 (green), 0.86 (magenta), and 1 (purple). The frequency dependent storage modulus $G'(\omega)$ (A) and complex viscosity $\eta^*(\omega)$ (B) with the dashed lines (A) corresponding to predictions from the Doi–Edwards model (purple, D–E) and double-folded lattice animal model (DFLA, grey), and the solid lines (B) showing power-law scaling $\eta^*(\omega) \sim \omega^{-x}$, with exponents listed. (C) The elastic plateau modulus G^0 (black), initial stress relaxation modulus G_N (blue), and shear-thinning exponent x (red) display non-monotonic dependence on ϕ_L, reaching maxima at $\phi_L = 0.68$. (D–G) Nonlinear OTM measurements performed on the same blends as in (A–C). (D) the maximum force $F_{\max}$ reached at the end of the 30 μm strain increases linearly with strain rate $\dot{\gamma}$ and depends non-monotonically on ϕ_L across all $\dot{\gamma}$ values. (E) Nonlinear viscosity η_{nl} determined from linear fits to $F_{\max}(\dot{\gamma})$ data shown in (D) display non-mónotonic dependence on ϕ_L. (F) Relaxation times, τ_1 (black squares), τ_2 (red circles), and τ_3 (blue triangles), as a function of ϕ_L, determined from fitting the force relaxation data to a sum of three exponentials, $F_R(t) = \sum_{i=1}^{3} C_i e^{-t/\tau_i}$, and averaging over all $\dot{\gamma}$. Upon averaging across ϕ_L, the timescales $\langle\tau_1\rangle$, $\langle\tau_2\rangle$, and $\langle\tau_3\rangle$ align with predicted values for τ_e, τ_R, and τ_D for linear chains. (G) The fractional amplitudes $c_i = C_i / \sum_{i=1}^{3} C_i$ of each exponential term in the fits to $F_R(t)$, denoting the relative weight of each mode in the overall relaxation, show that the slow relaxation is increasingly suppressed and fast relaxation becomes more dominant as $\dot{\gamma}$ increases. Adapted with permission from Peddireddy *et al* (2020a). Copyright (2020) by the American Physical Society.

The force relaxation profiles following nonlinear straining corroborate this physical picture. Specifically, the relaxation of the force on the probe is well described by a sum of three exponentials, similar to single-component DNA systems I describe in chapters 5 and 6 (Robertson and Smith 2007a, 2007c). The distinct relaxation timescales associated with each exponential decay, τ_1, τ_2, and τ_3, were shown to align with predicted values for, respectively, the entanglement time $\tau_{e,L} \simeq 30$ ms, Rouse time $\tau_{R,L} \simeq 0.1$ s, and disengagement time $\tau_{D,L} \simeq 1.8$ s for linear polymers (figure 7.2(F)), which are all much slower than the predicted values for rings, suggesting that it is the linear polymers that dominate the force relaxation rather than the slow de-threading or fast conformational relaxation of rings.

Finally, as the strain rate increased, the contribution, i.e., the fractional amplitude $c_i = C_i/[C_1 + C_2 + C_3]$, of the slow relaxation mode τ_3 decreased while the fast mode τ_1 increased (figure 7.2(G)), suggestive of reduced steric constraints that arise from the forced de-threading of rings and accumulation of linear chains at the leading edge of the probe.

Bulk rheology measurements on blends of the same $L \simeq 15\ \mu$m ring and linear DNA examined in figures 7.1 and 7.2, at concentrations of $c \simeq 0.8$, 1, and 2 mg mL^{-1} and $\phi_L \simeq 0.14$ and 0.5 (Kong *et al* 2022), showed qualitatively similar trends as the OTM measurements described above (Peddireddy *et al* 2020a). For example, bulk rheology measurements showed that all blends were in the rubbery plateau regime (figure 7.3(A)) and exhibited shear thinning (figure 7.3(B)) across the entire frequency range. Moreover, G^0 and x were shown to be higher for the $\phi_L = 0.5$ blend compared to $\phi_L = 0.14$ (figures 7.3(A) and (B)). However, bulk measurements reported that $G^0(\phi_L = 0.5)$ was ~2.5× higher than $G^0(\phi_L = 0.14)$, compared to the ~5× higher value measured using microrheology. Moreover, the bulk shear-thinning exponent was substantially higher than the microrheology result for $\phi_L = 0.14$ ($x_{\text{bulk}} \approx 0.75$ vs $x_{\text{micro}} \approx 0.35$) and modestly higher for $\phi_L = 0.5$ ($x_{\text{bulk}} \approx 0.88$ vs $x_{\text{micro}} \approx 0.65$).

These differences between measurements at different scales highlight the hierarchical and scale-dependent rheological properties of topologically-complex biopolymer blends and solutions. In addition, the stronger shear thinning and weaker ϕ_L-dependence observed in bulk rheology as compared to microrheology may also arise from the nature of the perturbation. Microrheology measurements are local, so the threading of a small fraction of rings (for e.g., $\phi_L = 0.14$) likely has less effect on bulk behavior due to the fact that very few local regions will contain a threaded ring; but instead will more often contain only co-entangled rings. As a result, the effect of threading may only strongly manifest when the fractions of rings and linear chains are comparable such that threaded rings pervade each local microscopic region. The few threaded rings can still contribute to the bulk rheology which senses the ensemble or average dynamics of the blend. This effect would lead to higher bulk values of G^0 and x compared to local values for $\phi_L = 0.14$, and similarly less increase in the values as the linear fraction is increased to $\phi_L = 0.5$. Likewise, the increased shear thinning in bulk rheology ($x_{\text{bulk}} > x_{\text{micro}}$) can be understood as due to more contributions from threaded rings, which is further amplified by the probes used in microheology being able to de-thread rings, thereby weakening shear alignment (Peddireddy *et al* 2020a).

Complementing OTM (figure 7.2) and bulk rheology (figures 7.3(A) and (B)) measurements on blends of ring and linear DNA of length $L \simeq 15\ \mu$m and varying linear fractions ϕ_L, microfluidics experiments measured the relaxation dynamics of ring DNA subject to planar extensional flow of in semidilute unentangled ring-linear blends ($c \simeq c_L^*$) of the same length $L \simeq 15\ \mu$m and similar blend fractions of $\phi_L \simeq 0.17$, $\phi_L \simeq 0.5$, and $\phi_L \simeq 0.83$ (figures 7.3(C)–(I)) (Zhou *et al* 2021a). Similar to the microrheology measurements on entangled blends (figure 7.2), microfluidics measurements exhibited a non-monotonic ϕ_L-dependence of conformational dynamics due to pervasive threading in blends with a sufficient number of linear chains. Specifically, the average fractional extension $\langle x \rangle / L_R$ was shown to decrease as the linear fraction increased from $\phi_L \simeq 0.17$ to $\phi_L \simeq 0.5$, following by a subsequent

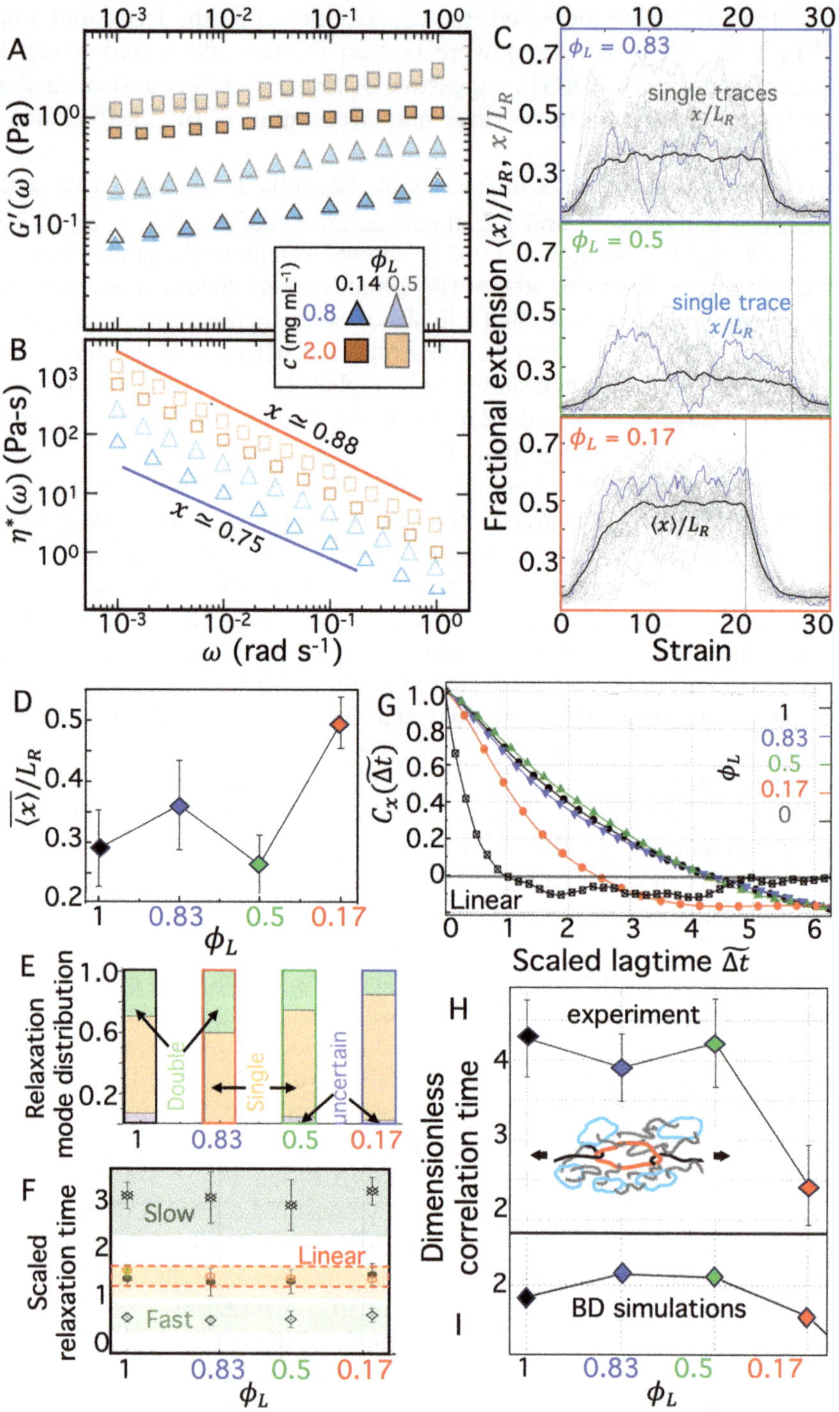

Figure 7.3. Bulk rheology and single-molecule extensional flow experiments on ring-linear DNA blends of varying linear fractions ϕ_L. (A, B) Bulk linear rheology measurements for entangled blends of ring and linear DNA of length $L \simeq 15\ \mu$m (45 kbp) at concentrations of $c = c_L + c_R \simeq 0.8$ mg mL^{-1} (blue triangles) and

2.0 mg mL^{-1} (orange rectangles), and DNA fractions $\phi_L = 0.14$ (dark shades, symmetric symbols) and 0.5 (light shades, elongated symbols). The frequency dependent (A) storage modulus $G'(\omega)$ and (B) complex viscosity $\eta^*(\omega)$ for blends with concentrations of 2 mg mL^{-1} (red) and 0.8 mg mL^{-1} (blue) and linear fractions $\phi_L = 0.5$ (light shades) and 0.8 mg mL^{-1}, $\phi_L = 0.14$ (dark shades) with color-coded solid lines showing power-law scaling $\eta^*(\omega) \sim \omega^{-x}$. (C–I) Microfluidic planar extensional flow experiments examining the fractional extension and conformational relaxation of ring DNA in semidilute blends of ring and linear DNA of length $L \simeq 15$ μm (45 kbp), concentration $c \simeq 50$ μg mL^{-1} ($\sim c_L^*$), and linear fractions $\phi_L = 0.17$ (red), 0.5 (green), 0.83 (blue), and 1 (black). (C) The population of fractional extensions of rings x/L_R (grey) during extensional flow of $Wi \simeq 1.5$ as a function of strain, with black and blue lines in each panel corresponding to the average of individual traces $\langle x \rangle / L_R$ and a representative single extension curve, respectively. The vertical dashed line in each panel indicates the cessation of flow. Data to the left and right of the line are averaged together to determine, respectively, the (D) strain-averaged fractional extension $\overline{\langle x \rangle}/L_R$ and (E) relaxation modes and timescales as functions of ϕ_L. (E) The fraction of extensional relaxations (data to the right of the curves in (C)) that are best described by a single (orange) or double (green) exponential; and the (F) corresponding relaxation timescales, color-coded as in E and normalized by the dilute limit value, as a function of ϕ_L. Crossed and open diamonds correspond to the slow and fast relaxation timescales for the double-mode population, and diamonds correspond to single-mode population timescales determined from experiments (black filled) and simulation (open red). Dashed red lines indicate mean and standard deviation of the linear DNA relaxation timescale determined from Hsiao *et al* (2017). (G) The autocorrelation $C_x(\Delta t)$ of the fractional extension of rings as a function of lag time Δt, non-dimensionalized by the strain rate, quantifies the timescale τ_c over which ring conformations remain correlated, indicated by the lag time Δt at which $C_x(\Delta t)$ crosses the horizontal line indicating $C_x(\Delta t) = 0$. (H, I) The ϕ_L-dependent conformational correlation timescales τ_c determined from the (H) experimental data shown in (G) or (I) simulation data (not shown) show similar trends. (A, B) Adapted with permission from Kong *et al* (2022). Copyright (2022) American Chemical Society. (C–I) Adapted from Zhou *et al* (2021a), with the permission of AIP Publishing.

deccrease from $\phi_L \simeq 0.5$ to $\phi_L \simeq 0.83$ (figures 7.3(C) and (D)). The larger linear fraction blends, $\phi_L \geqslant 0.5$, also exhibited a much broader range of fractional extensions with large peaks and valleys not seen at lower linear fractions or for linear DNA (figure 7.3(C)). These effects were attributed to transient threading and de-threading and stronger hydrodynamic interactions in $\phi_L \geqslant 0.5$ blends compared to primarily ring blends ($\phi_L \simeq 0.17$).

Moreover, following cessation of elongational flow, all blends were shown to exhibit two subpopulations, which both display exponential relaxation dynamics, but are delineated by having either one or two modes. While the former is expected for semidilute linear DNA, the latter, which is more prevalent for $\phi_L \geqslant 0.5$ blends, is indicative of fast relaxation of unconstrained rings and slow relaxation of threaded rings. These subpopulations further support the differences seen between microrheology and macrorheology, in which threading is only prevalent in a fraction of the ring population such that the effects may not be as evident in local measurements compared to bulk ensemble measurements. The molecular individualism that is uniquely observed for ring-linear blends is further indication of distinct topological interactions, such as ring-linear threading, which are only pervasive in blends with intermediate linear fractions (Zhou *et al* 2021b).

Further evidence of threading can be seen in the conformational autocorrelation $C_x(\Delta t)$ (figure 7.3(G)), which determines the lag time Δt over which the fractional extension of a stretched ring remains correlated, i.e., the conformational correlation time τ_c (figures 7.3(H) and (I)). Namely, $C_x(\Delta t)$ for the primarily ring blend decayed markedly faster than for higher ϕ_L blends, and the linear chain decorrelation time was likewise smaller. Simulations (figure 7.3(I)) showed that this effect was due to reduced hydrodynamic interactions between highly stretched linear DNA and adjacent (unthreaded) rings (Zhou *et al* 2021b). Conversely, enhanced hydrodynamic interactions between threaded rings and threading linear chains 'lock' the rings into more persistent conformations thus slowing conformational fluctuations.

The studies described above showcase the important role that ring-linear threading events play in the diffusion, relaxation, and rheology of ring-linear blends; and how their contributions vary depending on the lengthscale and timescale of the measurement. A natural question that arises from these findings is how an imposed local stress propagates from the molecular level to the bulk in ring-linear blends, and how enhanced flow alignment and conformational heterogeneity of threaded rings may lead to emergent propagation dynamics.

To address these questions, researchers integrated optical tweezers with differential dynamic microscopy (OpTiDDM), to couple force response to polymer dynamics, deformations, and stress propagation (figures 7.4(A)–(F)) (Peddireddy *et al* 2022). OpTiDDM experiments, consisting of cyclically moving a trapped probe at constant strain rates of $\dot{\gamma} \simeq 9.4–189\ s^{-1}$ (figure 7.4(A)) through a horizontal distance $s = 15\ \mu m$ while simultaneously measuring the force exerted on the probe (figure 7.4(B)) and the fluctuations of surrounding labeled DNA (figures 7.4(C) and (D)), were performed on $\phi_L = 0.5$ blends of ring and linear DNA of length $L \simeq 38\ \mu m$ (115 kbp) and concentrations $c \simeq 3c_e$ (0.5 mg mL^{-1}) and $c \simeq 4c_e$ (0.65 mg mL^{-1}) (figures 7.4(G)–(L)).

OT force measurements revealed strong $\dot{\gamma}$-dependent shear thinning for the $\sim 4c_e$ blend, indicated by a drop in the maximum force $F_M(t)$ over time (figure 7.4(G)), that was minimal for the $\sim 3c_e$ blend and most pronounced for $\dot{\gamma} \simeq 42\ s^{-1}$. This thinning behavior is consistent with enhanced shear thinning observed in rheology experiments on ring-linear DNA blends (figures 7.2(C), 7.3(B)) (Peddireddy *et al* 2020a, Kong *et al* 2022). The $\sim 4c_e$ blend also displayed pronounced elastic-like force retention following the relaxation phase, maintaining a non-zero residual force F_R that remained constant for the duration of the cyclic straining and was highest for $\dot{\gamma} \simeq 42\ s^{-1}$ (figure 7.4(H)). In contrast, the less entangled $\sim 3c_e$ blend initially maintained much less residual force as compared to $\sim 4c_e$ ($F_{R,0} \approx 1$ pN versus 4 pN), but $F_R(t)$ steadily increased during cyclic straining (figure 7.4(G) inset), suggestive of progressively slower relaxation due to increasing polymer buildup at the leading edge of the moving probe. Notably, the strain rate $\dot{\gamma} \simeq 42\ s^{-1}$ at which elasticity and shear thinning are maximized for $\sim 4c_e$, aligns with the predicted entanglement rate for the linear chains, $\tau_{e,L}^{-1}$, indicating that the most pronounced force response may occur when the deformation rate is resonant with the fastest relaxation rate of the system, i.e., the time at which the DNA feels the entanglement tube. This effect can be understood as arising from the chains being able to partially relax and reorient on the timescale of the strain for slower strain rates ($\dot{\gamma} < \tau_{e,L}^{-1}$), while for faster rates ($\dot{\gamma} \gg \tau_{e,L}^{-1}$) the DNA polymers do not feel the steric constraints (i.e., entanglements, threadings) from their neighbors, so can move more freely in response to straining. Both of these effects serve to facilitate force relaxation, and

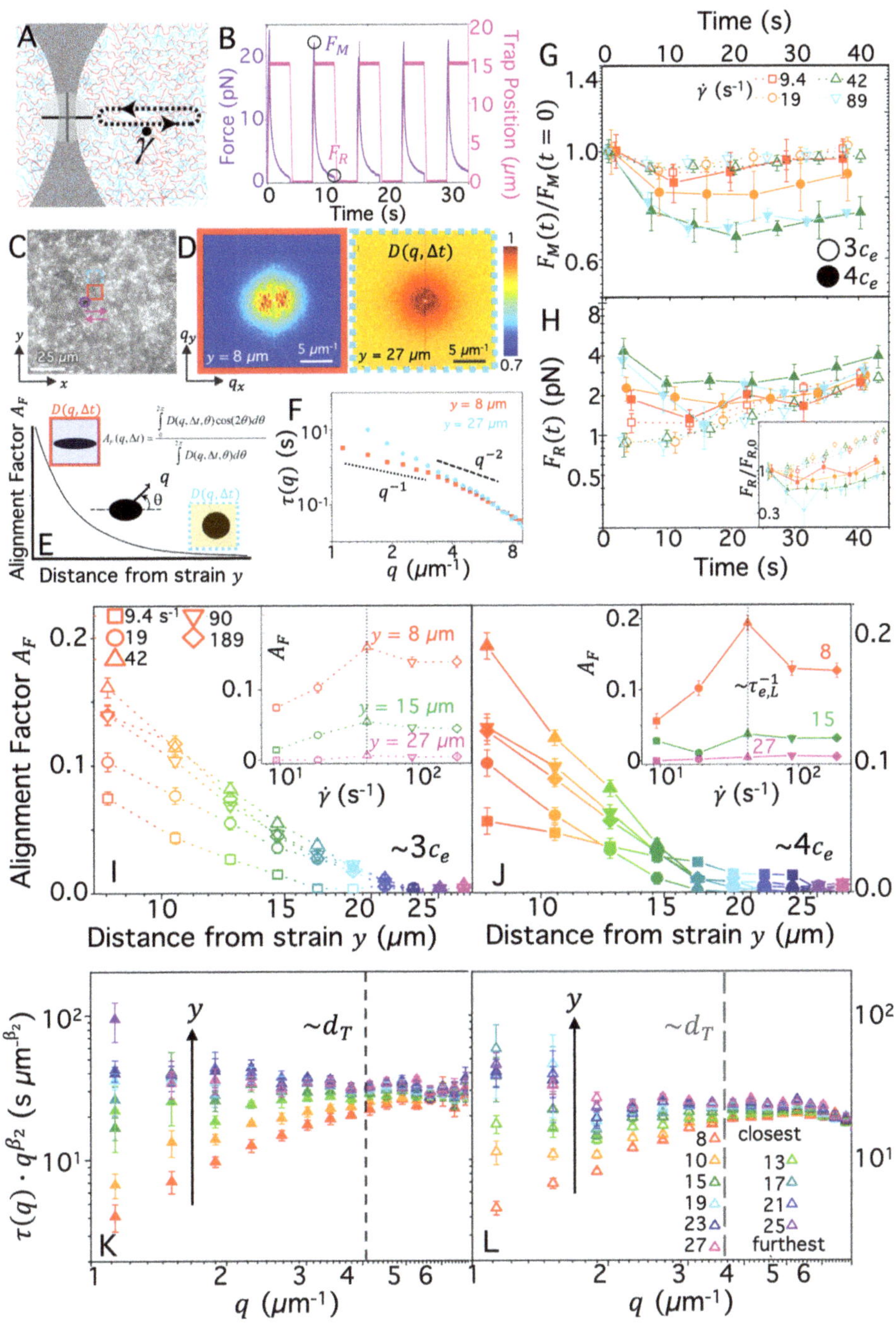

Figure 7.4. OpTiDDM shows enhanced elasticity, flow alignment, and stress propagation in $\phi_L = 0.5$ blends of ring and linear DNA. (A–F) Optical Tweezers integrating Differential Dynamic Microscopy (OpTiDDM) locally perturbs $\phi_L = 0.5$ blends of ring and linear DNA of length $L \simeq 38$ μm and concentrations $c \approx 3c_e$ and $c \approx 4c_e$ by (A) continuously sweeping an optically-trapped probe through the blends at varying strain rates

$\dot{\gamma} \simeq 9.4 - 189\ s^{-1}$ over (B) a distance of $s = 15\ \mu m$ (magenta, Trap Position) for 50 s, with each perturbation separated by a 3 s relaxation phase in which the probe is held fixed at the maximum stage position. The force exerted on the probe (purple) is measured during cyclic straining and the force reached at the maximum strain F_M and end of the relaxation phase F_R are evaluated. (C) During this probe (purple circle) motion (magenta arrows), a time-series of fluorescent-labeled DNA in the blends are recorded, after which the field-of-view is divided into smaller ROIs centered at 10 vertical distances of $y = 8\ \mu m$ (red border) to $y = 27\ \mu m$ (blue-dashed border) from the strain path, which are evaluated using DDM to determine the corresponding DDM image structure functions $D(\mathbf{q}, \Delta t)$, examples of which are shown in (D) for boxed-in ROIs in (C). (D) Near the strain ($y = 8\ \mu m$, red border), $D(\mathbf{q}, \Delta t)$ is anisotropic with two lobes that lie along the strain axis, while far from the strain ($y = 27\ \mu m$, cyan border), $D(\mathbf{q}, \Delta t)$ is radially symmetric. The colorscale indicates the magnitude of $D(\mathbf{q}, \Delta t)$, normalized by the corresponding maximum $D(\mathbf{q}, \Delta t)$ value. (F) From $D(\mathbf{q}, \Delta t)$, OpTiDDM computes the (E) alignment factor, $A_F(y)$, which quantifies the preferential alignment of the polymer motion with the strain path and (F) DDM decay times $\tau(q)$, which describe the macromolecular dynamics, and indicate diffusive and ballistic dynamics via the respective scalings $\tau(q) \sim q^{-2}$ and $\tau(q) \sim q^{-1}$. (E) $A_F(y)$, schematically portrayed, generally decreases with increasing y. (F) $\tau(q)$ determined by fitting $D(q, \Delta t)$ is shown for the ROIs evaluated in (D). (G, H) $F_M(t)$ and $F_R(t)$ measured for each cycle (the number of which depends on $\dot{\gamma}$) during the 50 s strain program, is plotted versus time t for $\dot{\gamma}(s^{-1}) \simeq 9.4$ (red squares), 19 (orange circles), 42 (green triangles), and 89 (cyan inverted triangles) and blend concentrations $c \approx 3c_e$ (open symbols) and $c \approx 4c_e$ (filled symbols). (G) $F_M(t)$ normalized by the initial value $F_M(t = 0)$ exhibits shear thinning that is most pronounced for $4c_e$ blends subject to a strain rate of $\dot{\gamma} = 42\ s^{-1} \simeq \tau_{e,L}^{-1}$. (H) $F_R(t)$ is generally higher for $4c_e$ blends compared to $3c_e$ blends and is maximized for $\dot{\gamma} = 42\ s^{-1}$. $F_R(t)$ normalized by the initial value (inset) shows residual force build up over time for the $3c_e$ blend that is absent at $4c_e$. (I, J) Alignment factor $A_F(y)$ versus vertical distance from the strain y for varying $\dot{\gamma}$ values listed in the legend, and (inset) plotted versus $\dot{\gamma}$ for select y values for $3c_e$ (I) and $4c_e$ (J) blends, with the vertical dashed line indicating the strain rate at which maximal alignment is reached, which corresponds to $\sim\tau_{e,L}^{-1}$ for $4c_e$. (K, L) $\tau(q)$ scaled by q^{β_2}, where β_2 is the scaling exponent that describes the power-law scaling $\tau(q) \sim q^{-\beta}$ for data to right of the dashed vertical line, which aligns with the predicted tube diameter d_T for $3c_e$ (K) and $4c_e$ (L) blends. Warm to cool colors indicate increasing distances y from the strain, listed in μm in the legend in K. Data for lengthscales $\lambda > d_T$, i.e., $q < 2\pi/d_T$, show a strong dependence on y, transitioning from superdiffusive to subdiffusive as y increases. Adapted from Peddireddy *et al* (2022). CC BY 4.0.

thus suppress elastic-like force retention and reduce the strain-induced entropic alignment that underlies shear thinning.

To test these hypotheses and correlate the force response with the DNA dynamics and deformations, DDM was performed on labeled DNA within local ROIs at different vertical distances y from the strain (figures 7.4(C) and (D)), from which the alignment factor A_F of the DDM image structure function was computed relative to the strain direction (figure 7.4(E)), with $A_F = 1$ and $A_F = 0$ signifying complete alignment and isotropy, respectively. This alignment of the DNA motion along the strain path was shown to decay with increasing distance y from the strain and be more pronounced for $4c_e$ blends (figure 7.4(J)) compared to $3c_e$ (figure 7.4(I)). Moreover, A_F was maximized at the same resonant strain rate of $\dot{\gamma} \simeq 42\ s^{-1} \simeq \tau_{e,L}^{-1}$ (figures 7.4(I) and (J) insets) at which shear thinning and elasticity were maximized (figures 7.4(G) and (H)), corroborating the connection between shear thinning and entropic stretching and alignment, and the prominent role that threading plays in enhancing these phenomena in ring-linear DNA blends.

These studies also examined the DDM decay time $\tau(q)$ to determine the nature of the DNA dynamics (i.e., diffusive, subdiffusive, superdiffusive, or ballistic) via the power-law scaling $\tau(q) \sim q^{-\beta}$, and how the dynamics depend on y and the lengthscale λ over which dynamics are measured (figures 7.4(K) and (L)). For all y distances and strain rates the DNA dynamics were distinct for lengthscales $\lambda = 2\pi q^{-1}$ above and below the predicted tube diameter d_T, i.e., below and above the crossover wave vector $q_c = 2\pi d_T^{-1}$ (figures 7.4(K) and (L)). For lengthscales $\lambda < d_T$ ($q > q_c$), the dynamics were shown to be modestly subdiffusive for all y distances, with an average scaling exponent of $\beta_2 \approx 2.7$ that corresponds to $\alpha \approx 0.73$, indicating that the strain does not impact the quiescent polymer dynamics at lengthscales below the entanglement lengthscale, because the polymers cannot couple to the strain. However, for lengthscales $\lambda > d_T$ ($q < q_c$), in which entanglements dominate, dynamics were shown to be nearly ballistic near the strain, indicating strain-induced stretching and flow; while strongly subdiffusive far from the strain, indicative of strong entanglement constraints (figures 7.4(K) and (L)) (Peddireddy *et al* 2022).

7.1.2 Ring-supercoiled blends

As I described at the beginning of this chapter, ring-linear polymer blends have been intensely researched since the 1980s using experimental, theoretical, and computational methods to study both synthetic polymers and DNA. While they continue to be a topic of intense debate and investigation, far less attention has been paid to blends containing supercoiled circular polymers, despite their physiological relevance. In chapter 6 I discuss the few theoretical and experimental studies performed on supercoiled polymer solutions, e.g., Smrek *et al* (2021). One reason for the dearth of studies on these systems is the difficulty in synthesizing supercoiled polymers at high concentrations. While bacterial plasmid DNA, the workhorse of biochemistry and molecular biology labs, naturally occurs in supercoiled circular topology, introducing supercoils into synthetic ring polymers or other biopolymers has proven elusive. Moreover, the purification methods used to extract and purify large quantities of plasmid DNA from cells often nick a fraction of the supercoiled constructs (figure 6.1), resulting in blends of torsionally relaxed rings and supercoiled constructs.

This common end product of large-scale DNA purification methods, namely blends of ring and supercoiled DNA, motivated particle-tracking and optical tweezers microrheology studies to measure the rheological properties of semidilute blends of ring and supercoiled DNA of length $L \simeq 17\ \mu\text{m}$ (50 kbp), fixed ratio $\phi_R{:}\phi_S \approx 3$ of ring to supercoiled DNA and concentrations, $\sim 0.5c^*$ to $\sim 2c^*$, that span the nominal dilute–semidilute crossover regime (figure 7.5) (Peddireddy *et al* 2020b).

Surprisingly, despite being well below the DNA entanglement concentration of $\sim 6c_L^*$, these studies revealed a crossover at $\sim c^*$ from dynamics that aligned with predictions for semidilute unentangled solutions to reptation model predictions for linear chains. Specifically, tracking of beads with diameter $2R_s = 1\ \mu\text{m}$ in the blends revealed a crossover to a rubbery $G' > G''$ regime for $c > c^*$ blends that was absent for $c \lesssim c^*$ blends (figure 7.5(A)). The elastic-dominated regime was paired with shear-thinning exponents of $x \approx 0.7$ for $c > c^*$, similar to those measured for

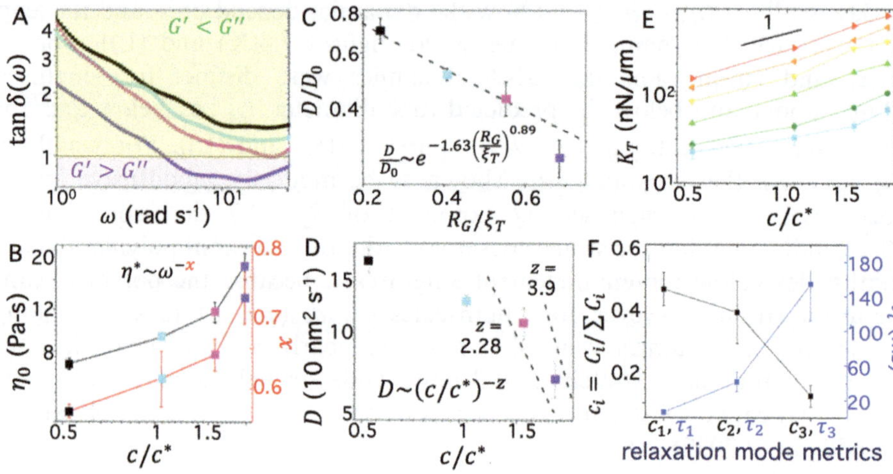

Figure 7.5. Optical tweezers and particle-tracking microrheology of semidilute blends of ring and supercoiled DNA at varying concentrations c/c^*. Particle-tracking (A–D) and optical tweezers (E, F) microrheology measurements on blends of DNA of fixed length $L \simeq 17\,\mu$m (50 kbp) and ratio of ring to supercoiled topologies $\phi_R{:}\phi_S \approx 3$, and varying total concentrations $\sim 0.5c^*$ (black), c^* (cyan), $1.5c^*$ (magenta), and $2c^*$ (purple). (A) The loss tangent $\tan\delta(\omega)$, determined from GSER analysis of MSDs of 1 μm beads, shows that the rheological properties for blends with $c \lesssim c^*$ are largely viscous (yellow region, $\tan\delta(\omega) > 1$) over the entire frequency range, but cross over to more elastic-dominated rheology for $c > c^*$ (purple region, $\tan\delta(\omega) < 1$). (B) The zero-shear viscosity η_0 (left axis, black connecting line) and shear-thinning exponent x (right axis, red connecting line) both show a crossover to steeper scaling with concentration c/c^* for $c > c^*$. (C) Diffusion coefficients D of 1 μm beads normalized by their dilute limit value D_0 plotted as a function of average radius of gyration of the blended DNA R_G scaled by the correlation blob size $\xi_T = R_G(c/c^*)^{-3/4}$ show agreement with the empirical relation shown that was previously reported for beads diffusing in semidilute unentangled linear PEG polymers (Kohli and Mukhopadhyay 2012). (D) Concentration dependence of diffusion coefficients (same data shown in C) for blends with $c > c^*$ (magenta, purple) show power-law scaling $D \sim (c/c^*)^{-z}$ that straddles predictions for beads diffusing in an entangled linear polymer solution with a tube diameter d_T that is larger ($z = 2.28$) or smaller ($z = 3.9$) than the bead diameter $2R_s$ (Pethrick 2004, Cai *et al* 2011). Data shown are for $2R_s \approx d_T$, in between these two scaling regimes. (E, F) Nonlinear OTM measurements show sustained elasticity with a terminal stiffness K_T scaling linearly with concentration c/c^* and increasing with increasing strain rates of $\dot\gamma$ (s^{-1}) $\simeq 19$ (cyan), 38 (dark green), 75 (light green), 113 (yellow), 151 (orange), and 189 (red). (F) Following nonlinear strains, the force relaxation is described by a sum of three exponentials with $\dot\gamma$-independent time constants of $\tau_1 \simeq 6$ ms, $\tau_2 \simeq 40$ ms, and $\tau_3 \simeq 150$ ms (blue, right axis) with fractional amplitudes of $c_1 \simeq 0.48$, $c_2 \simeq 0.40$, and $c_3 \simeq 0.12$ (black, left axis). Adapted from Peddireddy *et al* (2020b) with permission from the Royal Society of Chemistry.

entangled linear DNA and substantially larger than $x \approx 0.5$ measured for $c \lesssim c^*$ blends as well as semidilute unentangled linear DNA (Chapman *et al* 2014) (figure 7.5(B)). Corresponding bead diffusion coefficients for $c \lesssim c^*$ blends exhibited concentration dependence that matched the empirical relation $D/D_0 \sim e^{-1.63\,(R_G/\xi)^{0.89}}$ for semidilute unentangled linear polymer solutions (Kohli and Mukhopadhyay 2012), while $c > c^*$ blends displayed scaling $D \sim (c/c^*)^{-z}$ with z lying between predicted exponents $z = 2.28$ and $z = 3.9$ for beads of diameter $2R_s < d_T$ and $2R_s > d_T$, respectively, in entangled linear polymer solutions (Pethrick, 2004, Cai *et al* 2011). These results suggest that supercoiled polymers may thread rings when chains are overlapping to cause stronger constraints than observed for linear polymer counterparts at these concentrations to elicit entanglement-like dynamics.

Nonlinear optical tweezers measurements showed that blends exhibited sustained elastic-like force response, with terminal stiffness values K_T that were larger in magnitude than for entangled linear polymers, increased with increasing strain rate, and scaled linearly with c/c^* (figure 7.5(E)); features that are all suggestive of supercoiled-ring threadings. The force relaxation for nonlinear strains was well described by a sum of three exponentials $F_R(t) = \sum_{i=1}^{3} C_i e^{-t/\tau_i}$, with $\dot{\gamma}$-independent time constants of $\tau_1 \simeq 6$ ms, $\tau_2 \simeq 40$ ms, and $\tau_3 \simeq 150$ ms, which align closely with the Zimm time for supercoiled DNA ($\tau_1 \simeq \tau_{Z,S}$), and the Rouse time and disengagement time for ring DNA, respectively ($\tau_2 \simeq \tau_{R,R}$ and $\tau_3 \simeq \tau_{D,R}$) (figure 7.5(F)). This agreement with predictions for ring and supercoiled polymers is in opposition to the linear microrheology measurements (figures 7.5(A)–(D)) which more closely aligned with predictions for semidilute and entangled linear polymers. Moreover, the contribution of the disengagement timescale τ_3 was significantly lower than that for τ_1 and τ_2 (figure 7.5(F)), suggesting forced disentanglement or de-threading in the nonlinear regime. Taken together, the relaxation data indicate that nonlinear straining may de-thread supercoiled molecules from rings and allow rings to build up at the leading edge of the probe, enhancing the local concentration at the leading edge to more closely mimic the entangled regime. At the same time, the relaxation profiles exhibited signatures of dilute Zimm relaxation of the supercoiled constructs, which likely arise from the relaxation of the de-threaded supercoiled polymers that reside in the dilute wake of the probe.

This force-induced de-threading is similar to that described for ring-linear blends in the previous section; however, in the latter case it was the linear chains that gathered in front of the probe while the rings were 'left behind'. Generally, this may indicate that the larger and/or more easily deformed polymer gets pulled along with the probe while the more compact polymer with fewer degrees of freedom is not able to as easily move affinely with the strain.

7.2 Biopolymer composites

Beyond the access to multiple topologies that biopolymers afford, biopolymers are also unique in their wide range of stiffnesses, as described in chapter 1. For example, actin filaments have a persistence length $l_p \simeq 10$ μm that is $\sim$200× larger than that of DNA and $\sim$100× smaller than that of microtubules. At the same time, all three biopolymers span similar ranges of contour lengths and primitive path lengths, and entangled solutions thereof have comparable tube diameters and mesh sizes. Moreover, all three biopolymers are soluble in basic aqueous buffers making them ideal candidates for designing and understanding composites of flexible, semiflexible, and rigid polymers, which have been theoretically predicted to confer emergent high strength and low weight into materials for diverse industrial applications (Das and MacKintosh 2011, Thomas *et al* 2013, Golde *et al* 2018, Lopez-Menendez and Gonzalez-Torres 2019).

7.2.1 DNA–actin composites

To isolate the role that polymer flexibility plays in the dynamics of composites of flexible and stiff polymers, researchers designed composites of entangled DNA and actin in which the primitive path length, tube diameter, entanglement density, and entanglement time for the corresponding pure DNA and actin solutions were matched at $L_0 \approx 6\ \mu$m, $d_T \approx 760$ nm, $Z \approx 10$, and $\tau_e \approx 40$ ms, while the mass fraction of actin was varied as $\phi_A = 1 - \phi_{\rm DNA} = 0, 0.25, 0.5, 0.75, 1$ (figure 7.6(A)) (Fitzpatrick *et al* 2018). Optical tweezers microrheology measurements and Brownian Dynamics (BD) simulations together showed that DNA–actin composites exhibited enhanced stress-stiffening and prolonged elastic-like force response compared to single-component networks. Namely, all systems exhibited an initial increase in the effective stiffness K from the initial value K_0 to a maximum $K_{\rm max} > K_0$ after which softening ensued, with the stiffness reaching a terminal value $K_T < K_0$ (figure 7.6(B)). However, $K_{\rm max}/K_0$ and K_T/K_0 were both larger for composites than for $\phi_A = 0$ (pure DNA) and $\phi_A = 1$ (pure actin) networks and reached maxima for $\phi_A = 0.5$. Following strain, all systems displayed force relaxation curves that exhibited power-law decay with time, following an initial stalling period in which no relaxation was observed (figure 7.6(C)). The stalling time period $t_{0.9F_0}$ and terminal force F_T sustained at the end of the relaxation phase—both signatures of enhanced elastic memory—were shown to be maximized for composites (figure 7.6(C)), corroborating the strain response characteristics.

These results are quite surprising, given how much stiffer actin is compared to DNA. Despite replacing stiff actin with flexible DNA as ϕ_A is decreased from 1, the signatures of elastic strength and stiffening are actually enhanced, demonstrating that it is synergistic interactions between actin filaments and DNA that give rise to the emergent viscoelasticity. Moreover, all composites exhibit two distinct power-law decays, footprints of DNA and actin relaxation, respectively, compared to single-mode decay for pure DNA and actin networks (figure 7.6(C)).

BD simulations of the composites revealed that flexible DNA polymers drive actin filaments to form multi-filament bundles (figure 7.6(G)), while the entangled actin filaments provide a reinforcing scaffold to support the DNA mesh. These two features, both enhancing stiffness and elasticity, actually compete with one another. Namely, increasing bundling locally increases network stiffness, but also reduces the global connectivity of the actin scaffold by reducing the number of comprising fibers (now filament bundles rather than individual filaments). At comparable concentrations of actin and DNA, such as $\phi_A = 0.5$ composites, the favorable contributions from each of these processes are maximized without detrimental competition. Conversely, for lower ϕ_A values, bundling breaks actin network connections, thereby reducing stiffness; while for higher ϕ_A values, DNA-mediated depletion forces that drive actin bundling are reduced so the contribution of bundling to the emergent stiffening is reduced (figure 7.6(G)) (Fitzpatrick *et al* 2018).

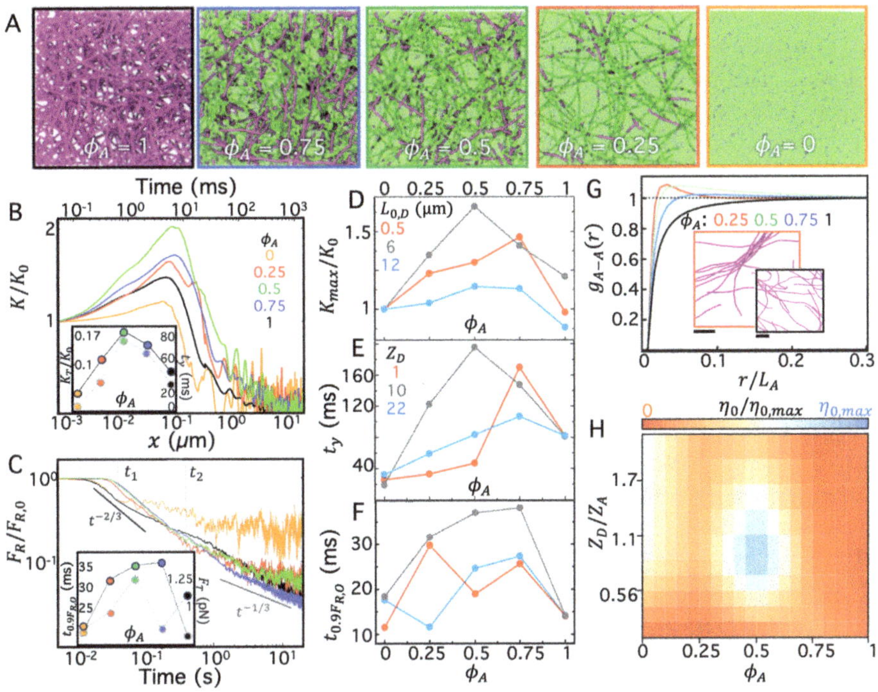

Figure 7.6. Entangled composites of actin and DNA exhibit emergent stress-stiffening and sustained elasticity. (A) Snapshots from BD simulations depicting composites of actin (purple) and DNA (green) of varying mass fractions of actin ϕ_A that maintain a primitive path length and entanglement density of both actin and DNA matched at $Z_D \approx Z_A \approx Z \approx 6\ \mu\text{m}$ and $L_{0,D} \approx L_{0,A} \approx L_0 \approx 10$. (B–E) Constant rate nonlinear OTM measurements with strain speed $v = 20\ \mu\text{m s}^{-1}$ and distance $s = 30\ \mu\text{m}$ for DNA–actin composites with $(L_0, Z) \approx (6\ \mu\text{m}, 10)$, as depicted in (A), as well as with additional DNA lengths that equate to $(L_{0,D}, Z_D) \approx (0.5\ \mu\text{m}, 1)$ (red) and $(L_{0,D}, Z_D) \approx (12\ \mu\text{m}, 22)$ (blue) (D–F). (B) Stiffness $K(x, t)$ normalized by the value K_0 measured at $(x, t) = (0{,}0)$ as a function of strain distance x and time t for $\phi_A = 0$ (orange), 0.25 (red), 0.5 (green), 0.75 (blue), and 1 (black) shows enhanced stiffening for composites as compared to single-component networks ($\phi_A = 0, 1$). (Inset) The fractional stiffness maintained at the end of the strain K_T/K_0 (left axis, black outlines) and the yield time $t_y = t(K = K_0/2e)$ at which the composite yields to more viscous-dominated response (right axis, grey outlines) both display non-monotonic dependence on ϕ_A. (C) The force relaxation following strain F_R, normalized by the initial value $F_{R,0}$, exhibits three distinct regions of power-law scaling $F_R \sim t^{-b}$ with $b \simeq 0$, $b \simeq 2/3$ and $b \simeq 1/3$ separated by timescales t_1 and t_2 (dashed lines). (Inset) The time $t_{0.9F_R}$ at which $F_R = 0.9F_{R,0}$ (left axis, black outlines), signifying the end of the initial elastic-like stalling period in which $b = 0$, and the residual force maintained at the termination of the relaxation phase F_T (right axis, grey outlines), both display non-monotonic dependence on ϕ_A. (D–F) The degree of stiffening $K_{\max}/K_0$ (D), yield time t_y (E), and stalling time $t_{0.9F_R}$ (F), as functions of ϕ_A, for composites with varying lengths of DNA listed in the legends in terms of L_0 and Z. The grey data are for the same composites shown in B, C. (G, H) BD simulations of the same composites examined in C–F show that (G) for $(L_{0,\text{D}}\ Z) \approx (6\ \mu\text{m}, 10)$, the correlation between actin filaments $g_{A-A}(r)$ separated by a distance r and plotted versus r/L_A exhibit $g_{A-A}(r) > 1$ peaks at short distances ($r/L_A < 0.1$), an indicator of increased self-association or bundling, that is absent for pure actin networks ($\phi_A = 1$, black) and most pronounced for $\phi_A = 0.5$ (green) and $\phi_A = 0.25$ (red) composites. Bundling or lack thereof is depicted in the inset simulation snapshots for $\phi_A = 0.25$ (red border) and $\phi_A = 1$ (black). This

enhanced bundling increases (H) the zero-shear viscosity η_0 above that of the single-component systems ($\phi_A = 0{,}1$). The heat map of $\eta_0/\eta_{0,\,\max}$ versus ϕ_A and Z/Z_A shows that η_0 is maximized when the DNA properties match those for actin: $\phi_A = \phi_D = 0.5$, $Z_D \approx Z_A$, $L_{0,D} \approx L_{0,A}$ (blue central region). (A, B, C, G) Adapted with permission from Fitzpatrick *et al* (2018). Copyright (2018) by the American Physical Society. (D, E, H) Adapted from Michieletto *et al* (2019) with permission from the Royal Society of Chemistry.

Follow-up studies examined the role of DNA length on the emergent phenomena, maintaining the same overall polymer concentration c, tube diameter d_T, and entanglement time τ_e as the studies described above (Michieletto *et al* 2019). By examining DNA constructs with shorter and longer primitive path lengths of $L_0 \approx 0.5\ \mu\text{m}$ and $L_0 \approx 12\ \mu\text{m}$, as compared to $L_0 \approx 6\ \mu\text{m}$ used in the original study, while maintaining the original actin parameters of $L_{0,A} \approx 6\ \mu\text{m}$ and $Z_A \approx 10$, the effect of DNA entanglement density $Z_D \approx L_0/d_T$ on the composite rheology was isolated. The same suite of measurements and simulations described above showed that the emergent non-monotonic dependence of stiffening and elastic retention on ϕ_A was robustly preserved for all DNA lengths, which spanned entanglement densities of $Z_D \approx 1-22$ (figures 7.6(D)–(F)). However, the degree of stiffening varied with Z_{DNA} due to differing abilities of the DNA to bundle or entangle with actin (figure 7.6(D)).

Surprisingly, the composite that displayed the strongest stiffening response and elastic retention was not that with the highest entanglement density, i.e., the composite with $L_{0,D} \approx 12\ \mu\text{m}$ and $Z_D \approx 22 \approx 2.2Z_A$, but rather the composite in which the entanglement densities of the two species were most strongly matched, i.e., for $L_{0,D} \approx L_{0,A} \approx 6\ \mu\text{m}$ and $Z_D \approx Z_A \approx 10$ (figures 7.6(D)–(F)). The coupling of dynamics between the two species allows for the optimum degree of bundling and entanglements, which compete with one another to stiffen the network locally and globally, respectively. BD simulations verified this competitive coupling by showing that the zero-shear viscosity was maximized for the $\phi_A = 0.5$ composite with $Z_D \approx Z_A$ (figure 7.6(H)).

DNA–actin composites at much higher total concentrations of $\rho = 5.5$ –12.5 mg mL^{-1}, compared to $\rho = 0.8$ mg mL^{-1} used in the studies described above, and fixed actin concentration that corresponded to $\phi_A \simeq 0.4-0.9$, were shown to phase separate into regions of nematically-aligned actin filaments and isotropically distributed DNA (Lai *et al* 2008). The actin domains spanned ~50–1000 μm in length and 1–20 μm in width, with the aspect ratio increasing with increasing DNA concentration, resulting in long thread-like regions of tightly bundled actin at high DNA concentrations. Notably, the domain sizes were reported to not depend on DNA length ($L \simeq 3.3\ \mu\text{m}$ versus $L \simeq 16\ \mu\text{m}$) or concentration. However, the addition of KCl decreased the domain sizes, due to charge screening, which ultimately led to mixing of the two phases for KCl concentrations above ~5 mM (Lai *et al* 2008).

The effect of microscale confinement on the structure of composites of DNA of length $L \simeq 55\ \mu\text{m}$ and actin was also examined by encapsulating composites with $\rho_D = 0.17$ mg mL^{-1} and $\rho_A = 0.065 - 1.05$ mg mL^{-1} in phospholipid-coated droplets with diameters $D \approx 6-60\ \mu$m (Negishi *et al* 2010). In bulk, as well as for droplets with $D > 16\ \mu$m and $\rho_A < 0.2$ mg mL^{-1}, composites lacked nematic alignment and exhibited structures similar to that reported in Lai *et al* (2008) under similar conditions. For the smallest droplets and highest actin concentrations, DNA was observed to be depleted to the surface of the droplets while actin both co-localized with DNA at the surface and filled the interior. When D increased and/or ρ_A decreased, actin became excluded from the DNA phase at the surface and remained entirely in the droplet interior (Negishi *et al* 2010).

7.2.2 DNA–microtubule composites

The studies described above highlight the important competing roles that microphase separation and bundling versus entanglements, connectivity and percolation play in dictating the rheology of biopolymer composites comprising two species with substantially different flexibilities. Important questions that follow are how important this competition is for composites in which the difference in flexibilities of the two polymeric species is even more substantial, and how the topology of the flexible polymer impacts this competition.

To address these questions, researchers performed OTM and confocal microscopy measurements on composites of microtubules and either linear or ring DNA of fixed length and concentration of $L \simeq 38\ \mu$m and $\rho_D = 0.65$ mg mL^{-1} (Peddireddy *et al* 2021) (figure 7.7). Varying concentrations of tubulin ($c_T = 0-7.5\ \mu$M) were incorporated into DNA solutions and allowed to polymerize in the presence of DNA. It is worth noting that this *in situ* polymerization process was optimized in the design of the DNA–actin composites described above (Fitzpatrick *et al* 2018, Michieletto *et al* 2019) to promote miscibility and isotropic network structure that mixing pre-formed filaments together can hinder (Lai *et al* 2008, Pelletier *et al* 2009).

OTM measurements showed that as the tubulin concentration increased from $c_T = 0$ to $\sim$7.5 μM, composites with ring DNA exhibited $\sim$3-fold and $\sim$40% monotonic increases in the elastic modulus ($G^0 \simeq 30$ mPa to $G^0 \simeq 100$ mPa) and shear-thinning exponent ($x \approx 0.65$ to $x \approx 0.85$), respectively (figure 7.7(A)). Both trends are indicative of increased elastic contributions to the stress response, as one may expect, as more rigid polymers are being added to the system. In contrast, for composites with linear DNA, G^0 increased by over an order of magnitude, from $G^0 \simeq 40$ mPa for $c_T = 0\ \mu$M, only slightly higher than that for the ring DNA system, to $G^0 \simeq 450$ mPa for $c_T = 2\ \mu$M (figure 7.7(A)). The shear-thinning exponent likewise increased from $x \approx 0.7$ to $x \approx 0.9$. However, as the tubulin concentration was increased further, in other words, more rigid rods were added to the DNA solution, G^0 and x surprisingly decreased. At $c_T = 7.5\ \mu$M, their values, $G^0 \simeq 65$ mPa and $x \approx 0.8$, were only slightly higher than for $c_T = 0\ \mu$M linear DNA solutions (no tubulin), and actually lower than for ring DNA solutions.

Similar topology-dependent trends were observed in response to nonlinear OTM strains of magnitude $\gamma = s/2R_s \simeq 6.7$ and $\dot{\gamma} \simeq 2.4-113$ s^{-1}. Namely, the maximum response force increased monotonically by a factor of $\sim$3 with increasing c_T for composites with ring DNA, but exhibited a non-monotonic dependence for those

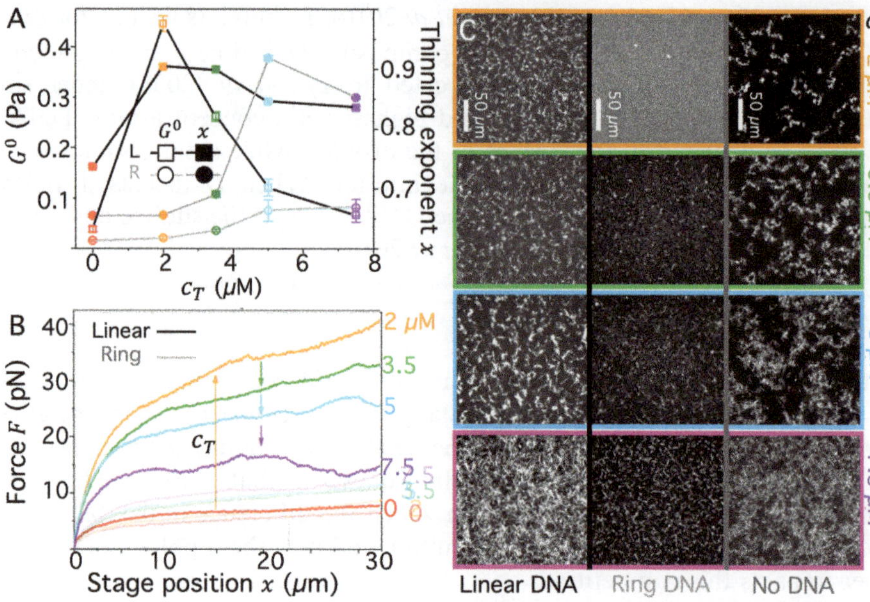

Figure 7.7. Composites self-assembled from microtubules polymerizing in the presence of linear or ring DNA exhibit topology-dependent rheology and structure. Linear OTM (A), nonlinear OTM (B), and confocal imaging (C) of composites of microtubules of varying concentrations, c_T (μM) = 0 (red), 2 (orange), 3.5 (green), 5 (cyan), 7.5 (purple), and DNA of length $L \simeq 38$ μm and concentration $\rho_D = 0.65$ mg mL^{-1} with either ring [circles (A), lighter shades (B)], or linear [squares (A), darker shades (B)] topology. (A) Elastic plateau modulus G^0 (open symbols, left axis, black lines) and shear-thinning exponent x (filled symbols, right axis, grey lines) as a function of tubulin concentration c_T for composites with ring (circles) or linear (squares) DNA. (B) The force $F(x)$ exerted by the composites to resist an optically-trapped bead moving through a distance of $s = 30$ μm at a rate of $\dot{\gamma} = 9.4$ s^{-1}. Arrows indicate the direction of increasing tubulin concentration, with color-coded c_T values listed to the right. Ring DNA values (lighter shades) are largely overlapping with each other due to the modest increase in $F(x)$ with increasing c_T. (C) Confocal microscopy images of labeled microtubules in composites with increasing c_T (top to bottom) and linear (left) and ring (middle) DNA, compared to microtubules polymerized in the absence of DNA (right). Adapted with permission from Peddireddy *et al* (2021). Copyright (2021) American Chemical Society.

with linear DNA, reaching a maximum value at $c_T = 2$ μM that was $\sim 8\times$ higher than without tubulin (figure 7.7(B)) (Peddireddy *et al* 2021).

Confocal imaging of microtubules in the composites revealed that the emergent topology-dependent stiffness and non-monotonic rheology was due to the different effects of ring and linear DNA on the polymerization of tubulin into microtubules (figure 7.7(C)). While the presence of DNA had no discernable impact on the polymerization kinetics or final steady-state composition of the actin in the DNA–actin composite studies described above (Fitzpatrick *et al* 2018, Michieletto *et al* 2019), the presence of linear DNA was found to promote microtubule polymerization while ring DNA actually inhibited polymerization. The polymerization enhancement by linear DNA may be expected as previous studies have shown that depletants or crowders can facilitate microtubule polymerization via entropic depletion interactions (Tseng and Graves 1998, Wieczorek *et al* 2013, Schummel *et al* 2017). While the inhibition by rings was more counterintuitive, previous studies have suggested that ring polymers can enhance the miscibility of blends and composites (Zhao and Choi 2006, Thomas *et al* 2013, Goh 2014, Kobayashi *et al* 2018).

The opposite effects of ring and linear DNA on microtubule polymerization led to very different steady-state composites at the same microtubule concentrations (figure 7.7(C)). At $c_T = 2\ \mu$M, a percolated network of co-entangled microtubules and linear DNA emerged, while in the presence of ring DNA, no discernible microtubule network was observed. In the absence of DNA, the resulting structure was intermediate between these two extremes, with tubulin assembling into disconnected clusters of microtubules. As c_T increased, microtubules began to emerge in the ring DNA composite but only appeared to form a connected network at $c_T \geqslant 5\ \mu$M, the same concentration at which an increase in the corresponding G^0 and x was observed (figure 7.7(A)). Conversely, microtubules in the linear DNA composites began to bundle and flocculate with increasing c_T, de-mixing from the DNA phase and reducing the microtubule network connectivity necessary for a strong elastic response. The result is a decrease in G^0 and x as microtubule entanglements are traded for larger/denser bundles, entropically driven by depletion interactions with the crowding linear DNA. This mechanism is analogous to the DNA-mediated actin bundling described above (Fitzpatrick *et al* 2018, Michieletto *et al* 2019) that led to non-monotonic dependence of stiffness on ϕ_A (figure 7.6). These studies further point to a generic mechanism underlying the emergent mechanical properties observed in composites: the synergistic coupling and competition between self-association, bundling, and de-mixing versus percolation, connectivity, and homogeneous mixing of distinct species.

7.2.3 DNA–dextran composites

Another key feature of many biopolymers is their ability to maintain structural and mechanical stability in a range of different ionic conditions and temperatures, and when mixed with synthetic polymers, colloids, phospholipids, hydrogels, or other macromolecules (Krajina *et al* 2018, Zhu *et al* 2020, Gao *et al* 2021, Nasirimarekani *et al* 2021, Clarke *et al* 2022). Dextran, Ficoll, and polyethylene glycol (PEG) are examples of synthetic polymers that are similar in size and structure to soluble proteins in cells that have been used to investigate the effect of cell-like crowding on the transport of tracer DNA and other biopolymers (Chapman *et al* 2015, Gorczyca *et al* 2015, Schummel *et al* 2017, Mardoum *et al* 2018, Aporvari *et al* 2022). However, fewer studies have examined composites of biopolymers and synthetic polymers, in which both constituents are present at significant fractions (rather than tracer concentrations).

Composites of DNA polymers with length $L \simeq 25$ kbp and dextran polymers with $M_W \simeq 500$ kDa, have been engineered with a fixed total concentration of polymers (DNA and dextran) of $11c^*$, and variable DNA volume fractions ($\phi_{\mathrm{DNA}} = 1 - \phi_{\mathrm{dex}}$) and topology (linear versus ring) (figure 7.8) (Khanal *et al* 2022). By coupling bulk rheology, DDM, and single-molecule tracking, researchers showed that bulk linear

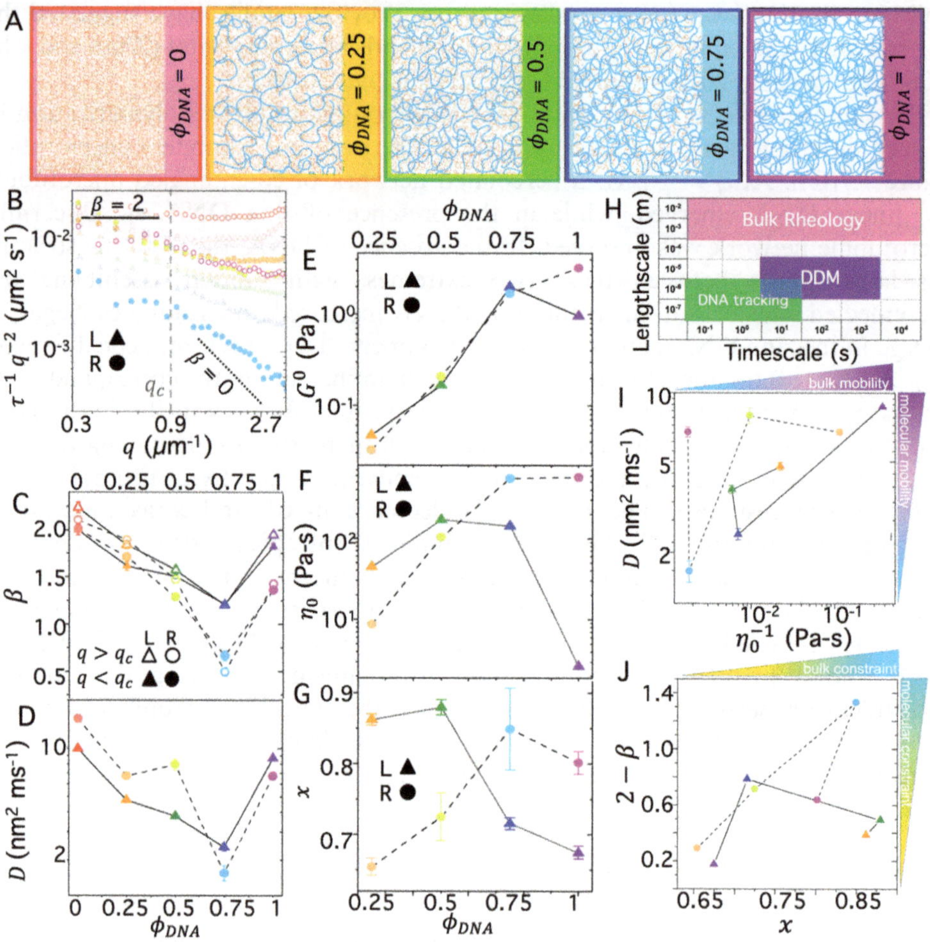

Figure 7.8. DDM and bulk rheology of composites of synthetic dextran polymers and either ring or linear DNA. (A) 11 c^* composites of dextran with $M_W \simeq 500$ kDa (red) and DNA of length $L \simeq 8.3$ μm (blue) with DNA volume fractions (indicated by color-coded borders) of $\phi_{\text{DNA}} = 0$ (red), 0.25 (orange), 0.5 (green), 0.75 (blue), and 1 (purple). The light/dark shades of each color indicate ring (light shades) or linear (dark shades) DNA at each ϕ_{DNA} in subplots B–G, I, and J. (B–D) DDM analysis of videos of fluorescent-labeled DNA in composites characterizes DNA diffusion by evaluating the (A) power-law scaling $\tau(q) \sim q^{-\beta}$ of the decay time $\tau(q)$ versus wave vector q to determine the (C) scaling exponent β that determines the deviation from normal diffusion ($\beta = 2$) and the (D) diffusion coefficient when approximating $\beta = 2$. (B) Plotting $\tau^{-1}q^{-2}$ gives a measure of diffusion via the relation $D = \tau^{-1}q^{-2}$ valid for normal diffusion in which $\beta = 2$, indicated by the horizontal black line. Negative slopes of $\tau^{-1}q^{-2}$ indicate halted motion or kinetic arrest ($\beta \to 0$). The dashed vertical line at $q_c = 0.9$ μm^{-1} denotes the lengthscale $\lambda_c = 2\pi q_c^{-1}$ at which DNA transport transitions from normal diffusion (left of the line, $\lambda > \lambda_c$, $q < q_c$) to subdiffusion (right of the line, $\lambda < \lambda_c$, $q > q_c$). Open symbols correspond to tracer linear (triangles) and ring (circles) DNA in pure dextran solutions ($\phi_{\text{DNA}} = 0$) and all $\phi_{\text{DNA}} > 0$ composites are filled triangles (linear DNA) or circles (ring DNA). (C) Scaling exponents β determined from fits of the data in (B) for $q < q_c$ (filled symbols) and $q > q_c$ (open symbols) to $\tau(q) \sim q^{-\beta}$ for composites with ring (circles, dashed lines) or linear (triangles, solid lines) DNA display non-monotonic dependence on ϕ_{DNA}, reaching a minimum at $\phi_{\text{DNA}} = 0.75$ that is more extreme for rings (circles, light shades) compared to linear DNA (triangles, dark shades). (D) Diffusion coefficients D, determined from fitting

$\tau(q < q_c)$ to $\tau(q) \sim D^{-1}q^{-2}$ exhibit similar non-monotonic dependence on ϕ_{DNA} as the scaling exponent β shown in (C). (E–G) Bulk rheology measurements of the linear viscoelastic moduli, $G'(\omega)$ and $G''(\omega)$ are evaluated to determine the (E) elastic plateau modulus $G^0 \approx G'[\omega(\tan \delta_{\min})]$, (F) zero-shear viscosity $\eta_0 \approx \eta^*(\omega \to 0)$, and (G) shear-thinning exponent x associated with the scaling relation $\eta^*(\omega) \sim \omega^{-x}$ versus ϕ_{DNA}. (H–J) The three techniques used to determine the metrics shown in (B–G) span 6 orders of spatiotemporal scales (H) to determine the extent to which signatures of (I) mobility and (J) constraints are consistent across scales or display hierarchical scale-dependence. (I) D, measured via DDM and DNA tracking, and η_0^{-1}, measured via bulk rheology, are molecular-level and bulk measures of mobility, respectively, with larger values indicating more mobile composite constituents. (J) $2 - \beta$, measured via DDM, and shear-thinning exponent x measured via bulk rheology, are molecular-level and bulk measures of constraints (e.g., entanglements), respectively, with larger values indicating stronger, more persistent constraints. (I–J) Data in the top-right and bottom-left of the plots indicate composites in which mobility and constraints are maximized and minimized, respectively, across scales. Off-diagonal composites exhibit emergent scale-dependent mobility and constraints. Adapted from Khanal *et al* (2022), with the permission of AIP Publishing.

viscoelastic properties and microscale DNA dynamics both exhibited non-monotonic dependence on ϕ_{DNA}, with exact trends tuned by the DNA topology (figure 7.8).

For both ring and linear DNA, the $\phi_{\text{DNA}} = 0.75$ composite exhibited the most pronounced subdiffusion, slowest effective diffusion coefficient D, and largest bulk zero-shear viscosity η_0, among the five ϕ_{DNA} values examined. The plateau modulus G^0 and shear-thinning exponent x were also maximized at $\phi_{\text{DNA}} = 0.75$ for the linear and ring DNA composites, respectively.

Importantly, while microscale and bulk metrics of mobility, D and η_0^{-1}, aligned with one another in some regions of the phase space, such as for $\phi_{\text{DNA}} = 0.75$ ring DNA and $\phi_{\text{DNA}} = 1$ linear DNA; in other cases, such as $\phi_{\text{DNA}} = 0.5$ and $\phi_{\text{DNA}} = 1$ ring DNA composites, the microscale mobility is relatively fast while the bulk mobility is slow. Similar scale dependence was observed for metrics of constraints, quantified as $2 - \beta$ at the microscale and x at the bulk scale. Specifically, $2 - \beta$, which is 0 for diffusive dynamics and increasingly positive with increasing subdiffusivity; and x, which is 0 for Newtonian behavior and approaches 1 for highly constrained polymer networks, were both minimized for $\phi_{\text{DNA}} = 0.25$ rings and maximized for $\phi_{\text{DNA}} = 0.75$ rings. Conversely, $\phi_{\text{DNA}} = 0.25$ and $\phi_{\text{DNA}} = 0.5$ linear DNA composites exhibited strong bulk constraints (i.e., x) but minimal microscale constraints (i.e., $2 - \beta$).

These topology-dependent and scale-dependent emergent properties were rationalized as arising from the different ways in which dextran alters the conformations and self-association of ring and linear DNA via depletion interactions, and the resulting constraints that arise from the altered conformations and interactions. Specifically, these data (figure 7.8) suggest that dextran causes linear DNA molecules to elongate from their native random coil configurations and bundle together, which either reduces DNA connectivity or creates a connected network of stiffer fibers (bundles) when ϕ_{DNA} is low or high, respectively. This phenomenon is similar to the DNA-driven bundling of cytoskeleton filaments (actin and microtubules) described in the previous sections, which leads to emergent enhanced stiffness at intermediate cytoskeletal protein concentrations. Alternatively, dextran either swells or compacts ring DNA when ϕ_{DNA} is either high ($\phi_{DNA} = 0.75$) or low ($\phi_{DNA} \leqslant 0.5$), respectively. Swelling promotes threading of rings by neighboring ring DNA and trace linear DNA contaminants, leading to the most suppressed mobility and enhanced elasticity among all composites.

7.2.4 Actin–microtubule composites

Another combination of polymer stiffness that can be examined using biopolymers, that is not easily accessible using synthetic polymers, is that of semiflexible and rigid rod polymers, of which actin and microtubules are the respective archetypes (Pelletier *et al* 2009, Ricketts *et al* 2018). Interacting networks of actin and microtubules are also of physiological significance as they are key to providing the cytoskeleton with its structural and mechanical properties (Fletcher and Mullins 2010, Pegoraro *et al* 2017, Dogterom and Koenderink 2019). However, systematic investigation of actin–microtubule composites *in vitro* was hampered until recently by the seemingly incompatible polymerization conditions (e.g., ionic strength, pH, temperature) of the two different proteins, despite their co-existence in cells.

Entangled composites. Early studies on actin-microtubule composites took advantage of Taxol stabilization to pre-form and stabilize microtubules that were then added to a polymerizing actin network to form the composite. The composite is then flowed into a sample chamber, a process that can introduce flow alignment, shearing, and bundling of filaments, as well as inconsistent mixing. Using this method, two-point particle-tracking microrheology experiments on roughly equimolar composites of actin ($c_A \simeq 23\ \mu\text{M}$) and microtubules ($c_T \simeq 22\ \mu\text{M}$) showed that the linear viscoelasticity of the composites was intermediate between that for corresponding single-component networks of actin and microtubules (Pelletier *et al* 2009). Moreover, while entangled actin solutions appeared incompressible, composites displayed a finite compressibility resulting from the high stiffness of microtubules (Pelletier *et al* 2009, Das and MacKintosh 2011).

Following this work, researchers designed hybrid polymerization conditions to enable *in situ* co-polymerization of both actin and microtubules in experimental sample chambers to reliably achieve isotropic filament orientation and mixing of the two species (Ricketts *et al* 2018, Ricketts *et al* 2020). This method also prevents shearing and flow alignment that may occur when pipetting pre-formed filaments and/or assembled networks into a sample chamber.

Using this *in situ* co-polymerization method, the mechanical properties of co-entangled composites of actin and microtubules at a total molar concentration of $c_A + c_T = 11.6\ \mu\text{M}$ and varying molar tubulin fractions $\phi_T = 1 - \phi_A$, were investigated using nonlinear OTM and two-color confocal microscopy (figure 7.9) (Ricketts *et al* 2018). Beyond the different stiffness of actin and microtubules, another important distinction that these studies highlighted was the differing mesh sizes of actin and microtubule networks at the same molarity. Because there are fewer subunits per unit length comprising actin filaments compared to microtubules, the mesh size of a microtubule network is $\sim 1.9\times$ larger than that for an actin network at the same molarity (i.e., $c_A = c_T$). Specifically, the mesh size of the actin

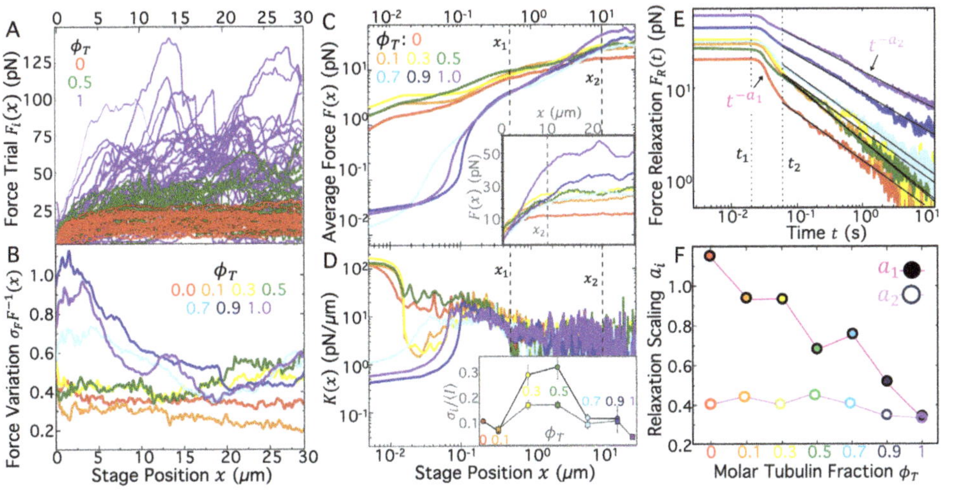

Figure 7.9. Co-entangled composites of actin filaments and microtubules exhibit stiffening, softening, and multi-phase power-law stress relaxation. Nonlinear optical tweezers microrheology measurements, with $s = 30\ \mu$m (stage positions $x = 0$ to s) and $v = 20\ \mu\text{m s}^{-1}$, performed on composites of actin filaments and microtubules at fixed overall concentration $c = 11.6\ \mu$M and varying molar fractions of actin ϕ_A and tubulin ϕ_T ($=1 - \phi_A$) $= 0$ (red), 0.1 (orange), 0.3 (yellow), 0.5 (green), 0.7 (cyan), 0.9 (blue), 1.0 (purple). (A) ~25 individual response force measurements $F_i(x)$ were performed for each ϕ_T, as shown for $\phi_T = 0$ (red), $\phi_T = 0.5$ (green), and $\phi_T = 1$ (purple), demonstrating increasing heterogeneity with increasing ϕ_T as quantified by (B) the force variation, defined as the standard deviation of F_i values across trials, normalized by their average $F = \langle F_i \rangle$, for each x value (x-axis) and ϕ_T (color-coded according to the legend). (C) Average response force $F(x)$ for each ϕ_T exhibits distinct behavior for composites that are microtubule-rich ($\phi_T > 0.5$, cyan, blue, purple) versus actin-rich ($\phi_T \leqslant 0.5$). Dashed vertical lines at $x_1 = 0.5\ \mu$m and $x_2 = 10\ \mu$m separate x ranges over which $F(x)$ curves display different functional forms and ϕ_T-dependence. Inset shows $F(x)$ on a linear scale to better show the large-x behavior. (D) Stiffness $K(x) = dF/dx$ versus x shows stiffening and softening for $\phi_T > 0.5$ and $\phi_T \leqslant 0.5$ composites, respectively. (Inset) Mobility $\sigma_I/\langle I \rangle$ of actin filaments (circles) and microtubules (squares), determined from the standard deviation of pixel intensities σ_I over the course of a confocal time-series, scaled by the average value $\langle I \rangle$, shows non-monotonic dependence on ϕ_T reaching a maximum at $\phi_T = 0.5$ (green). (E) Force relaxation F_R versus time t after the strain is halted exhibits an initial stalling period with constant F_R, followed by two phases of power-law relaxation $F_R \sim t^{-a_i}$ with distinct scaling exponents a_i plotted in (F). Dashed vertical lines at $t_1 = 20$ ms and $t_2 = 60$ ms separate the three phases. (F) Scaling exponents a_1 and a_2 versus ϕ_T determined via power-law fits to $F_R(t)$ for $\Delta t = 0 - t_1$ (filled symbols, magenta connecting lines) and $\Delta t = t_1 - t_2$ (open symbols, lavender connecting lines). Adapted from Ricketts *et al* (2018), Copyright (2018), with permission from Elsevier.

and microtubule networks comprising a composite can be computed via the relations

$$\xi_A \backsimeq 0.3\rho_A^{-1/2} \backsimeq 1.44 c_A^{-1/2} \tag{7.1}$$

$$\xi_{MT} \backsimeq 0.89\rho_T^{-1/2} \backsimeq 2.68 c_T^{-1/2} \tag{7.2}$$

where $\rho_{A/T}$ and $c_{A/T}$ are in units of mg mL^{-1} and μM.

From the single-component mesh sizes, an effective composite mesh size can be computed via

$$\xi_C \simeq (\xi_A^{-3} + \xi_{MT}^{-3})^{-1/3} \tag{7.3}$$

(Ricketts *et al* 2018).

These studies showed that the interplay between increasing mesh size (reduced network connectivity) and increasing polymer stiffness as ϕ_T goes from 0 to 1 (i.e., as actin filaments are replaced with microtubules), leads to emergent properties for composites with comparable molar concentrations of actin and tubulin, as I discuss below.

The response force $F(x)$ of composites subject to nonlinear OTM strains of $s = 30\ \mu$m and $v = 20\ \mu$m s^{-1} revealed that microtubule-rich composites ($\phi_T > 0.5$) exhibited substantially larger trial-to-trial variations as well as large x-dependent peaks and dips in each trial, both of which were reduced in actin-rich composites ($\phi_T \leqslant 0.5$) due to their smaller mesh size and ability of actin to bend in response to strain (figures 7.9(A) and (B)). The semiflexible actin mesh also supported microtubules against force-induced buckling, responsible for the large fluctuations observed in microtubule-rich composites (figure 7.9(A)), by partially absorbing and redistributing stresses, likewise reducing spatial heterogeneities. The trial-to-trial variation and x-dependence of this variation, quantified as the standard deviation $\sigma_F(x)$ of trial force values $F_i(x)$, scaled by the average $F(x)$, (figure 7.9(B)) demonstrates the suppression of large heterogeneities that results from trading microtubules for actin (reducing ϕ_T), as well as the small lengthscales, of order $\sim\xi_C$, over which the force variation is most apparent.

The average response force $F(x)$ for composites exhibited complex x-dependence that could largely be divided into two classes of behavior based on ϕ_T (figure 7.9(C)). At small strain distances, below $x_1 \approx 0.5\ \mu$m, actin-rich ($\phi_T \leqslant 0.5$) composites exhibited ~40-fold higher force values compared to microtubule-rich composites, which was shown to arise from faster poroelastic relaxation of stiffer and less connected microtubule-rich composites. Conversely, for strain distances above $x_1 \approx 10\ \mu$m, $\phi_T > 0.5$ composites exhibited substantially larger resistive forces than actin-rich composites, owing to the rigidity of the microtubules (figure 7.9(C) inset). Evaluating the stiffness $K(x) = dF/dx$ revealed that the small-x poroelasticity and large-x bulk rigidity was connected via a region of either stiffening $\frac{dK(x)}{dx} > 0$ for $\phi_T > 0.5$ or softening $\frac{dK(x)}{dx} < 0$ for $\phi_T \leqslant 0.5$ (figure 7.9(D)), due to the ability of microtubules to suppress actin bending modes necessary for softening.

This complex lengthscale-dependent response force was shown to arise from the emergent mobility of actin filaments and microtubules in composites with comparable concentrations of actin and tubulin ($\phi_T \simeq 0.5$), as measured via confocal microscopy (Ricketts *et al* 2018). Specifically, the standard deviation of pixel intensities σ_I in a given confocal time-series, scaled by the average value $\langle I \rangle$, gives a measure of how mobile the filaments are, revealing a non-monotonic dependence on ϕ_T with a maximum at $\phi_T = 0.5$ (figure 7.9(D) inset).

The force relaxation following strain F_R for all composites exhibited an initial stalling period for times $t < t_1 \approx 20$ ms, with no measurable force decay, followed by two phases of power-law decay described by $F_R \sim t^{-a_i}$, with different scaling exponents, a_1 and a_2, for times $t_1 < t < t_2 \approx 60$ ms and $t > t_2$ (figures 7.9(E) and (F)). This multi-modal power-law decay, similar to that observed in DNA–actin composites (Fitzpatrick *et al* 2018) and entangled DNA networks (Chapman and Robertson-Anderson 2014), is indicative of a broad spectrum of relaxation timescales. The three relaxation phases were shown to be dictated by poroelasticity ($F_R \sim t^0$, $t < t_1$), actin bending ($F_R \sim t^{-a_1}$, $t_1 < t < t_2$), and modified reptation ($F_R \sim t^{-a_2}$, $t > t_2$). Contributions from actin bending were progressively suppressed with increasing ϕ_T, seen as $a_1 \rightarrow a_2$ (figure 7.9(F)) while the scaling exponent describing the reptation regime a_2, which quantifies how quickly the force decays, displayed a non-monotonic dependence on ϕ_T, reaching a local maximum at $\phi_T = 0.5$ (figure 7.9(F)). This indicator of maximal mobility, corroborated by confocal microscopy mobility measurements (figure 7.9(D)), is evidence of the competition between increasing mesh size, that weakens the composite, and filament stiffness, that strengthens the composite. At equimolar ratios of actin and tubulin, the mesh size and flexibility are both sufficiently large to elicit the highest mobility. As ϕ_T increases or decreases, the flexibility or mesh size are respectively reduced to hinder mobility. This emergent behavior is similar in spirit to the competitive and synergistic mechanisms seen in other biopolymer composites, some of which are described above (Fitzpatrick *et al* 2018, Michieletto *et al* 2019, Peddireddy *et al* 2021, Khanal *et al* 2022).

Crosslinked composites. A useful feature of *in vitro* actin–microtubule composites is the ability to crosslink filaments with high specificity and versatility, allowing for actin–actin, microtubule–microtubule and actin–microtubule crosslinking with programmable molar ratios R of crosslinker to filamentous protein (Lin *et al* 2011, Francis *et al* 2019, Ricketts *et al* 2019, Farhadi *et al* 2020, Berezney *et al* 2022). Myriad physiological crosslinking proteins may be incorporated into composites to crosslink actin and/or microtubules. However, care must be taken in evaluating the contribution of these crosslinkers to composite dynamics, as they have different binding affinities, duty ratios, on/off rates, sizes, stiffnesses, and binding orientations that need to be considered (Tseng *et al* 2001, Strehle *et al* 2011, Yao *et al* 2011, Pringle *et al* 2013, Wang *et al* 2020).

An alternative 'synthetic' crosslinking method that eliminates many of these factors, to isolate the role of crosslinker ratio R on composite dynamics, is to incorporate biotinylated subunits (actin monomers and/or tubulin dimers) into the filaments (actin and/or microtubules), at a subunit fraction that can be tuned, and to use NeutrAvidin (NA), or another molecule in the avidin family, to form crosslinks between biotinylated subunits of different filaments (Ricketts *et al* 2020). By selectively incorporating biotinylated actin monomers, tubulin dimers, or both, and by pre-forming NA–biotin–subunit complexes, actin–actin crosslinks, microtubule–microtubule crosslinks, actin–microtubule crosslinks, or both actin–actin and microtubule–microtubule crosslinks can be incorporated into the same actin–microtubule composites discussed above (Ricketts *et al* 2020).

The biotin-NA bond can be considered static and permanent, such that crosslinking affinities and dynamics (i.e., on/off rates) can be neglected. Moreover, the length between crosslinks l_c, an important contributor to the mechanics and structure of the composites, can be computed directly for actin–actin, microtubule–microtubule, and actin–microtubule crosslinking via the respective relations:

$$l_{c,A} \simeq \frac{1}{2} l_{\text{mon}} \times R^{-1} \tag{7.4}$$

$$l_{c,MT} \simeq \frac{1}{2} (l_{\text{ring}}/13) \times R^{-1} \tag{7.5}$$

$$l_{c,A-MT} \simeq (l_{c,A} \times l_{c,MT})^{-1/2} \tag{7.6}$$

where $l_{\text{mon}} \simeq 2.7$ nm is the length that each actin monomer adds to an actin filament and $l_{\text{ring}} \simeq 7.8$ nm is the length that every ring of 13 tubulin dimers adds to a microtubule (Ricketts *et al* 2019).

Using this synthetic crosslinking approach, the effect of crosslinking on the mechanics and mobility of equimolar actin–microtubule composites, equivalent to the $\phi_A = 0.5$ composite in figure 7.9 (Ricketts *et al* 2018), have been characterized using linear and nonlinear OTM and two-color confocal microscopy (figure 7.10).

One such study examined the effect of crosslinking type—actin–actin ('actin'), microtubule–microtubule ('microtubule'), actin–microtubule ('co-linked'), and both 'actin' and 'microtubule' ('both', 'both 2×')—on the linear and nonlinear rheological properties of composites at fixed crosslinker ratio $R = 0.02$ (figure 7.10(A)), showing that all composites exhibited similar complex viscosity values $\eta^*(\omega)$ and thinning exponents $x \approx 0.5$ (figure 7.10(B)). Intriguingly, in the absence of crosslinkers, actin and microtubules displayed similar mobilities, $\sigma_I/\langle I \rangle$, as computed from confocal time-series (figure 7.10(A)), whereas all crosslinking types markedly suppressed the mobility of microtubules while having less impact on actin—even in composites with only actin crosslinking (figure 7.10(C)).

At mesoscopic scales ($x \gtrsim 1$ μm), the crosslinking motif played a more prominent role in the force response (figures 7.10(D)–(F)), with composites separating into two distinct classes of mechanical response when subject to nonlinear strains of $s = 10$ μm and $v = 10$ μm s^{-1} (figure 7.10(D)). Namely, 'actin' and 'both' crosslinking elicit viscoelastic stress-softening (figure 7.10(D)), i.e., $\frac{dK}{dx} < 0$, and similar x-averaged values of force $\langle F \rangle$ and stiffness $\langle K \rangle$ that are modestly larger than composites without crosslinkers ('none') (figure 7.10(E)). Conversely, 'microtubule', 'co-linked' and 'both 2×' motifs result in nearly elastic response, with a linear increase in force $F(x) \sim x$ and $\frac{dK}{dx} \approx 0$. The corresponding $\langle F \rangle$ and $\langle K \rangle$ values, similar among the three composites, were substantially larger than those for the class of softening composites (figure 7.10(E)). The force relaxation following strain likewise exhibits signatures of viscous dissipation for 'actin', 'both' and 'none' versus elastic storage for 'microtubule', 'co-linked' and 'both 2×', as quantified by the residual force $F_{R,\infty}$ sustained at the end of the relaxation phase, and the fractional force relaxation

$$\Delta f_R = (F_{R,0} - F_{R,\infty})/F_{R,0} \tag{7.7}$$

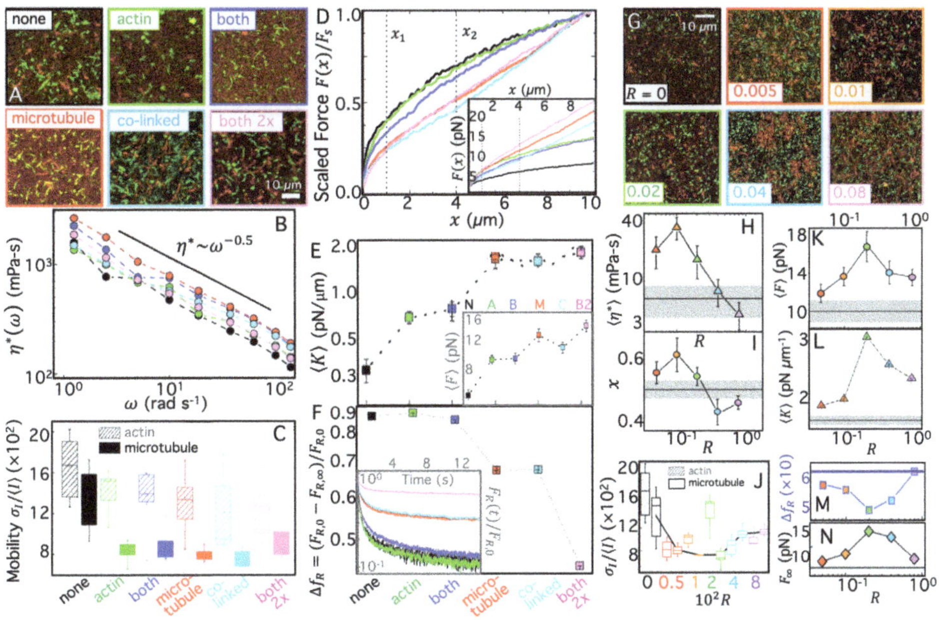

Figure 7.10. Composites of actin and microtubules with varying patterns and densities of biotin-NeutrAvidin crosslinking. Two-color confocal microscopy (A, G) and OTM (B–F, G–L) were used to characterize the linear viscoelasticity (B, H, I), nonlinear force response (D, E, J, K), stress relaxation (F, M), and quiescent filament mobility (C, L) of equimolar actin–microtubule composites with fixed concentration $c_T = c_A = 2.9$ μm and (A–F) varying types of crosslinking at fixed crosslinker:protein ratio $R = 0.02$ (shown/listed/color-coded in A) or (G–N) varying ratios of actin–actin crosslinking (shown/listed/color-coded in G). (A, G) Confocal micrographs of actin (green) and microtubules (microtubule, red) in composites with crosslinking of (A) no filaments (none, black border), actin to actin (green border), microtubules to microtubules, (red), actin to microtubules (co-linked, cyan), and both actin to actin and microtubules to microtubules at total $R = 0.02$ (both, blue) and $R = 0.04$ (both 2×, magenta); as well as (G) actin to actin at ratios $R = 0$ (black border), 0.005 (red), 0.01 (orange), 0.02 (green), 0.04 (cyan), and 0.08 (magenta). (B) Complex viscosity $\eta^*(\omega)$ versus oscillation frequency ω, determined from oscillatory OTM, exhibits shear thinning with exponent $x \simeq 0.5$ (solid black line) for all crosslinking types. (C) Mobility $\sigma_I/\langle I\rangle$ of actin filaments (hashed) and microtubules (filled), determined from the standard deviation in pixel intensities σ_I over the course of a confocal time-series, are suppressed by crosslinking of all types with the mobility of microtubules being more impacted than actin. (D) The response force $F(x)$, scaled by the value at the end of the $s = 10$ μm strain F_s, versus strain distance x, shows either elastic-like (microtubule, co-linked, 2× both) or more viscous-like (none, actin, both) response. Dashed vertical lines at $x_1 = 1$ μm and $x_2 = 4$ μm divide $F(x)$ into three Δx ranges with different functional forms. Inset shows unscaled $F(x)$. (E) The stiffness $K(x) = \frac{dF}{dx}$, averaged over all $x > x_2$, $\langle K\rangle$, for different crosslinking motifs quantifies the ~3-fold increased elasticity maintained in 'microtubule' (red), 'co-linked' (cyan), and 'both 2×' (magenta) composites compared to 'actin' (green) and 'both' (blue) composites. Inset shows the corresponding force averaged over $x > x_2$, $\langle F\rangle$, showing similar trends as $\langle K\rangle$. (F) The degree of force relaxation, quantified as the fractional difference between the force at the beginning $F_{R,0}$ and end $F_{R,\infty}$ of the relaxation phase, $\Delta f_R = (F_{R,0} - F_{R,\infty})/F_{R,0}$, with $\Delta f_R \to 0$ and 1 for complete elastic storage and viscous dissipation, respectively. (Inset) $F_R(t)$ curves from which Δf_R is computed. (H, I) Linear oscillatory OTM measurements of the (H) complex viscosity averaged over all measured frequencies $\langle\eta^*\rangle$ and (I) thinning exponent x from $\eta^*(\omega) \sim \omega^{-x}$ reveal non-monotonic dependence on crosslinker:actin ratio R, reaching maxima for $R = 0.01$. Horizontal black line and grey region in (H, I) indicate the corresponding average and standard error for $R = 0$. (J) Mobility of actin filaments (hashed boxes) and microtubules (open boxes), quantified by the fractional standard deviation of pixel intensities, $\sigma_I/\langle I\rangle$, as described in figure 7.9, show similar non-monotonic dependence on R, with microtubule mobility reaching a minimum at $R \approx 0.01$. (K, L) Response force (K) and stiffness (L),

averaged over all x values of a strain of $s = 10$ μm and $v = 10$ μm s^{-1}, both display non-monotonic dependence on R reaching a local maxima at $R = 0.02$. (M, N) The force relaxation following strain also exhibits non-monotonic dependence on R, with the (M) fractional dissipation Δf_R and (N) residual force $F_{R,\infty}$ reaching a local minimum and maximum, respectively, at $R = 0.02$. Blue (M) and black (N) horizontal lines indicate values for $R = 0$. (A–F) Adapted from Ricketts *et al* (2019). CC BY 4.0. (G–N) Adapted from Francis *et al* (2019) with permission from the Royal Society of Chemistry.

with $\Delta f_R \to 1$ and $\Delta f_R \to 0$ signifying complete dissipation and elastic storage, respectively. Namely, $F_{R,\infty}$ was lower and Δf_R was higher for 'actin', 'both' and 'none' composites compared to the elastic-like class of composites (figure 7.10(F)). These two distinct classes were shown to be dictated by the degree to which microtubules were crosslinked, and suggest that scale-dependent mechanics may play an important role in the ability of the cellular cytoskeleton to mediate a vast array of different mechanical processes.

To determine how these results depend on R, similar experiments were performed with the same equimolar actin–microtubule composites as in Ricketts *et al* (2019) (figures 7.10(A)–(F)), but focusing solely on actin crosslinking at varying crosslinker: actin ratios $R = 0.005 - 0.08$ (figure 7.10(G)) (Francis *et al* 2019). As I describe in chapter 5, many previous studies have shown that increasing R in actin networks increases elasticity and stiffness (e.g., Tseng *et al* 2001, Gardel *et al* 2004, Shin *et al* 2004, Wang *et al* 2020). In stark contrast, the results described in figures 7.10(G)–(N) for actin–microtubule composites reveal a non-monotonic dependence of viscoelasticity (figures 7.10(H) and (I)), nonlinear response force (figure 7.10(K)), stiffness (figure 7.10(L)), and elastic storage (figures 7.10(M) and (N)) on the crosslinker ratio. All of the metrics first increased from $R = 0$ to $R \approx 0.1$ then decreased as R continued to increase to $R = 0.8$, reaching a response similar to or even lower (figures 7.10(H) and (I)) than $R = 0$ composites.

For example, the average complex viscosity $\langle \eta^* \rangle$ was shown to decrease by nearly an order of magnitude as the crosslinker ratio increased from $R = 0.01$ to $R = 0.08$ (figure 7.10(H)), and the thinning exponent x likewise decreased over this R range, reaching values ~15% lower than the $R = 0$ composite (figure 7.10(I)) (Francis *et al* 2019). Moreover, the average force $\langle F \rangle$ and corresponding stiffness $\langle K \rangle$ measured in response to nonlinear strains ($s = 10$ μm, $v = 10$ μm s^{-1}) were shown to increase from $R = 0$ to $R = 0.02$, followed by a substantial decrease from $R = 0.02$ to $R = 0.08$ (figures 7.10(K) and (L)). These non-monotonic signatures of increasing or decreasing elastic storage and stiffening or softening for $0 \leqslant R \leqslant 0.02$ or $0.02 \leqslant R \leqslant 0.08$ were corroborated by the nonlinear force relaxation profiles, which showed the same non-monotonic dependence on the fractional dissipation Δf_R (figure 7.10(M)) and residual force $F_{R,\infty}$ (figure 7.10(N)), reaching a respective minimum and maximum at $R = 0.02$.

Unlike the effect of the crosslinking motif discussed above (figures 7.10(A)–(F)) (Ricketts *et al* 2019), the non-monotonic R dependence persisted from steady-state to nonlinear regimes and over micro- and mesoscopic scales. However, similar to these studies (figure 7.10(C)) (Ricketts *et al* 2019), steady-state mobility measurements showed that actin crosslinking had a stronger impact on the mobility of microtubules versus actin (figure 7.10(J)), indicating that it is the microtubule mobility that controls the composite stiffness. Namely, microtubule mobility is slowed most substantially when the actin network that scaffolds microtubules is both rigidly crosslinked and sufficiently dense, which occurs at intermediate R values. Too much crosslinking leads to actin bundling, thereby increasing the actin scaffold mesh size and thus allowing for more microtubule mobility. Conversely, too few crosslinks confer a dense but floppy scaffold that is insufficient to markedly suppress microtubule fluctuations.

Complementary nonlinear bulk rheology measurements were performed on composites of actin at $c_A \simeq 12$ μM and microtubules at varying concentrations of $c_T \simeq 1$ μM ($\phi_T = 0.08$), 2 μM ($\phi_T = 0.14$), and 4 μM ($\phi_T = 0.25$) (figure 7.11) (Lin

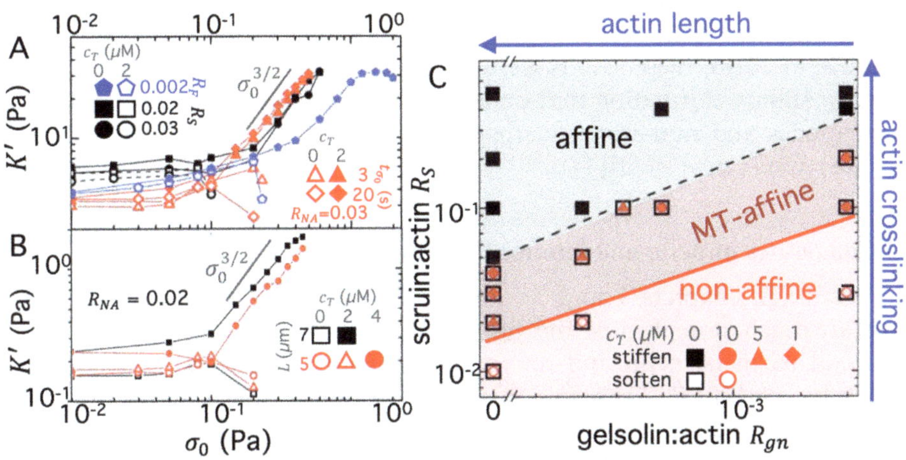

Figure 7.11. Nonlinear bulk rheological properties of actin–microtubule composites with varying microtubule concentrations and actin filament lengths. (A, B) Nonlinear bulk rheology measurements were performed on composites of actin at $c_A = 12$ μM and microtubules at $c_T = 1, 2,$ or 4 μM with varying ratios R_X and types X of crosslinkers (scruin: $X = S$, filamin: $X = F$, NeutrAvidin, $X = NA$). The actin length L was controlled by including varying gelsolin:actin ratios R_{gn}. (A) The bulk differential modulus $K' = d\sigma/d\gamma$ versus pre-stress σ_0 for actin networks ($c_T = 0$, open symbols) and composites with $c_T = 2$ μM (filled symbols) and crosslinked by filamin (blue), scruin (black) or NeutrAvidin (red) at crosslinker ratios of $R_F = 0.002$ (pentagons), $R_S = 0.02$ (squares), $R_S = 0.03$ (circles), or $R_{NA} = 0.03$ (triangles, diamonds). For NA-crosslinked composites, time in the pre-stress state also varied ($t_{\sigma_0} = 3$ s (triangles), $t_{\sigma_0} = 20$ s (diamonds). All composites exhibit power-law strain-stiffening $K' \sim \sigma_0^{3/2}$ (grey line) above a critical stress $\sigma_0 \sim 10^{-1}$ Pa, that is absent for actin networks (open squares and circles). (B) Reducing the actin filament length from $L \simeq 7$ μm (black squares) to $L \simeq 5$ μm (red symbols), in composites with $R_{NA} = 0.02$ and $c_T = 2$ μM (open triangles), eliminated the strain-stiffening behavior seen for composites with $L \simeq 7$ μm (black filled squares). Stiffening, with scaling $K' \sim \sigma_0^{3/2}$ (grey line), was recovered in composites with $L \simeq 5$ μm by increasing tubulin concentration to $c_T = 4$ μM (red filled circles). (C) Phase map of affine (black) and non-affine (red) deformation, underlying stiffening and softening, respectively, as functions of actin crosslinking (R_S, y-axis) and length (R_{gn}, x-axis). Without microtubules ($c_T = 0$, black squares), the dashed line separates affine (filled squares, black shaded region) and non-affine (open squares, red shaded region) regimes. Microtubules increase the stiffening/affine region of the phase space, indicated by the 'MT-affine' area with open (softening) black symbols overlapping with filled (stiffening) red symbols, and the lower red solid line that separates the affine and non-affine regions for composites. Data shown are for varying tubulin concentrations as listed in the legend. The positive slopes of the border lines show that increasing actin length (horizontal blue arrow, lowering R_{gn}) reduces the degree of crosslinking necessary for stiffening (vertical blue arrow, lowering R_S). Adapted from Lin *et al* (2011) with permission from the Royal Society of Chemistry.

et al 2011). The effect of actin crosslinking was investigated by incorporating physiological crosslinkers, scruin and filamin, as well as biotin-NeutrAvidin, at ratios $R = 0.005 - 0.08$ (figure 7.11(A)). For all crosslinkers, the presence of microtubules, even at less than 10% (i.e. $\phi_T = 0.08$) was sufficient to switch the nonlinear strain-softening behavior (i.e., $\frac{dK'}{d\sigma} < 1$) exhibited by weakly crosslinked actin networks to strain-stiffening (i.e., $\frac{dK'}{d\sigma} > 1$), with the critical microtubule concentration necessary to induce stiffening increasing with decreasing R (figures 7.11(A) and (B)). These studies also incorporated gelsolin at varying gelsolin:actin ratios R_{gn} to control the actin filament length L (figure 7.11(B)), and showed that the critical tubulin concentration c_T needed to switch the strain response from softening to stiffening increased with decreasing L (increasing R_{gn}) (figure 7.11(C)). Similar to (Ricketts *et al* 2018), these results were suggested to be caused by the microtubules facilitating affine deformation that underlies stress-stiffening, and suppressing actin bending modes and non-affine fluctuations that manifest as bulk stress-softening (figure 7.11(C)) (Lin *et al* 2011).

7.2.5 Composites of actin and intermediate filaments

As I describe in chapters 1 and 5, intermediate filaments, such as vimentin and keratin, are much more flexible and susceptible to counterion-crosslinking than their cytoskeletal partners, actin and microtubules (Herrmann *et al* 2007, Block *et al* 2015, Köster *et al* 2015). These unique properties suggest that *in vitro* composites of actin and intermediate filaments may exhibit emergent behavior that is quite different than that of the actin–microtubule composites discussed in section 7.2.4.

To investigate potential emergent properties, several studies have engineered and measured the rheological properties of actin–vimentin composites with varying actin and vimentin concentrations, actin crosslinker ratios and buffer conditions, reporting complex and conflicting results (Esue *et al* 2006, Jensen *et al* 2014, Golde *et al* 2018, Lopez-Menendez and Gonzalez-Torres 2019).

Bulk rheology measurements on actin–vimentin composites that were co-polymerized at a fixed overall protein concentration of $c_A + c_V = 24\ \mu$M and varying molar actin fractions $\phi_A = 0 - 1$, showed that composites exhibited significantly higher elastic modulus G' than single-component networks over four decades of frequency ω (figure 7.12(A)) (Esue *et al* 2006). At a given frequency, G' displayed a non-monotonic dependence on ϕ_A, reaching a maximum at $\phi_A = 0.25$ that was ~3-fold or ~4-fold larger than for single-component networks of vimentin ($\phi_A = 0$) or actin ($\phi_A = 1$), suggestive of increased elasticity (figure 7.12(B)). Counter to this observation, the power-law dependence of G' with ω, $G' \sim \omega^b$, increased monotonically with increasing ϕ_A, from $b = \frac{3}{40}$ for $\phi_A = 0$ to $b = \frac{15}{40}$ for $\phi_A = 1$ (figure 7.12(B) inset), indicating increasingly dissipative dynamics as vimentin is replaced with actin (Esue *et al* 2006).

These counterintuitive results were shown to arise from non-specific crosslinking between actin filaments and the tail domain of vimentin (figures 7.12(C) and (D)) (Esue *et al* 2006). Specifically, when full-length vimentin was replaced with a

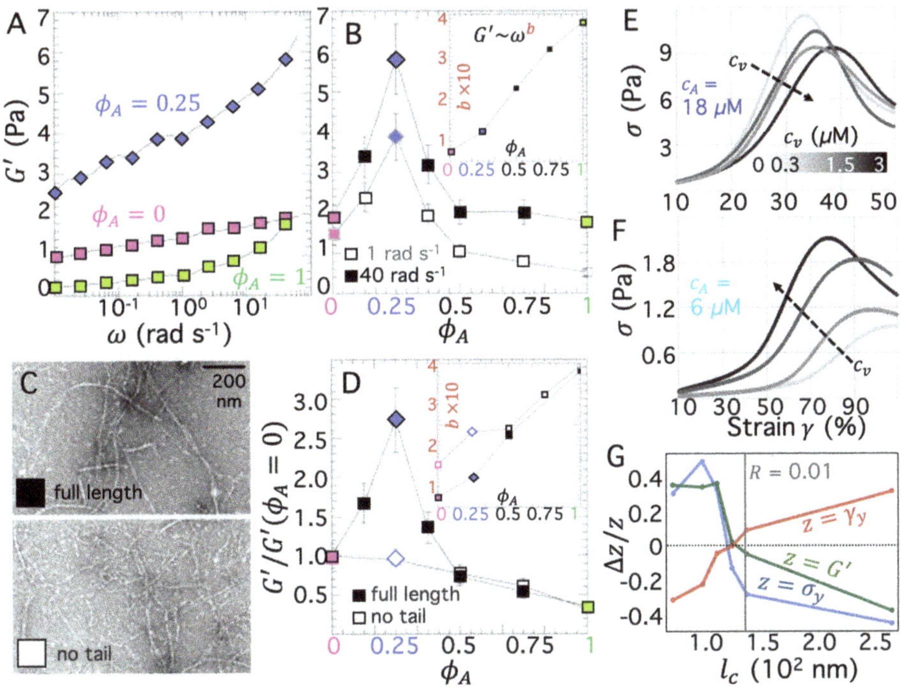

Figure 7.12. Actin–vimentin composites display emergent bulk rheological properties. (A) Bulk elastic modulus $G'(\omega)$ versus oscillation frequency ω for actin–vimentin composites with $c_A + c_V = 24\,\mu$M and molar actin fractions of $\phi_A = 0$ (vimentin only, magenta squares), $\phi_A = 1$ (actin only, green squares) and $\phi_A = 0.25$ (composite) blue diamonds). (B) G' measured at $\omega = 40$ rad s^{-1} (filled symbols) and $\omega = 1$ rad s^{-1} (open symbols) for the same composites in (A), color-coded accordingly, as well as for additional ϕ_A values, plotted as a function of ϕ_A. (Inset) G' follows power-law scaling $G' \sim \omega^b$ with an exponent that increases with increasing ϕ_A. (C) Electron micrographs of equimolar composites ($c_A = c_V = 1\,\mu$M) of actin and either full-length vimentin (top) or vimentin that is missing the tail domain suspected to interact with actin (bottom) show minimal structural difference. (D) Elastic modulus G' measured at $\omega = 1$ rad s^{-1} and normalized by the vimentin-only value $G'(\phi_A = 0)$ for composites with either full-length (filled symbols) or truncated (open symbols) vimentin shows that the emergent elasticity of composites is mediated by direct interactions between actin and the tail domain of vimentin. (Inset) Scaling exponent b that describes the scaling $G' \sim \omega^b$ is larger for truncated vimentin. (E, F) Bulk nonlinear stress $\sigma(\gamma)$ versus strain γ measured for composites of vimentin, with c_v (μM) = 0 (light grey), 0.3 (grey), 1.5 (dark grey), and 3 (black), and NeutrAvidin-crosslinked actin with $R = 0.01$ and either $c_A = 18\,\mu$M (E) or $c_A = 6\,\mu$M (F). (G) The fractional change in yield strain (red), linear elastic modulus (green), and yield stress (blue) upon co-polymerizing actin networks at $c_A = 15\,\mu$M with vimentin at $c_V = 3\,\mu$M (compared to no vimentin) as a function of length between crosslinkers l_c. (A–D) Adapted from Esue *et al* (2006). CC BY 4.0. (E–G) Jensen *et al* (2014), adapted by permission of the publisher (Taylor & Francis Ltd, http://www.tandfonline.com.).

construct that lacked the tail domain, the maximum in G' at $\phi_A = 0.25$ was eliminated and instead G' decreased monotonically with increasing ϕ_A (figure 7.12(D)). The frequency dependence of G' was likewise higher for $\phi_A < 0.5$ composites as compared to those with full-length vimentin (figure 7.12(D) inset). Electron micrographs of composites with full-length and truncated vimentin displayed no obvious structural differences, suggesting that the tail indeed mediates direct crosslinking with actin to increase elasticity, rather than altering the composite structure (figure 7.12(C)) (Esue *et al* 2006).

Following these findings, nonlinear bulk rheology measurements (Jensen *et al* 2014) of actin networks, crosslinked via biotin-NeutrAvidin at $R = 0.01$ and polymerized at concentrations of $c_A = 6-18\ \mu$M in the presence of varying concentrations of vimentin $c_V = 0.3-3\ \mu$M, showed that all composites exhibited linear elasticity, i.e., $\frac{d\sigma}{d\gamma} = 0$, at small strains ($\gamma \lesssim 20\%$), followed by stress-stiffening ($K' = \frac{d\sigma}{d\gamma} > 1$) then softening ($K' = \frac{d\sigma}{d\gamma} < 1$) (figure 7.12(E) and (F)). For $c_A < 12\ \mu$M, vimentin substantially increased the maximum stiffness $K'_{\max}$ and yield stress $\sigma_y = \sigma(K'_{\max})$ (figure 7.12(E)), while for $c_A > 15\ \mu$M, a decrease in both parameters was observed (figure 7.12(F)). Despite the substantial effect of vimentin on the nonlinear response of actin networks, varying c_V had little impact on the linear elasticity, quantified by $G' = K'(\gamma \to 0)$ (figures 7.12(E) and (F)).

This same study showed that this complex dependence on both c_V and c_T arose from the varying ratios of actin mesh size ξ ($\sim c_A^{-1/2}$) to crosslinker length l_c ($\sim R^{-1}$) in the composites (Jensen *et al* 2014). The addition of vimentin to sparsely crosslinked actin networks, with $l_c > \xi$, lowered the degree of actin crosslinking via steric interactions with vimentin that blocked available crosslinking sites, serving to reduce G' and σ_y and increase the yield strain γ_y (figure 7.12(G)). In the opposite limit of $l_c > \xi$, in which crosslinkers are abundant enough to ensure connections between actin filaments, even if some sites are blocked, steric entanglements with vimentin provide reinforcement to the actin network that suppresses the dissipative fluctuations that underlie stress-softening, leading to an increase in G' and σ_y and decrease in γ_y (figure 7.12(G)) (Jensen *et al* 2014).

A theoretical model based on a nonlinear continuum mechanics framework was proposed to describe the emergent nonlinear rheological behavior described above (figures 7.12(E)–(G)) (Jensen *et al* 2014, Lopez-Menendez and Gonzalez-Torres 2019). The key components of the model that could be tuned to capture the nonlinear stress-stiffening and yielding observed in experiments (figures 7.13(A) and (B)) are (i) a free energy term that describes the entropic elasticity associated with a transiently-crosslinked semiflexible polymer network and (ii) an energetic term that accounts for different interaction/coupling strengths between the two networks. Results of this modeling approach are detailed in figure 7.13 (Lopez-Menendez and Gonzalez-Torres 2019).

Similar to actin–microtubule composites, keeping the total protein concentration fixed in actin–IF networks and varying ϕ_A alters the mesh size of the composite as the dependence of ξ on concentration is different for vimentin compared to actin (Golde *et al* 2018, Ricketts *et al* 2018, Anderson *et al* 2019). This effect has been suggested to contribute to the emergent behavior reported in the studies above, and was the focus of another study that aimed to investigate the effect of varying fractions of vimentin and actin in composites with a fixed mesh size of $\xi \simeq 0.42\ \mu$m (Golde *et al* 2018).

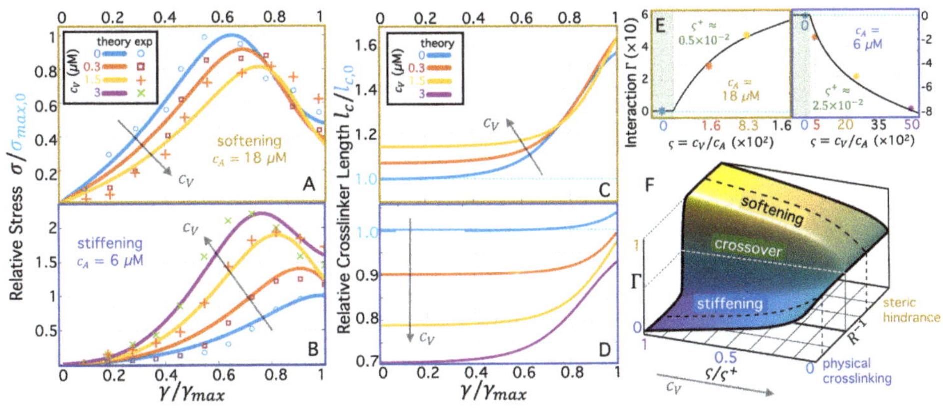

Figure 7.13. Theoretical modeling of nonlinear rheological properties of actin–vimentin composites. (A, B) Bulk nonlinear stress σ, normalized by its maximum for $c_V = 0$, $\sigma_{\max,0}$, versus strain γ, normalized by its maximum $\gamma_{\max}$, predicted via continuum mechanics modeling (solid lines) and experimentally measured (symbols) for composites of vimentin and crosslinked actin ($R = 0.01$) with c_V (μM) = 0 (blue line, light blue circles), 0.3 (orange line, red squares), 1.5 (yellow, orange crosses), and 3 (purple, green x's), and either $c_A = 18$ μM (A, yellow border) or $c_A = 6$ μM (B, blue border). (C, D) Crosslinker length l_c, normalized by its $c_V = 0$ value $l_{c,0}$ versus $\gamma/\gamma_{\max}$ for the same composites as in (A, B) show that for high c_A (C, yellow border), vimentin increases the crosslinker length by introducing steric interactions that block binding sites, whereas for low c_A (D, blue border), vimentin reduces l_c (i.e., enhances crosslinking) by providing a scaffold to reduce fluctuations. All composites exhibit an increase in l_c at large strains due to strain-induced crosslinker unbinding. (E) The actin–vimentin interaction parameter Γ as a function of $\varsigma = c_V/c_A$ for composites with c_V (μM) = 0 (blue), 0.3 (orange), 1.5 (yellow), 3 (purple), and either $c_A = 18$ μM (A, yellow border) or $c_A = 6$ μM (B, blue border), with the predicted functional form of $\Gamma(\varsigma)$ (black line) overlaid. The ς value at which $\Gamma(\varsigma)$ becomes non-zero ς^+ is listed. (F) Phase map of strengthening (blue, stiffening) and weakening (yellow, softening) behavior, as quantified by increasing or decreasing interaction parameter Γ (z-axis) for actin–vimentin composites as a function of ς/ς^+ (x-axis), which increases with increasing c_V and R^{-1} (y-axis), which scales as l_c. Adapted from Lopez-Menendez and Gonzalez-Torres (2019) Copyright (2019), with permission from Elsevier.

Recall that

$$\xi_A \simeq 0.3\rho_A^{-1/2} \tag{7.8}$$

$$\xi_V \simeq 0.42\rho_V^{-1/2} \tag{7.9}$$

for actin and vimentin, respectively, where ξ is in microns and ρ is in mg mL^{-1} (Herrmann *et al* 1996, Gardel *et al* 2003, Wickert *et al* 2005), such that single-component actin and vimentin networks with $\rho_A = 0.5$ mg mL^{-1} ($c_A = 11.9$ μM) and $\rho_V = 1$ mg mL^{-1} ($c_V = 17.5$ μM) have the same nominal mesh size $\xi_A \simeq \xi_V \simeq 0.42$ μm. Bulk rheology measurements showed that G' for the vimentin network at this mesh size was higher in magnitude and exhibited weaker frequency dependence than for actin, and its corresponding nonlinear response showed more pronounced stiffening (increasing K') and larger $K'_{\max}$ and σ_y values (Golde *et al* 2018).

Composites formed with varying volume fractions of these single-component networks ($\rho_{A,0} = 0.5$ mg mL^{-1} and $\rho_{V,0} = 1$ mg mL^{-1}) should maintain $\xi \simeq 0.42$ μm.

However, direct measurements of actin and vimentin mesh sizes in composites with varying volume fractions of $\rho_{A,0}$ actin and $\rho_{V,0}$ vimentin solutions, reported higher values of $\xi \simeq 0.8\ \mu$m to $\xi \simeq 1.6\ \mu$m for both actin and vimentin. Moreover, for any given volume fraction ratio, e.g., 25% actin ($0.25\rho_{A,0} = 0.125$ mg mL^{-1}), 75% vimentin ($0.75\rho_{V,0} = 0.75$ mg mL^{-1}), the respective mesh sizes were indeed comparable, i.e., $\xi_A \simeq \xi_V$ (Golde *et al* 2018).

Rheology measurements performed on composites that nominally maintained this matching mesh size with different volume fraction ratios exhibited G' values and scaling intermediate between $\phi_A = 1$ and $\phi_A = 0$ networks and monotonic increased with increasing c_A. The nonlinear rheological properties of composites were more complex than the linear regime with K' for the composites exhibiting multiple local maxima in K' and varying degrees of stiffening and softening that did not trend monotonically with c_A (Golde *et al* 2018).

These experimental results were shown to qualitatively agree with predictions from the glassy worm-like chain (GWLC) model (Semenov 1986, Kroy and Glaser 2007, 2009), which incorporates kinetic 'stickiness' of the polymers into the traditional WLC model by exponentially stretching the relaxation times of all modes with lengthscales larger than the interaction length associated with the stickiness. The agreement with GWLC predictions is consistent with vimentin exhibiting non-specific self-interactions but not crosslinking with actin, in contrast to the implications of Esue *et al* (2006). These discrepancies may be due to the higher concentrations of actin and vimentin used in Esue *et al* (2006), as well as higher salt concentration, both of which facilitate non-specific crosslinking.

Bulk rheology experiments similar to Golde *et al* (2018) were also performed for composites of actin and another ubiquitous intermediate filament, keratin, that has a mass per unit length that is comparable to that for actin (and smaller than vimentin) (Leitner *et al* 2012, Block *et al* 2015, Elbalasy *et al* 2021). The corresponding relation between mesh size and mass concentration for keratin

$$\xi_K \simeq 0.32\rho_K^{-1/2} \tag{7.10}$$

is therefore quite close to that for actin (equation (7.8)). As such, single-component actin and keratin networks with $\rho_{A,0} = 0.5$ mg mL^{-1} ($c_{A,0} = 11.9\ \mu$M) and $\rho_{K,0} = 0.6$ mg mL^{-1} ($c_{K,0} = 11.3\ \mu$M), respectively, have the same mesh size of $\xi \simeq 0.42\ \mu$m (Elbalasy *et al* 2021). These $\rho_{A,0}$ and $\rho_{K,0}$ values were used as the single-component boundary conditions, corresponding to actin mass fractions of $\Phi_A = 1$ and $\Phi_A = 0$, to examine the effect of varying ρ_A and ρ_K in composites that maintained a fixed mesh size of $\xi \simeq 0.42\ \mu$m.

Similar to the actin–vimentin studies described in figures 7.12(A)–(D) (Esue *et al* 2006), these studies showed that the loss tangent and frequency dependence of G', both indicators of increasing dissipation, increased monotonically as the actin mass fraction $\Phi_A = \rho_{A,0}/(\rho_{A,0} + \rho_{K,0})$ increased from $\Phi_A = 0$ and $\Phi_A = 1$ (figure 7.14(A)), whereas an emergent maximized elastic modulus G' and minimized data spread manifested at $\Phi_A = 0.22$ ($\rho_A = 0.125$ mg mL^{-1}, $\rho_V = 0.45$ mg mL^{-1}) (figure 7.14(B)).

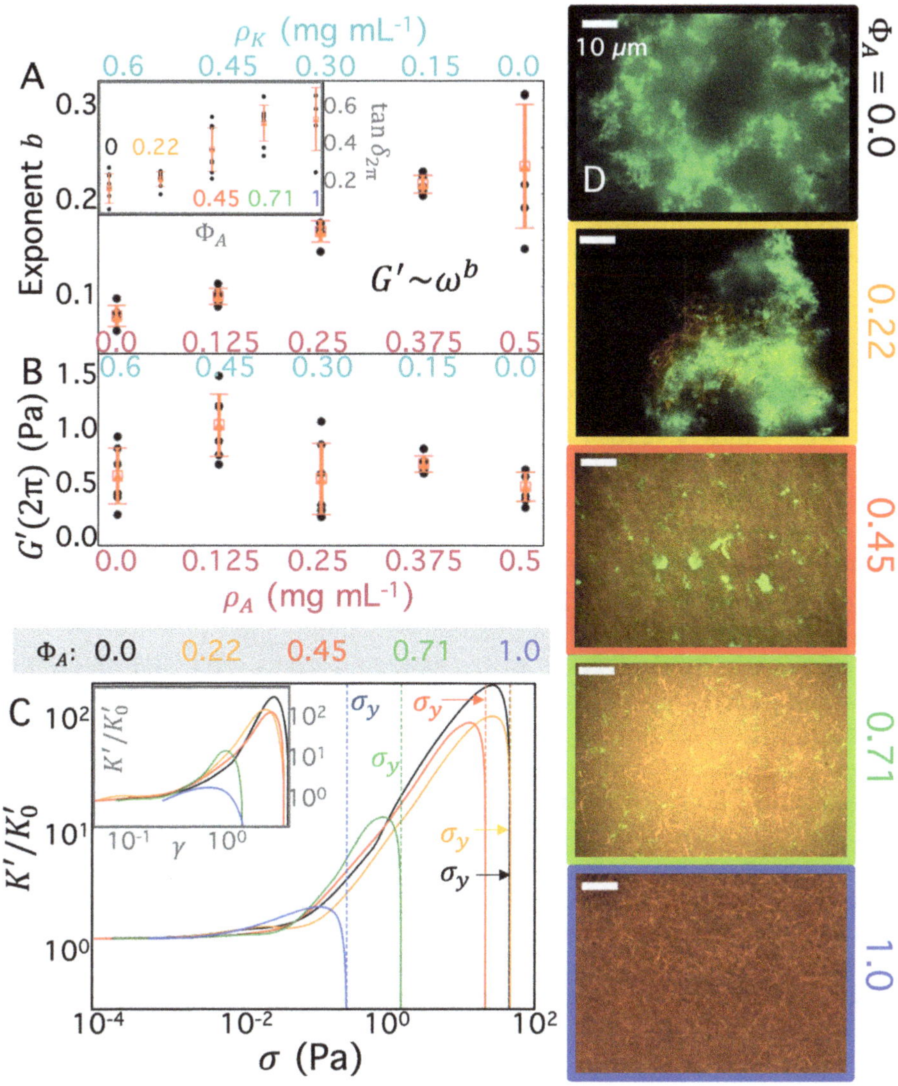

Figure 7.14. Bulk linear and nonlinear rheology of composites of actin and keratin with fixed mesh size and varying actin mass fractions Φ_A. Bulk linear (A, B) and nonlinear (C) rheology and two-color confocal microscopy (D) of composites of keratin (green) and actin (red) at varying combinations of actin and keratin mass concentrations of $\rho_A = 0 - 0.5$ and $\rho_K = 0.6 - 0$ (red and teal x-axis labels in A, B) paired to maintain a constant mesh size and equating to actin mass fractions of $\Phi_A = \rho_A / (\rho_A + \rho_K) = 0$ (black), 0.22 (gold), 0.45 (red), 0.71 (green), and 1 (blue). (A, B) Linear viscoelastic moduli $G'(\omega)$ and $G''(\omega)$ are analyzed to determine (A) the scaling exponent b that describes the relationship $G' \sim \omega^b$, (A inset) the loss tangent $\tan\delta$ evaluated at $\omega = 2\pi$ rad s^{-1}, and (B) elastic modulus G', also evaluated at $\omega = 2\pi$ rad s^{-1}, as functions of (ρ_A, ρ_K) and Φ_A. Data from individual trials (black) and their average and standard deviation (red) are shown for each Φ_A. (C) Nonlinear differential modulus K', scaled by its linear regime value K'_0, versus stress σ and (inset) strain γ for composites with $\Phi_A = 0$ (black), 0.22 (gold), 0.45 (red), 0.71 (green), and 1 (blue). Color-coded vertical dashed lines denote the yield stress σ_y for each Φ_A, which decreases with increasing Φ_A. (D) Two-color confocal micrographs of actin (red) and keratin (green) in composites with increasing Φ_A (top to bottom), with borders matching the color-coding in (A–C). Adapted from Elbalasy *et al* (2021). CC BY 3.0.

In the nonlinear regime, all composites exhibited strain-stiffening behavior that was substantially more pronounced than for similar actin–vimentin composites (Golde *et al* 2018), and was increasingly enhanced with decreasing Φ_A (increasing ρ_V) (figure 7.14(C)). Specifically, K' increased over two orders of magnitude from its linear regime value K_0' and reached yield stresses of $\sigma_y \simeq 43$ Pa (figure 7.14(C)) (Elbalasy *et al* 2021), compared to a $\lesssim$2-fold increase in K' and $\sigma_y \lesssim 3$ Pa for similar actin–vimentin composites (Golde *et al* 2018). Confocal microscopy images showed that keratin-rich composites exhibited tight bundling and heterogeneous clustering of keratin co-localized with actin, whereas actin-rich composites displayed more uniform mixing and homogeneous network formation (figure 7.14(D)) (Elbalasy *et al* 2021).

7.2.6 Composites of microtubules and intermediate filaments

A number of studies have focused on understanding molecular interactions between individual microtubules and various intermediate filaments, e.g., neurofilaments, vimentin, desmin, and keratin, which have reported co-localization and co-bundling of the two polymers via tubulin binding sites and electrostatic interactions (Gyoeva and Gelfand 1991, Liao and Gundersen 1998, Bocquet *et al* 2009, Uchida *et al* 2009, Huber *et al* 2015, Gan *et al* 2016). However, far fewer studies have examined composite *networks* of microtubules and intermediate filaments.

One previous study used TIRF microscopy, optical tweezers, and simulations to examine the polymerization and stability of microtubules, seeded at tubulin concentrations of $c_T = 20\ \mu$M and $c_T = 25\ \mu$M, in the presence of vimentin networks with $c_V = 2.3$ or $3.6\ \mu$M (figure 7.15) (Schaedel *et al* 2021).

These studies showed that tubulin polymerization and depolymerization rates were largely insensitive to vimentin concentration and instead were dictated solely by the tubulin concentration (figure 7.15(A)). Conversely, increasing vimentin concentration increasingly stabilized microtubules from catastrophic depolymerization (figure 7.15(B)), and increased their rescue rate, i.e., the rate at which depolymerized microtubules begin to polymerize again (figure 7.15(C)).

These results were coupled with OT measurements of the interaction force between microtubules and vimentin, as well as complementary theoretical modeling, to provide strong evidence for direct, transient interactions between microtubules and vimentin that were mediated by electrostatic and hydrophobic interactions (Schaedel *et al* 2021). Specifically, the addition of 18 mM $MgCl_2$, which promotes counterion crossbridging, increased the probability of microtubule–vimentin binding events and the strength of the microtubule–vimentin bond (figure 7.15(D)). Conversely, the addition of 0.1% TX100, a non-ionic detergent that disrupts hydrophobic interactions, reduced the microtubule–vimentin interaction probability nearly 2-fold (figure 7.15(D)) and likewise reduced the strength of those surviving bonds.

7.2.7 Vimentin–actin–microtubule composites

While the cytoskeleton consists of interacting actin, microtubules, and intermediate filaments, reconstituting composites of all three components has proven difficult due

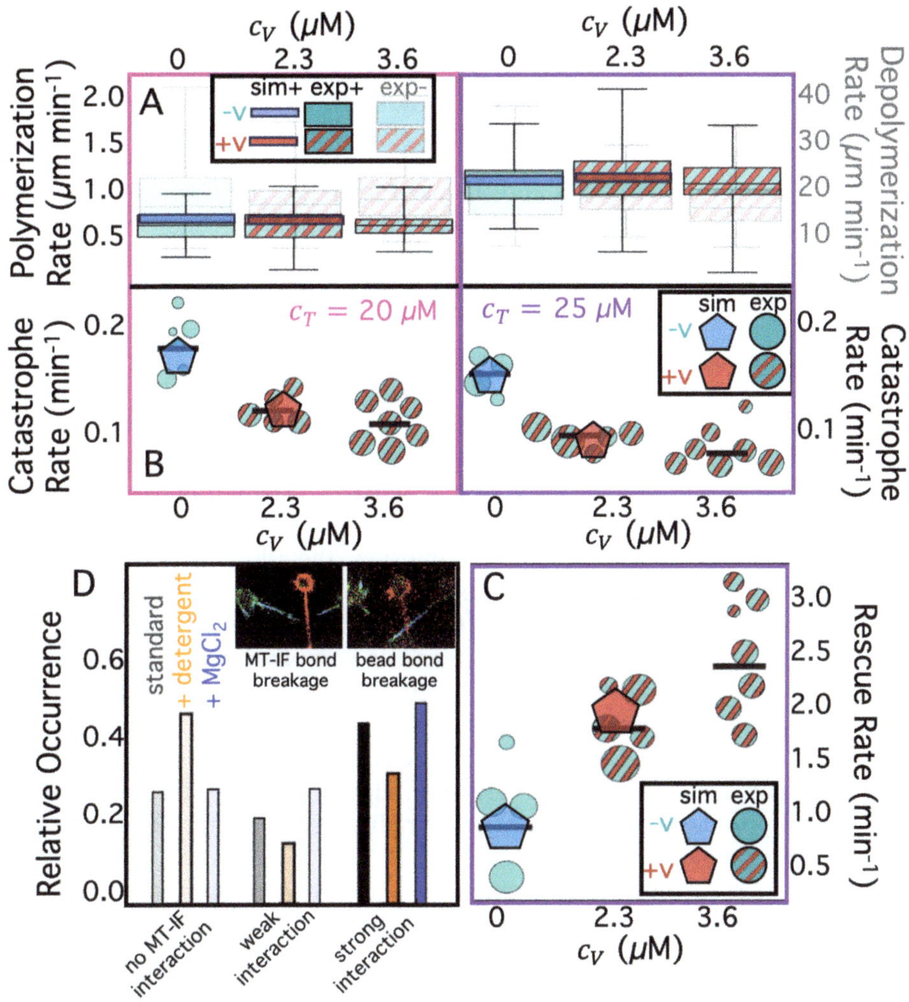

Figure 7.15. Effect of vimentin on the polymerization and stability of microtubules. (A, B, D) TIRF microscopy measurements of the (A) polymerization rate (left/black axis/labels, opaque bars) and depolymerization rate (right/grey axis/labels, translucent bars) of microtubules at concentrations of $c_T = 20\ \mu$M (left, magenta border) and $c_T = 25\ \mu$M (right, purple border) in the absence of vimentin ($c_V = 0$, $-$v, teal bars) or presence of vimentin at $c_V = 2.3\ \mu$M or $c_V = 3.6\ \mu$M (+v, teal/red hashed bars). Simulated polymerization rates are shown for $c_V = 0$ ($-$v, blue bar) and $c_V = 2.3\ \mu$M (+v, red bar). (B) Bubble chart of microtubule catastrophe rates for $c_T = 20\ \mu$M (left) and $c_T = 25\ \mu$M (right) determined from experiments (circles) and simulations (hexagons) without ($-$v, blue and teal) and with (+v, red/teal and red) vimentin at $c_V = 2.3\ \mu$M (sim and exp) or $c_V = 3.6\ \mu$M (exp only). Each circle is a unique experiment that contains data from multiple microtubules. The area of each circle scales with the sum of microtubule growth times for each experiment. Horizontal bars denote weighted averages. (C) Bubble chart of microtubule rescue rate with the same symbolization and composite parameters as in B. (D) Optical tweezers measurements of the relative occurrence of no interaction/bond between a microtubule and vimentin filament (left, light hues), breakage of a bond between microtubule and vimentin, indicative of weak MT–IF interaction (middle, intermediate hues), and breakage of a bond between the trapped microsphere and microtubule, indicative of strong MT–IF interaction

(dark hues, right). Relative occurrence of each interaction type was measured in standard conditions (left, greyscale bars), with non-ionic detergent 0.1% TX100 (middle, red shaded bars), and with 18 mM $MgCl_2$ (right, blue shaded bars). Inset TIRF images depict breakage of bond between microtubule (red) and vimentin (green) or bead (red circle). Adapted from Schaedel *et al* (2021). CC BY 4.0.

to incompatible buffer conditions and the need for many areas of expertise (Huber *et al* 2015). One previous study prepared actin–vimentin–microtubule (AVM) composites with equal mass concentration of actin and microtubules, $\rho_A = \rho_T = 1 \text{ mg mL}^{-1}$ ($c_A = 23.8\ \mu$M, $c_T = 9.1\ \mu$M), and varying vimentin concentrations of $\rho_V = 0-0.7 \text{ mg mL}^{-1}$ ($c_V = 0-13.2\ \mu$M) (figure 7.16(A)) (Shen *et al* 2021). For reference, these concentrations correspond to single-component network mesh sizes of $\xi_A \simeq 0.3\ \mu$M, $\xi_T \simeq 0.9\ \mu$M, and $\xi_V \simeq 0-0.5\ \mu$M.

Analysis of the displacements of embedded 1 microspheres ($R_s = 0.5\ \mu$m) in the composites revealed that the addition of vimentin to actin networks and actin–microtubule composites significantly suppressed particle motion, as evidenced by much narrower van Hove distributions (figure 7.16(B)). However, in line with previous studies on actin–microtubules composites, the addition of microtubules to networks of actin or vimentin, or actin–vimentin composites, only very slightly reduced the particle mobility (figure 7.16(B)), which was previously suggested to arise from their larger rigidity and mesh size as compared to actin and vimentin filaments and networks (Anderson *et al* 2019, Regan *et al* 2019). Multi-scale imaging, using transmission electron microscopy, scanning electron microscopy, and confocal microscopy, showed that all three components formed interpenetrating and co-entangled networks (figure 7.16(A)), suggesting that vimentin suppresses particle mobility in composites primarily by reducing the composite mesh size and increasing the entanglement density.

Two-point microrheology measurements further showed that this reduced mobility correlated with an order of magnitude increase in the disengagement time τ_D of AVM composites as c_V increased from 0 to 13.2 μM (figure 7.16(C)), following power-law scaling $\tau_D \sim c_V^{33}$ and further corroborating the role of vimentin in increasing entanglements and reducing the mesh size. The plateau modulus also increased monotonically with c_V but much more modestly, increasing less than ~2-fold, following to the scaling relation $G^0 \sim c_V^b$ with $b \simeq 0.5$. These results together suggest that the reduced mobility from increasing vimentin arises from dramatic slowing of relaxation timescales rather than increased elastic-like behavior (Shen *et al* 2021). This relative insensitivity of G^0 to increasing vimentin concentration may also indicate a competition between bundling and connectivity of actin and vimentin, as seen in several two-component composites described in previous sections, e.g., Fitzpatrick *et al* (2018), Francis *et al* (2019), Peddireddy *et al* (2021), and Khanal *et al* (2022).

Similar measurements were performed on actin–vimentin composites (no microtubules) with $c_V = 9.4\ \mu$M and $c_A = 2.4-47.6\ \mu$M, showing a power-law increase in G^0 with c_A, with an exponent $b \simeq 1.5$ that is ~3-fold larger than the dependence on c_V seen in AVM composites, but weaker than the scaling $b \simeq 2.2$ seen in actin-only

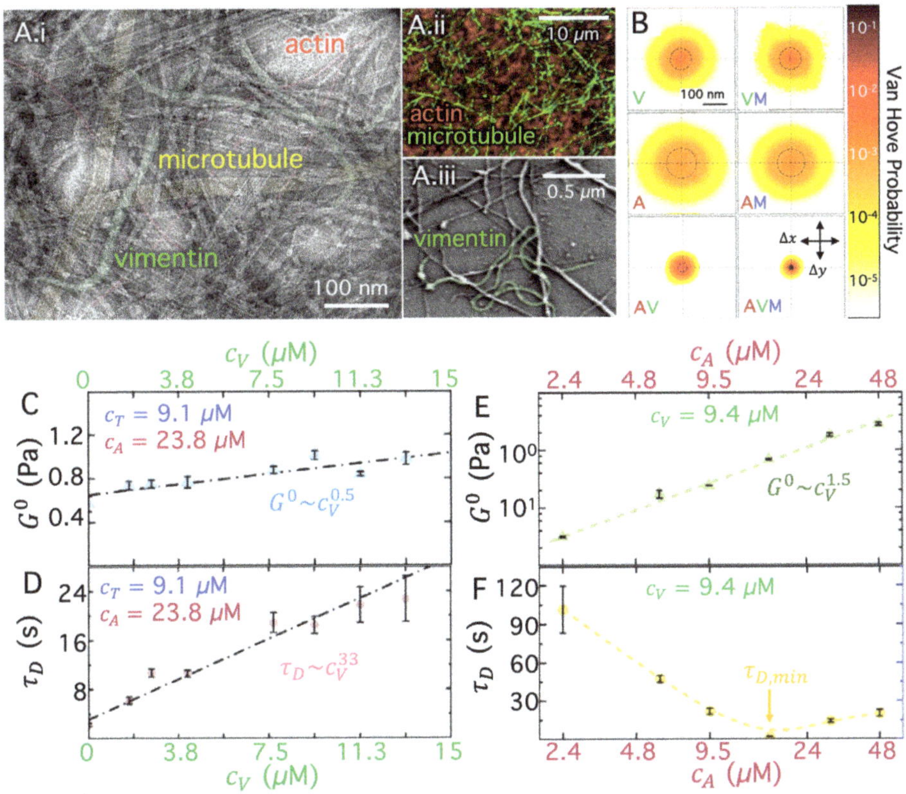

Figure 7.16. Imaging and microrheology of composites of actin, microtubules, and vimentin. (A) Images of a composite comprising actin, microtubules, and vimentin at concentrations of $c_A \simeq 23.8$ μM, $c \simeq 9.1$ μM and $c_V \simeq 9.4$ μM, using (i) transmission electron microscopy of actin (red), microtubules (yellow), and vimentin (green), (ii) confocal microscopy of actin (red) and microtubules (green), and (iii) scanning electron microscopy, with vimentin shown in green. (B) Two-dimensional van Hove probability distributions of displacements (Δx, Δy) of microspheres ($R_s = 0.5$ μm), displayed as heat maps with the color indicating the probability according to the scale, and the spread in (x, y) indicating displacements, as scaled by the 100 nm scale bar. Distributions are shown for composites with various combinations of vimentin at $\rho_V \simeq 8.75$ μM (green V, top and bottom rows), actin at $c_A \simeq 23.8$ μM (red A, bottom two rows), and microtubules at $\rho_T \simeq 9.1$ μM (blue M, right column). (C–F) Two-point microrheology measurements of the (C, E) plateau modulus G^0 and (D, F) disengagement time τ_D for (C, D) actin–microtubule–vimentin composites with varying vimentin concentrations (green, x-axis) and (E, F) actin–vimentin composites with varying actin concentrations (red, x-axis). Dashed lines in each panel indicate power-law scaling with exponents (C) $b \simeq 0.5$, (D) $b \simeq 33$, and (E) $y \simeq 1.5$; and (F) a spline fit that captures the non-monotonic dependence of τ_D on c_A. Adapted with permission from Shen *et al* (2021). Copyright (2021) by the American Physical Society.

networks (figure 7.16(E)) (Gardel *et al* 2004). Moreover, increasing c_A had a nearly opposite effect on the disengagement time at low actin concentrations, with τ_D decreasing ~20-fold as c_A increased to ~17 μM, rather than the increase measured for increasing c_V in AVM composites (figure 7.16(F)). After τ_D reached this local minimum, it then modestly increased. This complex dependence was suggested to arise from actin initially diluting actin–vimentin interactions (entanglements or crosslinks) as the actin molarity reaches that of vimentin (Shen *et al* 2021). This result may also indicate vimentin-driven actin bundling as more actin is added, thereby increasing the mesh size and reducing connectivity. The increase in τ_D seen for $c_A > c_V$ was suggested to arise from increased entanglement density as more polymers are being added to the composite, such that bundling no longer inhibits connectivity but rather promotes it (Shen *et al* 2021).

These intriguing results demonstrate a clear need for more studies on actin–IF–microtubule composites to span the parameter space and dissect the competitive and synergistic interactions between the different biopolymers.

7.3 Considerations and outlook

The blends and composites discussed in this section demonstrate the vast parameter space of possible multi-component systems that biopolymers afford, and the fascinating emergent properties that they display. The examples discussed in this chapter highlight the complex cooperative and competitive interactions that dictate the dynamics, rheology, and structure of biopolymer blends and composites, and the entropic and enthalpic contributions that drive these interactions. I also discussed design considerations, including advances that have been made to facilitate miscibility and co-entanglement of different biopolymers as well as methods to characterize the composites across scales.

To build on these studies, we should consider expanding efforts to engineer and investigate bio-synthetic composites comprising biopolymers and synthetic polymers to couple the resilience and toughness of synthetic components with the versatility and adaptability of biological components. Bridging synthetic and biological knowledge bases, approaches, and constituents will likely open up new areas of research in materials science, chemical engineering, and biophysics.

Another frontier in biopolymer composite research is the design of composites of biopolymers and non-polymeric inclusions such as colloids, cells, hydrogels, and carbon nanotubes. A large body of literature is devoted to understanding nano-polymer composites of synthetic polymers and nanoparticles, yet their extension to biopolymers and to other constituents beyond nanoparticles is limited at best. These systems will likely prove essential to advancing tissue engineering, designing healable materials, and understanding the intra- and inter-cellular space in living systems.

Moreover, there are very few examples of composites that comprise more than two components, despite the additional orthogonal tuning knob a third component offers. Of course, adding additional components increases the complexity of the system and the phase space of composite formulations many-fold, demanding theoretical models and simulations to parse the contributions from different constituents. However, the added complexity comes with more refined ability to tune the structure, rheology, and dynamics of the networks, and will likely give rise to new, emergent properties and physics that cannot be realized in two-component systems.

Finally, as I discuss in chapter 8, creating composite active matter is at the forefront of active matter physics and autonomous materials engineering research. By incorporating motors, enzymes, or responsive or triggerable components that can selectively 'activate' different constituents within a composite offers unprecedented programmability of active materials and non-equilibrium systems that can be harnessed to advance current efforts to design programmable, adaptable, and autonomously reconfigurable materials; and shed light on the complexities of cellular dynamics and intercellular transport.

References

Anderson S J, Matsuda C, Garamella J, Peddireddy K R, Robertson-Anderson R M and McGorty R 2019 Filament rigidity vies with mesh size in determining anomalous diffusion in cytoskeleton *Biomacromolecules* **20** 4380–8

Aporvari M S, Dang S, Marfai J, Coursey K, McGorty R and Robertson-Anderson R M 2022 Crowding and confinement act in concert to slow DNA diffusion within cell-sized droplets *iScience* **25** 105122

Berezney J, Goode B L, Fraden S and Dogic Z 2022 Extensile to contractile transition in active microtubule–actin composites generates layered asters with programmable lifetimes *Proc. Natl Acad. Sci.* **119** e2115895119

Block J, Schroeder V, Pawelzyk P, Willenbacher N and Köster S 2015 Physical properties of cytoplasmic intermediate filaments *Biochim. Biophys. Acta (BBA)—Mol. Cell Res., Mechanobiol.* **1853** 3053–64

Bocquet A, Berges R, Frank R, Robert P, Peterson A C and Eyer J 2009 Neurofilaments bind tubulin and modulate its polymerization *J. Neurosci.* **29** 11043–54

Cai L-H, Panyukov S and Rubinstein M 2011 Mobility of nonsticky nanoparticles in polymer liquids *Macromolecules* **44** 7853–63

Chapman C D, Gorczyca S and Robertson-Anderson R M 2015 Crowding induces complex ergodic diffusion and dynamic elongation of large DNA molecules *Biophys. J.* **108** 1220–8

Chapman C D, Lee K, Henze D, Smith D E and Robertson-Anderson R M 2014 Onset of non-continuum effects in microrheology of entangled polymer solutions *Macromolecules* **47** 1181–6

Chapman C D and Robertson-Anderson R M 2014 Nonlinear microrheology reveals entanglement-driven molecular-level viscoelasticity of concentrated DNA *Phys. Rev. Lett.* **113**

Chapman C D, Shanbhag S, Smith D E and Robertson-Anderson R M 2012 Complex effects of molecular topology on diffusion in entangled biopolymer blends *Soft Matter* **8** 9177–82

Clarke J *et al* 2022 Depletion-driven morphological control of bundled actin networks arXiv:2205.01864v2

Cosgrove T, Turner M J, Griffiths P C, Hollingshurst J, Shenton M J and Semlyen J A 1996 Self-diffusion and spin-spin relaxation in blends of linear and cyclic polydimethylsiloxane melts *Polymer* **37** 1535–40

Das M and MacKintosh F C 2011 Mechanics of soft composites of rods in elastic gels *Phys. Rev. E* **84** 061906

Dogterom M and Koenderink G H 2019 Actin–microtubule crosstalk in cell biology *Nat. Rev. Mol. Cell Biol.* **20** 38–54

Doi M and Edwards S F 1986 *The Theory of Polymer Dynamics* (Oxford: Oxford University Press)

Elbalasy I, Mollenkopf P, Tutmarc C, Herrmann H and Schnauß J 2021 Keratins determine network stress responsiveness in reconstituted actin–keratin filament systems *Soft Matter* **17** 3954–62

Esue O, Carson A A, Tseng Y and Wirtz D 2006 A direct interaction between actin and vimentin filaments mediated by the tail domain of vimentin *J. Biol. Chem.* **281** 30393–9

Farhadi L, Ricketts S N, Rust M J, Das M, Robertson-Anderson R M and Ross J L 2020 Actin and microtubule crosslinkers tune mobility and control co-localization in a composite cytoskeletal network *Soft Matter* **16** 7191–201

Fathizadeh A, Schiessel H and Ejtehadi M R 2015 Molecular dynamics simulation of supercoiled DNA rings *Macromolecules* **48** 164–72

Fitzpatrick R, Michieletto D, Peddireddy K R, Hauer C, Kyrillos C, Gurmessa B J and Robertson-Anderson R M 2018 Synergistic interactions between DNA and actin trigger emergent viscoelastic behavior *Phys. Rev. Lett.* **121** 257801

Fletcher D A and Mullins R D 2010 Cell mechanics and the cytoskeleton *Nature* **463** 485–92

Francis M L, Ricketts S N, Farhadi L, Rust M J, Das M, Ross J L and Robertson-Anderson R M 2019 Non-monotonic dependence of stiffness on actin crosslinking in cytoskeleton composites *Soft Matter* **15** 9056–65

Gan Z *et al* 2016 Vimentin intermediate filaments template microtubule networks to enhance persistence in cell polarity and directed migration *Cell Syst.* **3** 252–263.e8

Gao M, Krissanaprasit A, Miles A, Hsiao L C and LaBean T H 2021 Mechanical and electrical properties of DNA hydrogel-based composites containing self-assembled three-dimensional nanocircuits *Appl. Sci.* **11** 2245

Gardel M L, Shin J H, MacKintosh F C, Mahadevan L, Matsudaira P and Weitz D A 2004 Elastic behavior of cross-linked and bundled actin networks *Science* **304** 1301

Gardel M L, Valentine M T, Crocker J C, Bausch A R and Weitz D A 2003 Microrheology of entangled F-actin solutions *Phys. Rev. Lett.* **91** 158302

Goh S H 2014 Miscible polymer blends ed L A Utracki and C A Wilkie ed *Polymer Blends Handbook* (Dordrecht: Springer Netherlands) pp 1915–2151

Golde T, Huster C, Glaser M, Händler T, Herrmann H, Käs A and Schnauß J 2018 Glassy dynamics in composite biopolymer networks *Soft Matter* **14** 7970–8

Gorczyca S M, Chapman C D and Robertson-Anderson R M 2015 Universal scaling of crowding-induced DNA mobility is coupled with topology-dependent molecular compaction and elongation *Soft Matter* **11** 7762–8

Gyoeva F and Gelfand V 1991 Coalignment of vimentin intermediate filaments with microtubules depends on kinesin *Nature* **353** 445–8

Halverson J D, Grest G S, Grosberg A Y and Kremer K 2012 Rheology of ring polymer melts: from linear contaminants to ring-linear blends *Phys. Rev. Lett.* **108** 038301

Herrmann H, Bär H, Kreplak L, Strelkov S V and Aebi U 2007 Intermediate filaments: from cell architecture to nanomechanics *Nat. Rev. Mol. Cell Biol.* **8** 562–73

Herrmann H, Häner M, Brettel M, Müller S A, Goldie K N, Fedtke B, Lustig A, Franke W W and Aebi U 1996 Structure and assembly properties of the intermediate filament protein vimentin: the role of its head, rod and tail domains *J. Mol. Biol.* **264** 933–53

Hsiao K-W, Sasmal C, Ravi Prakash J and Schroeder C M 2017 Direct observation of DNA dynamics in semidilute solutions in extensional flow *J. Rheol.* **61** 151–67

Huber F, Boire A, López M P and Koenderink G H 2015 Cytoskeletal crosstalk: when three different personalities team up *Curr. Opin. Cell Biol., Cell Archit.* **32** 39–47

Hur K, Jeong C, Winkler R G, Lacevic N, Gee R H and Yoon D Y 2011 Chain dynamics of ring and linear polyethylene melts from molecular dynamics simulations *Macromolecules* **44** 2311–5

Iyer B V S, Lele A K and Shanbhag S 2007 What is the size of a ring polymer in a ring-linear blend? *Macromolecules* **40** 5995–6000

Jensen M H, Morris E J, Goldman R D and Weitz D A 2014 Emergent properties of composite semiflexible biopolymer networks *BioArchitecture* **4** 138–43

Kapnistos M, Lang M, Vlassopoulos D, Pyckhout-Hintzen W, Richter D, Cho D, Chang T and Rubinstein M 2008 Unexpected power-law stress relaxation of entangled ring polymers *Nat Mater* **7** 997–1002

Katsarou A F, Tsamopoulos A J, Tsalikis D G and Mavrantzas V G 2020 Dynamic heterogeneity in ring-linear polymer blends *Polymers* **12** 752

Kawaguchi D, Masuoka K, Takano A, Tanaka K, Nagamura T, Torikai N, Dalgliesh R M, Langridge S and Matsushita Y 2006 Comparison of interdiffusion behavior between cyclic and linear polystyrenes with high molecular weights *Macromolecules* **39** 5180–2

Khanal P, Peddireddy K R, Marfai J, McGorty R and Robertson-Anderson R M 2022 DNA topology dictates emergent bulk elasticity and hindered macromolecular diffusion in DNA–dextran composites *J. Rheol.* **66** 699–715

Kobayashi Y, Doi Y, Abdul Rahman S S, Kim E, Kim T-H, Takano A and Matsushita Y 2018 SANS study of ring topology effects on the miscibility of polymer blends *Macromolecules* **51** 1885–93

Kohli I and Mukhopadhyay A 2012 Diffusion of nanoparticles in semidilute polymer solutions: effect of different length scales *Macromolecules* **45** 6143–9

Kong D, Banik S, San Francisco M J, Lee M, Robertson Anderson R M, Schroeder C M and McKenna G B 2022 Rheology of entangled solutions of ring–linear DNA blends *Macromolecules* **55** 1205–17

Köster S, Weitz D A, Goldman R D, Aebi U and Herrmann H 2015 Intermediate filament mechanics *in vitro* and in the cell: from coiled coils to filaments, fibers and networks *Curr. Opin. Cell Biol., Cell Archit.* **32** 82–91

Krajina B A, Zhu A, Heilshorn S C and Spakowitz A J 2018 Active DNA olympic hydrogels driven by topoisomerase activity *Phys. Rev. Lett.* **121** 148001

Kroy K and Glaser J 2009 Rheological redundancy—from polymers to living cells *AIP Conf. Proc.* **1151** 52–5

Kroy K and Glaser J 2007 The glassy wormlike chain *New J. Phys.* **9** 416

Lai G H, Butler J C, Zribi O V, Smalyukh I I, Angelini T E, Purdy K R, Golestanian R and Wong G C L 2008 Self-organized gels in DNA/F-actin mixtures without crosslinkers: networks of induced nematic domains with tunable density *Phys. Rev. Lett.* **101** 218303

Leitner A, Paust T, Marti O, Walther P, Herrmann H and Beil M 2012 Properties of intermediate filament networks assembled from keratin 8 and 18 in the presence of Mg2+ *Biophys. J.* **103** 195–201

Liao G and Gundersen G G 1998 Kinesin is a candidate for cross-bridging microtubules and intermediate filaments: selective binding of kinesin to detyrosinated tubulin and vimentin *J. Biol. Chem.* **273** 9797–803

Lin Y-C, Koenderink G H, MacKintosh F C and Weitz D A 2011 Control of non-linear elasticity in F-actin networks with microtubules *Soft Matter* **7** 902–6

Lopez-Menendez H and Gonzalez-Torres L 2019 A theory to describe emergent properties of composite F-actin and vimentin networks *J. Mech. Phys. Solids* **127** 208–20

Mardoum W M, Gorczyca S M, Regan K E, Wu T-C and Robertson-Anderson R M 2018 Crowding induces entropically-driven changes to DNA dynamics that depend on crowder structure and ionic conditions *Front. Phys.* **6** 53

McKenna G B, Chen D, Mangalara S C H, Kong D and Banik S 2022 Some open challenges in polymer physics *Polym. Eng. Sci.* **62** 1325–55

McLeish T 2008 Polymer dynamics floored by the rings *Nat. Mater.* **7** 933–5

Michieletto D, Fitzpatrick R and Robertson-Anderson R M 2019 Maximally stiffening composites require maximally coupled rather than maximally entangled polymer species *Soft Matter* **15** 6703–17

Michieletto D, Marenduzzo D, Orlandini E, Alexander G P and Turner M S 2014 Threading dynamics of ring polymers in a gel *ACS Macro Lett.* **3** 255–9

Michieletto D, Marenduzzo D, Orlandini E and Turner M S 2017 Ring polymers: threadings, knot electrophoresis and topological glasses *Polymers* **9** 349

Michieletto D and Sakaue T 2021 Dynamical entanglement and cooperative dynamics in entangled solutions of ring and linear polymers *ACS Macro Lett.* **10** 129–34

Mills P J, Mayer J W, Kramer E J, Hadziioannou G, Lutz P, Strazielle C, Rempp P and Kovacs A J 1987 Diffusion of polymer rings in linear polymer matrices *Macromolecules* **20** 513–8

Nasirimarekani V, Strübing T, Vilfan A and Guido I 2021 Tuning the properties of active microtubule networks by depletion forces *Langmuir* **37** 7919–27

Negishi M, Sakaue T, Takiguchi K and Yoshikawa K 2010 Cooperation between giant DNA molecules and actin filaments in a microsphere *Phys. Rev.* E **81** 051921

O'Connor T C, Ge T and Grest G S 2022 Composite entanglement topology and extensional rheology of symmetric ring-linear polymer blends *J. Rheol.* **66** 49–65

Pan S, Nguyen D A, Dünweg B, Sunthar P, Sridhar T and Ravi Prakash J 2018 Shear thinning in dilute and semidilute solutions of polystyrene and DNA *J. Rheol.* **62** 845–67

Parisi D, Ahn J, Chang T, Vlassopoulos D and Rubinstein M 2020 Stress relaxation in symmetric ring-linear polymer blends at low ring fractions *Macromolecules* **53** 1685–93

Parisi D, Kaliva M, Costanzo S, Huang Q, Lutz P J, Ahn J, Chang T, Rubinstein M and Vlassopoulos D 2021 Nonlinear rheometry of entangled polymeric rings and ring-linear blends *J. Rheol.* **65** 695–711

Peddireddy K R, Clairmont R, Neill P, McGorty R and Robertson-Anderson R M 2022 Optical-tweezers-integrating-differential-dynamic-microscopy maps the spatiotemporal propagation of nonlinear strains in polymer blends and composites *Nat. Commun.* **13** 5180

Peddireddy K R, Lee M, Schroeder C M and Robertson-Anderson R M 2020a Viscoelastic properties of ring-linear DNA blends exhibit nonmonotonic dependence on blend composition *Phys. Rev. Res.* **2** 023213

Peddireddy K R, Lee M, Zhou Y, Adalbert S, Anderson S, Schroeder C M and Robertson-Anderson R M 2020b Unexpected entanglement dynamics in semidilute blends of supercoiled and ring DNA *Soft Matter* **16** 152–61

Peddireddy K R, Michieletto D, Aguirre G, Garamella J, Khanal P and Robertson-Anderson R M 2021 DNA conformation dictates strength and flocculation in DNA–microtubule composites *ACS Macro Lett.* **10** 1540–8

Pegoraro A F, Janmey P and Weitz D A 2017 Mechanical properties of the cytoskeleton and cells *Cold Spring Harb. Perspect. Biol.* **9** a022038

Pelletier V, Gal N, Fournier P and Kilfoil M L 2009 Microrheology of microtubule solutions and actin–microtubule composite networks *Phys. Rev. Lett.* **102** 188303

Pethrick R 2004 Polymer physics. Edited by Michael Rubinstein and Ralph H Colby Oxford University Press, Oxford, 2003. pp 440 *Polym. Int.* **53** 1394–5

Pringle J, Muthukumar A, Tan A, Crankshaw L, Conway L and Ross J L 2013 Microtubule organization by kinesin motors and microtubule crosslinking protein MAP65 *J. Phys. Condens. Matter* **25** 374103

Regan K, Ricketts S and Robertson-Anderson R 2016 DNA as a model for probing polymer entanglements: circular polymers and non-classical dynamics *Polymers* **8** 336

Regan K, Wulstein D, Rasmussen H, McGorty R and Robertson-Anderson R M 2019 Bridging the spatiotemporal scales of macromolecular transport in crowded biomimetic systems *Soft Matter* **15** 1200–9

Ricketts S N, Francis M L, Farhadi L, Rust M J, Das M, Ross J L and Robertson-Anderson R M 2019 Varying crosslinking motifs drive the mesoscale mechanics of actin–microtubule composites *Sci. Rep.* **9** 12831

Ricketts S N, Ross J L and Robertson-Anderson R M 2018 Co-entangled actin–microtubule composites exhibit tunable stiffening and power-law stress relaxation *Biophys. J.* **115** 1055–67

Ricketts S, Gurmessa B and M. Robertson-Anderson R 2020 Microscale mechanics of plug-and-play *in vitro* cytoskeleton networks *Parasitology and Microbiology Research* ed G Antonio Bastidas Pacheco and A Ali Kamboh (IntechOpen)

Robertson R M and Smith D E 2007a Direct measurement of the confining forces imposed on a single molecule in a concentrated solution of circular polymers *Macromolecules* **40** 8737–41

Robertson R M and Smith D E 2007 Self-diffusion of entangled linear and circular DNA molecules: dependence on length and concentration *Macromolecules* **40** 3373–7

Robertson R M and Smith D E 2007b Strong effects of molecular topology on diffusion of entangled DNA molecules *PNAS* **104** 4824–7

Robertson R M and Smith D E 2007c Direct measurement of the intermolecular forces confining a single molecule in an entangled polymer solution *Phys. Rev. Lett.* **99** 126001

Roovers J 1988 Viscoelastic properties of polybutadiene rings *Macromolecules* **21** 1517–21

Schaedel L, Lorenz C, Schepers A V, Klumpp S and Köster S 2021 Vimentin intermediate filaments stabilize dynamic microtubules by direct interactions *Nat. Commun.* **12** 3799

Schroeder C M, Shaqfeh E S G and Chu S 2004 Effect of hydrodynamic interactions on DNA dynamics in extensional flow: simulation and single molecule experiment *Macromolecules* **37** 9242–56

Schummel P H, Gao M and Winter R 2017 Modulation of the polymerization kinetics of α/β-tubulin by osmolytes and macromolecular crowding *Chem. Phys. Chem.* **18** 189–97

Semenov A N 1986 Dynamics of concentrated solutions of rigid-chain polymers. Part 1.—Brownian motion of persistent macromolecules in isotropic solution *J. Chem. Soc., Faraday Trans. 2* **82** 317–29

Shen Y *et al* 2021 Effects of vimentin intermediate filaments on the structure and dynamics of *in vitro* multicomponent interpenetrating cytoskeletal networks *Phys. Rev. Lett.* **127** 108101

Shin J H, Gardel M L, Mahadevan L, Matsudaira P and Weitz D A 2004 Relating microstructure to rheology of a bundled and cross-linked F-actin network *in vitro Proc. Natl Acad. Sci.* **101** 9636–41

Smrek J, Garamella J, Robertson-Anderson R and Michieletto D 2021 Topological tuning of DNA mobility in entangled solutions of supercoiled plasmids *Sci. Adv.* **7** eabf9260

Smrek J, Kremer K and Rosa A 2019 Threading of unconcatenated ring polymers at high concentrations: double-folded vs time-equilibrated structures *ACS Macro Lett.* **8** 155–60

Strehle D, Schnauß J, Heussinger C, Alvarado J, Bathe M, Käs J and Gentry B 2011 Transiently crosslinked F-actin bundles *Eur. Biophys. J.* **40** 93–101

Subramanian G and Shanbhag S 2008 Self-diffusion in binary blends of cyclic and linear polymers *Macromolecules* **41** 7239–42

Thomas S, Durand D, Chassenieux C and Jyotishkumar P 2013 *Handbook of Biopolymer-Based Materials: From Blends and Composites to Gels and Complex Networks* (New York: Wiley)

Tsalikis D G, Koukoulas T, Mavrantzas V G, Pasquino R, Vlassopoulos D, Pyckhout-Hintzen W, Wischnewski A, Monkenbusch M and Richter D 2017 Microscopic structure, conformation, and dynamics of ring and linear poly(ethylene oxide) melts from detailed atomistic molecular dynamics simulations: dependence on chain length and direct comparison with experimental data *Macromolecules* **50** 2565–84

Tsalikis D G and Mavrantzas V G 2014 Threading of ring poly(ethylene oxide) molecules by linear chains in the melt *ACS Macro Lett.* **3** 763–6

Tseng H-C and Graves D J 1998 Natural methylamine osmolytes, trimethylamine N-oxide and betaine, increase tau-induced polymerization of microtubules *Biochem. Biophys. Res. Commun.* **250** 726–30

Tseng Y, Fedorov E, McCaffery J M, Almo S C and Wirtz D 2001 Micromechanics and ultrastructure of actin filament networks crosslinked by human fascin: a comparison with α-actinin *J. Mol. Biol.* **310** 351–66

Ubertini M A, Smrek J and Rosa A 2022 Entanglement length scale separates threading from branching of unknotted and non-concatenated ring polymers in melts *Macromolecules* **55** 10723–36

Uchida A, Alami N H and Brown A 2009 Tight functional coupling of kinesin-1A and dynein motors in the bidirectional transport of neurofilaments *MBoC* **20** 4997–5006

von Meerwall E, Ozisik R, Mattice W L and Pfister P M 2003 Self-diffusion of linear and cyclic alkanes, measured with pulsed-gradient spin-echo nuclear magnetic resonance *J. Chem. Phys.* **118** 3867–73

Wang X, Zhu H, Lu Y, Wang Z and Kennedy D 2020 The elastic properties and deformation mechanisms of actin filament networks crosslinked by filamins *J. Mech. Behav. Biomed. Mater.* **112** 104075

Wickert U, Mücke N, Wedig T, Müller S A, Aebi U and Herrmann H 2005 Characterization of the *in vitro* co-assembly process of the intermediate filament proteins vimentin and desmin: mixed polymers at all stages of assembly *Eur. J. Cell Biol.* **84** 379–91

Wieczorek M, Chaaban S and Brouhard G J 2013 Macromolecular crowding pushes catalyzed microtubule growth to near the theoretical limit *Cel. Mol. Bioeng.* **6** 383–92

Xue K-L, Hu Y-F, Yu X-C and Hou J-X 2020 The diffusion properties of a ring polymer in a grid matrix *J. Polym. Res.* **27** 123

Yao N Y, Becker D J, Broedersz C P, Depken M, MacKintosh F C, Pollak M R and Weitz D A 2011 Nonlinear viscoelasticity of actin transiently cross-linked with mutant α-actinin-4 *J. Mol. Biol.* **411** 1062–71

Zhao L Y and Choi P 2006 A review of the miscibility of polyethylene blends *Mater. Manuf. Process* **21** 135–42

Zhou Y, Young C D, Lee M, Banik S, Kong D, McKenna G B, Robertson-Anderson R M, Sing C E and Schroeder C M 2021a Dynamics and rheology of ring-linear blend semidilute solutions in extensional flow: single molecule experiments *J. Rheol.* **65** 729–44

Zhou Y, Young C D, Lee M, Banik S, Kong D, McKenna G B, Robertson-Anderson R M, Sing C E and Schroeder C M 2021b Dynamics and rheology of ring-linear blend semidilute solutions in extensional flow: single molecule experiments *J. Rheol.* **65** 729–44

Zhu J, Lin H, Kim Y, Yang M, Skakuj K, Du J S, Lee B, Schatz G C, Van Duyne R P and Mirkin C A 2020 Light-responsive colloidal crystals engineered with DNA *Adv. Mater.* **32** 1906600

Part IV

Spatiotemporal Heterogeneity: from active matter to coacervates

IOP Publishing

Biopolymer Networks
Design, dynamics and discovery
Rae M Robertson-Anderson

Chapter 8

Active, responsive, and reconfigurable networks

The frontier of materials design and soft matter physics is active, responsive, and reconfigurable non-equilibrium materials, for which biopolymer networks are ideal candidates. In the cytoskeleton of cells, molecular motors generate forces and restructure networks of cytoskeletal biopolymers. In the nucleus, enzymes wind, unwind, cleave, and concatenate DNA, changing the viscoelastic properties of the crowded biopolymer network. Changes to the dynamics and structure of biopolymer networks (polymerization, bundling, etc) can also be triggered by variations in the chemical environment. In this chapter, I will discuss *in vitro* realizations of active biopolymer networks inspired by these biological feats, including network design, non-equilibrium dynamics, and mechanical properties. Key examples of active and responsive biopolymer networks that I will discuss include actomyosin networks, salt-mediated bundling of cytoskeleton networks, kinesin-microtubule active nematics, motor-driven cytoskeleton composites, and enzyme-driven DNA systems.

8.1 Motor-driven cytoskeleton networks

As I discuss in chapters 5 and 7, networks of actin filaments and microtubules have been extensively investigated in efforts to understand the role of polymer stiffness in polymeric systems, and shed light on the underlying structure, interactions, and dynamics that give rise to the mechanical properties of the cellular cytoskeleton. One of the most important properties of the cytoskeleton is its ability to restructure, move, and self-generate forces, via the action of motor proteins that push and pull on actin and microtubules (Liao and Gundersen 1998, Gatlin and Bloom 2010, Chanet *et al* 2017, Caridi *et al* 2018, Klemm *et al* 2018, Bashirzadeh *et al* 2022). As I describe below, motor-driven cytoskeleton networks have served as inspirational and model systems for understanding active matter research since its emergence in the 1990s (Needleman and Dogic 2017, Voth 2017, Ross *et al* 2019, Banerjee *et al* 2020, Swartz and Camley 2021, Kuçera *et al* 2022a).

doi:10.1088/978-0-7503-5037-2ch8

8.1.1 Actomyosin networks

Myosins are a family of ATP-fueled motor proteins that bind and walk along actin filaments (Sellers 2000, Alberts 2004, Fletcher and Mullins 2010, Sweeney and Houdusse 2010, Banerjee *et al* 2020, Robert-Paganin *et al* 2020). Myosin II motors, arguably the most widely studied of these, are dimers that polymerize into two-headed minifilaments at physiological salt concentrations (Conti and Adelstein 2008, Banerjee *et al* 2020, Grewe and Schwarz 2020). These minifilaments, $\sim$300 nm to 2 μm in length, comprising 10s to 100s of dimers, transiently crosslink actin filaments and slide antiparallel actin filaments past one another by taking non-processive steps along the paired filaments (Albert *et al* 2014, Murrell *et al* 2015, Linsmeier *et al* 2016a, Muresan *et al* 2022). This sliding action can generate contractile forces in bundles and networks of connected actin filaments if the filaments are of mixed polarity, i.e., the plus and minus ends of different filaments point in opposite directions (Murrell *et al* 2015, Linsmeier *et al* 2016a, Wollrab *et al* 2018). In this configuration, the unidirectional walking of the myosin heads toward the plus end of each filament causes the bound filaments to slide past each other (Mizuno *et al* 2007, Bendix *et al* 2008, Koenderink *et al* 2009).

The stepping motion of myosin II requires the hydrolysis of one bound ATP per step. However, it is actually the binding of ATP that releases myosin from actin filaments while myosin bound to ADP, or not bound to any nucleotide, binds actin filaments (more strongly without ADP and phosphate (P_i)) (Geeves 2016). As such, in the absence or at very low levels of ATP, myosin motors remain bound to actin filaments, acting as passive crosslinkers to rigidify the network (Humphrey *et al* 2002). In the presence of ATP, the nucleotide binds to actin-bound myosin and causes it to detach and hydrolyze the ATP, which allows the myosin-ADP-Pi to re-attach to the actin, release its P_i during the power-stroke, then release its ADP, pushing the undecorated myosin into a strong binding state that facilitates ATP binding and myosin release—and the cycle continues (Alberts 2004, Conti and Adelstein 2008, Fletcher and Mullins 2010). Because of the role of ATP in the myosin power stroke, increasing ATP concentration increases the stepping rate and can elicit stronger contractility (Silva *et al* 2011, Linsmeier *et al* 2016a). However, less intuitive is the fact that too much ATP can actually prevent actomyosin activity as it causes myosin to always be in the ATP-bound state which prevents binding actin (Mizuno *et al* 2007).

In muscle cells, myosin minifilaments synchronously pull on aligned mixed polarity bundles of actin filaments to generate macroscopic muscle contraction. However, in non-muscle cells, myosin II activity causes disordered actin networks to globally contract, locally contract into asters, undergo vortical and chaotic flow, and rip apart—dynamics that depend on the relative concentrations of actin, myosin, and passive crosslinkers, as well as surface interactions and confinement (Mizuno *et al* 2007, Bendix *et al* 2008, Murrell and Gardel 2012, Alvarado *et al* 2013, Murrell *et al* 2015, Linsmeier *et al* 2016a, Stam *et al* 2017, Wollrab *et al* 2018, Litschel *et al* 2021, Weirich *et al* 2021, Bashirzadeh *et al* 2022, Muresan *et al* 2022).

Entangled actomyosin networks. Early work on disordered actomyosin networks showed that, in the absence of passive crosslinkers, entangled actin networks ($c_A = 36\ \mu$M) exhibited markedly enhanced bulk fluidity in the presence of active myosin II at $c_m = 0.14\ \mu$M (myosin:actin ratio $R_m = 0.004$) (figure 8.1(A)) (Humphrey *et al* 2002). This effect, evidenced by a ~2.5× drop in G' (figure 8.1(B)) and two orders of magnitude faster relaxation time τ_D as compared to networks without myosin (figure 8.1(C)), was shown to arise from myosin motors releasing entanglements and promoting sliding of filaments past one another, causing network fluidization. In actomyosin networks without ATP, an opposite effect was seen whereby the viscoelastic actin network formed a bulk elastic gel (figure 8.1(A)). This gelation was quantified by a ~6-fold increase in G' and no apparent crossover frequency, $\omega_c \simeq 2\pi\tau_D^{-1}$ (figure 8.1(B)), indicating an immeasurably long relaxation timescale resulting from myosin acting as a passive crosslinker in the absence of ATP fuel (Humphrey *et al* 2002).

Myosin has also been shown to cause entangled actin networks to restructure into polar asters with motors focused in the center and actin filaments on the periphery (figures 8.2(A) and (B)), a result that has been suggested to arise from passive crosslinking of inactive myosin motors (i.e., 'deadheads') (Mizuno *et al* 2007, Silva *et al* 2011). Moreover, while it is generally accepted that passive crosslinkers are necessary for uniform contractility, at high enough myosin and actin concentrations, e.g., $c_A \simeq 23.8\ \mu$M and $R_m = 0.003$–0.02 ($10^2R = 3$–20), even active myosins may act similarly to transient passive crosslinkers to bundle filaments and enable short-range contractility, aster formation, and coalescence (figures 8.2(A) and (B)) (Silva *et al* 2011, Murrell and Gardel 2012, Linsmeier *et al* 2016a, Wollrab *et al* 2018, Weirich *et al* 2019, Lee *et al* 2021b). However, as I discuss below, introducing

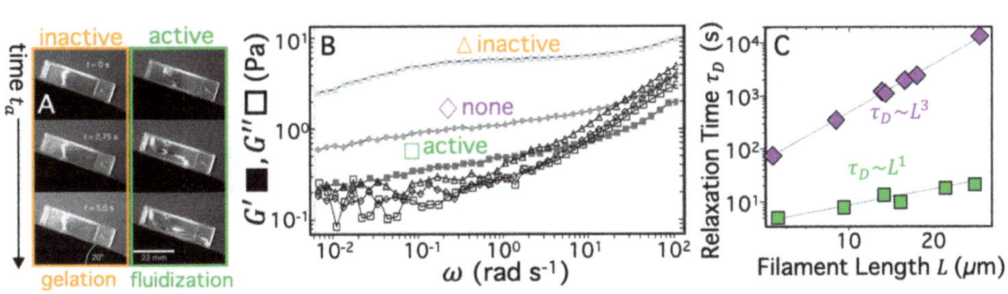

Figure 8.1. Seminal studies demonstrating myosin-mediated fluidization of entangled actin networks. (A) Cuvettes partially filled with networks of actin at $c_A = 36\ \mu$M and myosin at $c_m = 0.14\ \mu$M ($R_m = 0.004$) were tilted 70° from vertical and monitored over the course of 5.5 s to demonstrate myosin-driven gelation and fluidization of actin networks without ATP (inactive, orange) and with ATP (active, green), respectively. (B) Bulk linear viscoelastic moduli, $G'(\omega)$ (filled symbols) and $G''(\omega)$ (open symbols) for actin networks with active myosin (squares), inactive myosin (triangles), and no myosin (none, diamonds) confirm the gelation or fluidization of actin networks via interactions with inactive or active myosin. (C) The longest relaxation time τ_D, determined from the crossover frequency in B, as a function of actin filament length for actin networks without myosin (purple diamonds) and with active myosin (green squares). Power-law scaling $\tau_D \sim L^3$ for the actin network (purple) adheres to reptation model predictions while active network scaling $\tau_D \sim L^1$ aligns with sliding-dominated filament relaxation. Adapted from Humphrey *et al* (2002) Copyright (2002), with permission from Springer Nature.

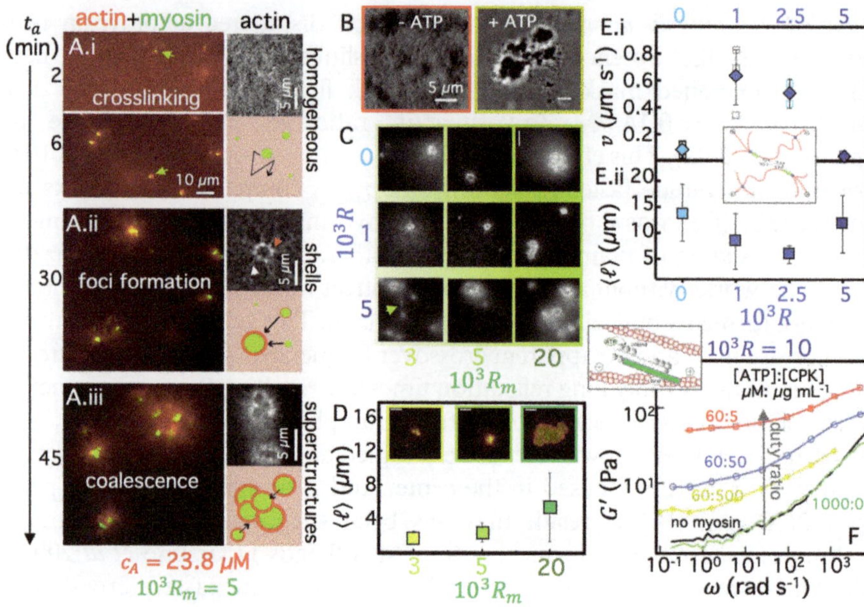

Figure 8.2. Active coarsening and condensation of actomyosin networks with and without biotin-streptavidin crosslinking. (A) Two-color confocal imaging of networks of actin (red) at $c_A = 23.8$ μM and myosin (green) at $R_m = 0.005$ ($10^3R_m = 5$) undergoing myosin-mediated (i) crosslinking, (ii) foci formation, and (iii) coalescence of foci as myosin activity time increases from $t_A = 2$ min to $t_A = 45$ min, resulting in a (i) homogeneous actin network, (ii) actin shells surrounding myosin-rich contractile foci, and (iii) superstructures of coalesced foci. To the right of each image is a zoom-in of the actin in the network (top) and a cartoon depiction of the process (bottom). Red and white arrows in ii show actin forming a ring around (red) and radiating outward from (white) the myosin-rich contractile core. (B) Differential interference contrast microscopy images of similar actomyosin networks as in A ($c_A = 23.8$ μM, $10^3R_m = 7$) without ATP (−ATP, red border) and with ATP (+ATP, green border), showing passive bundling of actin by inactive myosin and active contraction and coalescence by active myosin. (C) Introducing biotin-streptavidin crosslinkers at varying ratios $10^3R = 0$–5 (blue labels, vertical axis) alters the size and connectivity of condensates that form in actomyosin networks with $10^3R_m = 3$–20 (green labels, x-axis). (D) The average size of condensates $\langle \ell \rangle$ for networks with $10^3R = 2.5$ and myosin ratios shown in (C) increases with increasing R_m as visualized in the inset confocal images. (E) Speed v of moving condensates/foci (i) and foci size $\langle \ell \rangle$ (ii) versus crosslinker ratio 10^3R for networks with $10^3R_m = 20$ both show non-monotonic dependence on R, reaching minimal and maximal values, respectively, at intermediate R values $1 \leqslant 10^3R \leqslant 2.5$. (F) Linear optical tweezers microrheology measurements of $G'(\omega)$ for actomyosin networks with $10^3R = 10$ and $10^3R_m = 7$ and varying concentrations of ATP and ATP regeneration system CPK (creatine phosphokinase), listed next to the corresponding data as [ATP]:[CPK] in units of μM:μg mL^{-1}. At low levels of ATP (60 μM, yellow, blue, red), decreasing CPK increases the myosin duty ratio (grey arrow) to enhance elasticity, thereby increasing $G'(\omega)$. At high ATP levels (1000 μM, green) the network is indistinguishable from that without myosin (black) as the saturating ATP concentration prevents myosin processivity. (A, C–E) Adapted from Silva *et al* (2011) with permission of PNAS. (B, F) Modified from Mizuno *et al* (2007). © The American Association for the Advancement of Science.

additional passive crosslinkers, such as biotin-NeutrAvidin, fascin, filamin or α-actinin, alters the range and rate of contractility, in a manner that depends on the ratios of myosin, crosslinkers and actin, as well as the type of crosslinker (figures 8.2–8.5).

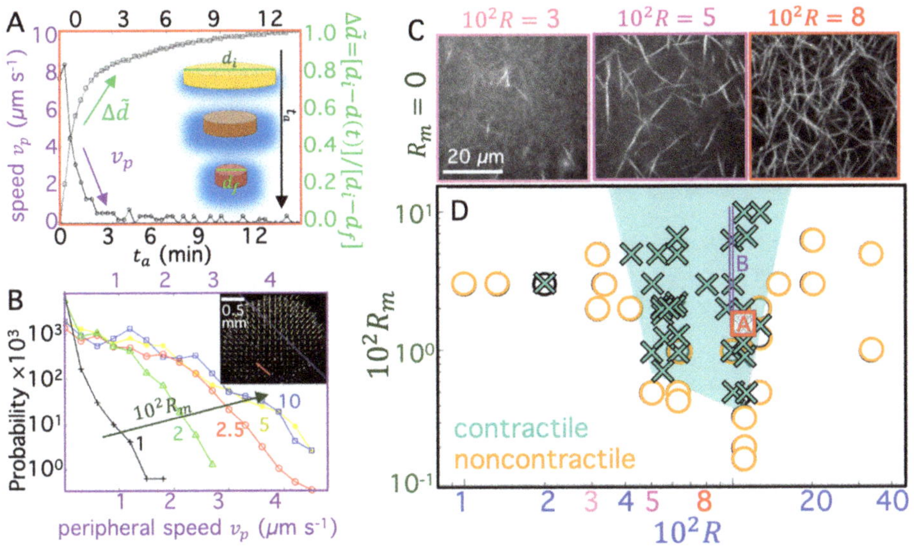

Figure 8.3. Contractile phase space of actomyosin networks crosslinked by α-actinin. (A, B) Bulk contraction of actomyosin networks with $c_A = 23$ μM and $10^3R_m = 20$ and crosslinked with α-actinin at $R = 0.11$. (A) Bulk contraction is quantified by measuring the time-dependent diameter $d(t_a)$ of the circular gel (cartoon depiction shown in inset) to determine the fractional contracted distance $\Delta d(t_a) = [d_i - d(t_a)]/[d_i - d_f]$ (green, squares) and contractile speed at the periphery $v_p(t_a)$ (purple, circles) over the course of myosin activity time t_A. (Inset) Cartoon depiction of actomyosin networks (orange) contracting within water droplets (blue) over time t_a. (B) Probability distribution of peripheral speeds v_p, determined via PIV (inset), are broadened with increasing myosin ratios of 10^2 $R_m = 1$ (black), 2 (green), 2.5 (red), 5 (yellow), and 10 (blue). (C) Collapse of 10 frames (5 μm) of a confocal z-stack of an actin network crosslinked at a ratio of 10^2 $R = 3$ (pink), 5 (magenta), and 8 (red). (D) Phase space of contractile (green x symbols) and noncontractile (orange circles) actomyosin networks as a function of myosin ratio R_m (y-axis), and crosslinker ratio (x-axis), with color-coded numbers matching corresponding image borders in (C). Green shaded region depicts contractile region of the phase space, and the red box and purple vertical lines demark the regions that correspond to the networks examined in (A, C) (red) and (B) (purple). Adapted from Bendix *et al* (2008) Copyright (2008), with permission from Elsevier.

Crosslinked actomyosin networks. Introducing biotin-NeutrAvidin crosslinkers into the coalescing actomyosin networks shown in figure 8.2(A), at ratios $1 \leqslant 10^3R \leqslant 5$, was reported to increase the connectivity between actomyosin clusters (figure 8.2(C)), and enable structures of increasing size $\langle \ell \rangle$ to form by increasing myosin:actin ratios from $10^3R_m = 3$ to $10^3R_m = 20$ (figures 8.2(C) and (D)). Interestingly, $\langle \ell \rangle$ displayed a non-monotonic dependence on passive crosslinking, reaching a minimum at $10^3R \approx 2$, that mirrored the non-monotonic dependence of the speed of moving foci v, which was maximized at a similar R value (figure 8.2(E)). These results suggest that the increased connectivity afforded by crosslinkers initially aids in contractility (increasing v) and favors linking together of small foci rather than more liquid-like coalescence (decreasing ℓ) (figure 8.2(C)), but eventually comes at a cost of increased friction and connections with the surrounding network that slow contractility (decreasing v) and enhance large-scale bundling and aggregation (increasing ℓ). These signatures of coarsening at high crosslinker ratios were also observed in seminal optical tweezers microrheology experiments on actomyosin networks with biotin-

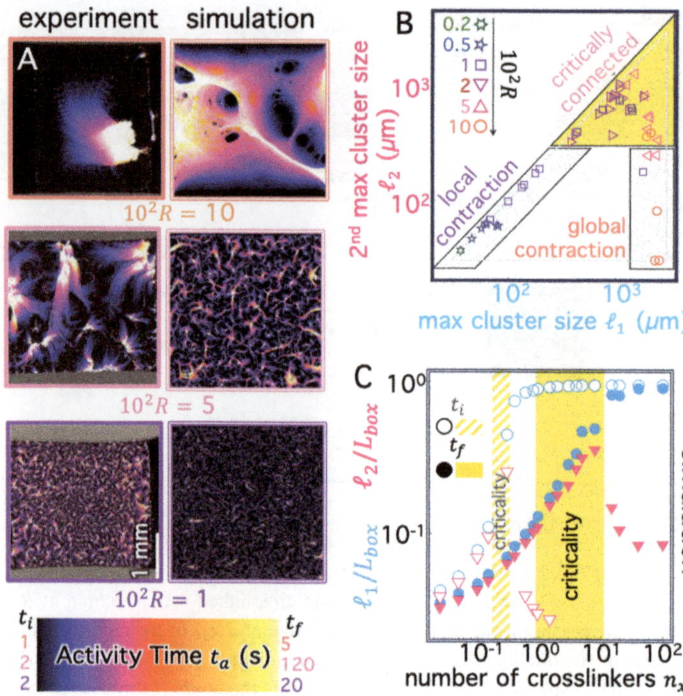

Figure 8.4. Experiments and simulations of actomyosin networks crosslinked with fascin show that interplay between activity and connectivity lead to a critically connected state. (A) Temporally color-coded projections of confocal (left) and simulated (right) time-series of labeled actin in actomyosin networks with $c_A = 12$ μM, 10^2 $R_m = 1$ and varying fascin:actin ratios 10^2 R= 10 (pink), 5 (magenta), and 1 (purple). Colors indicate time according to scale at bottom with $t_{a,i}$ and $t_{a,f}$ for each network listed in minutes to the left and right of the scale with matching color. (B) 2D plot of largest cluster size ℓ_1 (blue, y-axis) versus second largest cluster size ℓ_2 (magenta, x-axis) with data colors/symbols indicating increasing crosslinker ratios from $10^2 R = 0.2$ (green stars) to $10^2 R = 10$ (orange circles), as listed in the legend. Regions of the phase space that exhibit local contraction (purple), global contraction (orange), and critical connectivity (yellow triangle). (C) Simulated ℓ_1 (blue) and ℓ_2 (magenta) values, normalized by the simulation box size L_{box}, as a function of number of crosslinkers n_{xl} for networks before ($t_a = t_i$, open symbols, hashed yellow region) and after ($t_a = t_f$, filled symbols, solid yellow region) myosin activity. Myosin activity expands the region of the phase space in which criticality is observed. Adapted from Alvarado *et al* (2013) Copyright (2013), with permission from Springer Nature.

NeutrAvidin crosslinking at $10^3 R = 10$ with varying concentrations of ATP and the ATP regeneration agent creatine phosphokinase (CPK) (figure 8.2(F)) (Mizuno *et al* 2007). In the limit of high [ATP], the elastic modulus was indistinguishable from that of the passive actin network, indicating that the myosin remained in the ATP-bound state unable to bind to actin. At much lower levels of ATP and minimal CPK the network coarsened substantially, with G^0 increasing by nearly two orders of magnitude, suggestive of passive crosslinking of myosin with limited activity. As [CPK] was increased, the modulus decreased, owing to the lower myosin duty ratio afforded by more available ATP (figure 8.2(F)) (Mizuno *et al* 2007).

This complex interplay between passive crosslinking, myosin crosslinking, and myosin activity observed in actomyosin networks has been further investigated for

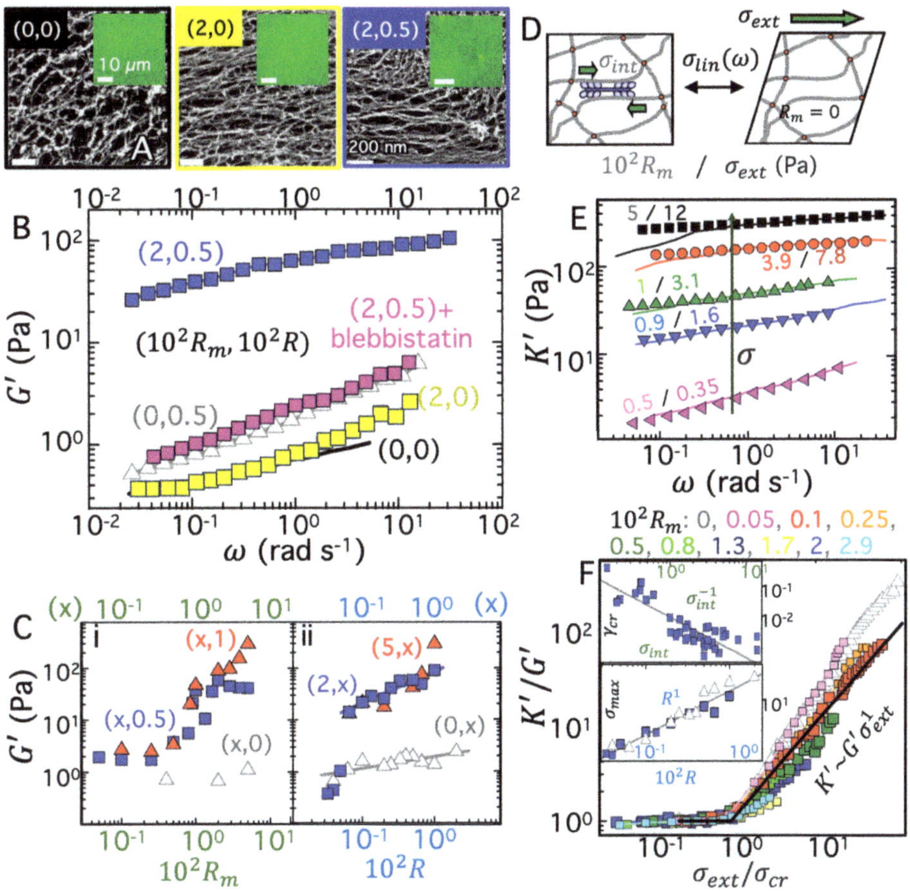

Figure 8.5. Linear and nonlinear bulk rheology of actomyosin networks crosslinked by filaminA. All data shown is for networks with $c_A = 23.8\ \mu$M and varying combinations of myosin:actin R_m and filaminA:actin R, color-coded and listed by each dataset as ($10^2 R_m$, $10^2 R$). (A) Confocal micrographs of (left) an entangled actin network, (middle) an actomyosin network, and (right) a crosslinked actomyosin network with insets showing zoomed-out view. Border colors match the corresponding ($10^2 R_m$, $10^2 R$) data shown in B. (B, C) Linear oscillatory rheology measurements of $G'(\omega)$ for actin networks with different combinations of $+/-10^2 R_m = 2$ and $+/-10^2 R = 0.5$ compared to networks without motors or crosslinkers (black) and networks with motors deactivated by the myosin inhibitor blebbistatin (magenta). (C) The elastic modulus G' measured at $\omega = 1$ rad s^{-1} as a function of (i) myosin concentration $10^2 R_m$ or (ii) filaminA concentration $10^2 R$ for networks with (i) $10^2 R = 0$ (grey triangles), 0.5 (blue squares), 1 (red triangles), or (ii) $10^2 R_m = 0$ (grey triangles), 2 (blue squares), 5 (red triangles). Solid lines in (ii) correspond to $G' \sim R^{0.17}$ (grey) and $G' \sim R^{0.79}$ (blue). (D) Schematic depicting nonlinear rheology measurements to compare the effects of internal pre-stress from myosin motors σ_{int} (left) and external pre-stress σ_{ext} (right) on the network response to linear oscillatory shearing $\sigma_{\text{lin}}(\omega)$. (E) Nonlinear modulus $K'(\omega)$ for actin networks subject to either internal (lines) or external (points) pre-stress quantified by, respectively, $10^2 R_m$ (left, light color-coded labels) and σ_{ext} (Pa) (right, dark color-coded labels). (F) K', normalized by the linear modulus G', versus σ_{ext}, normalized by the critical stress for the onset of nonlinearity σ_{cr} for actomyosin networks with $10^2 R = 0.5$ and varying myosin concentrations listed in the legend, collapse onto a master curve with power-law scaling $K' \sim G'\sigma_{\text{ext}}^1$ (black line). (Inset) The critical strain for nonlinearity decreases with increasing myosin-generated internal stress according to the power law $\gamma_{\text{cr}} \sim \sigma_{\text{int}}^{-1}$ (top), while the rupture stress $\sigma_{\max}$ increases with increasing crosslinking according to $\sigma_{\max} \sim R^1$ with (blue squares) and without (white triangles) myosin (bottom). Adapted from Koenderink *et al* (2009) with permission of PNAS.

different crosslinkers including α-actinin (Bendix *et al* 2008, Koenderink and Paluch 2018) (figure 8.3), fascin (figure 8.4) (Alvarado *et al* 2013, 2019, Stam *et al* 2017), and filamin (figure 8.5) (Koenderink *et al* 2009, Stam *et al* 2017).

Early work examining actomyosin networks with $c_A = 23\ \mu$M and $10^2 R_m = 2$, crosslinked by α-actinin at $R = 0.11$, demonstrated the formation of a macroscopic pancake-like gel that contracted to ~6% of its initial volume with a peripheral contractile speed v_p that rapidly slowed as the network shrunk and densified (figure 8.3(A)). Moreover, varying the myosin concentration showed that v_p increased with increasing R_m until reaching a saturating speed of $v_p \approx 4\ \mu\text{m s}^{-1}$ at $10^2 R_m = 5$ (figure 8.2(B)), generating forces of ~μN that correspond to ~100 pN per bundle (Bendix *et al* 2008, Koenderink and Paluch 2018).

This same study demonstrated that increasing the α-actinin:actin ratio R, in the absence of myosin, led to isotropic crosslinking followed by bundling (figure 8.3(C)), which resulted in a non-monotonic dependence of contractility on R (figure 8.3(D)). Namely, networks with too few ($10^2 R \lesssim 3$) or too many ($10^2 R \gtrsim 20$) crosslinkers inhibited contraction due to reduced connectivity from either too few crosslinkers to sufficiently connect filaments or too much bundling to maintain sufficient connections between bundles in the network (Bendix *et al* 2008, Silva *et al* 2011, Koenderink and Paluch 2018). Higher motor concentrations expanded the range of R values that allowed for contraction, likely by enhancing connectivity (important in the low R limit), and providing more force generation to counteract crosslinker friction (important in the high R limit).

To further investigate the interplay between motor activity and connectivity, and the underlying mechanisms and parameter space for actomyosin contraction, confocal imaging experiments examined the structure of actomyosin networks with $c_A \simeq 12\ \mu$M, $10^2 R_m = 1$ and varying fascin:actin ratios of $10^2 R = 0.2$–10 (figure 8.4) (Alvarado *et al* 2013). These studies confirmed that at very low levels of crosslinking ($10^2 R \lesssim 1$), actomyosin networks locally contract into clusters of sizes $\ell \approx 10^1$–$10^2\ \mu$m (figures 8.4(A) and (B)) (Alvarado *et al* 2013). As R increases, the contractility results in larger asters ($\ell \approx 10^2$–$10^3\ \mu$m) that break apart, forming a critically connected state in which the connection probability scales as a power law with the cluster area ℓ^2 (figures 8.4(A) and (B)). At even higher R values ($10^2 R \gtrsim 5$), when the network is maximally connected, the entire network globally contracts into a central network-spanning cluster of order $\ell \gtrsim 1$ mm (figures 8.4(A) and (B)). Complementary simulations were able to recapitulate these results and demonstrate that critical connectivity arises at an intermediate number of crosslinkers, below which small disconnected foci form, and above which global contraction ensues (figure 8.4(C)). These simulations also demonstrated that motor activity expands the criticality region of the phase space and shifts it to higher crosslinker densities (figure 8.4(C)) (Alvarado *et al* 2013).

Finally, these studies showed that contractility in the region of critical connectivity ($10^2 R = 2$) depended non-monotonically on R_m, with too few motors ($10^2 R_m \lesssim 0.2$) providing insufficient force to restructure the network while too many motors ($10^2 R_m > 5$) generate forces high enough to rupture connections between local asters, reducing the average cluster size proportionally. This counter-intuitive result, that increasing the density of force-generating units can hinder contractility, was supported by simulations that showed that cluster sizes scaled inversely with the force generated by the motors, $\ell \sim f_m^{-1}$. This suppressed contractility at high force was suggested to arise from breaking of crosslinker bonds and bending of filaments that violate the affine deformation criteria necessary for coordinated large-scale contraction (Alvarado *et al* 2013).

The studies discussed above were primarily focused on the effect of crosslinking on the structure and contraction rates of actomyosin networks, yet their results suggest similarly important roles of crosslinking and motor activity on the rheological properties of actomyosin networks. To investigate the impact of passive crosslinking and myosin-generated forces on rheological properties, bulk rheology measurements were performed on networks of actin at $c_A = 23.8\ \mu$M and varying concentrations of filamin ($0.05 \leqslant 10^2 R \leqslant 3$) and myosin ($0.1 \leqslant 10^2 R_m \leqslant 5$) (figure 8.5) (Koenderink *et al* 2009). Linear oscillatory measurements showed that without filamin crosslinking, myosin motors ($10^2 R_m = 2$) had negligible impact on the elastic modulus G' of the actin network. Moreover, adding crosslinkers without myosin, or with myosin and its inhibitor blebbistatin, both resulted in a similar modest increase in G'. However, G' measured for networks with both myosin and filamin was shown to be nearly two orders of magnitude higher than the passive actin network (figure 8.5(B)). This general result held for a range of myosin and filamin concentrations. Namely, increasing either R_m or R at a fixed R or R_m generally increases G' (figure 8.5(C)).

These same studies (Koenderink *et al* 2009) showed that passive networks pre-stressed by a large external stress σ_{ext} and active networks (presumably pre-stressed with σ_{int} by myosin motors) (figure 8.5(D)) exhibited similar frequency-dependence of the nonlinear modulus $K'(\omega)$; with motor-generated pre-stresses mapping nearly exactly to σ_{ext} (figure 8.5(E)). Moreover, the nonlinear modulus $K'(\sigma_{\text{ext}})$ of actomyosin networks with a wide range of myosin concentrations were shown to collapse to a single master curve described by the scaling $K' \sim G'\sigma_{\text{ext}}$ when σ_{ext} was scaled by the critical stress σ_{cr} for the onset of nonlinearity (figure 8.5(F)). Finally, while the rupture stress was shown to be independent of myosin concentration and scale linearly with crosslinker concentration (i.e., $\sigma_{\max} \sim R$), the critical strain for nonlinearity γ_{cr} was shown to be inversely proportional to motor-generated stress $\gamma_{\text{cr}} \sim \sigma_{\text{int}}^{-1}$, independent of R (figure 8.5(F) inset) (Koenderink *et al* 2009).

Theoretical modeling. Several theoretical models have been developed to shed light on the mechanisms driving contraction in different regions of the parameter space of actomyosin networks, considering contributions from filament bending (Lenz 2014, Stam *et al* 2017, Koenderink and Paluch 2018, Alvarado *et al* 2019), stretching (Lenz 2014, Stam *et al* 2017, Tam *et al* 2021), buckling (Koenderink and Paluch 2018, Wollrab *et al* 2018), and polarity sorting (Wollrab *et al* 2018), as well as friction from neighboring filaments, crosslinkers, and the viscous medium (Tam *et al* 2021) (figure 8.6).

Several models that have recapitulated experimentally observed actomyosin features have indicated that the robustly contractile (rather than extensile) action of myosin in disordered actin networks is due to the semiflexible nature of actin filaments, which allows for bending (figures 8.6(A)–(C)) (Lenz 2014, Tam *et al*

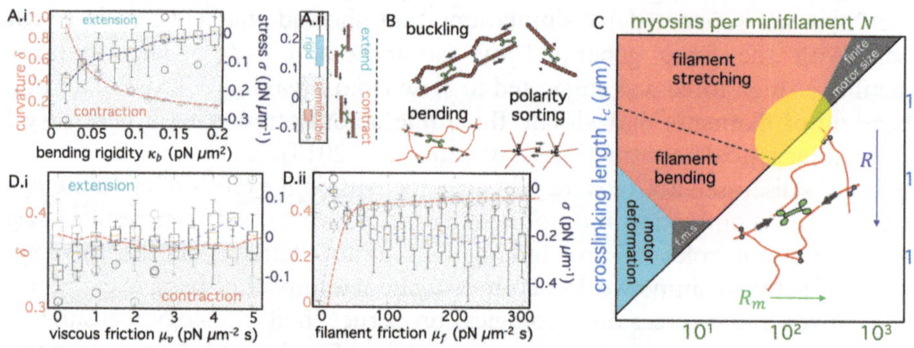

Figure 8.6. Simulations evaluating different potential contributions of buckling, polarity sorting, bending, stretching, and friction to actomyosin contractility. (A) Simulated networks of 50 semiflexible filaments and 10 force-generating motors are evaluated to determine (i) filament curvature δ (coral left axis) and network stress σ (cyan right axis) as a function of filament bending rigidity κ_b and (ii) average network stress σ for semiflexible (coral) and rigid (cyan) filaments. White regions ($\delta > 1$) indicate extension while grey regions ($\delta < 1$) indicate contraction. (B) Cartoon depiction of potential origins of contractility: filament buckling, bending, and polarity sorting. (C) Actomyosin parameter space, defined by the number of myosin heads per minifilament N (green x-axis) and length between crosslinkers l_c (blue y-axis), divided into regions with different predicted dominant mechanisms underlying contraction. Yellow area indicates experimentally investigated region of the parameter space. Filament bending and stretching dominate most of the parameter space with increasing R (blue arrow) and R_m (green arrow) pushing contractility towards bending and stretching, respectively. (D) Effect of (i) viscous friction and (ii) filament friction on the filament curvature δ (coral left axis) and network stress σ (cyan right axis) in simulated networks evaluated in (A) show that filament friction plays an important role in contractility. (A, D) Adapted from Tam *et al* (2021) Copyright (2021), with permission from Elsevier. (B) Adapted from Koenderink and Paluch (2018) Copyright (2018), with permission from Elsevier. (C) Adapted from Lenz (2014). CC BY 3.0.

2021). However, reducing the crosslinker density or increasing the rigidity of the filaments shifts the deformation to stretching-dominated by suppressing bending (figures 8.6(A) and (C)). Moreover, while filament friction from steric interactions (entanglements) or crosslinking does not, in and of itself, contribute to contractility, these steric hindrances enhance the filament bending that is presumed to be essential for global contraction (figure 8.6(D.i)). Conversely, viscous friction from the surrounding media has been suggested to modestly inhibit contraction (figure 8.6(D.ii)) (Tam *et al* 2021).

Other theoretical studies have suggested that for actomyosin networks that are highly bundled by passive crosslinkers, longitudinal buckling plays a more important role than transverse bending, owing to the increased stiffness of the fibers (figure 8.6(B)) (Stam *et al* 2017, Koenderink and Paluch 2018, Wollrab *et al* 2018). However, in this regime, at sufficiently low crosslinker densities and/or high motor concentrations contractility has been predicted to result from polarity sorting and dwelling of motors at the end of polar actin filaments (Wollrab *et al* 2018). This end-dwelling leads to preferential collection of motors at the centers of polar asters which act as contractile cores (Wollrab *et al* 2018).

Quasi-2D actomyosin networks. The experimental results described above are for disordered 3D networks confined in experimental sample chambers. However, numerous studies have been performed on quasi-2D actin networks, typically crowded to the surface by depletants such as methyl cellulose or PEG and selectively imaged using TIRF or confocal microscopy (Murrell and Gardel 2012, Linsmeier *et al* 2016a, Stam *et al* 2017). Similar to 3D networks, 2D networks exhibit organized contraction and local aster formation tuned by the concentrations of actin, crosslinkers, and motors. However, the regions of the parameter space where these distinct dynamics manifest differ from those of 3D networks (Linsmeier *et al* 2016a, Stam *et al* 2017, Wollrab *et al* 2018, Muresan *et al* 2022).

For example, previous studies on 2D actomyosin networks have shown that robust contractility can be achieved without crosslinkers, resulting in asters of locally contracted filaments or uniform contractility depending on the concentrations of actin and myosin (Linsmeier *et al* 2016a, Wollrab *et al* 2018) Selective activation of myosin in specific regions of the 2D network, with the use of myosin inhibitor blebbistatin (figure 8.7(A)), was shown to result in telescopic contractility in which the contraction speed scaled with the size of the activated region (figure 8.7(B)) (Linsmeier *et al* 2016a). The contractile dynamics in the activation zone were also shown to be dependent on the activation time t_a, increasing in speed and then becoming more ordered radially inward towards the contractile core (figure 8.7(C) inset). The divergence of the velocity field, ∇v, a measure of contraction, with more negative values indicating increasing contractility, was also shown to (negatively) increase over time until saturating at a maximum (negative) value at $t_a \approx 300$ s (figure 8.7(C)), after which coalescence or aggregation takes over as the primary mode of myosin-driven restructuring (Linsmeier *et al* 2016b).

This telescopic phenomenon was shown to scale primarily with the planar motor density Ω_m (figures 8.7(D) and (E)). Namely, the strain rate $\dot{\varepsilon}$ increased linearly with Ω_m, independent of changes to the filament stiffness (via bundling) or connectivity (via crosslinkers) (figure 8.7(D)) (Linsmeier *et al* 2016b). Contractility was also observed to be highly cooperative, switching from a minimal strain state to maximal strain state upon reaching percolation (Linsmeier *et al* 2016b). Specifically, fitting the maximum strain $\varepsilon_{\max}$ versus Ω_m to a Hill function yielded a cooperativity parameter of $n_{\text{Hill}} \approx 11$, indicating highly positive cooperativity, with a critical motor density for the onset of contractility of $\Omega_m = 0.56\ \mu\text{m}^{-2}$ (figure 8.7(E)). Isotropic active gel modeling and agent-based simulations were able to recapitulate the results to demonstrate that telescopic behavior can arise solely from viscoelasticity and active stresses (figures 8.7(D) and (E) insets).

Other studies on quasi-2D actomyosin networks have shown that contractile deformations can switch to uniaxial extension when the filaments are sufficiently bundled (via fascin), by making biaxial bending prohibitively costly (figures 8.7(F)–(H)) (Stam *et al* 2017). This uniaxial extensibility, suggested to arise from filament sliding, leads to local aster formation that is suppressed when the bundles are sufficiently crosslinked (via filamin) (figures 8.7(F) and (G)) (Stam *et al* 2017). Further increasing the crosslinking between bundles shifts the deformation again towards uniform contractility (figures 8.7(G) and (H)) (Lenz 2014, 2020, Stam *et al* 2017).

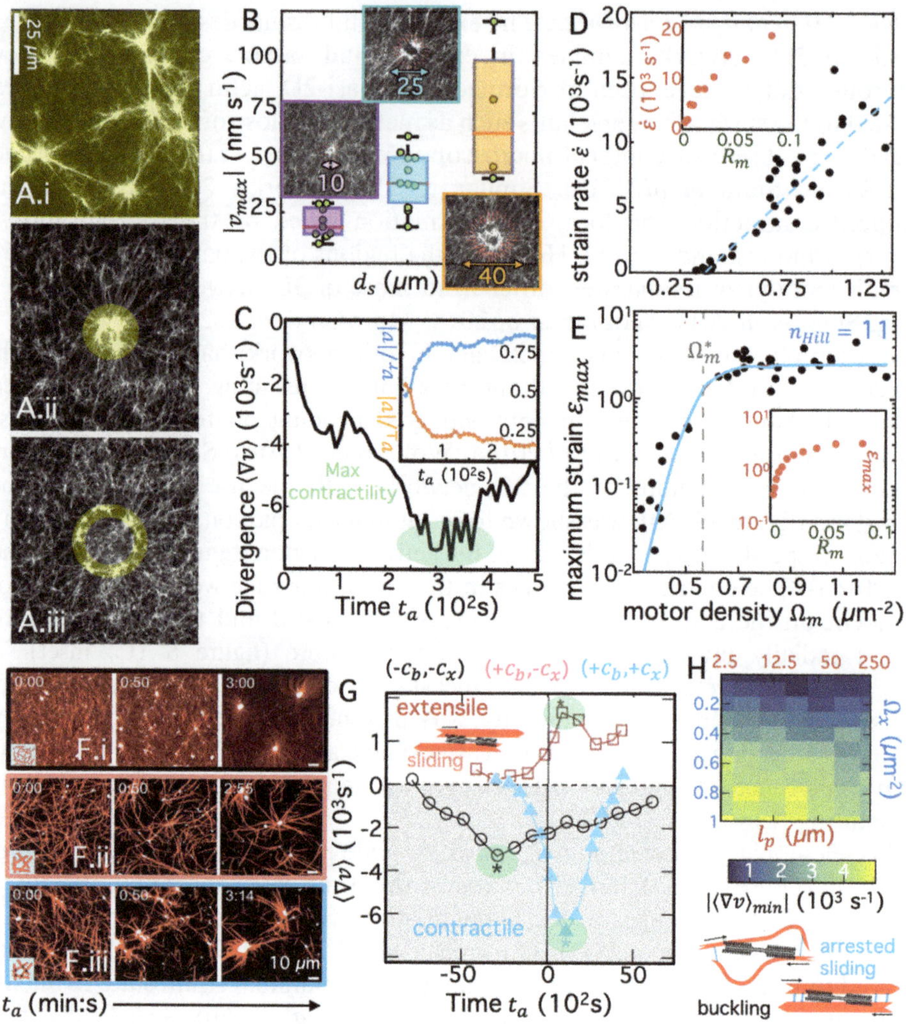

Figure 8.7. Confocal microscopy and PIV analysis of dynamics of quasi-2D contractile actomyosin networks. (A–E) Confocal imaging and PIV of quasi-2D actomyosin networks with $c_A = 1.3\ \mu$M and $10^2 R_m = 1.8$, crowded to a lipid bilayer membrane by methyl cellulose, in the presence of myosin inhibitor blebbistatin (20 nM). (A) Blebbistatin is deactivated, thereby activating myosin, by stimulation with 405 nm light, producing different patterns of contractility when (i) the entire FOV, (ii) a local circle, or (ii) local ring are illuminated (yellow). (B) Maximum contractile speed at the periphery $|v_{\max}|$ of stimulation zones of diameters d_s (μm) = 10 (purple), 25 (cyan), and 40 (orange) show that $|v_{\max}|$ increases with d_s. (C) Divergence of the velocity field averaged over the activation area $\langle \Delta v \rangle$, with more strongly negative values indicating more contractility, shows maximum contractility (green) reached at $t_a \approx 300$ s. (Inset) Fractional radial and tangential velocities $v_r/|v|$ (blue) and $v_\perp/|v|$ (orange) averaged over the activation area. (D) Contractile strain rate $\dot{\varepsilon}$ displays linear dependence (dashed blue line) on myosin minfilament number density Ω_m. (Inset) Agent-based simulation of $\dot{\varepsilon}$ shows similar linear dependence on R_m. (C) Maximum contractile strain $\varepsilon_{\max}$ versus Ω_m is well-fit to a Hill function (blue line) with a Hill coefficient $n_{\text{Hill}} = 11$ and critical myosin density $\Omega_m^* \simeq 56\ \mu\text{m}^{-2}$, above which networks undergo significant strain ($\varepsilon_{\max} > 1$). (Inset) Simulated $\varepsilon_{\max}$ versus R_m recapitulates experimental results. (F–H) Confocal imaging and PIV of quasi-2D networks of actin (red) at $c_A = 1\ \mu$M and myosin

(white) at $10^2 R_m = 7.7$ with (+) and without (−) bundling by fascin (c_b =100 nM) and/or crosslinking by filamin ($c_x = 2$ nM). (F) Actomyosin networks (i) without crosslinking or bundling ($-c_b$, $-c_x$) (black border), (ii) with bundling only ($+c_b$, $-c_x$) (coral border), and (ii) with both bundling and crosslinking ($+c_b$, $+c_x$) (blue border) contract over different spatiotemporal scales. Insets in left panels are cartoon depictions of actin network. (G) Divergence $\langle \Delta v \rangle$ versus myosin activity time t_a for networks shown in F show that crosslinking and bundling together ($+c_b$, $+c_x$) enhance contractility (blue triangles) compared to the ($-c_b$, $-c_x$) contractile network (open black circles), while bundling without crosslinking ($+c_b$, $-c_x$) leads to extensile deformation due to filament sliding (inset). Grey and white regions separated by dashed horizontal line denote contractile and extensile motion, respectively; and green circles denote maximum contractility or extensility. (H) Simulated maximum contractility, quantified as the magnitude of the minimum divergence $|\langle \Delta v \rangle_{\min}|$ (denoted by green regions in (G)), represented by the blue-yellow color scale, as a function of persistence length l_p of network fibers (filaments or bundles) and crosslinker number density Ω_x. Cartoon depiction of contractile mechanisms for crosslinked filaments that are flexible (buckling) or rigid (arrested sliding). (A–E) Adapted from Linsmeier *et al* (2016a). CC BY 4.0. (F–H) Adapted from Stam *et al* (2017) with permission of PNAS.

Moreover, in cases in which the filaments are very tightly bundled by non-compliant crosslinkers, motor gliding is slow and exhibits periods of stalling that results in larger force generation, in line with the results described above in which increased bundling leads to more pronounced contractility and force generation (Weirich *et al* 2021). Finally, studies on 2D actomyosin networks adhered to model cell membranes (Murrell and Gardel 2012) have investigated the impact of adhesion on the contractility, reporting that the dominant mechanism underlying contraction is filament buckling and severing. Increasing adhesion was shown to enhance local buckling and severing due to increased compressive stresses, while, at the same time, suppressing long-range global contraction due to increased adhesive drag (Murrell and Gardel 2012).

The above studies, as well as others (Koenderink and Paluch 2018, Burla *et al* 2019, Weirich *et al* 2021), have highlighted the importance of actin network architecture on the resulting network restructuring, focusing on the role of actin bundling and crosslinkers. Other studies have also investigated the role of filament length (Mizuno *et al* 2007, Lenz 2014, 2020), turnover (i.e., treadmilling) (Burla *et al* 2019, Malik-Garbi *et al* 2019, Tam *et al* 2021, Muresan *et al* 2022), and branching (Muresan *et al* 2022). For example, branching by the nucleating Arp 2/3 complex was reported to inhibit force generation and restructuring by inhibiting processivity of myosin motors along filaments (Muresan *et al* 2022).

Encapsulated actomyosin networks. Actomyosin networks encapsulated in lipid bilayer membranes, giant unilamellar vesicles (GUVs), or oil-in-water droplets have been investigated to determine the extent to which confinement and adhesion characteristics impact actomyosin network dynamics and architecture, revealing a range of architectures and dynamics that are not seen in bulk (Bashirzadeh and Liu 2019, Malik-Garbi *et al* 2019, Jahnke *et al* 2020, Litschel *et al* 2021, Bashirzadeh *et al* 2022).

For example, in the absence of crosslinkers or membrane anchoring, actomyosin networks confined in GUVs of diameters $D_{\mathrm{GUV}} \approx 10$–$60\ \mu$m were shown to uniformly contract to a central cluster for large GUVs ($D_{\mathrm{GUV}} \gtrsim 15\ \mu$m) or accumulate at the periphery for small GUVs ($D_{\mathrm{GUV}} < 15\ \mu$m) (figure 8.8(A)) (Bashirzadeh *et al* 2022). Incorporating fascin and/or α-actinin resulted in diverse

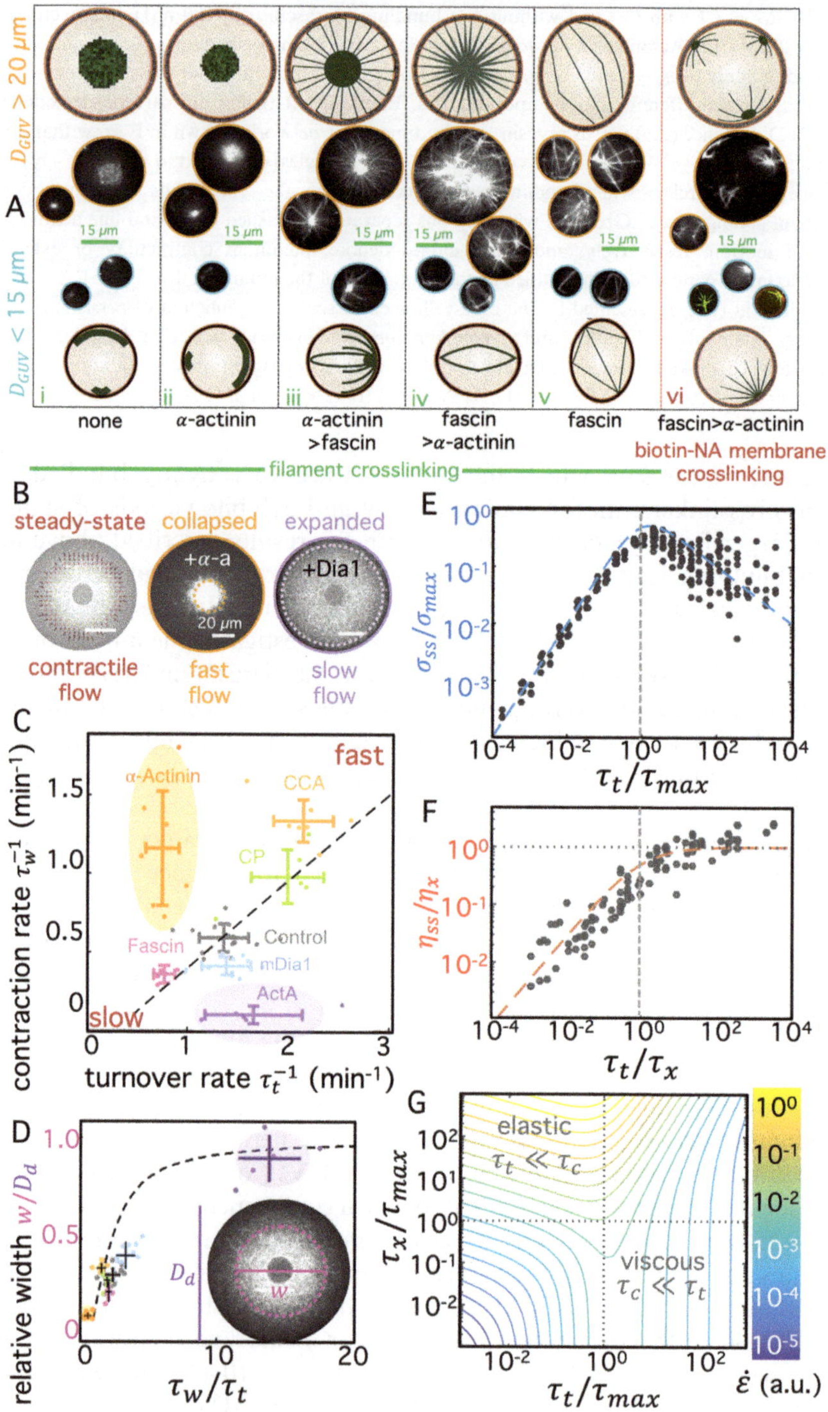

Figure 8.8. Structure and dynamics of encapsulated actomyosin networks depend on crosslinking, turnover, and membrane interactions. (A) Cartoons and confocal micrographs of actomyosin networks with $c_A = 5\ \mu$M

and $10^2 R_m = 1.26$, encapsulated in GUVs of varying diameters from $D_{GUV} < 15\ \mu$m (left, cyan borders) to $D_{GUV} > 20\ \mu$m (right, orange borders) show distinct structures in the presence of varying concentrations of α-actinin (ii–vi) and/or fascin (iii–vi) and without (green, i–v) or with (red, v) membrane adhesion via biotin-NA crosslinking. Green scale bars correspond to the confocal images of encapsulated actin. (B) Actomyosin networks formed by encapsulating Xenopus egg extract in water-in-oil droplets with diameter $D_d \approx 10^2\ \mu$m exhibit steady-state contractile flow directed radially inward (red, middle). The width of the contractile network w decreases and the contraction rate increases upon crosslinking with 10 μM α-actinin (orange, left), while branching using 1.5 μM ActA induces the opposite effect (purple, right). (B) Steady-state flow rates increase/decrease without altering the network structure by proportionally increasing/decreasing the rates of actin turnover τ_t^{-1} (x-axis) and contraction τ_w^{-1} (y-axis) (dashed line) using a variety of co-factors including: crosslinker fascin (pink, 2.6 μM), nucleator mDia (blue, 0.5 μM), depolymerizing capping protein (green, 0.5 μM), and depolymerizing cofilin/coronin/Aip1 (orange, 12.5/1.3/1.3 μM). Inclusion of α-actinin (10 μM, dark orange shaded region) or ActA (1.5 μM purple shaded region) alter the network structure as shown in A. (C) The network width w, depicted in the inset, normalized by the droplet diameter D_d as a function of the ratio between the rates of turnover and contraction τ_t^{-1}/τ_w^{-1} shows that increasing τ_w^{-1} generally shrinks the network while increasing τ_t^{-1} generally broadens it. (E–G) Computational modeling and simulations of actomyosin networks with crosslinking and turnover determine the role of turnover in sustaining long-range steady-state flows. (E) Steady-state stress exerted by the network at the boundaries σ_{ss}, normalized by the maximum predicted stress in the absence of turnover σ_{max}, versus the turnover time τ_t, normalized by the time τ_{max} to reach σ_{max}. Data for a range of different network parameters and turnover times collapse to a single curve that aligns with the predicted expression $\sigma_{ss} = \sigma_{max}/\left[\frac{\tau_t}{\tau_{max}} + \frac{\tau_{max}}{\tau_t}\right]$ (blue dashed line). (F) Steady-state viscosity η_{ss}, normalized by the value in the absence of turnover $\eta_x = 4\pi\mu_x\left[\frac{L}{l_c} - 1\right]^2$ where μ_x is the crosslink drag coefficient, versus turnover time τ_t, normalized by the time τ_x at which the response transitions from elastic to viscous. For $\tau_t < \tau_x$, network viscosity is controlled by the turnover time according to $\eta_{ss} = \eta_x\left[1 + \left(\frac{\tau_x}{\tau_t}\right)^{3/4}\right]^{-1}$ (red dashed line). (G) Phase map of the dependence of steady-state flow rate $\dot{\varepsilon}$, color-coded according to the unitless scale, on the elastic timescale τ_x (y-axis) and turnover time τ_t (x-axis). (A) Adapted from Bashirzadeh *et al* (2022) Copyright (2022), with permission from Elsevier. (B–D) Adapted from Malik-Garbi *et al* (2019) Copyright (2019), with permission from Springer Nature. (E–G) Adapted from McFadden *et al* (2017). CC BY 4.0.

structures ranging from connected meshworks, to stiff peripheral rings, to asters, depending on the crosslinker type and concentration as well as the GUV size (figure 8.8(A)). When filaments were anchored to the membrane via biotin-streptavidin, actomyosin activity resulted in peripheral contractile rings in the presence of α-actinin, which transitioned to peripheral asters with luminal protrusions when fascin was incorporated (figure 8.8(A)) (Bashirzadeh *et al* 2022). Moreover, the fraction of asters versus rings was reported to increase with increasing GUV size.

Network/GUV combinations that resulted in contractile actomyosin rings were shown to be most effective at deforming the GUVs via contraction (Bashirzadeh *et al* 2022), and the formation of such rings was shown to be the most probable when crosslinking filaments with talin and vinculin rather than α-actinin or fascin (Bashirzadeh and Liu 2019, Litschel *et al* 2021). These same studies showed that shorter filaments and smaller GUVs more readily produced rings, as opposed to asters or luminal networks, and that while membrane adhesion increased the probability of ring formation it was not a requirement (Litschel *et al* 2021).

Building on these works, researchers employed DNA linkers to specifically adhere encapsulated actin filaments to the periphery of droplets, and used UV-caged ATP to allow for light-controlled activity of myosin-coated microspheres (Jahnke *et al* 2020). These studies demonstrated that, upon photo-release of ATP, DNA-linked actomyosin networks formed asymmetric asters which preferentially localized to one side of the droplet, whereas in the absence of linkers the network contracted isotropically to a central cluster (Jahnke *et al* 2020).

While all of the studies discussed above employed phalloidin-stabilized actin filaments, other studies have investigated the role of filament turnover on actomyosin dynamics in cell-like confinement, using Xenopus egg extract encapsulated in water-in-oil droplets (figures 8.8(B)–(D)) (Malik-Garbi *et al* 2019). These studies showed that encapsulated extracts exhibited steady-state contractile flow towards the droplet center with the width of the network w and the contractile flow rate τ_w^{-1} remaining constant over time (figure 8.8(B)). Substantially increasing the contraction rate without altering the turnover rate τ_t^{-1}, achieved by incorporating high concentrations (10 μM) of α-actinin, shrunk the network width. Conversely, suppressing contractility by nucleating branched filaments with ActA, led to expanded networks (increased w) with slow flow (figure 8.8(B)). Beyond these extreme cases, incorporating a wide range of other nucleators, depolymerizing agents, and crosslinking proteins to selectively alter the turnover rate and network viscoelasticity, altered τ_w^{-1} and τ_t^{-1} proportionally, to maintain steady-state flow and network width (figure 8.8(C)). Moreover, the width was controlled by the ratio of turnover rate to contraction rate, with higher turnover rates relative to contraction resulting in larger widths (figure 8.8(D)).

Complementary simulations showed that the minimum requirements for continuous contractile flow are transient crosslinking and filament turnover, and that the balance of active stresses and viscoelastic resistance, which both scale with actin density, leads to a concentration-independent contraction rate for a wide range of crosslinker and motor concentrations (figures 8.8(E) and (F)) (McFadden *et al* 2017, Malik-Garbi *et al* 2019). Specifically, the steady-state stress σ_{ss} was shown to be dictated solely by the turnover rate according to the relation

$$\sigma_{ss} = \frac{\sigma_{\max}}{(\tau_t/\tau_{\max}) + (\tau_{\max}/\tau_t)} \tag{8.1}$$

where $\sigma_{\max}$ and $\tau_{\max}$ are the maximum stress achieved and the time at which $\sigma_{\max}$ is reached (figure 8.8(E)). Equation (8.1) reduces to linear scaling of the stress with the turnover rate in the fast τ_t^{-1} limit (i.e., $\sigma_{ss} \sim \tau_t^{-1}$). Alternatively, the steady-state viscosity was predicted to depend on the ratio of the turnover time τ_t and elastic crossover time τ_x according to

$$\eta_{ss} = \eta_x\left[1 + \left(\frac{\tau_x}{\tau_t}\right)^{3/4}\right]^{-1} \tag{8.2}$$

where

$$\eta_x = 4\pi\mu_x\left[\frac{L}{l_c} - 1\right]^2 \tag{8.3}$$

and μ_x is the crosslink drag coefficient (figure 8.8(F)) (McFadden *et al* 2017). In the limit of large turnover times, $\eta_{ss} \to \eta_x$ is dominated by the crosslinker density. Balancing active stresses and viscous resistance was shown to lead to two distinct modes of contractility for low and high turnover rates, respectively (figure 8.8(G)). The former supports flow by straining filaments to the elastic limit with effective viscosity scaling with crosslinker density and friction (equation (8.3)), while filaments in the latter case do not reach the elastic limit and effective viscosity scales with elastic stress and turnover time (equation (8.1)) (figure 8.8(G)) (McFadden *et al* 2017).

8.1.2 Other contractile actin networks

While the vast majority of studies on actomyosin networks have utilized myosin II minifilaments to generate stresses and active mechanics, several studies have investigated the role of other myosins, for example, myosin VI, which does not require polymerization into minifilaments to generate forces between actin filaments (Ennomani *et al* 2016). These studies demonstrated contractility of micropatterned 2D actomyosin rings with structure and dynamics that were dependent on the degree of bundling, crosslinking, and structural order of the network (figure 8.9(A)). TIRF microscopy was used to monitor the time-dependent perimeter of constricting rings of disordered networks, disordered bundles, or ordered bundles with and without α-actinin crosslinking (figures 8.9(A) and (B)). Crosslinking was shown to suppress contraction (shrinking) of ordered bundles and disordered networks, while disordered bundles did not contract without α-actinin (figure 8.9(B)). These seemingly opposite effects of crosslinking were shown to arise from a non-monotonic dependence of contraction speed on α-actinin concentration that was most pronounced for disordered bundles (figure 8.9(C)). This non-monotonicity, similar to reported trends in many of the myosin II studies discussed above, was suggested to arise from the same mechanism: too few crosslinkers are unable to provide sufficient connectivity for global contraction, while too many hinder contraction by increasing frictional drag and suppressing bending figure 8.9(D)) (Bendix *et al* 2008, Alvarado *et al* 2013, Linsmeier *et al* 2016a). Complementary simulations supported this conjecture by demonstrating that the mechanical energy, measured by the maximum deformation the network can impose on its substrate, displayed a similarly non-monotonic dependence on [α-actinin] that peaked at a critical intermediate connectivity value that was highest for disordered bundles (figure 8.9(D)) (Ennomani *et al* 2016).

Finally, the passive actin crosslinker, anillin, has been shown to induce contraction of actin bundles and constriction of bundled rings without ATP-consuming motors (figures 8.9(E)–(H)) (Kuçera *et al* 2021). TIRF microscopy was used to show that the initial perimeter p_0 of rings of actin crosslinked with anillin shrunk exponentially over time to a final perimeter value p_0 according to:

$$p(t) = p_0 e^{-t_a/\tau_\Delta} + p_f \tag{8.4}$$

where τ_Δ is the characteristic decay rate that was shown to be ~300 s, independent of the initial or final perimeter size (figure 8.9(F)). Introducing the depolymerizing agent, latrunculin, enhanced ring contraction, leading to a larger final fractional

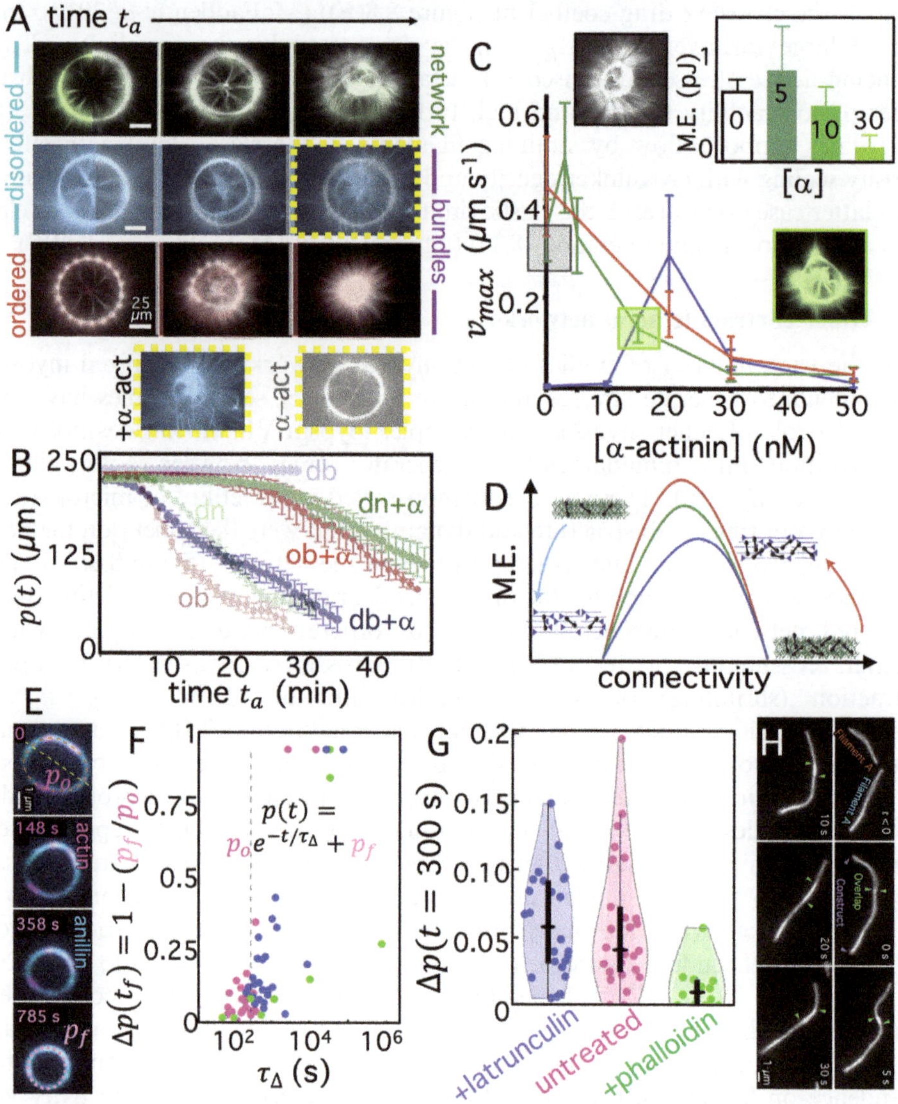

Figure 8.9. Contractile actin rings driven by myosin VI and anillin. (A–C) Rings of actin of initial perimeter $p_0 \approx 220\ \mu\mathrm{m}$, were assembled via surface micropatterning with actin promoting factor, into disordered branched networks (green, dn), disordered bundles (blue, db), and ordered bundles (red, ob), which contracted over time t_a due to myosin VI activity. (A) TIRF microscopy images of disordered networks (green) and bundles (blue) and ordered bundles (red) with α-actinin (false color images) and without (greyscale overlays). (B) Ring perimeters $p(t)$ for different architectures with α-actinin (dark hues) and without (light hues), color-coded and labeled as A, show that crosslinking induces contraction of disordered bundles (db, blue) but slows contractility for ordered bundles (ob, red) and disordered networks (dn, green). (C) Maximum perimeter velocity $v_{\max}$ versus α-actinin concentration for db (blue), ob (red), and dn (green) display peaks at different values of [α-actinin]. (Inset) Predicted maximal mechanical energy *ME* of the disordered network peaks at [α-actinin] = 5 μM, coinciding with peak $v_{\max}$. Grey and green translucent boxes indicate the parameters of the networks shown. (D) Qualitative relationship between *ME* and connectivity (controlled by crosslinking),

predicted from modeling, for db (blue), ob (red), and dn (green), determines the critical connectivity necessary to achieve peak contractility and force generation. (E–G) Rings of actin filaments (pink) contract via the passive crosslinker anillin (blue) increasing the overlap between neighboring filaments. (E) TIRF microscopy time-lapse images of an actin ring contracting from initial perimeter p_0 at $t_a = 0$ to final perimeter p_f at $t_a = 738$ s. (F) Maximum ring constriction $\Delta p = 1 - (p_f/p_0)$ versus time constant τ_Δ that characterizes the exponential decay from p_0 to p_f, $p(t) = p_0 e^{-t_a/\tau_\Delta} + p_f$, for rings of actin that are untreated (magenta), treated with lactrunculin that promotes depolymerization (blue), and phalloidin that stabilizes filaments against depolymerization (green). (Right) Distribution of Δp values at $t_a = 300$ s (indicated in left plot by dashed vertical line) show constriction is enhanced by latrunculin and suppressed by phalloidin. (G) Two actin filaments becoming crosslinked by anillin and subsequently increasing their overlap (indicated by green arrows) by transient crosslinking of anillin. (A–D) Adapted from Ennomani *et al* (2016) Copyright (2016), with permission from Elsevier. (E–H) Adapted from Kuçera *et al* (2021). CC BY 4.0.

perimeter change $\Delta p(t_f) = 1 - (p_f/p_o)$ (figures 8.9(F) and (G)). Conversely, the stabilizing agent, phalloidin, suppressed contraction, reducing $\Delta p(t_f)$ and increasing τ_Δ (figures 8.9(F) and (G)). This turnover dependent contraction was shown to arise from anillin maximizing the length of overlap of neighboring actin filaments to shorten filaments (figure 8.9(H)), a process facilitated by filament disassembly (Kuçera *et al* 2021).

8.1.3 Kinesin-microtubule networks

Kinesin dimers walk along microtubules to deliver cargo across cells. *In vitro*, researchers have shown that by crosslinking or connecting two kinesin dimers can connect neighboring microtubules and pull one relative to the other to impart contractile or extensile sliding of the two filaments, depending on their relative polarity, similar to the action of myosin II on actin (Ndlec *et al* 1997, Pinot *et al* 2009, Sanchez *et al* 2012, Henkin *et al* 2014, Wu *et al* 2017, Opathalage *et al* 2019, Lemma *et al* 2021).

Seminal experiments using this approach formed processive kinesin clusters by linking together biotinylated kinesin 401 dimers (88 kDa, k401-b) via streptavidin molecules. A kinesin:streptavidin ratio of $k{:}s = 4{:}1$ was shown to restructure quasi-2D networks of microtubules into diverse steady-state structures within minutes (Ndlec *et al* 1997, Surrey *et al* 2001a). At $c_T \simeq 2.5\ \mu$M, structures ranged from lattices of vortices at low kinesin concentrations ($c_k < 0.17\ \mu$M, $R_k \simeq 0.07$) to asters of varying sizes for $0.29\ \mu\text{M} < c_k < 0.43\ \mu\text{M}$ $(0.11 < R_k < 0.17)$ to thick bundles for $c_k \gtrsim 0.57\ \mu$M ($R_k \gtrsim 0.23$) (figure 8.10(A)). Similar structures were observed in networks of ~10-fold higher tubulin concentration ($c_T \simeq 26\ \mu$M) and $R_k > 0.03$, but at lower R_k values than reported in Ndlec *et al* (1997) (figure 8.10(B)) (Surrey *et al* 2001b).

Confinement to cylindrical and torus geometries led to the formation of vortical patterns rather than asters, while confinement in cell-sized droplets promoted aster formation over vortices (Ndlec *et al* 1997, Pinot *et al* 2009, Baumann and Surrey 2014, Bashirzadeh and Liu 2019). Similar networks encapsulated in droplets of diameter ~10 to ~30 μm restructured into central asters, cortical-like bundles, or rings for, respectively, large, intermediate, and small droplets (figure 8.10I) (Baumann and

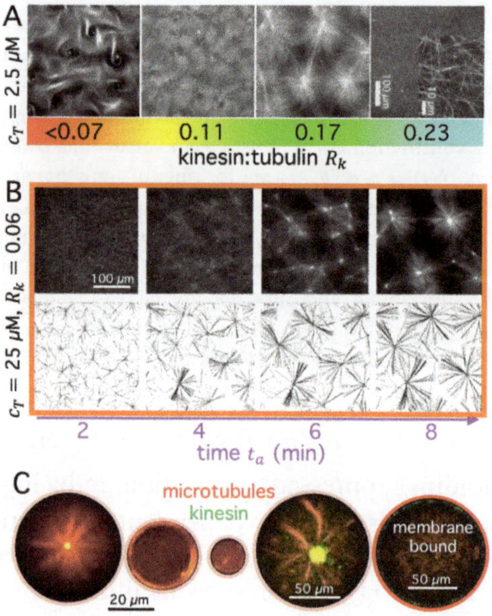

Figure 8.10. Self-organization of microtubules by kinesin clusters. (A) Dark-field microscopy images of Taxol-stabilized microtubules at $c_T \simeq 2.5\ \mu$M in the presence of varying kinesin:tubulin ratios of (left to right) $R_k \simeq 0.07$ (red), 0.11 (yellow), 0.17 (green), and 0.23 (cyan). (B) Experimental images (top) and simulations (bottom) of formation of microtubule asters over time (listed in minutes in purple) for networks with $c_T \simeq 2.5\ \mu$M and $R_k \simeq 0.06$. (C) Encapsulated microtubules (red) at $c_T \simeq 40\ \mu$M and kinesin (green) at $R_k \simeq 0.07$ form asters (left), cortical bundles (middle), and rings (right) for decreasing sizes of lipid monolayer droplets. (D) Central asters of microtubules ($c_T \simeq 2\ \mu$M) and kinesin ($R_k = 0.1$) formed in water-in-oil droplets are eliminated by anchoring kinesin to the membrane, allowing microtubules to instead glide along the inner membrane. (A) Adapted from Ndlec *et al* (1997) Copyright (1997), with permission from Springer Nature. (B) Modified from Surrey *et al* (2001a). © The American Association for the Advancement of Science. (C) Adapted from Baumann and Surrey (2014) (CC BY 4.0) and from Tsuji *et al* (2017). Copyright (2017) American Chemical Society.

Surrey 2014, Tsuji *et al* 2017). Adhering kinesin to the inner surface of emulsion droplets eliminated aster formation and localized microtubules to the inner surface (figure 8.10(C)), where they exhibited gliding and motility (Tsuji *et al* 2017).

This class of experiments demonstrated that kinesin could restructure microtubules into new steady-states. However, they could not control or characterize the dynamics of the networks en route to new steady-states, i.e., the active dynamics, which lasted for only ~3–20 min. To achieve kinesin-driven active matter with prolonged active lifetimes, researchers incorporated k401-b kinesin clusters into networks of microtubules that were assembled into bundles by depletants, e.g., PEG or pluronic, such that they remained in close proximity to one another and co-aligned, but could still slide past one another and extend because they were not physically crosslinked (figure 8.11(A) and (B)) (Sanchez *et al* 2012). This geometric constraint suppressed aster formation, clustering, and structural arrest. To prolong and enhance activity and flow, an ATP regeneration system was incorporated to maintain kinesin ATPase activity, and GTP was replaced with its non-hydrolyzable

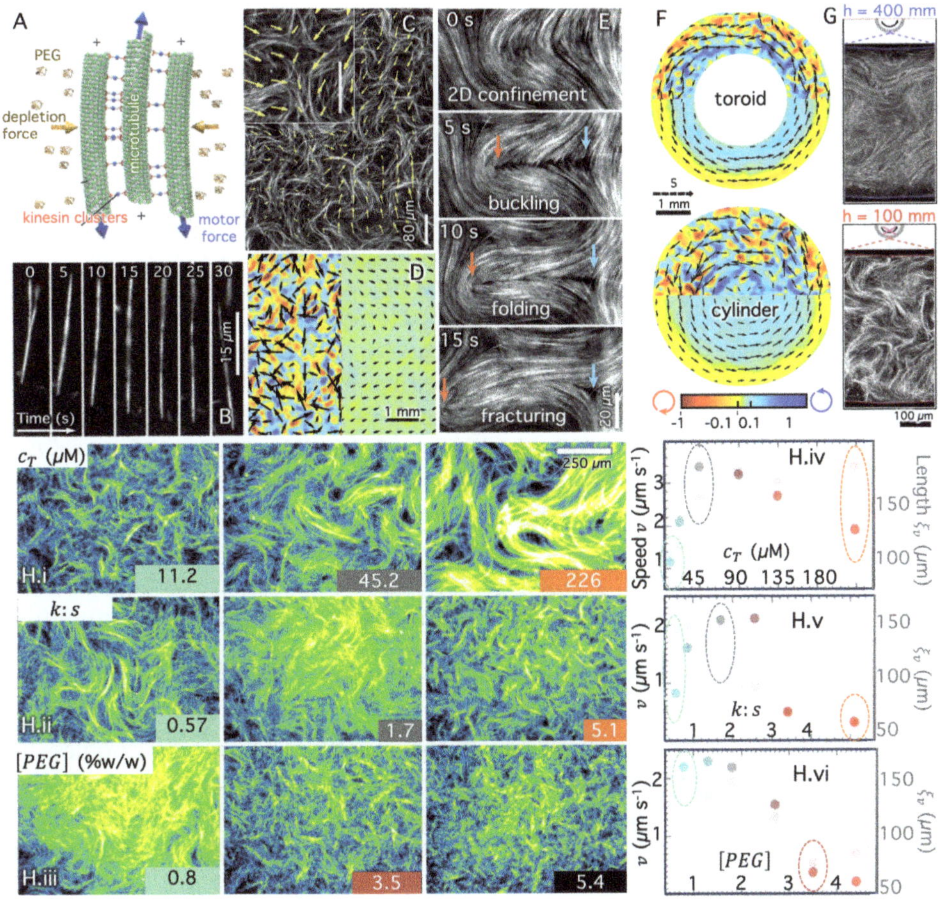

Figure 8.11. Dynamics and tunability of active networks of microtubule bundles driven by kinesin clusters. (A) Schematic of key components of microtubule-kinesin active matter that include depletants (PEG) to bundle microtubules and kinesin clusters that crosslink and walk along anti-aligned microtubules. (B) Microscope time-lapse of two microtubule bundles merging, extending, and falling apart. (C) Large-scale image of active microtubule network ($c_T \simeq 9.1\ \mu$M) with arrows indicating local velocity direction. Inset is zoom-in of top-left region of the FOV. (D) Instantaneous (left) and time-averaged (right) PIV flow field showing turbulent motion on the scale of millimeters, with arrows representing normalized velocity vectors and heat maps indicating the local vorticity direction according to the color scale in F (red = CW, blue = CCW). (D) A monolayer of bundled microtubules forms a liquid-crystalline phase of nematically aligned bundles exhibiting fast streaming flows with oppositely paired disinclination line defects (red and blue arrows) that arise from repeated cycles of buckling, folding, and fracturing over time. (F) Toroidal or cylindrical confinement support coherent circular flows as seen in the time-averaged PIV flow fields (bottom halves). Vorticity color maps and arrow lengthscales are shown and match D. (G) Coherent (top) and incoherent (bottom) motion of microtubule bundles in toroids with heights $h = 400$ mm (blue) and $h = 100$ mm (red). (H) Varying structure (i–iii), speed v (left axis, iv–vi), and velocity pair correlation lengthscale ξ_v (right axis, iv–vi) of kinesin-microtubule networks with varying microtubule concentration c_T (i, iv), kinesin:streptavidin ratio $k{:}s$ (ii, v), or depletant concentration $[PEG]$ (iii, vi). (i–iii) False color confocal images of kinesin-microtubule networks after reaching steady-state, with varying c_T (top), $k{:}s$ (middle), and $[PEG]$ (bottom), as listed in the bottom right of each image in units listed in the first column. Background color of labels match the conditions of the circled data in (iv–vi). Unless noted, system parameters are $c_T \simeq 9.1\ \mu$M, $c_k \simeq 410$ nM ($10^2 R_k \simeq 4.5$), $k{:}s = 1.7$, and $[PEG] = 0.8\%$.

(iv–vi) v (left axes, dark shaded symbols) and ξ_v (right axes, light shaded symbols) for kinesin-microtubule networks as functions of c_T (iv), $k{:}s$ (v), and $[PEG]$ (vi). (A–C, E) Adapted from Sanchez *et al* (2012) Copyright (2012), with permission from Springer Nature. (D, F, G) Modified from Wu *et al* (2017). © The American Association for the Advancement of Science. (H) Adapted from Henkin *et al* (2014). © 2014 The Author(s) Published by the Royal Society. All rights reserved.

analog GMPCPP to stabilize microtubules and produce atypically short filaments ($L \approx 1.5\,\mu$m) (Sanchez *et al* 2012, Henkin *et al* 2014). Finally, the k401-b: streptavidin ratio was lowered from $k{:}s = 4$ to $k{:}s = 1.7$, which was shown to enhance active dynamics (Sanchez *et al* 2012, Henkin *et al* 2014).

This basic construction results in successive extension, bending, buckling, fracturing, and reforming of bundles to produce sustained, steady vortical flows (figure 8.11(C)) that can persist for up to two days and extend to millimeter scales (figure 8.11(D)) (Sanchez *et al* 2012, Henkin *et al* 2014). These general features of the bundled active networks (BANs) are insensitive to the concentrations of ATP (0.01–3 mM), tubulin (~4.6–46 μM), kinesin (~0.02–1.36 μM), and PEG (0.4–10%). When confined to 2D, the active microtubule bundles formed a liquid-crystalline monolayer of locally-aligned bundles that exhibited streaming flows with disinclination line defects that were continuously created and annihilated (figure 8.11(E)). Notably, the typical microtubule bundle curvature spanned tens of microns while the run lengths of the stress-generating kinesins have been shown to be less than a micron (Nasirimarekani *et al* 2022).

Under cylindrical or toroidal confinement, the signature turbulent directionless flows of the 3D bulk kinesin-microtubule networks transitioned to more ordered coherent flow that was oriented with the confinement geometry (figure 8.11(F)) (Wu *et al* 2017). Notably, coherence was eliminated for confinement geometries with large ratios of width to height, i.e. quasi-2D, demonstrating that coherence is a 3D phenomenon (figure 8.11(G)) (Wu *et al* 2017). Moreover, under confinement in cell-sized oil-in-water droplets that were squeezed between two surfaces, kinesin-driven network flow was shown to be sufficient to propel the droplets (Sanchez *et al* 2012). Similar self-propulsion was observed when encapsulating kinesin and microtubules in dextran-rich droplets formed from water–water phase separation of aqueous solutions of dextran and PEG (Sakuta *et al* 2023). In these studies, microtubules co-localized on the inner droplet periphery and kinesin-crosslinked microtubules formed small aggregates in the interior. Upon addition of ATP, aggregates and asters began to grow and undergo vortical flow with speeds that scaled with the kinesin concentration (Sakuta *et al* 2023).

While these general features of BANs described above have been shown to be reproducible across a wide parameter space, the network structure and flow speed v, as well as the velocity correlation lengthscale ξ_v, which defines the characteristic lengthscale over which correlated flow persists, can be tuned by varying, e.g., the microtubule concentration c_T, kinesin:streptavidin ratio $k{:}s$, and depletant concentration $[PEG]$ (figure 8.11(H)) (Henkin *et al* 2014). Similar to the previously reported non-monotonic dependence of actomyosin contraction rate on myosin concentration (e.g., figures 8.2, 8.3), kinesin-microtubule networks have been shown to undergo maximal flow at intermediate kinesin:tubulin ratios R_k, with too few motors not being able to generate enough force for maximal flow while too many motors introduce steric hindrances that slow motion (Henkin *et al* 2014). For example, for a network with $c_T \simeq 13.3\ \mu\text{M}$, a peak speed of $v \approx 3\ \mu\text{m s}^{-1}$ was reported with $10^2 R_k \simeq 0.4$, while $v \approx 1\ \mu\text{m s}^{-1}$ was measured for higher values of $10^2 R_k \simeq 1.0$–3.5 (Henkin *et al* 2014, Chandrakar *et al* 2022). Similar non-monotonic dependence was also reported for: (1) microtubule concentration, with a peak speed of $v \approx 4\ \mu\text{m s}^{-1}$ reported for $c_T \simeq 46\ \mu\text{M}$ (figure 8.11(Hi,iv)); (2) kinesin:streptavidin ratio, with peak speed $v \approx 2\ \mu\text{m s}^{-1}$ occurring at $k{:}s = 1.7$ (figure 8.11(Hii,v)); and (3) PEG concentration, with peak speed of $v \approx 2\ \mu\text{m s}^{-1}$ reported for $[PEG] = 1.2\%$ and nearly stalling when $[PEG]$ increased to 4.4% (figure 8.11(Hiii,vi)) (Henkin *et al* 2014).

To expand the phase space and tunability of the dynamics and structure of BANs, several modifications have been introduced, including replacing the processive clusters of k401-b kinesin dimers (figures 8.12(A)) with either non-processive clusters of k365-b kinesin monomers (figures 8.12(B, D, E)), or k560-b kinesin dimers permanently bound to microtubules via covalent bonding of their non-motor terminus (Chandrakar *et al* 2022). These studies also investigated the effects of bundling microtubules with a passive, transient crosslinker, protein regulator of cytokinesis 1 (PCR1), as compared to bundling with a depletant, 2% pluronic. Both full-length PCR1, as well as a truncated version, PCR1-NSΔC (figures 8.12(F)–(H)), which is expected to be more stable against degradation due to the lack of a C-terminus, were evaluated.

These studies first corroborated the k401-b dynamics reported previously (figure 8.11) (Sanchez *et al* 2012, Henkin *et al* 2014), showing that the flow speed reached a pronounced maximum of $v \approx 3\ \mu\text{m s}^{-1}$ at $10^2 R_k \simeq 0.4$ ($c_k \simeq 50$ nM) followed by a ~2–3-fold drop upon increasing R_k (figure 8.12(D)). Also, in line with previous studies on k401-b, the flow correlation length ξ_v was reported to decrease over the sample lifetime T_a, which likewise decreased with increasing motor concentration (figure 8.12(D)), suggestive of motor interference (Chandrakar *et al* 2022).

Replacing k401-b with non-processive k365-b motors eliminated the non-monotonic dependence of v on kinesin concentration, instead maintaining an average value of $v \approx 3.5\ \mu\text{m s}^{-1}$ up to the highest measured R_k value (figure 8.12(D)). The correlation length ξ_v also maintained nearly constant values over the course of ~9 hours (figure 8.12(E)), indicating more stable and constant dynamics compared to their k401-b counterparts. Conversely, the decay in T_a with increasing kinesin concentration was similar for both k401-b and k365-b (figure 8.12(D)).

Interestingly, using permanently-bound k560 motors caused the flow speed to increase monotonically with motor concentration before reaching an R_k-independent plateau, similar to k365-b motors. However, the structural correlation lengths decayed significantly over time, similar to freely diffusing k401-b. Moreover, k401-b networks in which microtubules were bundled with PCR1 crosslinkers instead of depletants (figures 8.12(F)–(H)) were able to achieve similar lifetimes and non-monotonic dependence of v as the original k401-b system, but with less consistency and greater sensitivity on system parameters such as crosslinker and kinesin concentrations (Chandrakar *et al* 2022). Replacing PCR1 with its more stable truncated version PCR1-NSΔC allowed for higher flow speeds and longer lifetimes that increased linearly with increasing crosslinker concentration (figure 8.12(H)), as opposed to the

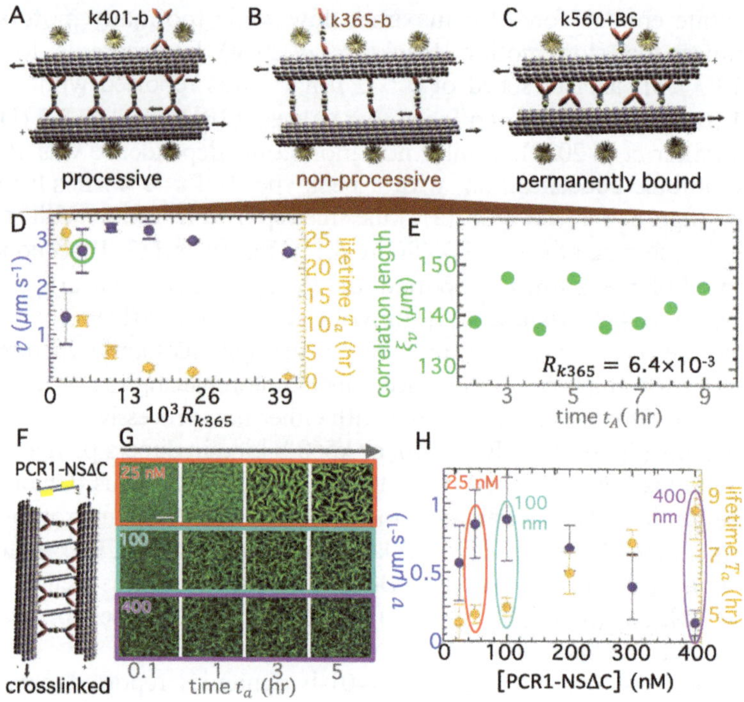

Figure 8.12. Engineering stability and longevity into kinesin-microtubule networks by varying kinesin constructs and bundling agents. (A–C) Schematic of microtubules, bundled by 2% pluronic (yellow stars), being pulled in opposite directions by (A) processive clusters of k401-b kinesin dimers, (B) non-processive clusters of k365-b kinesin monomers (maroon text), and (C) permanently-bound k560 kinesin dimers. (D, E) Non-processive k365-b motors show the most robust and persistent activity, quantified by (D) flow speed v (blue circles and axis labels) and lifetime T_a (yellow circles and axis labels) versus kinesin:tubulin ratio 10^3R_k, and (E) flow correlation length ξ_v (green circles) versus activity time t_a shown for the ratio circled in green in D. (F–G) Effect of microtubule bundling by truncated passive crosslinker PCR1-NSΔC. (G) Time-lapse confocal images of kinesin-microtubule networks undergoing restructuring over the course of activity time $t_a = 0.1$–5 h (left to right) in the presence of PCR1-NSΔC at concentrations of 25 nM (red, top), 100 nM (middle, cyan), and 400 nM (bottom, purple). (H) Flow speed v (blue circles and axis labels) and lifetime T_a (yellow circles and axis labels) versus concentration of PCR1-NSΔC. Circled data correspond to color-matched time-lapse images shown in G. All data are for tubulin concentration $c_T = 13.3\ \mu$M. Adapted from Chandrakar *et al* (2022) with permission from the Royal Society of Chemistry.

decrease seen with PCR1. This increased lifetime was coupled with less restructuring over time (figure 8.12(G)) (Chandrakar *et al* 2022).

In the studies described above, the kinesin motors were continuously consuming ATP and acting on microtubules, with no way to turn on or off or spatially pattern the activity. In actomyosin networks, this photo-control is achieved by using the photo-deactivatable myosin inhibitor, blebbistatin, as shown in, e.g., figures 8.5, 8.7. However, there is no simple analog to this inhibitor for kinesin. Instead, to photo-control kinesin activity, researchers have employed caged ATP that is released upon UV illumination (figures 8.13(A)–(C)) to spatially pattern activity and mix inactive and active regions of kinesin-microtubule networks (Bate *et al* 2022).

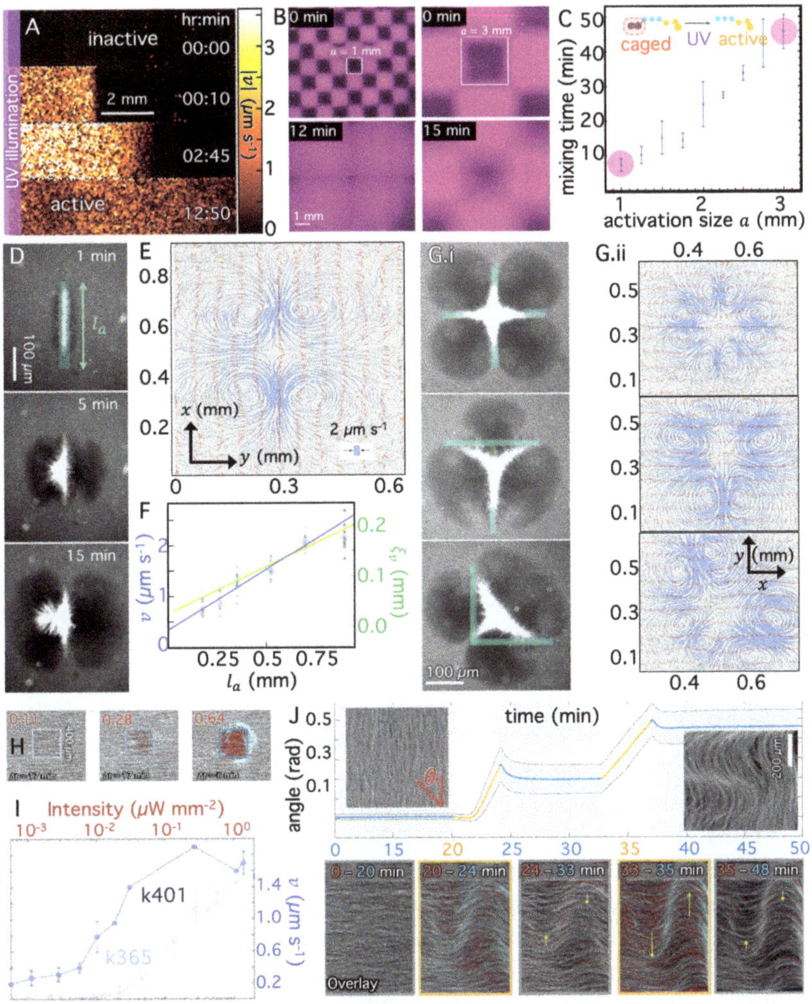

Figure 8.13. Photo-activation, control, and patterning of kinesin-microtubule active nematics. (A–C) Caged ATP is used to selectively activate k401-b kinesin clusters ($10^3 R_k \simeq 10$) bound to microtubule bundles ($c_T \simeq 11.8\ \mu$M) to locally fluidize the crosslinked kinesin-microtubule gel via UV illumination that releases ATP. (A) Speed distribution over time (top to bottom panels) of tracer microspheres embedded in a kinesin-microtubule network illuminated at the left end (purple bar) to activate the motors. Speeds are color-coded according to the scale at right. Over time the active phase expands into the inactive phase, thereby self-mixing the sample. (B) Checkerboard patterned UV illumination mixes the active fluid faster when the grid size is smaller (left column). UV-caged fluorescent dyes that emit fluorescence (magenta) upon UV illumination are visualized. An even distribution of magenta intensities indicates complete mixing. The same regions shown in the top images are shown at a later time in the corresponding bottom images. (C) Mixing time scales linearly with the checkerboard grid size a, depicted in B. The dark and light pink circles denote small and large grid systems shown in B. Inset shows the schematic of UV release of caged ATP. (D–G) k401-iLID and k401-Micro at $c_{ki} \simeq c_{kM} \simeq 0.1\ \mu$M are incorporated into networks of microtubule bundles with $c_T \simeq 2\ \mu$M ($10^3 R_k \simeq 50$) to create spatiotemporal patterning of advective fluid flow and contraction by selectively illuminating small regions of a FOV (cyan bars in D, G). (D) Fluorescence microscopy images of microtubules contracting towards the central illumination bar over time (top to bottom). Initially the microtubules are evenly

distributed, producing a grey background, but then successively accumulate (bright white regions) in the illumination region, and create voids (black regions) in the near surroundings. (E) Streamline plot of background buffer flow during the contraction shown in D, determined by tracking embedded microspheres ($R_s = 1$ μm). Streamline thickness represents speed according to the 2 μm s^{-1} calibration bar and red arrows indicate local flow direction. (F) Average maximum flow speed $|v_{\max}|$ (left/blue axis, dark grey symbols) and spatial correlation lengthscale ξ_v (right/green axis, light grey symbols) increase linearly with activation bar length l_a. Blue and green lines are linear fits to $|v_{\max}|$ and ξ_v, respectively. (G) Superposition of activation bars with different l_a and orientation (horizontal or vertical) create distinct (i) contractile patterns of microtubules and (ii) corresponding flow fields. (H–J) Kinesin-microtubule networks with $c_T \simeq 4.6$ μM were prepared with photo-responsive k365-iLID and k365-Micro motors at $10^3 R_k \simeq 66$ and activated by 488-nm illumination (H) in small regions of the FOV (cyan boxes), (I) at varying laser powers (listed in red in H and I), and (J) in periodic intervals of illumination (orange) and dark (blue) with initial and final times of each interval listed by the first (red) and last (cyan) time point. Microscopy images are overlays of the colorized first and last frame over the listed time period. Grey regions indicate no motion. (J) Average microtubule orientation angle versus time is shown with the corresponding images. (A–C) Adapted from Bate *et al* (2022). CC BY 4.0. (D–G) Adapted from Ross *et al* (2019a) Copyright (2019), with permission from Springer Nature. (H–J) Adapted from Lemma *et al* (2023). CC BY 4.0.

Another important advance towards photo-control of kinesin activity is the engineering of k401 kinesin dimers that are fused with either a photo-activated dimerizing domain, iLID (improved Light-Induced Dimer), or its binding partner, Micro (Guntas *et al* 2015, Ross *et al* 2019). Illumination with 488-nm light induces a conformational change in iLID to increase its binding affinity for Micro (Guntas *et al* 2015, Ross *et al* 2019). This photo-activated dimerization forms kinesin clusters similar to the k401-b-streptavidin kinesin clusters, but that only remain connected when exposed to light (Ross *et al* 2019, Lemma *et al* 2023). By combining k401-iLID and k401-Micro at equal molarity, researchers have been able to mimic the active crosslinking of the widely used k410-b clusters with spatial and temporal control, and demonstrate the ability to localize and spatiotemporally pattern active stresses and dynamics (figures 8.13(D)–(J)) (Ross *et al* 2019, Lemma *et al* 2023). This technology has also been extended to photo-activate k365 kinesin monomers, which were shown to enhance the lifetime and stability of active flows, to spatiotemporally control the extensile flow of kinesin-microtubule networks (Lemma *et al* 2023).

In the active nematics realized above, the density of active crosslinkers (i.e. kinesin motors) was low enough such that individual microtubule bundles were assumed to be disconnected and could thus easily slide and flow past one another (Sanchez *et al* 2012). To explore the other limit of a fully percolated network of active crosslinkers, researchers designed kinesin-microtubule networks with $c_T \simeq 36$ μM, $c_k \simeq 0.3$–0.75 μM ($10^3 R_k \simeq 8.3$–21), and microtubules of length $L \approx 6$ μm (Fürthauer *et al* 2019), all significantly larger than the parameters used in the active fluid experiments described above (Chandrakar *et al* 2022). Moreover, the kinesins used were XCTK2 kinesin-14 motors that can crosslink and slide aligned microtubules without the need to form tetrameric clusters (Hentrich and Surrey 2010). In these experiments, the entire network was observed to globally contract to a nematically aligned state within ~10 min, which persisted for ~1 hour until the network buckled and displayed complex dynamics for hours longer. In the nematically aligned state, microtubules slid past each other at a speed of $v \simeq 20\ \text{nm s}^{-1}$, comparable to the rate at which the motors walked along the microtubules, and independent of motor concentration and microtubule polarity (Fürthauer *et al* 2019). At lower and higher kinesin concentrations, the network either did not contract and align or buckled instantly. The steady self-straining state was shown to arise from a balance between active stresses and viscous drag (Fürthauer *et al* 2019).

8.1.4 Motor-driven cytoskeleton composites

As described above, motor-driven networks of either actin or microtubules have been investigated for decades, revealing wide-ranging non-equilibrium phenomena. More recently, researchers have succeeded in designing motor-driven composites of actin and microtubules (Lee *et al* 2021a, Berezney *et al* 2022, Sheung *et al* 2021, 2022, McGorty *et al* 2023).

8.1.4.1 Myosin-driven composites

For example, incorporating myosin II minifilaments at a concentration $c_M \simeq 0.24\ \mu\text{M}$ ($10^3 R_M \simeq 80$) into equimolar composites of co-entangled actin and microtubules ($c_A \simeq c_T \simeq 2.9\ \mu\text{M}$), was shown to produce steady uniform contraction of both actin and microtubules, characterized by ballistic motion (rather than diffusive, subdiffusive, or superdiffusive) (figures 8.14(B) and (C)) (Lee *et al* 2021b). Moreover, actin and microtubules contracted at the same speed of $v_A \simeq v_{\text{MT}} \simeq 11\ \text{nm s}^{-1}$, measured via DDM; and exhibited correlated contractility as characterized via PIV (figures 8.14(B) and (C)). In the absence of microtubules, actin dynamics were turbulent and incoherent with ~7× faster speeds, resulting in local asters and rupturing similar to previous studies on actomyosin networks without crosslinkers (figures 8.14(B) and (C)). The dynamics were also substantially more heterogeneous across different regions of the sample, with a ~43% spread (i.e., σ_v/v) in measured speeds as compared to $\sigma_v/v \simeq 8\%$ for composites (figure 8.14(C)).

Subsequent studies showed that varying the molar fraction of actin ($\phi_A = c_A/[c_A + c_T]$) or myosin concentration c_M did not alter the ballistic and coordinated motion of the actin and microtubules, but did alter the average contractile speed from $v \simeq 2\ \text{nm s}^{-1}$ to $v \simeq 85\ \text{nm s}^{-1}$ (figures 8.14(A) and (D)) (Lee *et al* 2021a). The time dependence of the composite structure, quantified by the structural correlation length ξ (figure 8.14(E)), and contractile speed, determined via DDM, were also shown to be tuned by ϕ_A (figure 8.14(F)). Specifically, for large actin fractions and myosin concentrations ($\phi_A > 0.5$, $c_M > 0.24$) composites exhibited acceleration and structural decoupling of actin and microtubules ($\xi_{MT} > \xi_A$), whereas for $\phi_A < 0.5$ and $c_M < 0.24$, there was minimal detectable restructuring and modest deceleration over time (figures 8.14(E) and (F)). Complementary mathematical modeling based on rigidity percolation theory demonstrated that the shear modulus G' of the active composites was largest with high concentrations of microtubules (low ϕ_A) or myosin (high c_M) (figures 8.14(D) and (F)), with the former arising from the steady-state rigidity of the microtubules while the latter was due to motor-driven coarsening of an initially floppy network (Lee *et al* 2021a). This effect

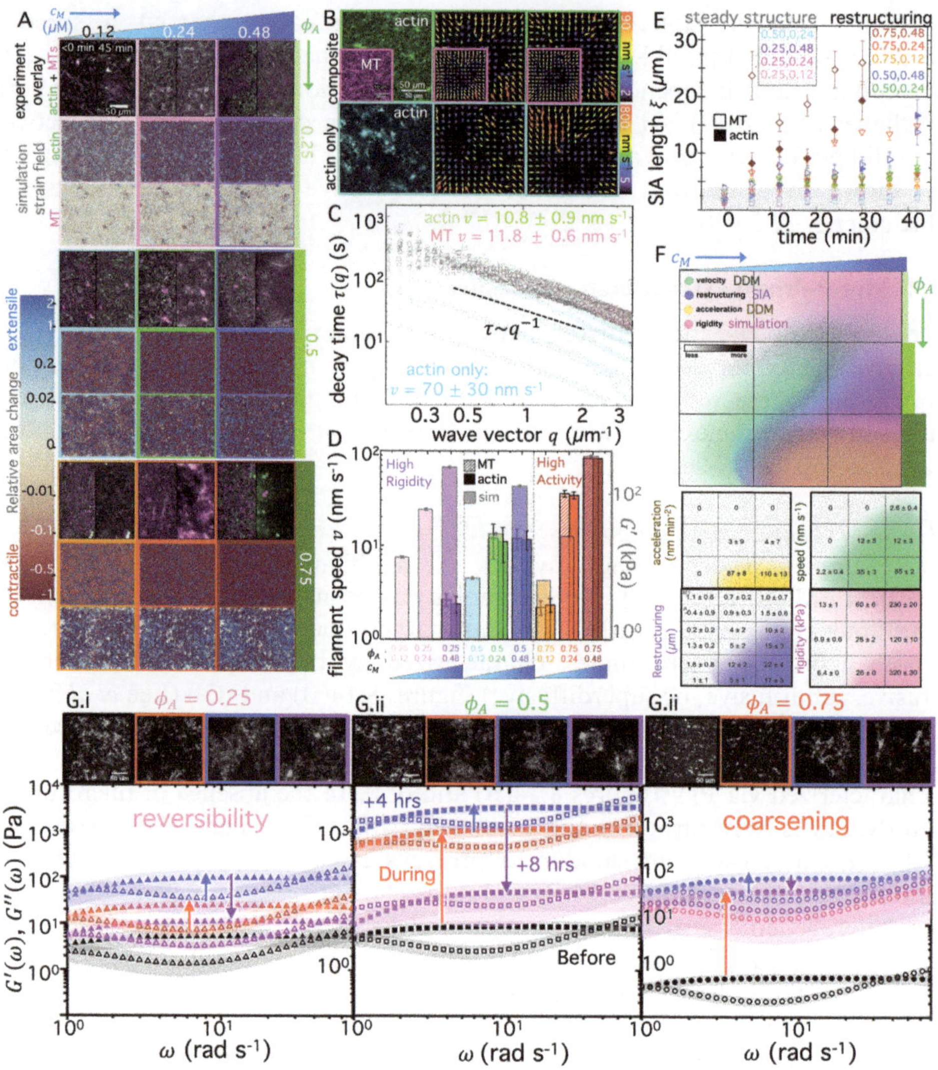

Figure 8.14. Co-entangled composites of actin and microtubules driven by myosin motors to undergo controlled and tunable contractile dynamics. All data shown are for composites with a total molar concentration of $c_A + c_T = 5.8\,\mu$M, with varying molar actin fractions $\phi_A = 0.25$, 0.5, 0.75 (green) and myosin concentrations (blue) c_M (μM) = 0.12, 0.24, 0.48. Myosin activity was photo-controlled by blebbistatin. (A) Confocal microscopy images of actin (green) and microtubules (magenta) in composites before myosin activity (left half of panels) and after 45 min of activity (right half of panels) for increasing c_M (left to right) and ϕ_A (top to bottom). Below each microscope image is a corresponding simulated strain field for actin (top) and microtubules (bottom) in the composite. Strain map colors indicate the degree to which the strain is contractile (red) or extensile (blue). (B) Confocal micrographs before myosin stimulation ($t_a = 0$) (left), and PIV velocity vector fields at $t_a = 30$ s (middle) and $t_a = 6$ min (right), for (top row) actin (green) and microtubules (magenta, insets) in an equimolar ($\phi_A = 0.5$) composite with $c_M = 0.24\,\mu$M, compared to (bottom) the same network without microtubules (actin only). The magnitude of the velocity vectors are color-coded according to scales at right. (C) DDM decay time $\tau(q)$ versus wave vector q for actin (green) and microtubules (magenta) in the composite, and actin in the actin-only network (cyan) shown in B. All data

exhibit ballistic motion signified by $\tau(q) \sim q^{-1}$ scaling, with the average speeds listed. Multiple data sets shown in each color represent different trials. (D) Speed v of actin (filled) and microtubules (hashed) measured via DDM (left/black axis, bright shaded bars), and shear modulus G' computed from simulations (right/grey axis, translucent bars) for composites grouped by ϕ_A (separated by dashed vertical lines). Myosin concentration c_M increases from left to right for each group (blue triangles). (E) Structural correlation length ξ determined from SIA (see chapter 4) versus activity time for composites of varying (ϕ_A, c_M) combinations, listed and color-coded in the legend, show that composites can be divided into those that undergo minimal restructuring (grey shaded region, steady structure, grey legend) and those that undergo substantial restructuring (white region, black bordered legend). (F) Phase map of composite formulations, defined by ϕ_A (x-axis) and c_M (y-axis) and the degree to which they exhibit high velocity (green), acceleration (yellow), restructuring (blue), and/or rigidity (pink). Below the composite map are individual maps with values for each quantity listed. (G) Linear optical tweezers microrheology measurements of $G'(\omega)$ (filled symbols) and $G''(\omega)$ (open symbols) for active composites with $c_M = 0.24\ \mu$M and $\phi_A = 0.25$ (i, triangles), 0.5 (ii, squares), and 0.75 (iii, circles), collected before myosin photo-activation (black), during activity (red), and 4 hours (blue) and 8 hours (purple) after ceasing photo-stimulation. Arrows indicate the direction of the change in $G'(\omega)$ after the interval of the same color, showing that $\phi_A = 0.25$ composites can reversibly return to their starting state (downward arrows are comparable to upward arrows) and $\phi_A = 0.75$ composites can undergo substantial coarsening (large upward arrows, minimal downward arrows). $\phi_A = 0.50$ composites exhibit both reversibility and coarsening. Confocal images above plots show microtubules in the composites at each time point that moduli are measured, with matching border colors. (A, D–F) Adapted with permission from Lee *et al* (2021a) with permission from the Royal Society of Chemistry. (B, C) Modified from Lee *et al* (2021b). © The Authors, some rights reserved; exclusive licensee AAAS. (G) Adapted with permission from Sheung *et al* (2021) Copyright (2021) American Chemical Society.

was further corroborated and characterized by computing the strain field of simulated composites and evaluating the extent to which actin and microtubules exhibited contractile or extensile strain (figure 8.14(A)). This analysis revealed that for low ϕ_A, microtubules in the composites remain largely undeformed while the actin exhibits local regions of contractile and extensile deformation. Conversely, for high ϕ_A, the strain fields for actin and microtubules are decorrelated from one another, with actin and microtubules exhibiting, respectively, high contractility and more extensile strains. At equimolar conditions the strain fields of both networks are correlated and contractile, with contractility increasing with increasing c_M (figure 8.14(A)) (Lee *et al* 2021a).

To investigate the force response of the light-activated actomyosin-microtubule composites described above, OTM was used to measure the linear and nonlinear rheological properties of composites with $c_M = 0.24\ \mu$M and ϕ_A= 0.25, 0.5, and 0.75 (figure 8.14(G)) (Sheung *et al* 2021). The motor concentration and strain rates were chosen to ensure that the measurement timescale was fast compared to the motor-driven active dynamics, such that the composites could be considered in quasi-steady-state during each measurement (Sheung *et al* 2021). This decoupling allowed the use of GSER to extract G' and G'' from thermal fluctuations of the trapped bead, and to evaluate the nonlinear force response in terms of the quasi-static structure of the composites, which is dictated by ϕ_A and c_M (Sheung *et al* 2021).

These studies measured G' and G'' for composites at distinct time points relative to myosin activity, including before myosin activation (via blebbistatin deactivation), during myosin activity, and 4 and 8 hours after activity. All composites exhibited entanglement-like dynamics dominated by an elastic plateau for all times relative to activity. However, the magnitude of the plateau modulus G^0 strongly depended on composite composition and time, with motor activity increasing G^0 by over two orders of magnitude for $\phi_A \geqslant 0.5$ composites by active restructuring of both actin and microtubules (figure 8.14(G)). This restructuring persisted for up to 4 hours after ceasing motor stimulation, leading to a continued increase in G^0, followed by a decrease back towards their pre-activity states only after 8 hours. Moreover, microtubule-rich composites were shown to enable to most pronounced drop in G^0 while actin-rich composites exhibiting minimal reduction in G^0. The equimolar composite uniquely exhibited both a strong response to activity, i.e., the largest increase in G^0, as well as ample relaxation back to its initial state. These results, coupled with time-lapse confocal images of microtubules in the composites (figure 8.14(G)), suggest that the non-monotonic dependence of mechanical response on ϕ_A arises from the synergistic effects of added stiffness from the microtubules and sufficient motor substrate for pronounced activity (Sheung *et al* 2021).

8.1.4.2 Double-motor composites

Building on this work, researchers incorporated k401-b kinesin clusters ($c_k = 0.35\ \mu$M, $R_k = 0.1$) into co-entangled composites of actin ($c_A = 2.3\ \mu$M) and microtubules ($c_T = 3.5\ \mu$M) with and without myosin II ($c_M = 0.47\ \mu$M, $R_M = 0.2$) (figure 8.15(A)) (McGorty *et al* 2023), and used confocal microscopy (figures 8.15(B) and (D)), PIV (figure 8.15(C)), and DDM (figures 8.15(C) and (F)) to quantify the dynamics of the actin and microtubules in the composites. Similar to the myosin-driven composites described above (figure 8.14), both actin and microtubules exhibited ballistic dynamics with comparable speeds that reached maximum values of $v_{\max} \approx 7$ nm s^{-1} (figures 8.15(C.i) and (F)). However, the nature of the ballistic motion was more variable than the single mode of organized contraction observed across the parameter space of myosin-driven composites (Lee *et al* 2021a). Specifically, the dynamics across all composite formulations and activity times, generally displayed three classes of behavior: (i) slow, isotropic, local restructuring, (ii) fast, unidirectional flow, and (iii) multi-mode dynamics that exhibited both directional flow and local restructuring (figures 8.15(B) and (C)).

Moreover, the filament speed in all composites initially increased, reaching a maximum value $v_{\max}$, after which deceleration ensued (figure 8.15(F)). Surprisingly, the addition of myosin substantially delayed the onset of the acceleratory phase but only modestly reduced $v_{\max}$ from ~7 to ~6 nm s^{-1} (figure 8.15(F)) (McGorty *et al* 2023). Dual motor activity also suppressed de-mixing of the actin and microtubule networks and restructuring of the composites, as evidenced by time-lapse confocal imaging that showed more co-localization and reduced aggregation (figure 8.15(D)). SIA analysis supported this result by showing that double-motor composites had reduced structural correlation lengthscales (ξ_{MT}, ξ_A) and stronger coupling between ξ_{MT} and ξ_A (Sasanpour *et al* 2022, McGorty *et al* 2023). Complementary mathematical modeling of composites (figure 8.15(E)) suggested that this antagonistic interaction between myosin and kinesin arose from the competing contractile versus extensile nature of the motors; as well as the competition between motors driving

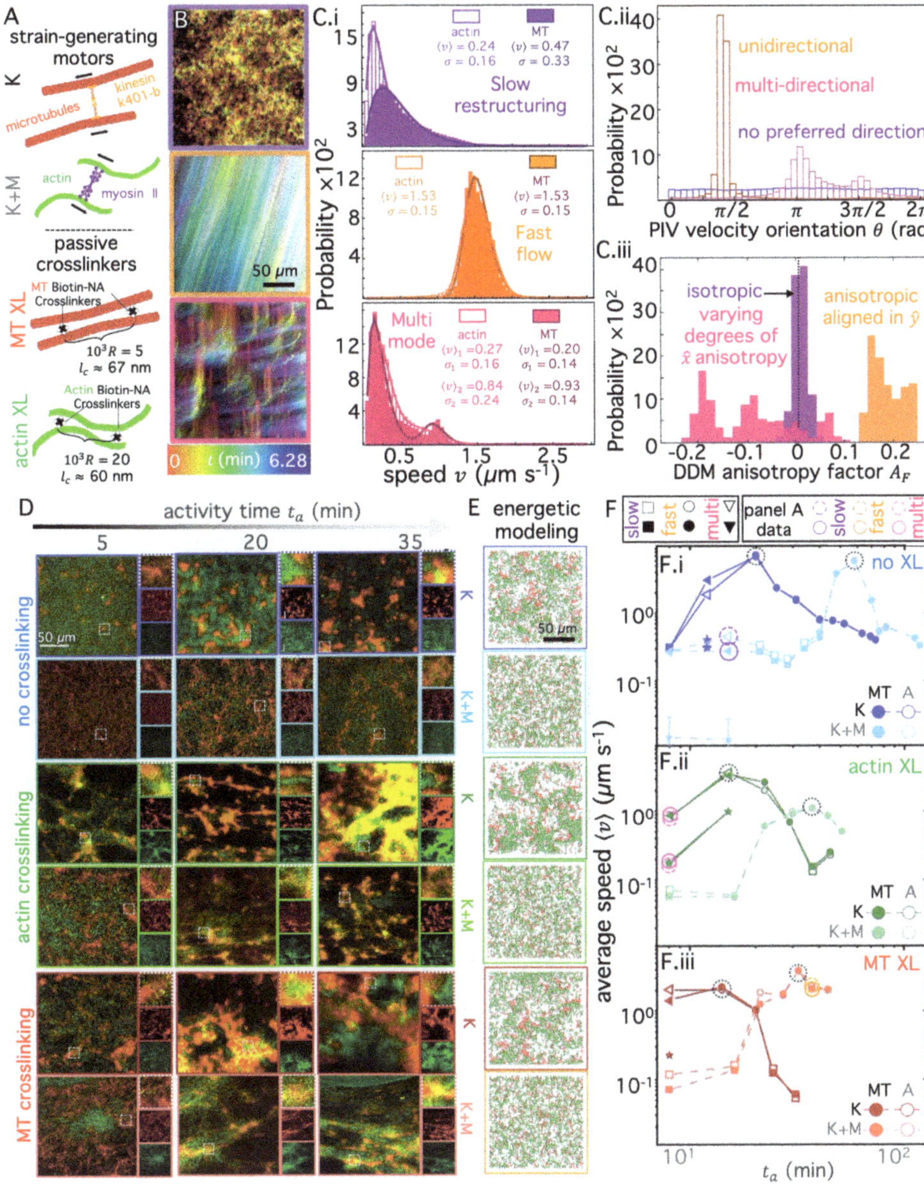

Figure 8.15. Dynamics of actin-microtubule composites driven by kinesin and myosin motors exhibit motor antagonism and a strong dependence on crosslinking. (A) Schematic of components of active composites including strain-generating motors, k401-b kinesin clusters (orange, $c_K = 0.35\ \mu$M) that act on microtubules (red, $c_T = 3.5\ \mu$M), and myosin II minifilaments (purple, $c_M = 0.47\ \mu$M) that act on actin filaments (green, $c_A = 2.3\ \mu$M). Composites with kinesin only (K) and both motors (K+M) were engineered without passive crosslinkers (no XL), with microtubules crosslinked by biotin-NeutrAvidin at $R = 0.005$ (MT XL) or with actin crosslinked by biotin-NeutrAvidin at $R = 0.02$ (Actin XL). (B) Sample color-coded projections of the time-series of microtubules in composites show three distinct classes of dynamics: slow restructuring (top, purple border), fast unidirectional flow (middle, orange border), and multi-mode dynamics (bottom, magenta

border). (C) Probability distributions of (i) speeds v of actin (open bars) and microtubules (filled bars) for the time-series shown in (B), determined via PIV. Solid lines show fits of the data to Schulz distributions, with mean $\langle v \rangle$ and standard deviation σ_v for each distribution listed. Multi-mode distributions (magenta) are fit to a sum of two Schulz distributions with distinct $\langle v \rangle$ and σ_v values. (ii) Distributions of actin velocity orientations θ, determined via PIV performed on the same data analyzed in (i), for slow (purple), fast (orange), and multi-mode (magenta) dynamics that exhibit, respectively, no preferred direction, a single direction, or multiple resolvable peaks in different directions. (iii) Anisotropy factor A_F determined from DDM performed on the microtubules in the composites shown in B determines the extent to which the dynamics deviate from isotropic motion ($A_F = 0$) and display directed motion along $\hat{x}$ ($A_F < 0$) or $\hat{y}$ ($A_F > 0$). Slow data (purple) show isotropic motion, fast data (orange) show motion strongly aligned in $\hat{y}$, and multi-mode data (magenta) show a combination of isotropic and $\hat{x}$-aligned motion. (D) Confocal images of actin (green) and microtubules (red) restructuring over activity time t_a (defined as the time that kinesin motors are added, listed in minutes above each image) in composites with no crosslinking (blue borders, rows 1, 2), actin crosslinking (green borders, rows 3, 4), and microtubule crosslinking (red borders, rows 5, 6); and kinesin (K, dark shades, rows 1, 3, 5), or kinesin and myosin (K+M, rows 2, 4, 6). To the right of each two-color image are the corresponding single-color images for actin and microtubules, as well as a zoom-in of the area denoted by the white dashed line box. (E) Energy-minimizing modeling of composites recapitulates the restructuring seen in experimental images. (F) Average speed of actin (open symbols) and microtubules (filled symbols), measured via DDM, versus t_a for kinesin only (K, dark shades, solid connecting lines) and double motor (K+M, light shades, dashed connecting lines) composites with (i) no crosslinking, (ii) actin crosslinking, and (iii) microtubule crosslinking. The solid and dashed outline circles correspond to the data shown in (B) and the different symbols correspond to data classified as slow (squares), fast (circles), or multi-mode (triangles). Adapted from McGorty *et al* (2023). CC BY 4.0.

like filaments together and co-entanglements between unlike filaments providing frictional drag against the motor stresses (McGorty *et al* 2023).

Incorporating biotin-NeutrAvidin crosslinking of either actin or microtubules at $R_A = 0.02$ or $R_{MT} = 0.005$ (figure 8.15(A)) had a nearly opposite effect on the dynamics and structure as incorporating myosin (figures 8.15(D)–(F)). Namely, both types of crosslinking increased the rate at which composites accelerated to $v_{\max}$ and decelerated to a new steady-state (figure 8.15(F)). Crosslinking also enhanced de-mixing and aggregation of actin and microtubules (figures 8.15(D) and (E)), opposite to the increased miscibility of the two networks afforded by myosin (Sasanpour *et al* 2022, McGorty *et al* 2023). Crosslinking also reduced the maximum speeds reached to $v_{\max} \approx 1$–$4\ \mathrm{nm\ s^{-1}}$, with and without myosin, and increased the propensity to exhibit unidirectional bulk flow as compared to slow isotropic restructuring (figure 8.15(F)) (Sasanpour *et al* 2022, McGorty *et al* 2023). These collective features were suggested to arise from the decreased degrees of structural freedom of the filaments and enhanced like-filament connectivity (Sasanpour *et al* 2022, McGorty *et al* 2023).

8.1.4.3 Kinesin-driven composites

Actin has also been incorporated into the bundled kinesin-microtubule active matter platform described in section 8.1.3, in which short microtubules bundled by PCR1 generate extensile flows driven by k401-b clusters (figures 8.11–8.13) (Henkin *et al* 2014, Chandrakar *et al* 2022). In these studies, interpenetrating networks of actin and microtubules are formed by adding actin monomers and the non-hydrolyzable ATP analog, AMP-PCP, to pre-formed microtubule bundles ($c_T \simeq 16.4\ \mu$M) and allowing them to polymerize for 2 hours before adding kinesin clusters and UV-caged ATP (Berezney *et al* 2022). As actin concentration increased from $c_A \simeq 3\ \mu$M to $c_A \simeq 50\ \mu$M, composites were reported to transition from mixed networks with fluid-like extensile dynamics, to contractile layered asters of actin and microtubules, to a percolated bulk contractile network. In the aster-forming regime, increasing actin concentration increased the finite lifetime of the asters and promoted more microtubule-rich asters, with actin being squeezed out into the surrounding space (Berezney *et al* 2022). Similarly, in the bulk contractile regime, actin and microtubules initially contract together but eventually phase separate, leaving the contractile region largely void of actin. Increasing the ATP concentration from 50 μM to 300 μM, generally shifted the phase diagram towards more extensile behavior at any given actin concentration.

The active composites described above have all employed phalloidin, Taxol, and/or non-hydrolyzable nucleotide analogs to produce stabilized actin filaments and microtubules. This stabilization suppresses polymerization, depolymerization, and treadmilling of the filaments, such that motor-filament interactions are the only source of non-equilibrium dynamics. More recently, researchers have designed surface-localized composites of gliding microtubules and polymerizing actin filaments (Kuçera *et al* 2022a). In the absence of actin, adhering kinesin-1 motors to a passivated cover glass, and flowing in microtubule nucleation 'seeds' and tubulin dimers, enabled *in situ* microtubule polymerization and gliding of kinesin-bound microtubules to form a network of nematically aligned microtubule bundles that reach steady-state global structure. Alternatively, in the absence of microtubules, actin filaments polymerized from surface-bound nucleation seeds formed stable networks of filaments that lack preferred orientation (Kuçera *et al* 2022a). Combining these two systems caused actin networks to become more organized and align with the microtubules. In turn, the increasingly ordered actin filaments guided the gliding microtubules and supported their alignment and growth, resulting in a composite of persistent co-aligned actin and microtubules. These same studies showed that the actin network provided microtubules with structural memory such that they were able to reform in the same oriented state following depolymerization in the presence of actin. Moreover, the alignment of actin filaments with the microtubules was maintained even after destroying the microtubule network (Kuçera *et al* 2022a).

A similar study investigated the role of actin network architecture on the gliding motility of microtubules, comparing the effects of entangled linear filaments versus branched networks formed by Arp2/3 (Kuçera *et al* 2022b). In this study, the microtubules did not form bundles or self-renewing nematic structures because they were stabilized with GMPCPP prior to adding to the sample chamber with affixed kinesin motors. Microtubule motility was shown to be substantially slowed by both actin network architectures due to friction from steric filament interactions and the crowding of the filaments to the surface. However, similar to (Kuçera *et al* 2022a), the linear actin network facilitated guiding of microtubules, which in turn, caused the actin network to become nematically aligned. Conversely, branched actin networks were unable to steer or order microtubules, so, likewise, remained structurally isotropic (Kuçera *et al* 2022b).

8.2 Chemically-triggered biopolymer networks

The above studies have all generated non-equilibrium activity by incorporating molecular motors to generate stresses internally and autonomously in networks. Another key mechanism that biology uses to alter the structure and mechanics of its myriad networks is chemical responsiveness. Namely, biopolymer networks can undergo dramatic structural and mechanical changes in response to variations in their chemical environment, such as the concentration and valency of salts, concentrations and types of nucleotides, and pH. These triggered networks are an important class of responsive materials with properties and rates of variations that can be precisely tuned by user-controlled changes to buffer conditions.

8.2.1 Salt-triggered bulk contraction

In chapter 6, I describe the effect of salt on the structure and aging dynamics of DNA nanostars and their networks (figure 6.10) (Nguyen and Saleh 2017, Jeon *et al* 2018). These experiments were performed using semipermeable microfluidic perfusion chambers, pioneered in Park *et al* (2016), to allow for controlled buffer exchange via diffusion rather than flow, to ensure that the networks remain mechanically undisturbed. In brief, using these devices, researchers demonstrated that networks of crosslinked DNA nanostars formed at high [Na^+] underwent contraction upon lowering the salt concentration via microfluidic-enabled buffer exchange (Nguyen and Saleh 2017). Subsequent cycling between high and low salt conditions caused the networks to continue to irreversibly contract and eventually rupture. A nearly opposite effect was seen when modulating Mg^{2+} instead of Na^+ whereby the network expanded rather than contracted upon lowering salt concentration, and then contracted back and reversibly re-expanded under subsequent cycling (figure 6.10) (Nguyen and Saleh 2017).

Similar experiments, using microfluidic chambers adapted from Park *et al* (2016), were performed on entangled actin networks ($c_A = 5.8\ \mu\text{M}$) and equimolar composites of actin and microtubules ($c_A = c_T = 2.9\ \mu\text{M}$) (figures 8.16(A)–(C)) (Ricketts *et al* 2020). Namely, networks were formed in the microfluidic devices in the presence of normal 'low-salt' polymerization buffer containing 2 mM Mg^{2+}. After 30 min, the salt concentration was increased to 20 mM Mg^{2+} which was maintained for 90 min, after which the 'high-salt' buffer was exchanged for the initial low-salt buffer. As shown in figure 8.16(A), introducing high-salt conditions caused the actin network to contract, no longer filling the sample chamber, and steadily shrink in width for the entire high-salt period (figures 8.16(A) and (B)). Similar to the effect of Na^+ on DNA nanostar networks (Nguyen and Saleh 2017), lowering the Mg^{2+} concentration back to the initial low-salt conditions caused the actin network to continue to contract rather than expand, albeit at a slower rate (figures 8.16(B) and (C)).

Similar initial and final conditions were observed for actin-microtubule composites, with both networks and composites monotonically shrinking to ~10% of their initial width (figure 8.16(C)) (Ricketts *et al* 2020). However, the time course of contraction was notably different for composites compared to actin networks, with composites exhibiting a pronounced delay in contractile dynamics and subsequently

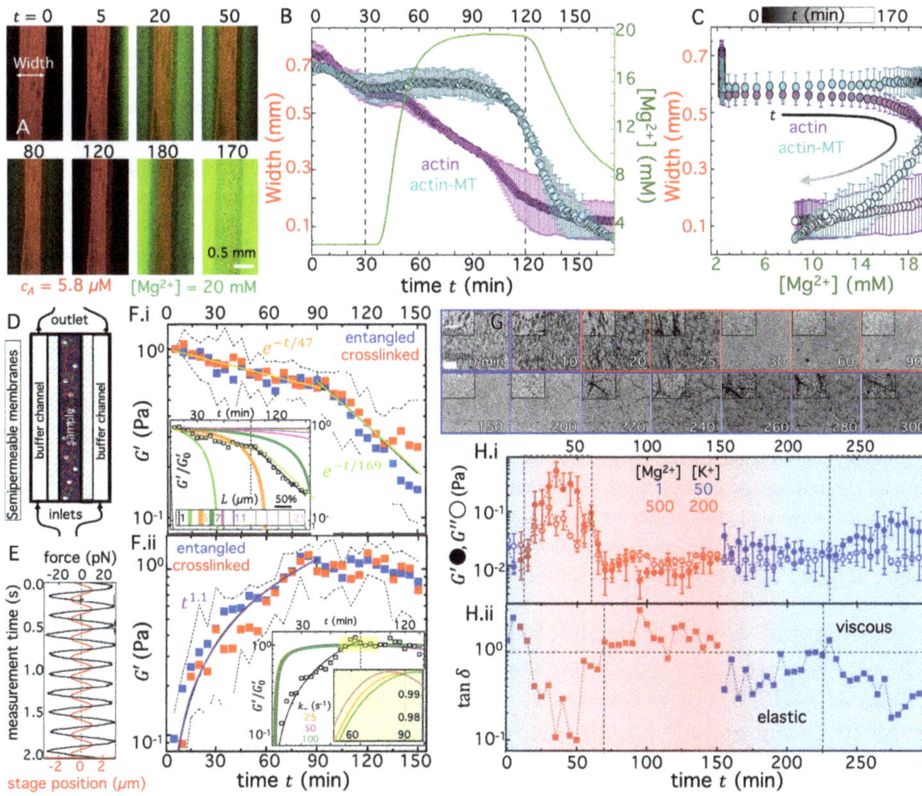

Figure 8.16. Chemically-triggered actin networks and actin-microtubule composites undergo bulk contraction and microrheological state changes. (A–C) Bulk contraction of entangled actin networks ($c_A = 5.8\ \mu$M) and equimolar composites of actin and microtubules ($c_A = c_T = 2.9\ \mu$M) mediated by increasing concentration of Mg^{2+} from 1 mM (low salt) to 20 mM (high salt) over the course of 90 minutes. Microfluidic perfusion chambers depicted in D allow for *in situ* exchange of low and high [Mg^{2+}] buffers through semipermeable membranes that flank the network on the left and right sides. (A) Confocal images of actin network (red) contracting over time t after initiating exchange of low to high salt buffer (listed in mins). Increasing concentration of [Mg^{2+}] is visualized, using fluorescein salt, as increasing intensity of green background. (B) Width (left red axis) of actin network (purple) and actin-microtubule composite (cyan) versus time with error bars representing standard deviation across replicates. [Mg^{2+}] (right green axis, green curve) versus time is also shown, with vertical dashed lines indicating the times at which high salt and low salt buffers are introduced. (C) Data shown in C plotted versus [Mg^{2+}], with time indicated by dark to light shades according to the scale at top. (D) Schematic of microfluidic perfusion chambers with semipermeable membranes flanking the sample and inlets and outlets for introducing new buffer and removing existing buffer through the buffer channels. (E) Sample oscillatory optical tweezers measurement used to determine $G'(\omega)$ and $G''(\omega)$ in F, H. The force (black, top axis) exerted on an optically trapped microsphere and the stage position (red, bottom axis) controlling the oscillation profile for a microsphere ($R_s = 2.25\ \mu$m) oscillating with an amplitude of 1 μm through a network confined in a perfusion chamber depicted in D. (F) G', averaged over oscillation frequency, versus time for entangled (blue) and crosslinked (red) actin networks ($c_A = 11.6\ \mu$M) (i) during exchange from polymerization buffer to buffer lacking ATP and Mg^{2+} and including Ca^{2+} to induce depolymerization, and (ii) subsequent exchange back to polymerization buffer. Symbols are averages over all frequencies and dashed lines indicate standard deviation. Lines denote fits of the data to (i) exponential functions with scaling $G' \sim e^{-t/47}$ (orange) and $G' \sim e^{-t/169}$ (green), where time constants are in mins, and (ii) power-law function

$G' \sim t^{1.1}$. Insets show corresponding modeling results as lines and experimental data as symbols with black fit lines, where entangled and crosslinked network data are averaged together: (i) G', normalized by the $t = 0$ value G_0, for crosslinked networks of varying actin lengths $L = 1–25\ \mu m$, indicated by colors in the legend, that reflect the distribution of experimentally measured lengths. Line thickness is proportional to the weight of each length L in the experimental distribution, calibrated by the 50% scale bar shown. (ii) G'/G_0 for crosslinked networks with varying depolymerization rates k_- (s^{-1}) = 25 (orange), 50 (magenta), and 100 (green). The yellow shaded inset is a zoom-in of the crossover region from power law to plateau behavior, likewise shaded in yellow, and centered on the dashed vertical line at $t_c \approx 90$ min. (G, H) The effect of *in situ* increase of salt, similar to experiments in (A–C), on the microstructure (G) and microrheology (H) of actin networks ($c_A = 5.8\ \mu M$) crosslinked by inactive myosin II minifilaments. Buffer conditions are switched from [Mg^{2+}], [K^+] = 1, 50 mM (low salt, blue) to [Mg^{2+}], [K^+]= 500, 200 mM (high salt, red) and back to low salt (blue) by initiating buffer exchange at $t = 5$ min (low to high) and $t = 150$ min (high to low) indicated by colors of image borders (G) and plot backgrounds (H). (G) Inverted intensity confocal images of actin networks at different times, listed in mins, during the salt modulation program indicated by the border colors of each image. Insets show zoom-ins of the images. (H) Microrheology measurements, depicted in E, showing (i) $G'(t)$ (filled circles), $G''(t)$ (open circles), and (ii) tan $\delta(t)$ (filled squares) during the same salt modulation program as in G, denoted by the background shades and symbol colors. Dashed vertical lines mark key transition points in the rheological data that signify state changes. Horizontal dashed line in (ii) denotes tan $\delta = 1$ ($G' = G''$). (A–C) Adapted from Ricketts *et al* (2020). CC BY 4.0. (E, F) Adapted from Gurmessa *et al* (2018) with permission from the Royal Society of Chemistry. (D, G, H) Adapted from Gurmessa *et al* (2021). CC BY 4.0.

~2× more rapid contraction that was, surprisingly, most pronounced once the composite was re-introduced to low-salt conditions (figures 8.16(B) and (C)) (Ricketts *et al* 2020). In other words, the actin network was able to more quickly respond to changing salt conditions, undergoing fast contraction during high-salt conditions and slower contraction in the subsequent low-salt phase, whereas the composite required a much longer time to initiate contraction, but then contracted at a substantially faster rate than for the actin network (figures 8.16(B) and (C)). The initial delay was rationalized as arising from the slower relaxation timescales for microtubules compared to actin. At the same time, the larger mesh size of the composite compared to the actin network allowed for more rapid 'squeezing' of the network pores once the microtubules had sufficient time to configurationally respond to the changing conditions (Ricketts *et al* 2020). The irreversibility and continued contraction following reintroduction of low-salt conditions was suggested to arise from configurational free energy minimization that occurs on a slower timescale than the electrostatic-driven crosslinking and clustering of filaments (Ricketts *et al* 2020).

8.2.2 Microrheology of chemically-triggered cytoskeleton networks

Building on the bulk studies described above, researchers incorporated similar microfluidic chambers into an optical tweezers platform to allow for linear oscillatory OTM measurements during buffer exchange (figures 8.16(D)–(H)) (Gurmessa *et al* 2018, 2021). By tuning the chemical modulation to be slow on the timescale of each ~2 s measurement, the viscoelastic moduli could be determined for each measurement using a quasi-steady-state assumption. Specifically, in these measurements trapped beads are oscillated over a range of frequencies from which the measured amplitudes of the force response and stage position, as well as the phase angle between them are used to determine the elastic and viscous moduli (figure 8.16(I)) (Brau *et al* 2007, Chapman *et al* 2014). These measurements are identical to those I describe in chapter 3 and used for data shown in figures 5.2(D) and (I) and in Chapman *et al* (2014) and Gurmessa *et al* (2019).

This microfluidic-OTM platform was used to determine the time-varying rheological properties of entangled and crosslinked actin networks undergoing disassembly and re-assembly via triggered filament depolymerization and re-polymerization (figure 8.16(F)) (Gurmessa *et al* 2018). Specifically, networks of entangled actin filaments ($c_A = 11.6\ \mu$M) in buffer conditions that support polymerization, namely, 50 mM KCl, 1 mM $MgCl_2$, and 0.4 mM ATP, were formed in microfluidic chambers and triggered to depolymerize via buffer exchange to conditions that destabilize actin filaments (i.e., addition of 0.1 mM $CaCl_2$; removal of KCl, $MgCl_2$, ATP).

Linear oscillatory OTM measurements performed for 150 min following initiating of this exchange showed that the time-dependent elastic modulus $G'(t)$ dropped by an order of magnitude for both entangled and crosslinked networks over the course of the experiment (figure 8.16(F.i)). This reduction in $G'(t)$ exhibited two phases of exponential decay, an initial slow decay up to $t_c \approx 90$ min, with a time constant $\tau_1 \simeq 167$ min, followed by a steeper decay, with $\tau_2 \simeq 47$ min, that persisted up to $t_f \approx 150$ min (figure 8.16(Fi.)). Upon re-introducing polymerization-amenable buffer conditions, $G'(t)$ began to increase back to its original value over time (figure 8.16(F.ii)), returning to a state with indistinguishable elastic properties compared to before depolymerization (Gurmessa *et al* 2018). Moreover, $G'(t)$ exhibited an initial nearly linear increase with time, namely $G' \sim t^{1.1}$ until $t_c \approx 90$ min, followed by a steady-state plateau value with no discernible time dependence ($G' \sim t^0$) (figure 8.16(F.ii)).

Importantly, while crosslinking the actin network via biotin-NeutrAvidin at $10^3R = 7$ (the upper limit for forming isotropic crosslinked networks) increased the value of G' for all times, it had no measurable impact on the time course of $G'(t)$ (figure 8.16(F)), indicating that crosslinking does not alter (de)polymerization kinetics; and it is, in fact, (de)polymerization that drives the time-varying rheology. Moreover, while the crossover time t_c was similar for both polymerization and depolymerization dynamics, suggesting similar state transitions, the functional forms of the two phases were different, indicative of different underlying mechanisms driving each phase (Gurmessa *et al* 2018).

Mathematical modeling of this process, using rigidity percolation theory coupled with Master equations (figure 8.16(F) insets), showed that this two-phase behavior arose from a rigidity percolation phase transition from a percolated rigid network to a floppy weakly-connected network, or vice versa, for depolymerization or re-polymerization, respectively (Gurmessa *et al* 2018). The exponential decays during depolymerization, rather than a discrete drop in $G'(t)$ at t_c was shown to arise from the distribution of filament lengths that comprise the network, with shorter filaments depolymerizing faster than longer ones, effectively 'smearing out' the transition (figure 8.16(F.i)). During re-polymerization, the linear increase, which was markedly slower than model predictions (figure 8.16(F.ii)), was suggested to arise from competing processes of nucleation, elongation, fragmentation, and annealing, the latter two of which are not accounted for in the toy model (Gurmessa *et al* 2018).

Using this same technique, the impact of varying salt concentration on the rheology of actin networks crosslinked with inactive myosin II minifilaments was investigated to parse the competing contributions of crosslinking (via myosin) and bundling (via salt) to network connectivity and rigidity (figures 8.16(G) and (H)) (Gurmessa *et al* 2021). These studies showed that increasing salt initially increased G' dramatically, but subsequently induced a drop as the increased bundling broke the percolation of the network (figures 8.16(G) and (H)). Only upon re-introducing low-salt conditions did a percolated network reform and again exhibit the ability to elastically resist stresses (figure 8.16(H)). However, the final network was distinct from the initial network, exhibiting more bundling and elastic-like contributions to the rheology, indicative of irreversible filament interactions (figure 8.16(H)) (Gurmessa *et al* 2021).

8.3 Non-equilibrium DNA networks

8.3.1 Motor-driven DNA networks

Inspired by actomyosin active matter, researchers have used DNA and its motor protein FtsK50C, used in cell division and chromosomal segregation (Aussel *et al* 2002, Crozat and Grainge 2010), to engineer a DNA-based network that emulates the active dynamics of actomyosin networks (figure 8.17) (Bertrand *et al* 2012). To mimic actin filaments, ~12–14 single-stranded DNA oligos were assembled into cylindrical bundles or 'nanotubes' with ~10 nm diameter, $L \approx 5$–$10\ \mu$m, and $l_p \approx 5\ \mu$m (all similar properties to actin) (figure 8.17(A)). Decorating nanotubes with ssDNA sticky ends, at a 4:1 nanotube:ssDNA ratio enabled crosslinking via basepair-specific binding of DNA strands of length $L \approx 1.8\ \mu$m (5.8 kbp), with complementary single-stranded overhangs, to attach to the sticky ends (figure 8.17(A)). The resulting passive network of crosslinked nanotubes at $c_{NT} \simeq 0.2\ \mu$M exhibits gel-like properties (figures 8.17(B) and (E)). Incorporating FtsK50C and ATP creates an active network by FtsK50C binding to different segments of the DNA linkers and pulling them together, forming a DNA loop that brings the attached nanorods together (figure 8.17(C)), simulating the action of two actin filaments pulled together by myosin. While some FtsK motors were shown to transiently bind and unbind linkers, repetitively pulling and releasing, the majority of the motors in the network held linkers in the contracted state for extended periods of time, leading to bulk contraction of the nanotube gel. These active dynamics were characterized by tracking microspheres attached to both passive and active networks, showing behavior similar to actomyosin networks (figures 8.17(D) and (E)) (Bertrand *et al* 2012, Sheung *et al* 2022). Specifically, the van Hove distributions of microsphere displacements Δx in passive networks were Gaussian (figure 8.17(D)); and the MSDs were extremely subdiffusive ($\alpha \approx 0.5$), and reached a finite size plateau $\langle \Delta x^2 \rangle_{\Delta t > 0.1} \sim \Delta t^0 \approx 10^3$ nm^2, related to the network mesh size, at $\Delta t \approx 0.1$ (figure 8.17(E)). Conversely, active networks exhibited van Hove distributions with exponential large displacement tails (figure 8.17(D)) and less subdiffusivity ($\alpha \approx 0.8$)

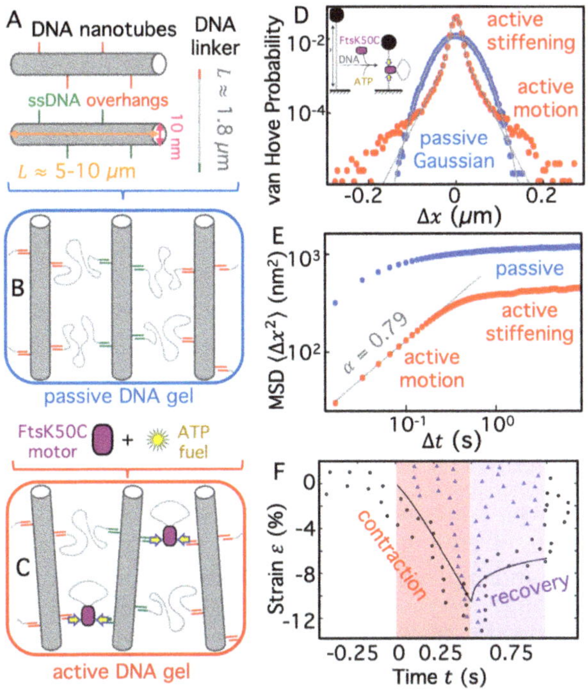

Figure 8.17. Motor-driven networks of DNA nanotubes exhibit active motion and stiffening. (A–C) An active DNA network with properties similar to actomyosin networks is achieved by (A) decorating DNA nanotubes, assembled from ~12–14 DNA oligos, with two different ssDNA sticky ends (red and green) and incorporating dsDNA linkers with complementary ssDNA overhangs to bind to the sticky ends; resulting in (B) a passive crosslinked network of DNA nanorods with gel-like properties (blue). (C) Adding the DNA motor, FtsK50C, and its fuel, ATP, to the passive network results in an active contractile network (red). (D, E) Tracking beads attached to passive (blue) and active (red) networks (depicted in inset in D). (D) The van Hove distribution of particle displacements, Δx, at $\Delta t = 1$ s is expectedly Gaussian for the passive network (blue), while the active network distribution (red) exhibits pronounced large displacement tails, indicative of active motion, and strong caging, from active stiffening of the network. Grey fit lines are a Gaussian function (passive) or sum of Gaussian and exponential (actI). (E) Mean-squared displacements of beads $\langle \Delta x^2 \rangle$ versus Δt show that particles in the passive network (blue) can explore a larger surrounding space than the active network (red), i.e. $\langle \Delta x^2 \rangle_p > \langle \Delta x^2 \rangle_a$, at large lag times, due to the contraction and stiffening of the network by motor activity. At short times, the active network allows for more mobility of the particles, driven by motor activity, manifesting as weaker subdiffusion compared to the passive case, with an anomalous scaling exponent α that is higher and persists for longer lag times. (F) Mathematical modeling of an active contracting gel (solid lines) recapitulates experimental results (circles, triangles) for the bulk strain ε as a function of time t, where $t = 0$ s indicates the onset of contraction. The model captures both the contraction phase (red) and recovery phase (purple) that active DNA nanorod networks exhibit. (A–E) Adapted from Bertrand *et al* (2012) with permission of PNAS. (F) Adapted from Bacca *et al* (2019) with permission from the Royal Society of Chemistry.

that extended to longer times ($\Delta t \approx 0.5$ s) before $\langle \Delta x^2 \rangle$ reached a plateau (figure 8.17(E)), due to non-thermal motor-driven displacements. The stiffening of the gel via motor-driven contraction manifested as larger zero-displacement peaks in the van Hove distributions (figure 8.17(D)) and a lower MSD plateau value

($\langle \Delta x^2 \rangle_{\Delta t > 0.5} \approx 300\ \text{nm}^2$) (figure 8.17(E)) compared to passive networks (Bertrand *et al* 2012).

Notably, while motor activity stiffened the network, the ~10-fold stiffening was much less than the ~100-fold stiffening reported in actomyosin networks (Mizuno *et al* 2007, Koenderink *et al* 2009, Bertrand *et al* 2012), which was suggested to arise from the flexibility of the linkers on which the motors act. A generalized theory for motor-driven contraction of polymer gels was able to reproduce these experimental results, including the contraction and recovery periods from attachment and detachment of the motors (figure 8.17(F)) (Bacca *et al* 2019). Finally, simulations of FtsK motors acting on single DNA strands of different branching architectures, showed that bulk contraction of the gel arose from coordinated action of the motors due to their unique force responsiveness (Lu and Chen 2022).

8.3.2 Topologically-active DNA networks

In chapter 6, I discussed the important role that polymer topology plays in the rheological properties of entangled biopolymer solutions, as demonstrated extensively for ring, linear and supercoiled DNA (Robertson and Smith 2007, Peddireddy *et al* 2020a, 2020b, 2022, 2023, Smrek *et al* 2021, Khanal *et al* 2022, Kong *et al* 2022). More recently, researchers have exploited this topological dependence, along with the suite of commercially available enzymes that convert different DNA constructs from one topology to the other, to create 'topologically-active' DNA networks that exhibit time-dependent rheological properties mediated by enzymatically-driven topological conversion of the comprising DNA (Krajina *et al* 2018, Michieletto *et al* 2022, Marfai *et al* 2023).

The seminal demonstration of topologically-active DNA solutions (Michieletto *et al* 2022) focused on concentrated solutions of supercoiled DNA of length $L \simeq 2\ \mu\text{m}$ (6 kbp) undergoing linearization via the single-site restriction enzyme, BamHI (figures 8.18(A)–(H)); and linear λ DNA ($L \simeq 16\ \mu\text{m}$, 48.5 kbp) undergoing fragmentation via five different multi-site enzymes that cut the linear DNA into 5, 6 or 141 fragments of varying lengths (figures 8.18(I)–(K)). The time-varying viscosity $\eta(t_a)$ of the solutions undergoing digestion, determined from MSDs of embedded microspheres, showed that linearization of supercoiled DNA generally thickened the solutions over time (increasing $\eta(t_a)$) (figures 8.18(B) and (E)) while fragmentation of linear DNA led to viscous-thinning over time (decreasing $\eta(t_a)$) (figure 8.18(J)).

Specifically, enzymatic linearization of supercoiled DNA was shown to steadily increase $\eta(t_a)$ over the course of ~240 min, with the degree and rate of viscous thickening increasing with both the enzyme:DNA stoichiometry, $S \simeq 0.05\ \text{U}\ \mu\text{g}^{-1}$, $0.1\ \text{U}\ \mu\text{g}^{-1}$, $0.5\ \text{U}\ \mu\text{g}^{-1}$, and DNA concentration, $c \simeq 1.5\ \text{mg mL}^{-1}$, $3\ \text{mg mL}^{-1}$, $6\ \text{mg mL}^{-1} \simeq 2c_S^*, 4c_S^*, 8c_S^*$ (Peddireddy *et al* 2020b, Michieletto *et al* 2022) (figures 8.18(B) and (E)).

While the dependence on stoichiometry may be intuitive as more enzymes would allow more DNA to be digested in a given time interval, according to Michaelis–Menten (MM) kinetics, the dependence on DNA concentration is less obvious. To parse these different contributions to the time-varying viscosity $\eta(t_a)$, time-

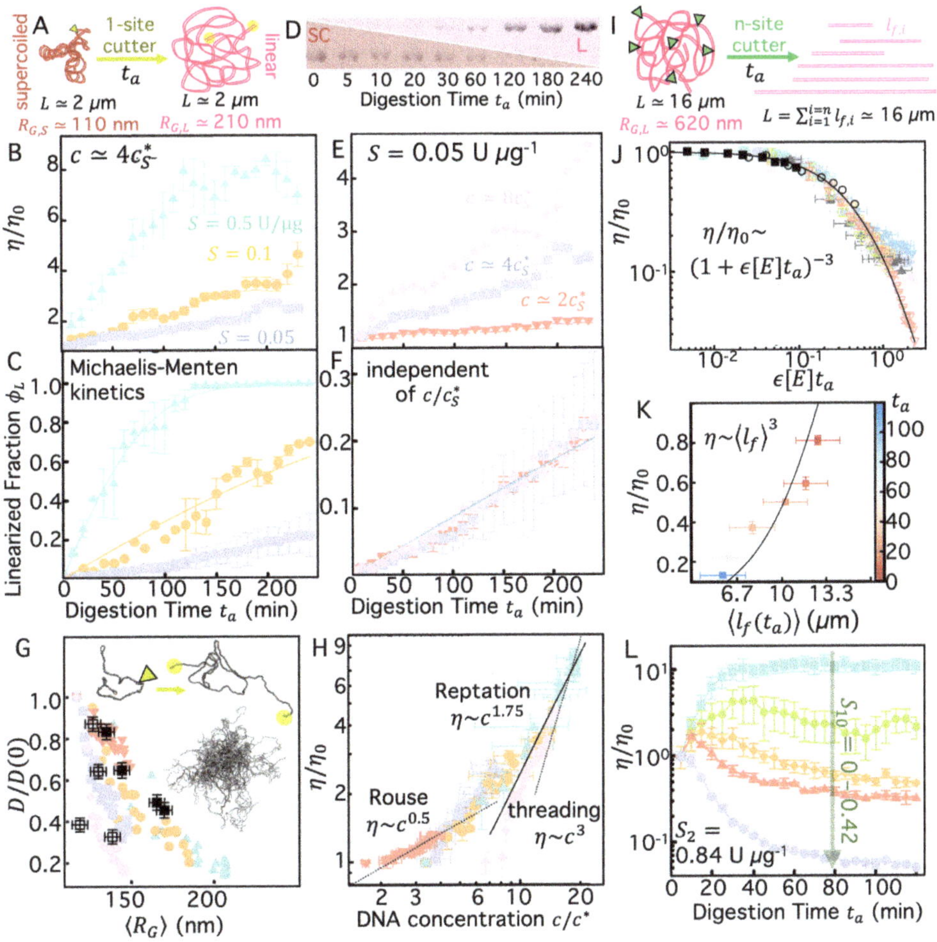

Figure 8.18. Topologically-active DNA solutions undergoing viscous thickening and thinning via enzymatic digestion. (A–H) Linearization of supercoiled DNA causes viscous thickening. (A) Supercoiled DNA (red) is cleaved by a single-cutter enzyme BamHI (yellow triangle), generating a linear strand (magenta) with two free ends (yellow circles) over activity time t_a. Linear and supercoiled DNA have the same contour length ($L_L = L_S \simeq 2\ \mu$m) but different radii of gyration ($R_{G,L} \simeq 2R_{G,S}$). (B, C) The scaled viscosity η/η_0 (B) and fraction of linearized DNA ϕ_L (C) versus t_a for DNA solutions with concentration $c \simeq 3$ mg mL$^{-1} \simeq 4c_S^* \simeq 19c_L^*$ and enzyme:DNA stoichiometries S (U μg^{-1}) $\simeq$ 0.5 (cyan), 0.1 (orange), and 0.05 (lilac). Solid lines in C are fits to Michaelis–Menten scaling with varying digestion rates. (D) Gel electrophoresis of supercoiled DNA (SC, red) undergoing linearization (L, pink) over the course of ~4 hours. Band intensity analysis of gels is used to compute the fraction of linear DNA ϕ_L as a function of t_a. (E, D) Same parameters as plotted in B and C for fixed stoichiometry $S = 0.05$ U μg^{-1} and varying DNA concentrations of c (mg mL^{-1} | c_S^*) $\simeq$ 1.5 | 2 (coral), 3 | 4 (lilac), 6 | 8 (pink). (G) Brownian dynamics simulations of experiments, with a simulated cleaving event and densely packed supercoiled (black) and linearized (grey) DNA depicted in inset, measure DNA diffusion coefficients D normalized by the $t_a = 0$ value D_0 as a function of average radius of gyration $\langle R_G \rangle$ (which depends on t_a) for solutions with DNA concentration $c \simeq c_S^*$ (filled black squares) and $c \simeq 15c_S^*$ (open black squares). Simulation data are overlaid on experimental data plotted in (B) and (E), showing good agreement across the parameter space. (H) Scaled viscosity η/η_0 (same data as in (B) and (E)) plotted versus scaled DNA concentration $c/[c^*(t_a)]$ show universal

collapse with three regimes of power-law scaling $\eta/\eta_0 \sim (c/c^*)^x$ with $x \simeq 0.5$, 1.75, and 3, in line with predictions for, respectively, Rouse dynamics, reptation, and threading. (I–K) Fragmentation of linear DNA exhibits universal thinning. (I) Linear λ-DNA (magenta) of length $L \simeq 16\ \mu$m is cleaved at $n > 1$ sites by an n-site cutting enzyme (green triangles) to produce n fragments of varying lengths l_f (pink) that sum to L. (J) Scaled viscosity η/η_0 versus scaled digestion time $\tilde{t}_a = \epsilon[E]t_a$ for solutions of λ DNA at $c \simeq 20c^*$ undergoing fragmentation via five different n-site cutters, where $n = 5$, 6 or 141, at stoichiometries $S = 0.27$–5.5 U μg^{-1}. All n, S combinations, denoted by different colors, collapse onto a universal curve described by $\eta/\eta_0 \sim (1 + \epsilon[E]t_a)^{-3}$ (black line). (K) η/η_0 versus time-dependent average fragment length $\langle l_f(t_a)\rangle$, determined via gel electrophoresis, with color denoting t_a, follows scaling $\eta/\eta_0 \sim \langle l_f\rangle^3$ (black line) predicted by the reptation model. (L) η/η_0 versus t_a for solutions of ring DNA ($L \simeq 14.7\ \mu$m, $c/c^* \simeq 17$) undergoing linearization and fragmentation via a 2-site cutter at constant stoichiometry $S_2 = 840$ U mg^{-1} and 10-site cutter at S_{10}(U mg^{-1}) $= 0$ (cyan), 2.1 (green), 21 (orange), 84 (red), 420 (lilac). Linearization from a constant S_2 causes all solutions to exhibit initial thickening, while increasing S_{10} leads to increasing thinning following initial thickening. Adapted from Michieletto *et al* (2022). CC BY 4.0.

resolved gel electrophoresis experiments (figure 8.18(D)) were analyzed to correlate the active digestion time t_a with the fraction of linearized (digested) DNA in solution ϕ_L (figures 8.18(C) and (F)). This analysis verified the expected MM dependence of digestion, quantified by $\phi_L(t_a)$, on stoichiometry S. It also surprisingly revealed that DNA concentration had no impact on $\phi_L(t_a)$ (figure 8.18(F)), despite the strong dependence it had on the degree of thickening (figure 8.18(E)).

To shed light on this intriguing phenomenon, complementary Brownian dynamics simulations considered the effect of the changing average radius of gyration $\langle R_G\rangle$ during digestion (figure 8.18(G)) (Michieletto *et al* 2022). The empirical relation $R_{G,L} \simeq 2R_{G,S}$ (Robertson *et al* 2006) implies that as linearization of supercoiled DNA proceeds, $\langle R_G\rangle$ of the molecules in solution should increase, which was verified by direct measurements of $\langle R_G\rangle$ in simulations (Michieletto *et al* 2022). Moreover, the dependence of the particle diffusion coefficients on $\langle R_G\rangle$, determined from simulations and experiments, agreed remarkably well for both entangled ($8c_S^*$) and semidilute ($4c_S^*$) solutions (figure 8.18(G)), suggesting that the time-varying $\langle R_G\rangle$ may play an important role in the concentration dependence of $\eta(t_a)$. To test this conjecture, the viscosity was evaluated as a function of DNA concentration, scaled by the time-dependent overlap concentration $c^*(t_a)$, which was computed via the scaling

$$c^*(t_a) \sim \langle R_G\rangle^{-3} \tag{8.5}$$

(figure 8.18(H)). While the absolute concentration c does not change over time, $c^*(t_a)$ increases, such that c/c^* for any given DNA concentration decreases (Michieletto *et al* 2022). This rescaling led to data collapse for all concentrations and stoichiometries, with power-law scalings of $\eta/\eta_0 \sim (c/c^*)^x$ that aligned with predictions for Rouse relaxation ($x \simeq 0.5$), reptation ($x \simeq 1.75$), and constraint release ($x \simeq 3$), for $c/c^* < 6$, $6 < c/c^* < 10$, and $c/c^* > 10$, respectively (figure 8.18(H)). The concentration regimes over which the different relaxation modes appear to dominate are consistent with previous findings that the critical entanglement concentration for DNA is $\sim 6c^*$ (Robertson and Smith 2007), and that markedly slower dynamics observed for DNA rings in ring-linear blends above $\sim 10c^*$ are due to threading (Robertson and Smith 2007).

In this same work, similar experiments performed on entangled linear λ DNA ($c/c^*(t_a = 0) \simeq 20$) undergoing fragmentation (figure 8.18(I)), displayed a universal decrease in viscosity under the action of five different multi-site cutting enzymes that cleaved the DNA into 5, 6 or 141 fragments with ends that are either blunt or have sticky overhangs (figure 8.18(J)). By rescaling the digestion time by the enzyme concentration $[E]$, based on stoichiometries of $S = 0.27\text{–}5.5\ \text{U}\ \mu\text{g}^{-1}$, and an enzyme-independent constant ϵ, i.e.,

$$t_a \rightarrow \tilde{t}_a = \epsilon[E]t_a \tag{8.6}$$

the time-dependent viscosity $\eta(t)/\eta_0$ for all cases collapsed to a single master curve that could be described by the thinning function

$$\eta/\eta_0 \sim (1 + \epsilon[E]t_a)^{-3} \tag{8.7}$$

(figure 8.18(J)). This scaling aligns with predictions from living polymer theory in which $\epsilon[E]$ is a measure of the digestion rate (Cates 1987, Michieletto 2020, Michieletto *et al* 2022). By determining the time-dependent mean fragment length $\langle l_f(t_a) \rangle$ from gel electrophoresis, the viscosity was shown to scale with the fragment length as

$$\eta/\eta_0 \sim \langle l_f \rangle^3 \tag{8.8}$$

(figure 8.18(K)), in line with predicted reptation model scaling (Doi and Edwards 1986, Rubinstein and Colby 2003).

Finally, both viscous thickening and subsequent thinning were realized in a solution of ring DNA of length $L \simeq 14.7\ \mu\text{m}$ (44 kbp) and concentration $c = 1.4\ \text{mg mL}^{-1}$ ($c/c^* \simeq 17$) digested with a 2-cutter enzyme XhoI at $S_2 = 840\ \text{U mg}^{-1}$ and $\sim$400× to $\sim$2× lower stoichiometry of a 10-cutter enzyme EcoRI ($S_{10} = 2.1\text{–}420\ \text{U mg}^{-1}$) (figure 8.18(L)). In the absence of the 10-cutter ($S_{10} = 0$), η/η_0 increased $\sim$10-fold over the course of the first hour ($t_a \approx 60$ min), followed by a t_a-independent plateau, similar to the single-cutter linearization experiments (figure 8.18(B)). Conversely, for all $S_{10} > 0$ cases, the solutions initially thickened, with η/η_0 reaching a peak value η_{max}/η_0 at a specific gating time t_{gate}, after which η/η_0 immediately decreased, eventually reaching a plateau value η_{min}/η_0 that ranged from $\sim$2× larger than $\eta/\eta_0(t_a = 0)$ for $S_{10} = 2.1\ \text{U mg}^{-1}$ to $\sim$50× smaller for $S_{10} = 420\ \text{U mg}^{-1}$, (figure 8.18(L)). The metrics for this thickening and gated thinning, e.g., η_{max}/η_0, η_{min}/η_0, t_{gate}, followed power-law scaling with S_{10} (Michieletto *et al* 2022).

Building on this realization of non-monotonic time dependence of microrheological properties, subsequent work (Marfai *et al* 2023) aimed to determine the extent to which this non-equilibrium behavior manifests at the bulk scale and if it is robust to mixing with synthetic systems such as the dextran solutions and DNA-

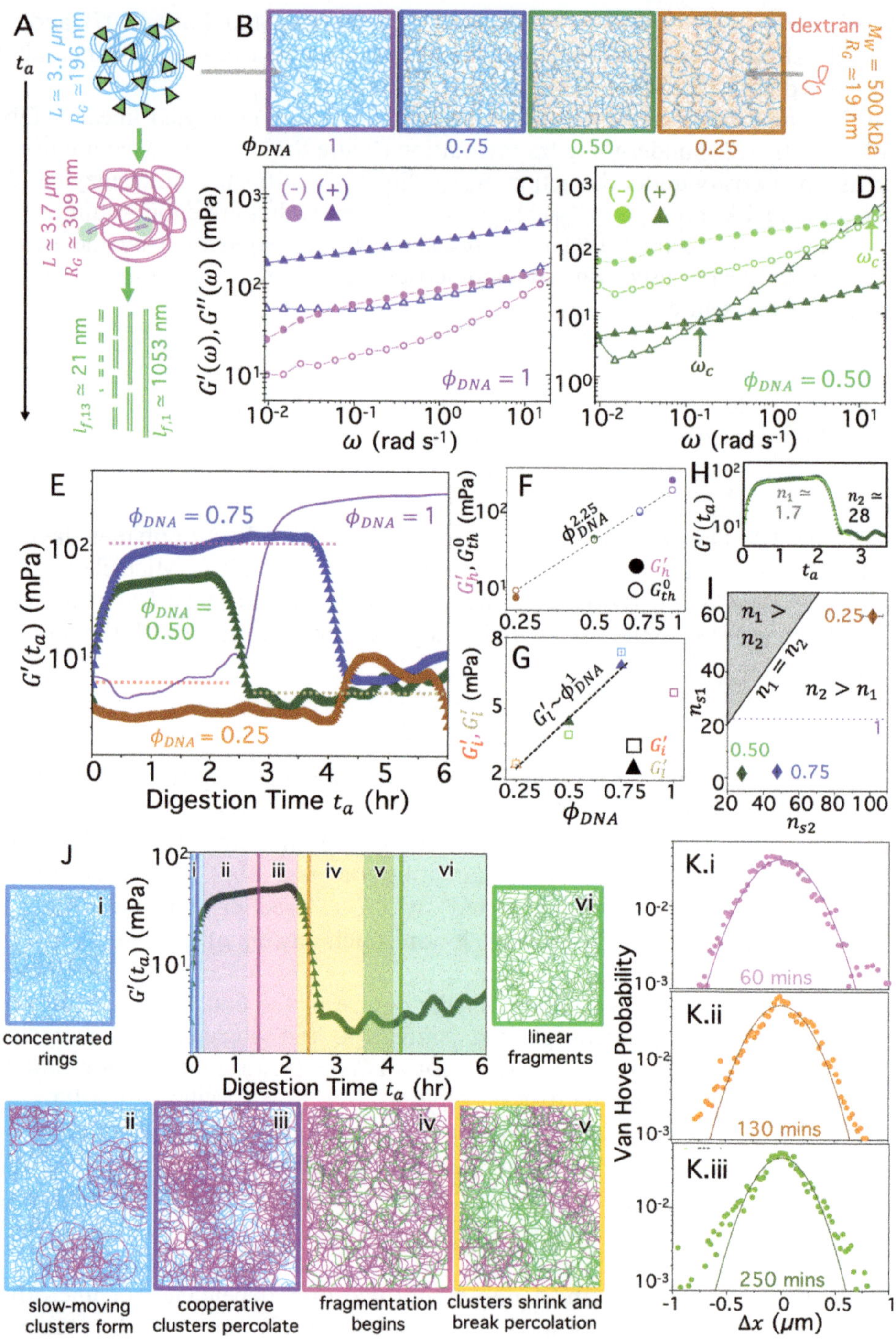

Figure 8.19. Bulk rheological state-switching of topologically-active composites of DNA and dextran. (A) A 13-cutter enzyme (ApoI, green triangles) cleaves ring DNA (blue) at 13 sites to linearize the DNA (magenta)

with the first cut, then successively cleave the linear chain into 13 fragments (green) of varying lengths l_f over time t_a (black arrow). (B) The enzymatic digestion process depicted in A is incorporated into $11c^*$ composites of ring DNA and dextran (orange) at varying DNA volume fractions $\phi_{DNA} = 1$ (100% DNA, purple), 0.75 (blue border), 0.5 (green), 0.25 (orange) to create topologically-active bio-synthetic composites. (C, D) $G'(\omega)$ (filled symbols) and $G''(\omega)$ (open symbols) measured after 6 h with ((+), triangles) and without ((−), circles) ApoI for $\phi_{DNA}= 1$ (C) and $\phi_{DNA}= 0.5$ (D). (E) The elastic modulus G', measured at $\omega = 1$ rad s^{-1}, as a function of ApoI activity time t_a for $\phi_{DNA} < 1$ composites (symbols) and the $\phi_{DNA} = 1$ DNA solution (purple line) show abrupt state-switching from initial low-elasticity states with $\langle G'(t_a)\rangle = G'_i$, depicted for $\phi_{DNA} = 1$ by the dashed red line, to high-elasticity states with $\langle G'(t_a)\rangle = G'_h$ (shown for $\phi_{DNA} = 0.75$ by magenta dashed line), and finally back to low-elasticity states $\langle G'(t_a)\rangle = G'_l$ (shown for $\phi_{DNA} = 0.5$ by gold dashed line). (F) G'_h (filled circles) and theoretically predicted entanglement plateau modulus G^0_{th} (open circles) versus ϕ_{DNA} with predicted reptation model scaling $G^0_{th} \sim \phi^{2.25}_{DNA}$ (dashed line). (G) G'_i (open squares) and G'_l (filled triangles) versus ϕ_{DNA} with predicted scaling for the semidilute unentangled regime $G' \sim \phi^1_{DNA}$ (dashed line). (H) Fits (light green lines) of $G'(t_a)$ for $\phi_{DNA} = 0.5$ (also shown in E) to effective Hill functions (equation (8.8)) for the time ranges that span each transition period, with the corresponding cooperativity parameters n_1 and n_2 listed. (I) n_1 versus n_2 for all composites (color-coded diamonds), with the dashed purple line denoting n_1 for the $\phi_{DNA} = 1$ system, which does not exhibit a second transition (no n_2). The grey and white areas denote regions of the parameter space in which $n_1 > n_2$ (where no data reside) and $n_2 > n_1$ (where all composite data lie). The black line is the phase line separating the two regimes. (J) Cartoon depiction of cooperative model, inspired by glass transitions, that captures the discrete state-switching behavior seen in E. (K) van Hove probability distributions for DNA tracked in the composites at different times t_a that correlate with (i) normal Gaussian dynamics at $t_a = 60$ min, and (ii, iii) heterogenous dynamics with exponential tails and super-Gaussian peaks at $t_a = 130$ min and 250 min. Adapted from Marfai *et al* (2023).

dextran composites studied in Khanal *et al* (2022), as I describe in chapter 7. To this end, researchers performed bulk rheology measurements on composites of circular DNA of length $L \simeq 3.7$ μm (11 kbp) and dextran of $M_w = 500$ kDa, with fixed total concentration of $11c^*$ ($\sim$5.28 mg mL^{-1} for DNA, $\sim$318 mg mL^{-1} for dextran) (Khanal *et al* 2022, Marfai *et al* 2023) and varying volume fractions of the DNA solution, ϕ_{DNA} (0, 0.25, 0.5, 0.75, 1). To push the composites out of equilibrium, the 13-site cleaving enzyme, ApoI, was incorporated (figures 8.19(A) and (B)). ApoI first cuts each DNA ring into a linear strand then successively cleaves the full-length linear strand into 13 smaller linear fragments with 13 distinct lengths in the range $l_f \simeq 21$–1053 nm (figure 8.19(A)). For all composites, the stoichiometry was fixed at $S_{13} = 50$ U mg^{-1} to allow for digestion to proceed slowly and steadily over the course of $\sim$2–4 hours, as confirmed via time-resolved gel electrophoresis (Marfai *et al* 2023).

The bulk frequency-dependent viscoelastic moduli, measured with and without ApoI digestion, revealed that for pure DNA ($\phi_{DNA} = 0$), digestion surprisingly increased $G'(\omega)$ and $G''(\omega)$ (figure 8.19(C)), despite the DNA being fragmented into much smaller chains. Conversely, for $\phi_{DNA} < 1$ composites, the viscoelastic moduli generally decreased following digestion (figure 8.19(D)). This difference was shown to arise from the extent to which the DNA fragments, with a mean length $\langle l_f \rangle \simeq 285$ nm and corresponding entanglement concentration $c_{e,\langle l_f \rangle} \approx 6c^*_{\langle l_f \rangle} \approx 5.1$ mg mL^{-1}, are entangled at the end of digestion for each composite (Marfai *et al* 2023). For $\phi_{DNA} = 1$, the DNA concentration $c_{DNA} \simeq 5.28$ mg mL^{-1} equates to $\sim 1.04 c_{e,\langle l_f \rangle}$, so one may expect entanglements of linear chains to dominate the rheology, causing the increase in $G'(\omega)$ (figure 8.19(C)). Conversely, DNA concentrations in $\phi_{DNA} = 0.75, 0.5, 0.25$ composites correspond to $\sim 0.8c_{e,\langle l_f \rangle}$, $\sim 0.5c_{e,\langle l_f \rangle}$ and $\sim 0.3c_{e,\langle l_f \rangle}$ respectively, suggesting that entanglements are largely lost by fragmentation, causing $G'(\omega)$ to drop (figure 8.19(D)).

To investigate the time course of the viscoelastic moduli en route from the initial to digested states, researchers measured the viscoelastic moduli continuously at $\omega = 1$ rad s^{-1} for $t_a = 0$–6 hours, which gel electrophoresis experiments showed was at least 1 hour longer than the time for the DNA in all composites to be fully digested (Marfai *et al* 2023). In contrast to the steady increase and decrease in microviscosity reported in Michieletto *et al* (2022), bulk measurements of $G'(t_a)$ for all composites showed an abrupt jump from an initial, relatively constant value G'_i to a higher time-independent one G'_h, with values ~5× to ~200× higher than G'_i, depending on ϕ_{DNA} (figure 8.19(E)). The magnitude of G'_h aligned closely with the theoretically predicted value and scaling for the elastic plateau modulus G^0_{th} for linear DNA at concentrations corresponding to each ϕ_{DNA} (i.e., $G'_h \approx G^0_{th} \sim \phi^{2.25}_{DNA}$) (figure 8.19(F)) (Rubinstein and Colby 2003). This agreement suggests that in the high-elasticity state, the entangled DNA, which is primarily linear, dominates the rheology, with little impact of dextran. Moreover, while pure DNA remains in the G'_h state for the remainder of the 6 hours, all composites displayed a subsequent, equally sharp drop to a state characterized by a lower elastic modulus G'_l that scaled as $G'_l \sim \phi^1_{DNA}$ (figure 8.19(G)), in accord with predictions for the stress relaxation modulus of unentangled semidilute polymers (Rubinstein and Colby 2003). The initial modulus values followed more complex and non-monotonic dependence on ϕ_{DNA}, owing to the varying contributions of dextran-mediated bundling and swelling of linear and ring DNA, along with enhanced ring-linear threading in $\phi_{DNA} = 0.75$ composites (figure 8.19(G)).

The robust sigmoid-like functional dependence of $G'(t_a)$ during the transitions for all composites (figure 8.19(E)) is generically reminiscent of cooperative transitions in two-state systems in which the cooperativity of many molecular-level constituents and mechanisms is necessary to impart large-scale structural changes to the system (Ruckenstein and Nagarajan 1981, Ivanov *et al* 2005, Zhou *et al* 2008, Bauer *et al* 2013, Bercy and Bockelmann 2015, Pazmiño Betancourt *et al* 2015, Linsmeier *et al* 2016a, Michieletto *et al* 2017). In these cases, the steeper the sigmoid, the more cooperative the process that drives the switch from state 1 to state 2, which can be quantified using a Hill function

$$P_2(f) = \left[1 + \left(\frac{\mathcal{F}_s}{f}\right)^n\right]^{-1} \tag{8.9}$$

where P_2 is the probability to be in state 2, f is the parameter that dictates which state the system is in, $\mathcal{F}_s$ is the characteristic value of f at which $P_2 = P_1 = 0.5$, and n is the Hill coefficient, or cooperativity term, that quantifies the steepness of the transition, with $n > 0$ and $n < 0$ indicative of cooperative and antagonistic processes, respectively (Alberts 2004, Hill 2013).

Adapting equation (8.9) to describe the time-dependent elastic modulus in the transition regime (figure 8.19(E)), yields

$$G'(t_a) = G'_1 + \frac{G'_2 - G'_1}{1 + (\tau_s/t_a)^n} \tag{8.10}$$

where G'_1 and G'_2 are the elastic moduli in the initial and final states flanking the transition and τ_s is the characteristic switching time. By fitting $G'(t_a)$ for the time ranges over which the (1) initial jump ($G' \rightarrow G'_h$) and (2) subsequent drop ($G'_h \rightarrow G'_l$) occur (figure 8.19(H)), the cooperativity strengths (n_1, n_2) and switching times (τ_{s1}, τ_{s2}) were determined, revealing that all transitions exhibited positive cooperativity with n_2 always being substantially larger n_1 (figure 8.19(I)).

The underlying cooperative mechanism was suggested to be analogous to that for glass transitions, in which the transition to bulk glass-like dynamics is only achieved when discrete clusters of slow-moving constituents grow and connect enough to reach percolation throughout the network (Chaudhuri *et al* 2007, Bauer *et al* 2013, Pazmiño Betancourt *et al* 2015, Zhong *et al* 2022). In traditional glass transitions, this abrupt phase transition occurs by steadily decreasing the temperature, and, upon increasing the temperature, glassiness remains until the average cluster size becomes smaller than the system size such that percolation is broken. By analogy (figure 8.19(J)), as the rings are linearized, local 'slow' clusters of entangled linear chains form and grow with little impact on bulk rheology until the clusters percolate, causing an abrupt jump from G'_i to G'_h. As the linear chains are chopped into smaller and smaller fragments there is little effect on the rheology until the average fragment length drops below the critical entanglement length, thus breaking percolation and causing the discrete drop from G'_h to G'_l (figure 8.19(J)). Complementary DNA tracking experiments confirmed this physical picture by demonstrating that the van Hove distributions of DNA displacements during the transitions were non-Gaussian with exponential large displacement tails (figure 8.19(K)), which have been shown to be a universal signature of glass transitions (Chaudhuri *et al* 2007, Michieletto *et al* 2017, Marfai *et al* 2023).

As I describe in chapter 6 (see figure 6.7), a complementary approach to engineering topologically-active DNA networks, has been to use Topoisomerase II (T2) to transiently link and unlink ring DNA to form dynamic concatemers, coined 'Olympic rings' (Krajina *et al* 2018). This action was shown to induce either fluidization in the presence of ATP, by disentangling linked or entangled rings, or gelation in the absence of ATP by preventing unlinking of concatemers. Specifically, researchers performed DLS microrheology to measure the viscoelastic moduli of highly concentrated solutions ($c \simeq 6$ mg mL$^{-1} \approx 200c*$) of nicked circular DNA of length $L \simeq 7.5$ μm (22.6 kbp), in the absence or presence of T2, at a concentration corresponding to ~0.4 T2 dimers per DNA ring. Without T2 or ATP, $G'(\omega)$ and $G''(\omega)$ exhibited frequency dependence in line with reptation model predictions, with a disengagement time $\tau_D \approx 2$ s, determined from the crossover frequency $\omega_c \approx 0.5$ s^{-1} (figure 6.7) (Krajina *et al* 2018).

Addition of T2 and ATP increased the crossover frequency by ~4× to $\omega_c \approx 2$ s^{-1}, corresponding to a longest relaxation time of $\tau_{T2} \approx 0.5$ s, which is indicative of the linking and unlinking timescale of T2. Because T2 can break and reseal rings, it effectively acts to evade entanglement constraints so τ_D no longer controls the crossover to terminal flow regime. Rather, complete relaxation of the system can be achieved over the shorter timescale τ_{T2} of T2 linking/unlinking. This fluidization also manifested as a ~2.25× lower plateau modulus, indicating that the effective entanglement density was proportionally reduced (recall $G_N^0 \sim N_e^{-1}$). Following 1 hour of dynamic concatenation, researchers 'froze' the network in its concatenated state by inactivating the T2 via chelation of divalent cations with EDTA (Krajina *et al* 2018). This action eliminated the terminal flow regime (figure 6.7), indicating that the longest relaxation timescale was well above 10 s ($\omega \approx 0.1$ s^{-1}) demonstrating that both disengagement and unlinking were prohibited. However, the plateau modulus and the high-frequency scaling of $G'(\omega)$ and $G''(\omega)$ remained similar to the active T2 case, confirming that the dynamics controlling this faster regime (timescales shorter than τ_{T2}) are those of single chains and chain segments which do not 'feel' the steric linking constraints (Krajina *et al* 2018).

8.4 Considerations and outlook

The systems, physical properties and underlying mechanisms I have discussed in this chapter are intended to provide a broad overview of recurring patterns of emergent phenomena that active biopolymer networks exhibit, and the governing physical principles that drive their non-equilibrium behavior. I have not attempted to encompass the expansive and rapidly growing body of literature on active matter or *in vivo* and cellular active matter. I instead focused on several model active biopolymer platforms that may be harnessed to design more complex systems and to understand the behavior of other out-of-equilibrium systems.

Some frontier areas in active and non-equilibrium biopolymer networks that require investigation and design considerations include:

Reversibility: The majority of the activity and dynamics I discussed are irreversible processes, e.g., contraction or fragmentation, that prevent the system from returning to its starting state or undergoing multiple cycles of activity. While this irreversibility is driven by the energy dissipation on which active matter systems rely, biology is able to overcome this dissipation to produce periodic, recoverable, and reversible dynamics, such as circadian rhythms. Designing systems that can exhibit such periodicity, reversibility, and/or healing, and understanding the system requirements for such activity, is an important next step in biopolymer network research.

Multi-engine systems: Most active biopolymer systems to date have relied on the action of a single motor, enzyme, or other 'engine' to push the system out of equilibrium. How multiple active components acting on the same or different substrates impact the dynamics and structure of biopolymer networks is an important research area that will likely reveal new emergent physics.

Bio-synthetic composites: Incorporating the dynamic force-generating capabilities of biopolymer systems into synthetic materials is a major challenge and goal in materials research. Coupling the 'living' nature of biopolymers with the resilience and reproducibility of synthetic systems can provide a powerful platform for designing autonomous, reconfigurable, responsive materials capable of moving, morphing, and self-healing.

References

Albert P J, Erdmann T and Schwarz U S 2014 Stochastic dynamics and mechanosensitivity of myosin II minifilaments *New J. Phys.* **16** 093019

Alberts B 2004 *Molecular Biology of the Cell* (Garland)

Alvarado J, Cipelletti L and Koenderink, G. H 2019 Uncovering the dynamic precursors to motor-driven contraction of active gels *Soft Matter* **15** 8552–65

Alvarado J, Sheinman M, Sharma A, MacKintosh F C and Koenderink G H 2013 Molecular motors robustly drive active gels to a critically connected state *Nat. Phys.* **9** 591–7

Aussel L, Barre F-X, Aroyo M, Stasiak A, Stasiak A Z and Sherratt D 2002 FtsK is a DNA motor protein that activates chromosome dimer resolution by switching the catalytic state of the XerC and XerD recombinases *Cell* **108** 195–205

Bacca M, Saleh O A and McMeeking R M 2019 Contraction of polymer gels created by the activity of molecular motors *Soft Matter* **15** 4467–75

Banerjee S, Gardel M L and Schwarz U S 2020 The actin cytoskeleton as an active adaptive material *Annu. Rev. Condens. Matter Phys.* **11** 421–39

Bashirzadeh Y and Liu A P 2019 Encapsulation of the cytoskeleton: towards mimicking the mechanics of a cell *Soft Matter* **15** 8425–36

Bashirzadeh Y, Moghimianavval H and Liu A P 2022 Encapsulated actomyosin patterns drive cell-like membrane shape changes *iScience* **25** 104236

Bate T E, Varney M E, Taylor E H, Dickie J H, Chueh C-C, Norton M M and Wu K-T 2022 Self-mixing in microtubule-kinesin active fluid from nonuniform to uniform distribution of activity *Nat. Commun.* **13** 6573

Bauer T, Lunkenheimer P and Loidl A 2013 Cooperativity and the freezing of molecular motion at the glass transition *Phys. Rev. Lett.* **111** 225702

Baumann H and Surrey T 2014 Motor-mediated cortical versus astral microtubule organization in lipid-monolayered droplets *J. Biol. Chem.* **289** 22524–35

Bendix P M, Koenderink G H, Cuvelier D, Dogic Z, Koeleman B N, Brieher W M, Field C M, Mahadevan L and Weitz D A 2008 A quantitative analysis of contractility in active cytoskeletal protein networks *Biophys. J.* **94** 3126–36

Bercy M and Bockelmann U 2015 Hairpins under tension: RNA versus DNA *Nucleic Acids Res.* **43** 9928–36

Berezney J, Goode B L, Fraden S and Dogic Z 2022 Extensile to contractile transition in active microtubule–actin composites generates layered asters with programmable lifetimes *Proc. Natl Acad. Sci.* **119** e2115895119

Bertrand O J N, Fygenson D K and Saleh O A 2012 Active, motor-driven mechanics in a DNA gel *Proc. Natl Acad. Sci.* **109** 17342–7

Brau R R, Ferrer J M, Lee H, Castro C E, Tam B K, Tarsa P B, Matsudaira P, Boyce M C, Kamm R D and Lang M J 2007 Passive and active microrheology with optical tweezers *J. Opt. A: Pure Appl. Opt.* **9** S103

Burla F, Mulla Y, Vos B E, Aufderhorst-Roberts A and Koenderink G H 2019 From mechanical resilience to active material properties in biopolymer networks *Nat. Rev. Phys.* **1** 249–63

Caridi C P *et al* 2018 Nuclear F-actin and myosins drive relocalization of heterochromatic breaks *Nature* **559** 54–60

Cates M E 1987 Reptation of living polymers: dynamics of entangled polymers in the presence of reversible chain-scission reactions *Macromolecules* **20** 2289–96

Chandrakar P *et al* 2022 Engineering stability, longevity, and miscibility of microtubule-based active fluids *Soft Matter* **18** 1825–35

Chanet S, Miller C J, Vaishnav E D, Ermentrout B, Davidson L A and Martin A C 2017 Actomyosin meshwork mechanosensing enables tissue shape to orient cell force *Nat. Commun.* **8** 1–13

Chapman C D, Lee K, Henze D, Smith D E and Robertson-Anderson R M 2014 Onset of non-continuum effects in microrheology of entangled polymer solutions *Macromolecules* **47** 1181–6

Chaudhuri P, Berthier L and Kob W 2007 Universal nature of particle displacements close to glass and jamming transitions *Phys. Rev. Lett.* **99** 060604

Conti M A and Adelstein R S 2008 Nonmuscle myosin II moves in new directions *J. Cell Sci.* **121** 11–8

Crozat E and Grainge I 2010 FtsK DNA translocase: the fast motor that knows where it's going *Chem. Bio. Chem.* **11** 2232–43

Doi M and Edwards S F 1986 *The Theory of Polymer Dynamics* (Oxford: Oxford University Press)

Ennomani H, Letort G, Guérin C, Martiel J-L, Cao W, Nédélec F, De La Cruz E M, Théry M and Blanchoin L 2016 Architecture and connectivity govern actin network contractility *Curr. Biol.* **26** 616–26

Fletcher D A and Mullins R D 2010 Cell mechanics and the cytoskeleton *Nature* **463** 485–92

Fürthauer S, Lemma B, Foster P J, Ems-McClung S C, Yu C-H, Walczak C E, Dogic Z, Needleman D J and Shelley M J 2019 Self-straining of actively crosslinked microtubule networks *Nat. Phys.* **15** 1295–300

Gatlin J C and Bloom K 2010 Microtubule motors in eukaryotic spindle assembly and maintenance *Semin. Cell Dev. Biol.* **21** 248–54

Geeves M A 2016 Review: the ATPase mechanism of myosin and actomyosin *Biopolymers* **105** 483–91

Grewe J and Schwarz U S 2020 Mechanosensitive self-assembly of myosin II minifilaments *Phys. Rev.* E **101** 022402

Guntas G, Hallett R A, Zimmerman S P, Williams T, Yumerefendi H, Bear J E and Kuhlman B 2015 Engineering an improved light-induced dimer (iLID) for controlling the localization and activity of signaling proteins *Proc. Natl Acad. Sci.* **112** 112–7

Gurmessa B, Francis M, Rust M J, Das M, Ross J L and Robertson-Anderson R M 2019 Counterion crossbridges enable robust multiscale elasticity in actin networks *Phys. Rev. Res.* **1** 013016

Gurmessa B J, Bitten N, Nguyen D T, Saleh O A, Ross J L, Das M and Robertson-Anderson R M 2018 Triggered disassembly and reassembly of actin networks induces rigidity phase transitions *Soft Matter* **15** 1335–44

Gurmessa B J, Rust M J, Das M, Ross J L and Robertson-Anderson R M 2021 Salt-mediated stiffening, destruction, and resculpting of actomyosin network *Front. Phys.* **9** 760340

Henkin G, DeCamp S J, Chen D T N, Sanchez T and Dogic Z 2014 Tunable dynamics of microtubule-based active isotropic gels *Philos. Trans. Royal Soc. A: Math., Phys. Eng. Sci.* **372** 20140142

Hentrich C and Surrey T 2010 Microtubule organization by the antagonistic mitotic motors kinesin-5 and kinesin-14 *J. Cell Biol.* **189** 465–80

Hill T L 2013 *Cooperativity Theory in Biochemistry: Steady-State and Equilibrium Systems.* (Springer Science & Business Media)

Humphrey D, Duggan C, Saha D, Smith D and Käs J 2002 Active fluidization of polymer networks through molecular motors *Nature* **416** 413–6

Ivanov V, Piontkovski D and Zocchi G 2005 Local cooperativity mechanism in the DNA melting transition *Phys. Rev.* E **71** 041909

Jahnke K, Weiss M, Weber C, Platzman I, Göpfrich K and Spatz J P 2020 Engineering light-responsive contractile actomyosin networks with DNA nanotechnology *Adv. Biosyst.* **4** 2000102

Jeon B, Nguyen D T, Abraham G R, Conrad N, Fygenson D K and Saleh O A 2018 Salt-dependent properties of a coacervate-like, self-assembled DNA liquid *Soft Matter* **14** 7009–15

Khanal P, Peddireddy K R, Marfai J, McGorty R and Robertson-Anderson R M 2022 DNA topology dictates emergent bulk elasticity and hindered macromolecular diffusion in DNA-dextran composites *J. Rheol.* **66** 699–715

Klemm A H, Bosilj A, Glunc ic M, Pavin N and Tolic I M 2018 Metaphase kinetochore movements are regulated by kinesin-8 motors and microtubule dynamic instability *MBoC* **29** 1332–45

Koenderink G H, Dogic Z, Nakamura F, Bendix P M, MacKintosh F C, Hartwig J H, Stossel T P and Weitz D A 2009 An active biopolymer network controlled by molecular motors *Proc. Natl Acad. Sci.* **106** 15192–7

Koenderink G H and Paluch E K 2018 Architecture shapes contractility in actomyosin networks *Curr. Opin. Cell Biol., Cell Archit.* **50** 79–85

Kong D, Banik S, San Francisco M J, Lee M, Robertson Anderson R M, Schroeder C M and McKenna G B 2022 Rheology of entangled solutions of ring–linear DNA blends *Macromolecules* **55** 1205–17

Krajina B A, Zhu A, Heilshorn S C and Spakowitz A J 2018 Active DNA olympic hydrogels driven by topoisomerase activity *Phys. Rev. Lett.* **121** 148001

Kuçera O, Gaillard J, Guérin C, Théry M and Blanchoin L 2022a Actin–microtubule dynamic composite forms responsive active matter with memory *Proc. Natl Acad. Sci.* **119** e2209522119

Kuçera O, Gaillard J, Guérin C, Utzschneider C, Théry M and Blanchoin L 2022b Actin architecture steers microtubules in active cytoskeletal composite *Nano Lett.* **22** 8584–91

Kuçera O, Siahaan V, Janda D, Dijkstra S H, Pilátová E, Zatecka E, Diez S, Braun M and Lansky Z 2021 Anillin propels myosin-independent constriction of actin rings *Nat. Commun.* **12** 4595

Lee G, Leech G, Lwin P, Michel J, Currie C, Rust M J, Ross J L, McGorty R J, Das M and Robertson-Anderson R M 2021a Active cytoskeletal composites display emergent tunable contractility and restructuring *Soft Matter* **17** 10765–76

Lee G, Leech G, Rust M J, Das M, McGorty R J, Ross J L and Robertson-Anderson R M 2021b Myosin-driven actin-microtubule networks exhibit self-organized contractile dynamics *Sci. Adv.* **7** eabe4334

Lemma L M, Norton M M, Tayar A M, DeCamp S J, Aghvami S A, Fraden S, Hagan M F and Dogic Z 2021 Multiscale microtubule dynamics in active nematics *Phys. Rev. Lett.* **127** 148001

Lemma L M, Varghese M, Ross T D, Thomson M, Baskaran A and Dogic Z 2023 Spatio-temporal patterning of extensile active stresses in microtubule-based active fluids *PNAS Nexus* **2** pgad130

Lenz M 2020 Reversal of contractility as a signature of self-organization in cytoskeletal bundles *eLife* **9** e51751

Lenz M 2014 Geometrical origins of contractility in disordered actomyosin networks *Phys. Rev.* X **4** 041002

Liao G and Gundersen G G 1998 Kinesin is a candidate for cross-bridging microtubules and intermediate filaments: selective binding of kinesin to detyrosinated tubulin and vimentin *J. Biol. Chem.* **273** 9797–803

Linsmeier I, Banerjee S, Oakes P W, Jung W, Kim T and Murrell M P 2016a Disordered actomyosin networks are sufficient to produce cooperative and telescopic contractility *Nat. Commun.* **7** 12615

Linsmeier I, Banerjee S, Oakes P W, Jung W, Kim T and Murrell M P 2016b Disordered actomyosin networks are sufficient to produce cooperative and telescopic contractility *Nat. Commun.* **7** 12615

Litschel T, Kelley C F, Holz D, Adeli Koudehi M, Vogel S K, Burbaum L, Mizuno N, Vavylonis D and Schwille P 2021 Reconstitution of contractile actomyosin rings in vesicles *Nat. Commun.* **12** 2254

Lu D and Chen B 2022 Coordinated motion of molecular motors on DNA chains with branch topology *Acta Mech. Sin.* **38** 621225

Malik-Garbi M, Ierushalmi N, Jansen S, Abu-Shah E, Goode B L, Mogilner A and Keren K 2019 Scaling behaviour in steady-state contracting actomyosin networks *Nat. Phys.* **15** 509–16

Marfai J, McGorty R J and Robertson-Anderson R M 2023 Cooperative rheological state-switching of enzymatically-driven composites of circular DNA and dextran *Adv. Mater.* **35** e2305824

McFadden W M, McCall P M, Gardel M L and Munro E M 2017 Filament turnover tunes both force generation and dissipation to control long-range flows in a model actomyosin cortex *PLoS Comput. Biol.* **13** e1005811

McGorty R J *et al* 2023 Kinesin and myosin motors compete to drive rich multiphase dynamics in programmable cytoskeletal composites *PNAS Nexus* **2** pgad245

Michieletto D 2020 Non-equilibrium living polymers *Entropy* **22** 1130

Michieletto D, Nahali N and Rosa A 2017 Glassiness and heterogeneous dynamics in dense solutions of ring polymers *Phys. Rev. Lett.* **119** 197801

Michieletto D, Neill P, Weir S, Evans D, Crist N, Martinez V A and Robertson-Anderson R M 2022 Topological digestion drives time-varying rheology of entangled DNA fluids *Nat. Commun.* **13** 4389

Mizuno D, Tardin C, Schmidt C F and MacKintosh F C 2007 Nonequilibrium mechanics of active cytoskeletal networks *Science* **315** 370–3

Muresan C G, Sun Z G, Yadav V, Tabatabai A P, Lanier L, Kim J H, Kim T and Murrell M P 2022 F-actin architecture determines constraints on myosin thick filament motion *Nat. Commun.* **13** 7008

Murrell M, Oakes P W, Lenz M and Gardel M L 2015 Forcing cells into shape: the mechanics of actomyosin contractility *Nat. Rev. Mol. Cell Biol.* **16** 486–98

Murrell M P and Gardel M L 2012 F-actin buckling coordinates contractility and severing in a biomimetic actomyosin cortex *PNAS* **109** 20820–5

Nasirimarekani V, Subramani S, Herzog S, Vilfan A and Guido I 2022 Active bending of disordered microtubule bundles by kinesin motors *ACS Omega* **7** 43820–8

Ndlec F J, Surrey T, Maggs A C and Leibler S 1997 Self-organization of microtubules and motors *Nature* **389** 305–8

Needleman D and Dogic Z 2017 Active matter at the interface between materials science and cell biology *Nat. Rev. Mater.* **2** 1–14

Nguyen D T and Saleh O A 2017 Tuning phase and aging of DNA hydrogels through molecular design *Soft Matter* **13** 5421–7

Opathalage A, Norton M M, Juniper M P N, Langeslay B, Aghvami S A, Fraden S and Dogic Z 2019 Self-organized dynamics and the transition to turbulence of confined active nematics *Proc. Natl Acad. Sci. USA* **116** 4788–97

Park C-Y, Jacobson D R, Nguyen D T, Willardson S and Saleh O A 2016 A thin permeable-membrane device for single-molecule manipulation *Rev. Sci. Instrum.* **87** 014301

Pazmiño Betancourt B A, Hanakata P Z, Starr F W and Douglas J F 2015 Quantitative relations between cooperative motion, emergent elasticity, and free volume in model glass-forming polymer materials *Proc. Natl Acad. Sci.* **112** 2966–71

Peddireddy K R, Clairmont R, Neill P, McGorty R and Robertson-Anderson R M 2022 Optical-tweezers-integrating-differential-dynamic-microscopy maps the spatiotemporal propagation of nonlinear strains in polymer blends and composites *Nat. Commun.* **13** 5180

Peddireddy K R, Clairmont R and Robertson-Anderson R M 2023 Polymer threadings and rigidity dictate the viscoelasticity of entangled ring-linear blends and their composites with rigid rod microtubules *J. Rheol.* **67** 125–38

Peddireddy K R, Lee M, Schroeder C M and Robertson-Anderson R M 2020a Viscoelastic properties of ring-linear DNA blends exhibit nonmonotonic dependence on blend composition *Phys. Rev. Res.* **2** 023213

Peddireddy K R, Lee M, Zhou Y, Adalbert S, Anderson S, Schroeder C M and Robertson-Anderson R M 2020b Unexpected entanglement dynamics in semidilute blends of supercoiled and ring DNA *Soft Matter* **16** 152–61

Pinot M, Chesnel F, Kubiak J Z, Arnal I, Nedelec F J and Gueroui Z 2009 Effects of confinement on the self-organization of microtubules and motors *Curr. Biol.* **19** 954–60

Ricketts S N, Khanal P, Rust M J, Das M, Ross J L and Robertson-Anderson R M 2020 Triggering cation-induced contraction of cytoskeleton networks via microfluidics *Front. Phys.* **8** 596699

Robert-Paganin J, Pylypenko O, Kikuti C, Sweeney H L and Houdusse A 2020 Force generation by myosin motors: a structural perspective *Chem. Rev.* **120** 5–35

Robertson R M, Laib S and Smith D E 2006 Diffusion of isolated DNA molecules: dependence on length and topology *PNAS* **103** 7310–4

Robertson R M and Smith D E 2007 Strong effects of molecular topology on diffusion of entangled DNA molecules *PNAS* **104** 4824–7

Robertson R M and Smith D E 2007 Self-diffusion of entangled linear and circular DNA molecules: dependence on length and concentration *Macromolecules* **40** 3373–7

Ross T D, Lee H J, Qu Z, Banks R A, Phillips R and Thomson M 2019 Controlling organization and forces in active matter through optically defined boundaries *Nature* **572** 224–9

Rubinstein M and Colby R H 2003 *Polymer Physics* (Oxford, New York: Oxford University Press)

Ruckenstein E and Nagarajan R 1981 Critical micelle concentration and the transition point for micellar size distribution *J. Phys. Chem.* **85** 3010–4

Sakuta H, Nakatani N, Torisawa T, Sumino Y, Tsumoto K, Oiwa K and Yoshikawa K 2023 Self-emergent vortex flow of microtubule and kinesin in cell-sized droplets under water/water phase separation *Commun. Chem.* **6** 1–9

Sanchez T, Chen D T N, DeCamp S J, Heymann M and Dogic Z 2012 Spontaneous motion in hierarchically assembled active matter *Nature* **491** 431–4

Sasanpour M, Achiriloaie D H, Lee G, Leech G, Currie C, Lindsay K A, Ross J L, McGorty R J and Robertson-Anderson R M 2022 Reconstituting and characterizing actin-microtubule composites with tunable motor-driven dynamics and mechanics *JoVE* **186** e64228

Sellers J R 2000 Myosins: a diverse superfamily *Biochim. Biophys. Acta (BBA)–Mol. Cell Res.* **1496** 3–22

Sheung J Y *et al* 2021 Motor-driven restructuring of cytoskeleton composites leads to tunable time-varying elasticity *ACS Macro Lett.* **10** 1151–8

Sheung J Y, Garamella J, Kahl S K, Lee B Y, McGorty R J and Robertson-Anderson R M 2022 Motor-driven advection competes with crowding to drive spatiotemporally heterogeneous transport in cytoskeleton composites *Front. Phys.* **10** 1055441

Silva M S E, Depken M, Stuhrmann B, Korsten M, MacKintosh F C and Koenderink G H 2011 Active multistage coarsening of actin networks driven by myosin motors *PNAS* **108** 9408–13

Smrek J, Garamella J, Robertson-Anderson R and Michieletto D 2021 Topological tuning of DNA mobility in entangled solutions of supercoiled plasmids *Sci. Adv.* **7** eabf9260

Stam S, Freedman S L, Banerjee S, Weirich K L, Dinner A R and Gardel M L 2017 Filament rigidity and connectivity tune the deformation modes of active biopolymer networks *Proc. Natl Acad. Sci.* **114** E10037–45

Surrey T, Nédélec F, Leibler S and Karsenti E 2001a Physical properties determining self-organization of motors and microtubules *Science* **292** 1167–71

Swartz D W and Camley B A 2021 Active gels, heavy tails, and the cytoskeleton *Soft Matter* **17** 9876–92

Sweeney H L and Houdusse A 2010 Structural and functional insights into the myosin motor mechanism *Annu. Rev. Biophys.* **39** 539–57

Tam A K Y, Mogilner A and Oelz D B 2021 Protein friction and filament bending facilitate contraction of disordered actomyosin networks *Biophys. J.* **120** 4029–40

Tsuji M, Rashedul Kabir A M, Ito M, Inoue D, Kokado K, Sada K and Kakugo A 2017 Motility of microtubules on the inner surface of water-in-oil emulsion droplets *Langmuir* **33** 12108–13

Voth G A 2017 A multiscale description of biomolecular active matter: the chemistry underlying many life processes *Acc. Chem. Res.* **50** 594–8

Weirich K L, Dasbiswas K, Witten T A, Vaikuntanathan S and Gardel M L 2019 Self-organizing motors divide active liquid droplets *PNAS* **116** 11125–30

Weirich K L, Stam S, Munro E and Gardel M L 2021 Actin bundle architecture and mechanics regulate myosin II force generation *Biophys. J.* **120** 1957–70

Wollrab V, Belmonte J M, Baldauf L, Leptin M, Nédeléc F and Koenderink G H 2018 Polarity sorting drives remodeling of actin-myosin networks *J. Cell Sci.* **132** jcs219717

Wu K-T, Hishamunda J B, Chen D T N, DeCamp S J, Chang Y-W, Fernández-Nieves A, Fraden S and Dogic Z 2017 Transition from turbulent to coherent flows in confined three-dimensional active fluids *Science* **355** eaal1979

Zhong Y, Yu L and Huang Q 2022 Investigating the linear viscoelastic behaviour at high frequencies in the transition to glassy regime for polystyrene melts and solutions *Rheol. Acta* **61** 689–700

Zhou H-X, Rivas G and Minton A P 2008 Macromolecular crowding and confinement: biochemical, biophysical, and potential physiological consequences *Annu. Rev. Biophys.* **37** 375–97

Chapter 9

Self-assembly and phase separation

In crowded biological cells, entropically-driven depletion interactions, cooperativity, and hydrophobic interactions drive biopolymer networks to self-assemble into heterogeneous structures over different lengthscales and timescales. These interactions also lead to phase separation of interacting biopolymer networks, as in the widely-studied phenomenon of liquid–liquid phase separation (LLPS) of biopolymers and other macromolecules. This chapter focuses on the underlying kinetics and thermodyamics of LLPS and the physical properties of the biomolecular condensates that form during the process. I will highlight key examples of biopolymer LLPS, the associated mechanical and structural properties of the condensates, and the role of various tuning parameters including: biopolymer size, charge, and stiffness, as well as crowding and ionic conditions. I will close the chapter with a brief discussion of other phenomena related to LLPS and frontier topics of interest.

9.1 Beyond local heterogeneity

In chapters 6–8, I discuss examples of microscale spatiotemporal heterogeneities in biopolymer networks, such as bundling and flocculation of microtubules and actin in the presence of DNA (Fitzpatrick *et al* 2018, Peddireddy *et al* 2021), DNA aggregation induced by dextran crowding (Gorczyca *et al* 2015, Khanal *et al* 2022), and motor-driven aster formation and de-mixing of actin and microtubules in active composites (Berezney *et al* 2022, McGorty *et al* 2023). In these cases, beyond a critical lengthscale, the heterogeneities could be neglected when considering the ensemble bulk properties. Motor-driven systems have also been shown to form disconnected asters and aggregates that span dozens of microns (Silva *et al* 2011, Alvarado *et al* 2013, Koenderink and Paluch 2018, Weirich *et al* 2019). But the disconnected nature of such aggregates prevents them from substantially contributing to the bulk rheology, which instead is dictated by the surrounding percolated network of filaments or bundles (Alvarado *et al* 2013, Stam *et al* 2017, Peddireddy

doi:10.1088/978-0-7503-5037-2ch9

et al 2021, Marfai *et al* 2023). Moreover, motor-driven or depletion-driven aggregates and clusters that I discuss in previous chapters are typically rigid, solid-like structures that contain very little interstitial fluid and adopt amorphous or nematic geometries (Ndlec *et al* 1997, Silva *et al* 2011, Henkin *et al* 2014, Stam *et al* 2017, Weirich *et al* 2019, Peddireddy *et al* 2021). These coarse structures also tend to be stable and irreversible in the absence of chemical fuel or perturbation.

Here, I discuss systems in which the dominant structural feature is phase separation, and I focus on the kinetics and thermodynamics of phase separation (Hyman *et al* 2014, Alberti *et al* 2019, Lee *et al* 2021), the bulk properties of the droplets or aggregates (Aarts *et al* 2005, Riback *et al* 2020, Ghosh *et al* 2021, Shimobayashi *et al* 2021, Fonin *et al* 2022), and the dynamics and structure of the biopolymer network(s) comprising each phase (Miyagi *et al* 2008, Harmon *et al* 2017, Sing and Perry 2020, Abyzov *et al* 2022, Guseva *et al* 2023, Sahu *et al* 2023).

9.2 Introduction to liquid–liquid phase separation (LLPS)

Perhaps the most widely-studied phase separation phenomenon in biology is liquid–liquid phase separation (LLPS), in which a homogeneous biopolymer network separates into dense liquid-like droplets of biopolymers, also referred to as condensates or coacervates, that are surrounded by a contiguous 'gas' phase that is typically much more dilute. LLPS underlies the self-assembly of recently discovered membrane-less organelles that cells use for various functions such as compartmentalization and catalysis, and is more generally recognized as a key driver of the spatial organization of cells (Brangwynne *et al* 2015, Banani *et al* 2017, Shin *et al* 2018, Strom and Brangwynne 2019, Lyon *et al* 2021, Lee *et al* 2022).

In vitro, LLPS occurs in single-component biopolymer networks via weak non-covalent polymer–polymer association (e.g., electrostatic attraction, hydrogen bonding, etc), leading to biopolymer-rich droplets surrounded by primarily solvent (figure 9.1(A)) (Hyman *et al* 2014, Alberti *et al* 2019, Gouveia *et al* 2022, Sahu *et al* 2023). Binary biopolymer composites can also self-assemble into coacervates that contain both species, in which case LLPS is driven by, e.g., charge attraction of an anionic nucleic acid and cationic protein (Lu and Spruijt 2020, Sing and Perry 2020). Depending on the properties of the constituents, composites can also separate into dense condensates of one species surrounded by dense solution of the other species via entropic depletion and repulsive interactions (Biswas *et al* 2012, Delarue *et al* 2018, André and Spruijt 2020). The role of constituent properties, salt, pH, and crowding conditions have also been shown to impact the nucleation, assembly, and stability of coacervates, which often undergo aging, coarsening, and coalescence over time (Jeon *et al* 2018, Alberti *et al* 2019, McCarty *et al* 2019, Riback *et al* 2020, Sing and Perry 2020, Shimobayashi *et al* 2021, Conrad *et al* 2022, Gouveia *et al* 2022, Sahu *et al* 2023).

Despite these complexities, at the very basic level, the phase map predicting the existence of liquid–liquid phase separation in a polymer–solvent system (figure 9.1(A)) can be described by the Flory–Huggins model (Rubinstein and Colby 2003)

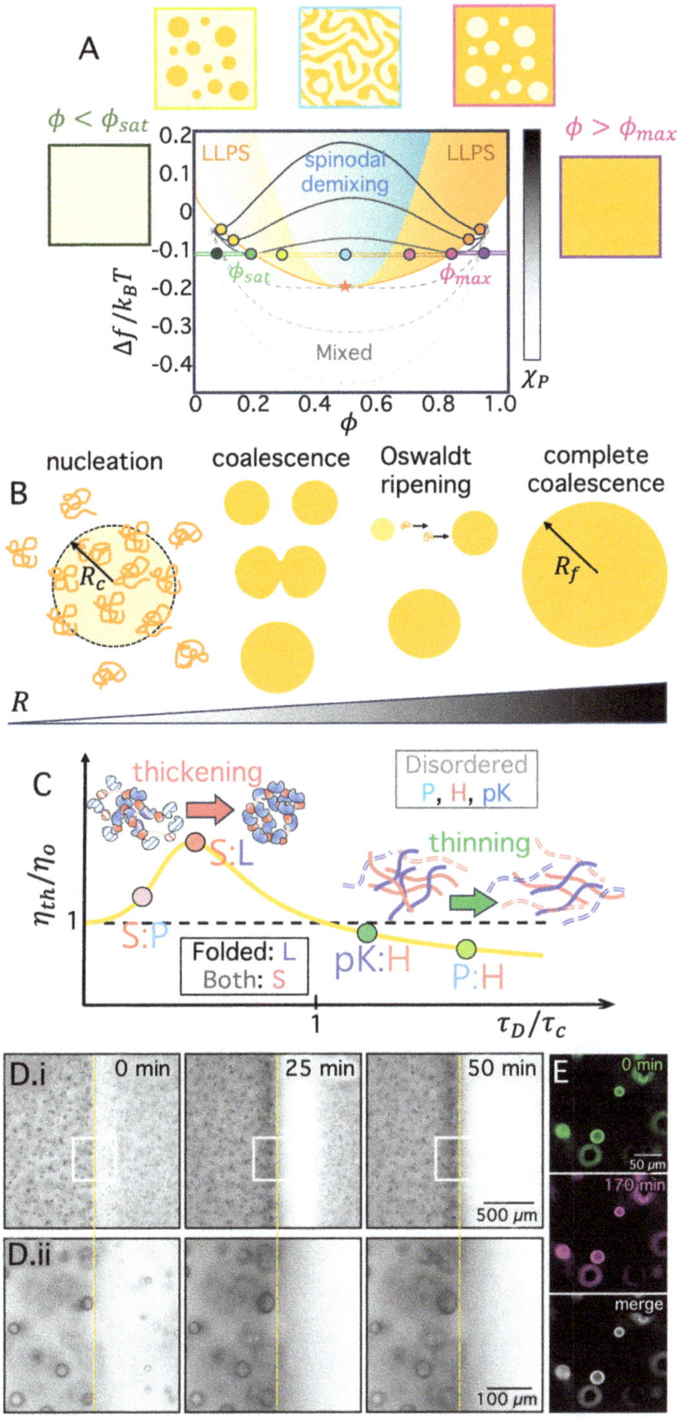

Figure 9.1. Physics of liquid–liquid phase separation from nucleation to coalescence and ripening. (A) State diagram for a polymer–solvent system with varying volume fraction ϕ (x-axis) and free energy density

difference $\Delta\hat{f}$ (y-axis) which depends on ϕ and the interaction parameter χ_P. The lines of different greyscale shades denote systems with different χ_P values (increasing according to greyscale), with dashed lines denoting χ_P values in which LLPS is energetically prohibited. The orange line is the binodal that denotes the co-existence phase where mixed and de-mixed states are equally probable. The orange regions mark the low (light shade) and high (dark shade) ϕ regions that favor LLPS, depicted in the cartoons at top-left (light-green border) and top-right (magenta border). The blue region denotes the de-mixed phase dominated by spinodal decomposition (depicted by the cyan-bordered cartoon). The horizontal double-line is the tie line that connects the low-ϕ and high-ϕ limits of LLPS at the given $\Delta\hat{f}$. All ϕ values that lie in the orange regions along the tie line will undergo LLPS. Examples of low-ϕ (light-green circle and bordered cartoon) and high-ϕ (magenta circle and bordered cartoon) states are shown, as well as states that do not support LLPS in the low-ϕ ($\phi < \phi_{\text{sat}}$, dark green circle and bordered cartoon) and high-ϕ ($\phi > \phi_{\text{max}}$, purple circle and bordered cartoon). The red star denotes the critical point. (B) The process of LLPS is (left) initiated by nucleation of individual polymers that form a metastable condensed liquid droplet when the droplet radius reaches R_c; (middle) condensates grow over time (indicated by scale at bottom) by undergoing coalescence and Ostwald ripening until (right) a single large condensate forms, at which point the system is in a stable phase-separated state. (C) The coalescence time for condensates that are viscoelastic, displaying either shear thickening (pink, S:P, S:L) or shear thinning (pK:H, P:K), is determined by the shear relaxation time τ_D rather than the Newtonian coalescence time τ_c. The viscosity in the dense condensate phase η_{th}, scaled by the Newtonian viscosity η_0 versus τ_D/τ_c shows that the non-Newtonian coalescence time is either shorter or longer than τ_c for thickening (pink) or thinning (green) condensates, respectively. Condensates shown are formed from oppositely-charged proteins that are either folded (L), disordered (P, H, pK), or have both folded and unfolded domains (S), with more ordered/disordered systems giving rise to thickening/thinning. (D) Nucleation and ripening over time (left to right) of oil droplets in a synthetic polymer gel that is divided into softer (left half) and stiffer (right half) phases show elastic ripening of droplets that dissolve in the stiff phase and reform in the soft phase. Zoom-ins of the boxed regions in (i) are shown in (ii). (E) A homogenous polymer network, soft enough to support droplet nucleation, prevents droplet ripening and growing, as shown by the similar sizes of droplets at 0 and 170 min. (C) Adapted from Ghosh *et al* (2021). CC BY 4.0. (D) Adapted from Rosowski *et al* (2020) Copyright (2020), with permission from Springer Nature.

that provides an expression for the change in free energy Δf between mixed (one bulk phase) and de-mixed (phase separation) states

$$\frac{\Delta f}{k_B T} = \left(\frac{\phi}{N}\right) \log \phi + (1 - \phi) \log (1 - \phi) + \chi_P \phi (1 - \phi) \tag{9.1}$$

where ϕ is the volume fraction of polymer in solution, N is the degree of polymerization, and χ_P is the interaction term associated with polymer–polymer interactions, with larger values shifting the system towards phase separation (figure 9.1(A)) (Rubinstein and Colby 2003, Brangwynne *et al* 2015).

The interface created by LLPS is also an important consideration, both for its biological role in compartmentalization and force generation, as well as its use as a model system for understanding interfacial capillary forces and surface tension in soft matter systems (Yanagisawa *et al* 2014, Wang and McGorty 2019, Gouveia *et al* 2022).

The pressure difference at the LLPS interface, i.e., the capillary pressure

$$\Delta p = 2Y/R \tag{9.2}$$

is determined from the condensate radius R and the surface tension Y associated with the cost of a molecule residing on the surface instead of the interior bulk (Gouveia *et al* 2022). Typical LLPS surface tension values of $Y \approx 10^{-4}$–10^{-7} N m^{-1} (Feric *et al* 2016,

Caragine *et al* 2018, Jawerth *et al* 2018, Narayanan *et al* 2019, Ijavi *et al* 2021) dictate a minimum condensate size

$$R_c = 2Y/\Delta\hat{f} \tag{9.3}$$

where $\Delta\hat{f} = \frac{\Delta f}{k_B T}$ is the free energy density difference between the condensed and bulk phases (figure 9.1(A)) (Kashchiev 2000). Below R_c, the surface tension renders the surface area to volume ratio of the condensate too great to be energetically favorable, causing the droplet to dissolve into the bulk phase. This relation, together with the minimum concentration for condensate nucleation ϕ_{sat} (figure 9.1(A)) (Kashchiev 2000, Hyman *et al* 2014, Shimobayashi *et al* 2021, Gouveia *et al* 2022), are lead factors controlling the onset of LLPS.

While R_c sets the minimum requirement for condensate formation (figure 9.1(B)), the energetic cost of maintaining an interface with Δp drives condensates to reduce their surface area to volume ratio $\frac{R^2}{R^3} \sim R^{-1}$, by increasing R. This free energy minimization underlies two widely-observed LLPS phenomena that increase R: (i) coalescence, in which two similarly sized condensates merge to form one droplet (figure 9.1(B)); and Ostwald ripening, in which a small droplet dissolves and its constituents get absorbed by a larger droplet (figure 9.1(B)).

The surface tension, along with the viscosity of the liquid-like condensate η_c, has also been shown to control the coalescence speed

$$v_c = Y/\eta \tag{9.3}$$

and timescale

$$\tau_c = \eta R_c / Y \tag{9.4}$$

(Eggers *et al* 1999, Aarts *et al* 2005, Feric *et al* 2016).

However, recent optical tweezers measurements showed that a variety of protein condensates exhibit viscoelastic shear thinning or thickening over the coalescence timescale, calling into question the validity of the Newtonian viscosity model for v_c (Ghosh *et al* 2021). These studies demonstrated that the key timescale governing coalescence is the shear relaxation timescale $\tau_D = 2\pi/\omega_c$, when $G'(\omega_c) = G''(\omega_c)$, which is dictated by network reconfiguration and is either longer or shorter than τ_c for shear thickening or thinning condensates, respectively (figure 9.1(C)) (Ghosh *et al* 2021).

Other work has shown that when the viscosity of the surrounding dilute 'gas' phase η_d is higher than η_c, then the relevant viscosity in equation (9.3) is η_d rather than η_c (Kashchiev 2000). Finally, droplets that form in the presence of heterogeneous polymer networks have been shown to undergo a process termed 'elastic ripening' in which droplets dissolve in stiff regions and reform in soft regions (figure 9.1(D)) (Rosowski *et al* 2020). Conversely, homogenous polymer networks can either stabilize droplets against Ostwald ripening and coalescence, or suppress LLPS entirely, above a critical network elasticity (Rosowski *et al* 2020). While these results were observed for purely synthetic systems of polymers and oil droplets, they are likely relevant to cell-like environments that comprise viscoelastic polymer networks (e.g., cytoskeleton) and liquid-like droplets (e.g., membrane-less organelles).

9.3 Crowding and liquid–liquid phase separation

Macromolecular crowding, a hallmark of the intracellular environment where biomolecular condensates form (Brangwynne *et al* 2015, André and Spruijt 2020), has been shown to both facilitate and hinder LLPS, as well as alter the state diagram and condensate properties through depletion interactions, co-condensation, and/or alteration of solvent conditions. A number of protein-based LLPS systems have been shown to require ~10% inert crowders, such as PEG, dextran, Ficoll, or BSA, to form condensates (Delarue *et al* 2018, Guo *et al* 2019, Vega *et al* 2019, André and Spruijt 2020, Yang *et al* 2020). Others have shown shifting of the state diagram towards condensate formation, i.e. lowering ϕ_{sat}, with increasing crowder concentration (Lin *et al* 2015, Kaur *et al* 2019, Yang *et al* 2020). Conversely, crowding by BSA and lysozymes have been shown to destabilize several protein condensates as a result of the similar partitioning coefficients of the crowder and protein as well as potential attractive interactions (Protter *et al* 2018, Ghosh *et al* 2019).

These examples highlight the important role that the properties of the crowders play in condensate formation, including their size, structure, and interactions with the condensing biopolymer and solvent (Ghosh *et al* 2019, André and Spruijt 2020). For example, coacervates of anionic polyU-RNA and cationic spermine, which only form above a critical spermine:PolyU ratio $[s{:}P]_{sat} \simeq 0.14$ in the absence of crowding, were shown to form at decreasing ratios in the presence of increasing PEG ($M_w \simeq 8$ kDa), reaching $[s{:}P]_{sat} \simeq 0.10$ for 20 w/w% PEG (figure 9.2(A)) (Marianelli *et al* 2018). Conversely, Ficoll ($M_w \simeq 70$ kDa) had minimal impact on $[s{:}P]_{sat}$ (figure 9.2(B)). Interestingly, their small molecule analogs, EG and sucrose, too small to serve as entropic crowders that drive depletion interactions, showed similar trends as their polymer counterparts. Similar crowder-dependent effects were seen for the critical temperature T_c required for polyU-spermine condensation, with PEG lowering T_c from ~22 °C to ~16 °C, while Ficoll had negligible effect (figure 9.2(C)). These results were coupled with observations the Ficoll co-localized in the condensates while PEG was excluded (figure 9.2(D)).

These crowder-dependent effects were shown to arise from PEG (and EG) destabilizing, i.e., opening up, the folded polyU-RNA, via exclusion of water, to facilitate association with spermidine (Marianelli *et al* 2018). Moreover, the co-localization of Ficoll in the droplet phase (figure 9.2(D)) hindered its ability to drive condensation via depletion interactions.

The degree to which crowders are enriched in or excluded from condensates has also been shown to depend on the crowder size, as demonstrated by studies on the intrinsically disordered RGG domain of the LAF-1 protein, that undergoes LLPS at salt-dependent concentrations $c_{sat} \gtrsim 1.5$–11 μM (figure 9.2(E)) (Schuster *et al* 2018). These studies showed that the extent to which dextran crowders co-localized in the condensate phase decreased with increasing molecular weight, with $M_w \simeq 4.4$ kDa dextran being entirely enriched in droplets, $M_w \simeq 10$ kDa being only partially enriched, and $M_w \simeq 70$ kDa dextran being entirely excluded (figure 9.2(F)) (Schuster *et al* 2018).

Finally, crowding has been shown to coarsen droplets and induce sol–gel transitions in otherwise liquid-like condensates (Lin *et al* 2015, Molliex *et al* 2015,

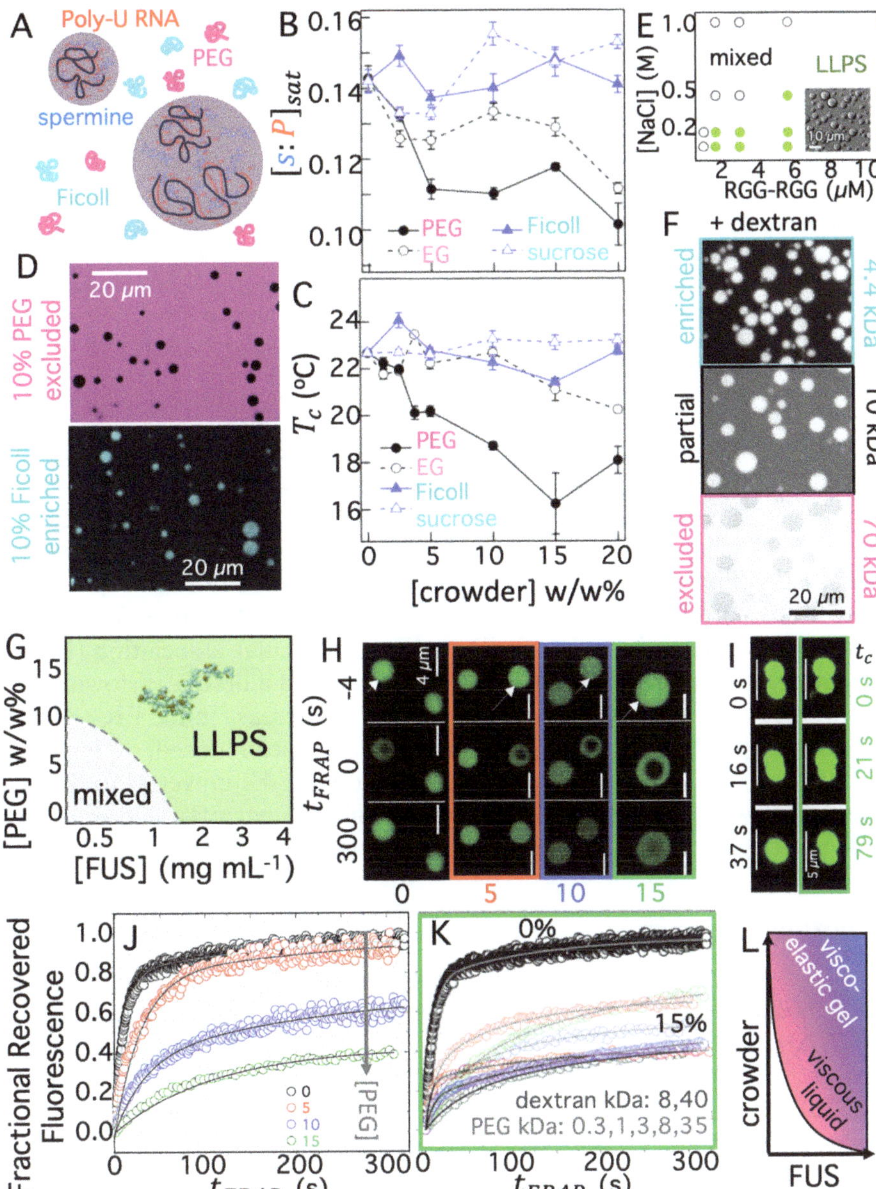

Figure 9.2. The effect of crowding on liquid–liquid phase separation. (A–D) Condensates formed from PolyU-RNA (red) and spermine (blue) are affected differently by different crowders, PEG (magenta) or Ficoll (cyan). (A) Cartoon depiction of the system. (B and C) The effect of crowder concentration (x-axis) on the minimum critical (B) spermine:PolyU ratio $[s\colon P]_{\mathrm{sat}}$ and (C) temperature T_c for LLPS. Polymeric crowders, PEG (filled black circles) and Ficoll (filled blue triangles) and their corresponding small molecule subunits, EG (open black circles) and sucrose (open blue triangles). (D) Confocal micrographs of condensates in the presence of fluorescent-labeled PEG (magenta) or Ficoll (cyan) show PEG is excluded while Ficoll is enriched in the droplet phase. (E and F) Condensates formed from tandem RGG domains of LAF-1 (E) form droplets (inset) in the absence of crowders for a range of concentrations of RGG-RGG and NaCl (green filled circles), with higher [NaCl] promoting dissolution

(empty circles); and (F) uptake (shown as brighter condensates than solvent background) or exclude dextran crowders (shown as brighter background than condensates) depending on the dextran molecular weight [4.4 kDa (cyan, uptake), 10 kDa (black, partial uptake), 70 kDa (magenta, exclusion)]. (G–K) LLPS of the ribonucleoprotein, FUS, crowded by PEG or dextran. (G) State diagram of FUS condensation as a function of [PEG] and [FUS]. (H) Confocal images of FUS droplets (green) taken before (−4 s), immediately after (0 s) and 300 s after photobleaching when crowded by PEG at weight percentages of 0 (black), 5 (red), 10 (blue), and 15 (green) show reduced recovery for higher [PEG]. (I) Coalescence of droplets crowded by 0% (black) or 15% (green) PEG. (J and K) Fractional recovered fluorescence after photobleaching versus t_{FRAP} for FUS droplets without crowders (black bordered circles) and with different (J) [PEG], color-matched to H, and (K) molecular weights of PEG (lighter shades) and dextran (darker shades) at 15%. (L) State diagram showing dependence of [FUS] and [crowder] on condensates exhibiting liquid-like (pink) or gel-like (blue) properties. (B–D) Adapted from Marianelli *et al* (2018) with permission from the Royal Society of Chemistry. (E, F) Adapted from Schuster *et al* (2018). CC BY 4.0. (H–K) Adapted from Kaur *et al* (2019). CC BY 4.0.

Kaur *et al* 2019). This effect manifests as slowing and arrest of condensed proteins, quantified using fluorescence recovery after photobleaching (FRAP) (Taylor *et al* 2019) as well as examining coalescence times (André and Spruijt 2020). For example, LLPS of the ribonucleoprotein FUS was shown to be facilitated by 8 kDa PEG crowding, shifting ϕ_{sat} from ~1.5 μM without PEG to ~0.5 μM in the presence of 10% PEG (figure 9.2(G)), which was suggested to arise from enhanced excluded volume interactions that facilitated intermolecular association (Kaur *et al* 2019). However, these enhanced interactions also caused a dramatic slowing of FUS proteins in the condensate phase, as measured by an increase in the FRAP time and recovery fraction (figure 9.2(H)), which was more pronounced at higher PEG concentrations. This signature of gelation was shown to be universal for a range of PEG molecular weights, as well as for dextran, and was corroborated by showing a dramatic prolonging of the coalescence time (figure 9.2(I)) (Kaur *et al* 2019).

9.4 Complex coacervates

The first discovery of liquid–liquid phase separation was the electrostatic association of two oppositely-charged biopolymeric species, e.g., a nucleic acid and protein (figure 9.2(A)), that drove separation into a biopolymer-rich liquid-like phase, termed a complex coacervate, and a polymer-poor solvent phase (Tiebackx 1911, de Jong and Kruyt 1930). Most biopolymeric complex coacervates that have been investigated to date comprise RNA and protein, but DNA–protein and protein–protein coacervates have also been realized *in vitro* and implicated in cellular function (Hyman *et al* 2014, Kayitmazer 2017, Alberti *et al* 2019, Sing and Perry 2020).

LLPS via complex coacervation occurs when the energetic cost of charge separation outweighs the entropic cost of association, which was first described by the Voorn–Overbeek model (Overbeek and Voorn 1957) that treats polyelectrolytes as independent point charges and accurately predicts that increasing salt concentration hinders coacervation via charge-screening.

However, experiments have shown that coacervation is actually entropically rather than enthalpically driven (Priftis *et al* 2012, Fu and Schlenoff 2016, Chang *et al* 2017, Kayitmazer 2017), and that salt concentration is higher in the condensate than the dilute phase (Liu *et al* 2017, Radhakrishna *et al* 2017, Li *et al* 2018)—both at odds with Voorn–Overbeek theory and motivating new theoretical models. The key theoretical frameworks that have been proposed to overcome the limitations of the Voorn–Overbeek model include:

(i) Polymer field theories (figure 9.3(A)), such as the reptation model, that treat surrounding polymers as an effective field potential (de Gennes 1979, Castelnovo and Joanny 2001, Kudlay and Olvera de la Cruz 2003, Qin and de Pablo 2016);

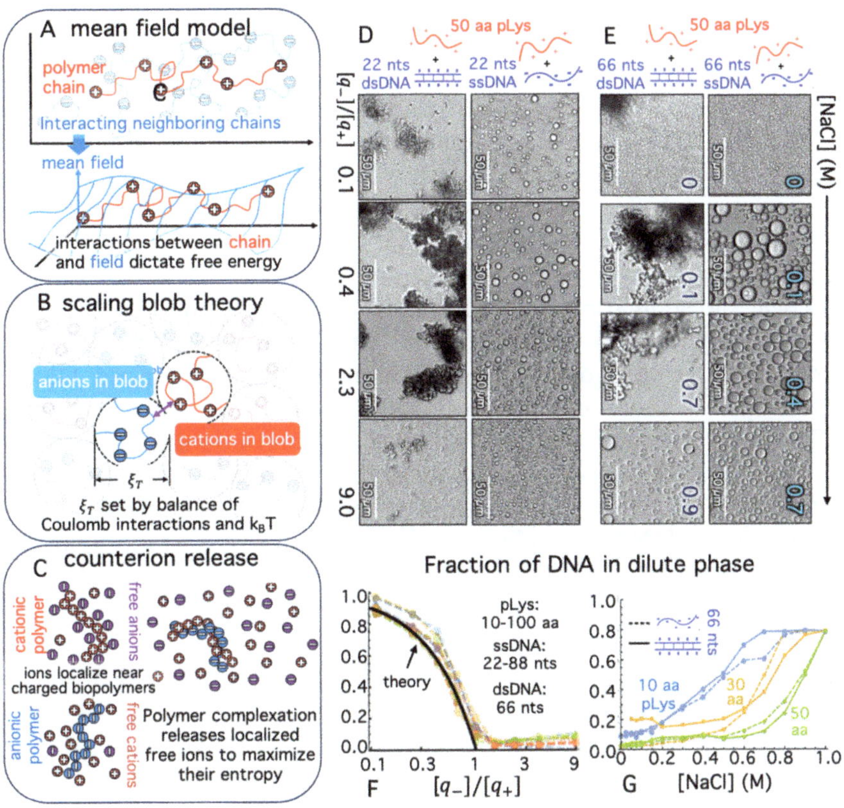

Figure 9.3. Complex coacervation: theoretical approaches and the role of polymer stiffness. (A–C) Different models used to describe and predict the state diagram and underlying physics of complex coacervation include: (A) mean-field approaches similar to the reptation model, (B) scaling theories that coarse-grain the system to the correlation blob size ξ_T, and (C) counterion release theory that describes the entropic release of free ions localized near charged polymers. (D–F) Cationic poly(L)lysine (red) and either double-stranded (left columns in D and E) or single-stranded (right columns in D and E) anionic DNA form either liquid-like coacervates (ssDNA) or solid-like precipitates (dsDNA) with properties that depend on the (D) pLys:DNA charge ratio $[q_-]/[q_+]$ and (E) NaCl concentration; but have universally similar dependence of complexation probability, measured by the fraction of the DNA in the dilute phase (y-axis), on (F) $[q_-]/[q_+]$ and (G) [NaCl] for a range of sizes of DNA (22–88 nt) and pLys (10–100 amino acids). (A–C) Adapted from Sing and Perry (2020) with permission from the Royal Society of Chemistry. (D–G) Adapted with permission from Vieregg *et al* (2018). Copyright (2018) American Chemical Society.

(ii) Scaling theory or blob theory (figure 9.3(B)) (described in chapter 2) (Shusharina *et al* 2005, Wang and Rubinstein 2006, Rubinstein *et al* 2018, Rumyantsev and de Pablo 2019);
(iii) Counterion release theory (figure 9.3(C)), i.e., entropically-driven expulsion of opposite-charged polyelectrolytes during complexation (Record *et al* 1978, Zhang and Shklovskii 2005, Salehi and Larson 2016, Lytle and Sing 2017, Adhikari *et al* 2018).

Scaling and field theory approaches (figures 9.3(A) and (B)) typically more accurately describe coacervation of polymers in the limit of low linear charge density, where charge repulsion along a single chain counteracts the drive to condense, but can be overcome by thermal fluctuations that bring opposite-charged segments in close proximity (Castelnovo and Joanny 2001, Shusharina *et al* 2005, Qin and de Pablo 2016, Sing 2017, Rubinstein *et al* 2018). In the limit of high charge density, the strength of self-repulsion is too strong to allow for fluctuation-driven condensation, so instead coacervation is predicted to occur via counterion expulsion (figure 9.3(C)) (Manning 2003, Salehi and Larson 2016, Lytle and Sing 2017, Adhikari *et al* 2018).

Theoretical and simulation studies have also suggested that increased biopolymer stiffness suppresses coacervation (Lytle and Sing 2018, Shakya *et al* 2020), in line with experimental results on the complexation of double-stranded DNA versus single-stranded DNA with cationic poly(L)lysine (figures 9.3(D–G)) (Vieregg *et al* 2018). These studies showed that for a given salt concentration, ssDNA more readily formed liquid-like coacervates while dsDNA formed solid-like precipitates (figure 9.3(D)). This effect was independent of the lengths of DNA and poly(L) lysine, as well as the DNA:pLys charge ratio $[q_-/q_+]$ (figure 9.3(D)). Despite the very different properties of the condensed phases for ssDNA and dsDNA, the fraction of DNA that remained in the dilute phase for any given set of conditions was invariant to these differences (figures 9.3(F) and (G)) (Vieregg *et al* 2018). Moreover, increasing the concentration of NaCl in solution to $\sim$700 mM was shown to 'melt' the dsDNA precipitates into liquid-like droplets that resembled their single-stranded counterparts (figure 9.3(E)). In line with these results, rheological measurements of a range of complex coacervates have shown universally that decreasing salt content smoothly shifts the rheological properties from fluid-like to solid-like (Spruijt *et al* 2010, 2013, Wang and Schlenoff 2014, Liu *et al* 2017), with a broad range of salt concentrations in which coacervates exhibit viscoelastic rather than purely viscous properties, similar to figures 9.2(J)–(L).

9.5 LLPS of intrinsically disordered proteins

Arguably the most celebrated and ubiquitous biopolymer LLPS systems are biomolecular condensates of intrinsically disordered proteins (IDPs) (Brangwynne *et al* 2015, Shin *et al* 2018, McCarty *et al* 2019, Fonin *et al* 2022, Spruijt 2023). As I discuss in chapter 1 (see section 2.4 and figure 1.2(J)), unlike typical small soluble proteins, which are intricately folded to hide their hydrophobic patches, IDPs have large sections of unstructured polypeptides and adopt a variety of marginally stable structures (figures 1.2(J) and 9.4(A)). A primary route that IDPs use to improve stability and reduce hydrophobicity is to self-assemble into coacervates (figure 9.4(C)), as seen for, e.g., amyloid disease proteins such as tau and FUS (figures 9.2(G)–(L)) (Shin and Brangwynne 2017, McCarty *et al* 2019). Theoretical models of IDP condensates describe each IDP as a chain of stickers separated by spacers (figure 9.4(A)) in which the stickers are the attractive patches that allow for IDP crosslinking and spacers are non-interacting flexible chains (Choi *et al* 2011, 2020, McCarty *et al* 2019, Zeng *et al* 2020). This repeating pattern of (non) interacting segments, as well as multivalent interactions, i.e., more than one associative interaction per IDP, has been shown to be essential to LLPS (Harmon *et al* 2017, Borcherds *et al* 2021).

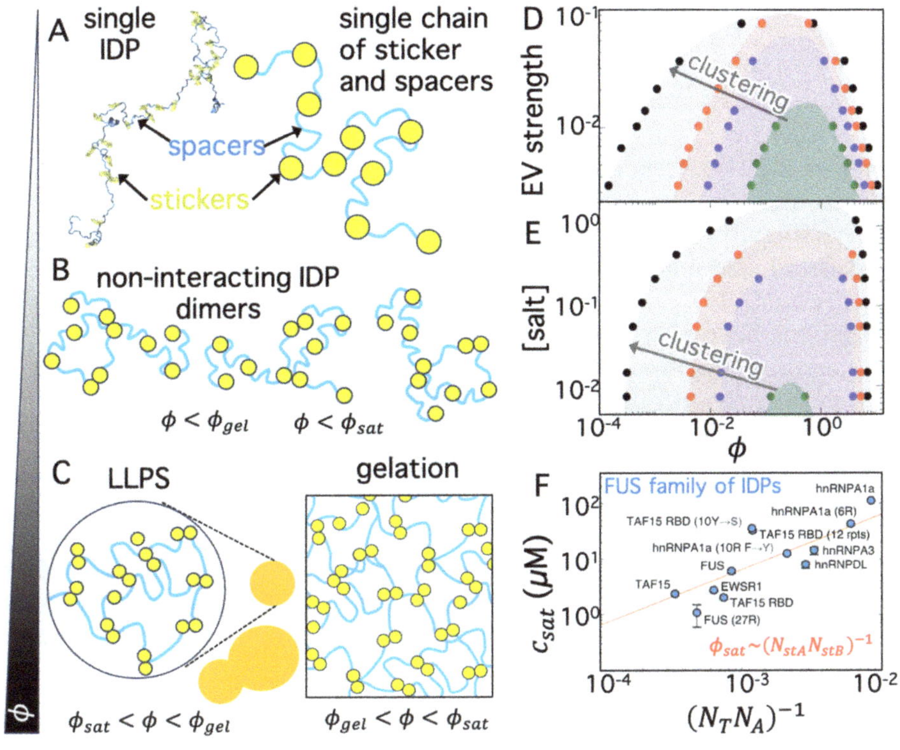

Figure 9.4. Phase separation of intrinsically disordered proteins. (A–C) Modeling an IDP as a chain of stickers (yellow) separated by flexible linkers (blue) predicts (B) the formation of isolated dimers dissolved in the solvent for $\phi < \phi_{sat}$ and $\phi < \phi_{gel}$, followed by (C) either liquid–liquid phase separation for $\phi > \phi_{sat}$ (left) or bulk gelation for $\phi > \phi_{gel}$ (right) if $\phi_{sat} < \phi_{gel}$ (left) or $\phi_{gel} < \phi_{sat}$ (right). (D, E) The effect of (D) excluded volume interactions (i.e., solvent conditions) and (E) salt concentration on the range of IDP concentrations ϕ that support LLPS (shaded regions). The different colors denote increasing sticker clustering in the direction of the grey arrow: green, blue, red, black. (F) Critical LLPS concentration c_{sat} ($\sim\phi_{sat}$) for 11 different IDPs in the FUS family versus the inverse product of the number per chain of tyrene and arginine residues, N_T and N_A, which are sticker pairs, show scaling that aligns with predictions (equation (9.6)). (D, E) Adapted with permission from McCarty *et al* (2019). Copyright (2019) American Chemical Society. (F) Adapted from Wang *et al* (2018) Copyright (2018), with permission from Elsevier.

Computational studies have shown that the physical properties of both stickers and spacers impact the ability for IDPs to form condensates (Harmon *et al* 2017, Choi *et al* 2020). In particular, the extent to which polymeric spacers are swollen, ideal, or condensed random coils controls the ability to phase separate or undergo bulk gelation. The propensity for spacers to adopt these distinct conformations is driven by the relative strength and sign of polymer–polymer interactions χ_P versus polymer–solvent interactions χ_{PS} (Choi *et al* 2011, 2020, Harmon *et al* 2017).

Good solvent conditions, in which $\chi_{PS} < 1$ and excluded volume (EV) interactions are high, result in swollen coil linkers with negative global cooperativity that hinders droplet formation, i.e., makes the critical saturation concentration ϕ_{sat} prohibitively high (figure 9.4(D)). Instead, IDPs undergo bulk gelation without LLPS at a critical concentration $\phi_{gel} < \phi_{sat}$ (figure 9.4(C)) (Harmon *et al* 2017). Conversely, spacers in poor solvent conditions, with $\chi_{PS} > 1$ and minimal EV interactions, are condensed coils that exhibit positive global cooperativity, driving LLPS for concentrations above ϕ_{sat}, which is below ϕ_{gel} (figures 9.4(C) and (D)). In cases in which LLPS increases the concentration in the dense phase beyond ϕ_{gel}, the droplet undergoes a sol–gel transition instead of remaining in a liquid-like state (Harmon *et al* 2017). Related to the effect of solvent condition on phase separation of IDPs, is the impact of increasing salt concentration. Similar to the effect seen in figures 9.2(E) and 9.3(E), increasing salt concentration has been shown to increase ϕ_{sat} and shrink the region of the phase space that supports LLPS (figure 9.4(E)) (McCarty *et al* 2019).

Simulations have also predicted a finite range of linker lengths that allow for phase separation (Harmon *et al* 2017). Very short spacers lead to locally positive but globally negative cooperativity, resulting in discrete dimers of IDPs (figure 9.4(B)), whereas very long linkers result in zero global and local cooperativity, in which case bulk gelation is favored over LLPS, i.e., $\phi_{gel} < \phi_{sat}$ (figure 9.4(C)) (Harmon *et al* 2017, McCarty *et al* 2019).

In addition to the spacer length, other factors with obvious impact on liquid–liquid phase separation of IDPs are the sticker association strength χ_{st}, degree of clustering θ_{st} (figures 9.4(D) and (E)), and valence N_{st} (i.e., number of stickers per chain). For example, the saturation concentration for the onset of LLPS is predicted to scale as

$$\phi_{sat} \sim N_{st}^{-2} \tag{9.5}$$

or

$$\phi_{sat} \sim (N_{stA}N_{stB})^{-1} \tag{9.6}$$

for single-species or pair interactions, respectively, as seen in experiments (figure 9.4(F)) (Wang *et al* 2018, Borcherds *et al* 2021). Moreover, uniformly distributed stickers (minimal clustering) have been predicted to increase ϕ_{sat} and shrink the LLPS region of the phase space below that of randomly distributed and clustered stickers which strengthen interactions (figures 9.4(D) and (E)) (Borcherds *et al* 2021). Similarly, field theory simulations and experiments have shown that clusters of like-charged residues broaden the LLPS region of the phase space, lowering ϕ_{sat} and increasing ϕ_{max} (figure 9.1A) (Nott *et al* 2015, Das *et al* 2018a, 2018b). However, in the limit of high sticker clustering, the resulting condensate takes the form of a stiff solid-like aggregate rather than a liquid-like droplet due to the increased lifetime and strength of the binding interactions (Choi *et al* 2020, Martin *et al* 2020). Note that a requirement for liquid-like behavior is for interactions to be transient and weak to allow for fluid-like rearrangement.

Despite maintaining liquid-like properties, the conformational dynamics of IDPs in coacervates have been shown to be dramatically slowed as compared to dilute and crowded bulk conditions (Abyzov *et al* 2022, Guseva *et al* 2023). For example, NMR studies on the disordered domain of the measles virus nucleoprotein showed that in dilute conditions, three principal relaxation modes dominate the dynamics–fast librational motion, intermediate segmental motion, and slow whole-chain motion—with the slow mode exhibiting the smallest relative amplitude (Abyzov *et al* 2016, Guseva *et al* 2023). Bulk crowding by PEG ($M_w = 10$ kDa) slowed the intermediate and slow modes, but had minimal impact on both the fast relaxation timescale and the relative amplitudes of the different relaxation modes (Guseva *et al* 2023). Conversely, in condensates, all three modes were markedly slowed down and the amplitude of the fast mode became lower than that of the two slower modes, suggesting that strong interchain interactions suppressed librational freedom (Abyzov *et al* 2022).

On larger spatiotemporal scales, the diffusion coefficients of IDPs within condensates have been measured using a variety of techniques including FRAP (Taylor *et al* 2019), NMR, fluorescence correlation spectroscopy (FCS) (Elson 2011), DLS (Stetefeld *et al* 2016), and dark-field microscopy (Pan *et al* 2021). These measurements have also been used to infer the viscoelastic properties of condensates (figures 9.5(A)–(D)) (Abyzov *et al* 2022). FRAP, NMR diffusometry, and particle-tracking experiments have measured IDP diffusion coefficients of $D_c \approx 10^{-3}$–$1\ \mu\text{m}^2\ \text{s}^{-1}$, which are over 10^2-fold lower than the dilute phase value of $D_0 \approx 250\ \mu\text{m}^2\ \text{s}^{-1}$, and which equate to viscosities of $\eta_c \approx 1$–10^3 Pa s (Burke *et al* 2015, Nott *et al* 2015, Brady *et al* 2017, Murthy *et al* 2019, Taylor *et al* 2019, Abyzov *et al* 2022). The broad range of values reflects the dependence on the IDP properties, salt concentration, and presence of other biopolymers such as RNA (figures 9.5(A) and (B)) (Abyzov *et al* 2022).

For example, ultrafast scanning FCS measurements of nanospheres in LAF-1 condensates showed that increasing [NaCl] universally decreased the viscosity of the condensates (figure 9.5(A)), whereas the addition of short RNA fragments (15–30 nucleotides) and long RNA chains (~3000 nucleotides (nts)), respectively, decreased and increased the coacervate viscosity (figure 9.5(B)) (Wei *et al* 2017). Moreover, the viscosity of most IDP condensates increases over time, as determined by decreasing D_c values (figures 9.5(C) and (D)), as the condensates expel fluid, coarsen, and eventually become stiff aggregates (Lin *et al* 2015, Boeynaems *et al* 2018, Babinchak and Surewicz 2020). This liquid-to-solid aging process can last several hours to days depending on the IDP and environmental conditions (figures 9.5(C–E)) (Ray *et al* 2020, Abyzov *et al* 2022); and can also be probed by measuring coalescence events, which decrease as the droplets coarsen (Abyzov *et al* 2016, Jawerth *et al* 2018).

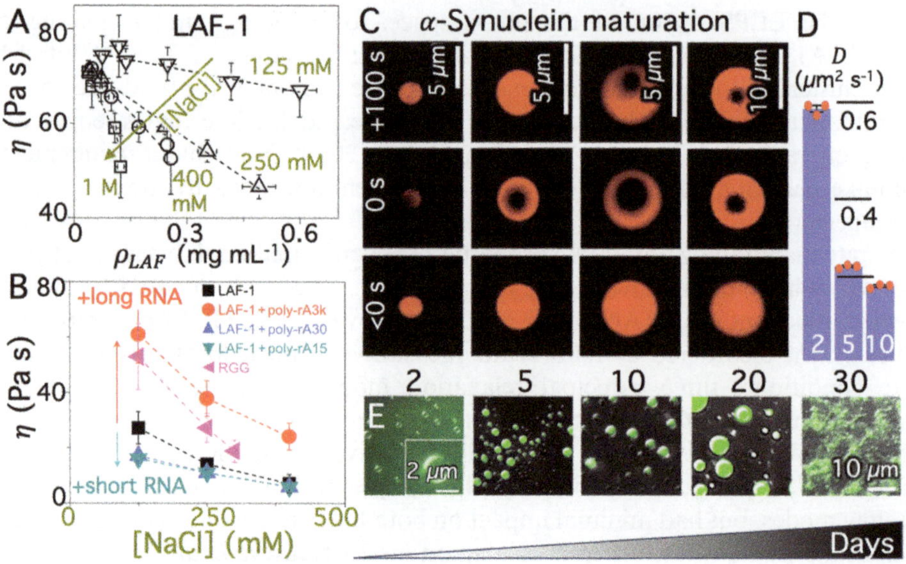

Figure 9.5. Dynamics of IDPs in condensates. (A and B) The viscosity η of LAF-1 condensates as a function of (A) LAF-1 mass concentration ρ_{LAF} for varying concentrations of NaCl (green labels and arrow); and (B) [NaCl] for condensates of the RGG domain (purple triangles), full length LAF-1 (black squares), and LAF-1 with polyU-RNA of increasing lengths: 15 nts (teal inverted triangles), 30 nts (blue triangles), and 3000 nts (red circles). (C–E) Maturation of α-Synuclein condensates. (C) FRAP images taken before (bottom row, <0 s), immediately after (middle row, 0 s), and 100 s after (top row) photobleaching for condensates of increasing ages (left to right, listed in days). (D) Diffusion coefficients of α-Synuclein determined from FRAP experiments on condensates after 2, 5, and 10 days. (E) Overlaid differential interference contrast (DIC) images of condensates (greyscale) and fluorescence images of labeled α-Synuclein (green) show growth of condensates followed by maturation into solid-like fibrils. (A, B) Adapted from Wei *et al* (2017) Copyright (2017), with permission from Springer Nature. (C–E) Adapted from Ray *et al* (2020) Copyright (2020), with permission from Springer Nature.

9.6 LLPS of nucleic acids

DNA nanostars, which I discussed in chapter 6 in the context of branched biopolymer networks (figure 6.10), have been shown to form liquid droplets when the crosslinking overhangs on the arms of the stars are sufficiently flexible (figure 6.10(A)) (Biffi *et al* 2013, Nguyen and Saleh 2017, Jeon *et al* 2018, Conrad *et al* 2019, Nguyen *et al* 2019). In these symmetric, 4-armed double-stranded DNA constructs (20 nucleotides per arm), the overhangs are made flexible by including a 6 nt unpaired single-stranded segment before the overhang. Making the arms flexible by similar modification at the central joint of the star, was not sufficient for condensation if the overhangs remained stiff (figure 6.10(B)). Moreover, due to the relative stiffness of the nanostar arms, even the highest nanostar concentrations in condensates are well below the volume fractions necessary for other LLPS systems ($\sim$1% versus 10–30% for typical IDPs) (Nguyen *et al* 2019, Conrad *et al* 2022).

Interestingly, salt has an opposite effect on DNA nanostar coacervates as compared to most other biomolecular condensates, with increasing salt facilitating rather than hindering condensation (figures 9.2(E), 9.3(G), 9.4(E)), and causing droplets to densify rather than dissolve (figures 9.3(E) and (G) and 9.5(C)) (Nguyen and Saleh 2017, Jeon *et al* 2018). Specifically, increasing [NaCl] from 0.25 M to 1 M was shown to increase the concentration of DNA in the coacervates from $\rho_c \approx 19$ mg mL^{-1} to $\rho_c \approx 35$ mg mL^{-1}, independent of the initial DNA concentration before phase separation ($\rho_0 \approx 5$–15 mg mL^{-1}) (Jeon *et al* 2018); and likewise increase the surface tension, also at odds with other LLPS systems. The increased surface tension followed scaling predictions based on the salt-dependent Gibbs free energy ΔG for overhang hybridization

$$|\Delta G| \sim \ln[\text{NaCl}] \tag{9.7}$$

and considering that the surface tension is the energetic cost of increasing the surface area by the area of a single nanostar

$$Y \sim |\Delta G| V_{\text{mol}}^{-2/3} \tag{9.8}$$

where V_{mol} is the volume a nanostar occupies in the bulk phase. Combining these relations yields the empirical result

$$Y V_{\text{mol}}^{2/3} \sim \ln[\text{NaCl}] \tag{9.9}$$

(figure 9.6(B)) (Jeon *et al* 2018). Complementary particle-tracking microrheology measurements showed that droplet viscosity η increased from 24 to 90 Pa-s with increasing [NaCl], and diffusion coefficients likewise decreased (figure 9.6(C)). However, the condensates remained primarily viscous rather than viscoelastic, as demonstrated by the linear scaling of MSD with lag time. These salt-dependent effects were attributed to stabilization of the overhang bonds that increases the energetic cost of bond breakage at the surface (figure 9.6(B)) and hinders DNA mobility (figure 9.6(C)).

Moreover, at high enough concentrations, above the valence saturation limit (when all arms of all nanostars can form a connection), the structural connectivity in the coacervate was shown to become heterogeneous, with highly connected local clusters loosely connected to one another (Biffi *et al* 2013, Jeon *et al* 2018). This cluster formation (Bauer *et al* 2013 Liu *et al* 2017) led to a stronger than expected decrease in D with increasing η as compared to the Stokes constant $D\eta$ (figure 9.6(C)), indicating that measurements of D corresponded to the collective diffusion coefficient of the cluster at higher salt concentrations (Jeon *et al* 2018). Moreover, the heterogeneous structure, similar to that observed in glass transitions, lowered the surface tension, as most bonds are oriented towards cluster centers rather than the interface so the cost of being at a surface is lower (figure 9.6(B)).

Similar to other biomolecular condensates, nanostar condensates have been shown to both uptake and exclude crowders depending on the properties of the crowder (Nguyen *et al* 2019, André and Spruijt 2020). For example, the uptake of dextran by nanostar condensates has been shown to depend on the hydrodynamic radius of dextran $R_{H,d}$ relative to the mesh size of the condensed nanostar network ξ_{ns} (figure 9.6(D)) (Nguyen *et al* 2019). An equal concentration of dextran in the coacervate and gas phases, corresponding to a partition coefficient $P = 0.5$, was

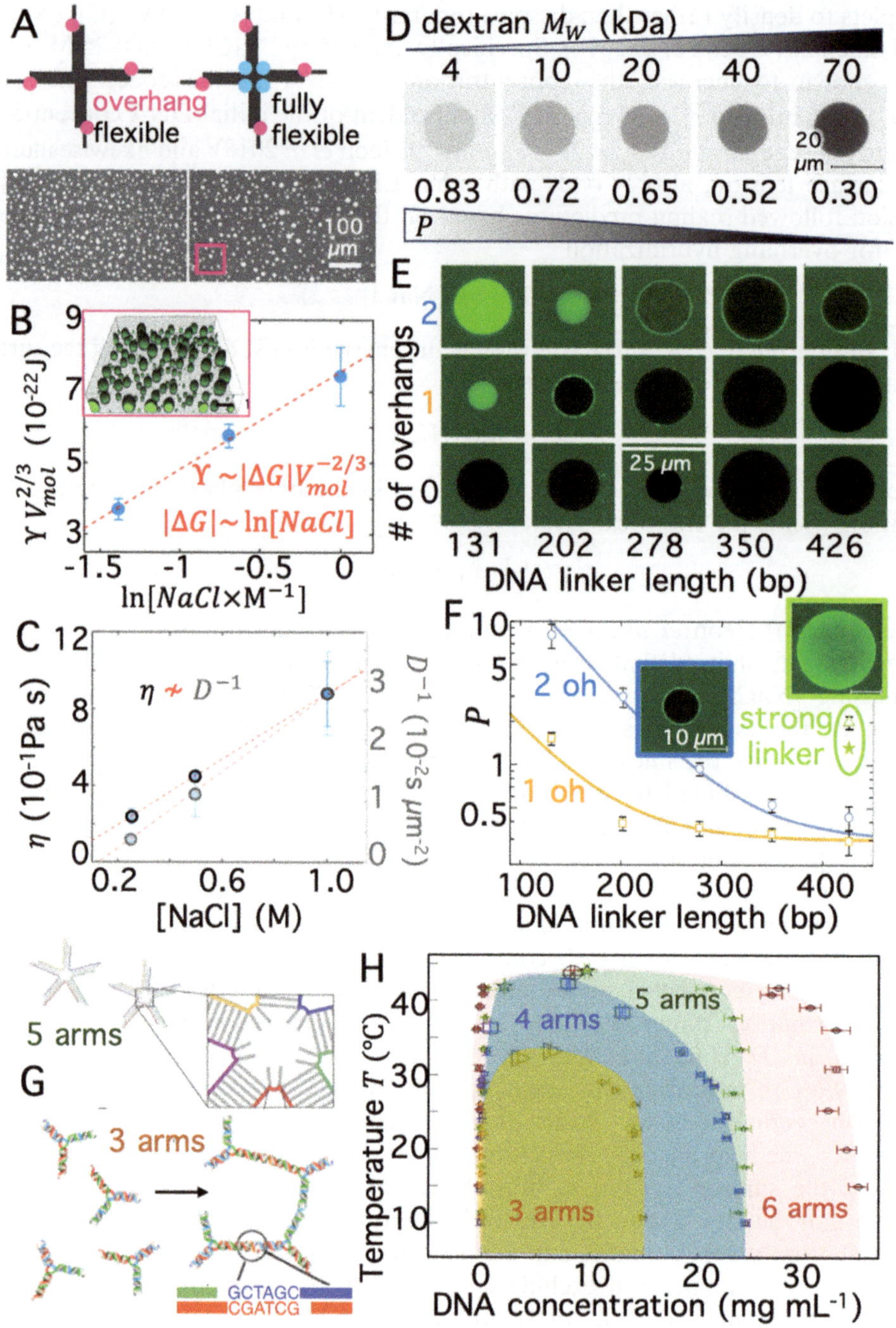

Figure 9.6. Liquid–liquid phase separation of DNA nanostars. (A–D) LLPS of 4-arm DNA nanostars with flexible overhangs. (A) Cartoon of stars with flexible overhangs (magenta) and either stiff or flexible (cyan) joints that phase separate as shown in fluorescence images below. (B) Surface tension Y scaled by the surface area that a nanostar on the surface of a droplet occupies $V_{\mathrm{mol}}^{2/3}$ versus the natural log of [NaCl] shows the predicted scaling (red dashed line) $\mathrm{Y} \sim |\Delta G|\ V_{\mathrm{mol}}^{2/3}$ where $|\Delta G| \sim \ln[\mathrm{NaCl}]$ is the Gibbs free energy of overhang hybridization. (Inset)

3D confocal reconstruction of the magenta enclosed region in A. (C) Viscosity η (black/left axis, black bordered circles) and inverse diffusion coefficient D^{-1} (grey/right axis, grey bordered circles) versus [NaCl] with linear fits (red dashed line) showing that the product $D\eta$ decreases with increasing [NaCl] (D^{-1} increases more steeply than η). (D) Fluorescence images of nanostar condensates with labeled dextran of increasing molecular weight (left to right) show that co-partitioning of dextran in droplets decreases (droplets become darker) with increasing dextran molecular weight. This molecular weight dependence is quantified by the partition coefficient P that decreases with increasing dextran molecular weight. (E and F) 4-arm nanostars and long DNA linkers form condensates that co-partition to varying degrees depending on the number of linker overhangs, linker length, and binding affinity. (E) Images of droplets with fluorescent-labeled linkers show that uptake increases with increasing number of overhangs (bottom to top) and decreasing linker length (right to left). Excluded linkers with overhangs preferentially co-localize on the droplet exterior rather than the bulk solution. (F) Partition coefficient versus DNA linker length for linkers with 2 overhangs (blue), 1 overhang (orange), or with strengthened overhang binding affinity (green, circled). (G and H) Nanostars with varying numbers of arms (valency), depicted in G, show a broadening of the LLPS regime (shaded regions) with increasing valency, as shown by (H) the temperature versus DNA concentration phase diagram for nanostars with 6 (red), 5 (green), 4 (blue), and 3 (orange) arms. (A–C) Adapted from Nguyen and Saleh (2017) and Jeon *et al* (2018) with permission from the Royal Society of Chemistry. (D–F) Adapted with permission from Nguyen *et al* (2019). Copyright (2019) American Chemical Society. (G, H) Adapted from Conrad *et al* (2019) and Biffi *et al* (2013) with permission of PNAS.

shown to occur for 40 kDa dextran in which $2R_{H,d} \approx \xi_{ns}$ ($\sim$9 nm) (figure 9.6(D)). Increasing the dextran size to $M_w = 70$ kDa reduced its uptake to $P \simeq 0.3$ while lowering to $M_w = 4$ kDa increased uptake to $P \simeq 0.83$ (figure 9.6(D)).

To investigate the ability for larger biopolymers to be co-partitioned in nanostar condensates, researchers designed long DNA strands of length $L = 131$–462 bp, $\sim$3–12× longer than the 46 bp nanostars, with 0, 1, or 2 overhangs capable of linking to the nanostars (figures 9.6(E) and (F)) (Nguyen *et al* 2019). All DNA linker lengths that lacked linking overhangs were excluded from the nanostar liquid phase, whereas 131 bp single-linker and double-linker strands were taken up, as well as 262 bp double-linker strands (figures 9.6(E) and (F)). While larger strands were excluded from the coacervate interior, they preferentially accumulated on droplet interfaces rather than the dilute phase (figure 9.6(E)). Increasing the linker strength by extending the overhang length and including a cytosine/guanine pair in the nanostar/linker, allowed for longer DNA strands to be taken up by the droplets (figure 9.6(F)), owing to the increased energetic gain of binding that outweighs the entropic cost of confinement.

The nanostar valence, i.e., the number of arms, has also been shown to play an important role in phase separation, with increasing valence leading to a wider region of the phase space that supports LLPS, higher dissolution temperature $T_{\max}$, and higher sustained DNA concentration $\phi_{\max}$ (figures 9.6(G) and (H)) (Biffi *et al* 2013, Conrad *et al* 2022).

Researchers have also created *in vitro* coacervates of single-stranded DNA (ssDNA) by high-temperature annealing and condensation of palindromic domains, followed by cooling and hybridization, to form well-defined structures via kinetic trapping (figures 9.7(A)–(C)) (Merindol *et al* 2018). With this approach, condensates formed for DNA lengths above $\sim$100 basepairs (figure 9.7B) and divalent salt concentration above $\sim$20 mM (figure 9.7(C)).

LLPS of complementary double-stranded DNA constructs has also been demonstrated by adding an associative side group to two different dsDNA oligomers with

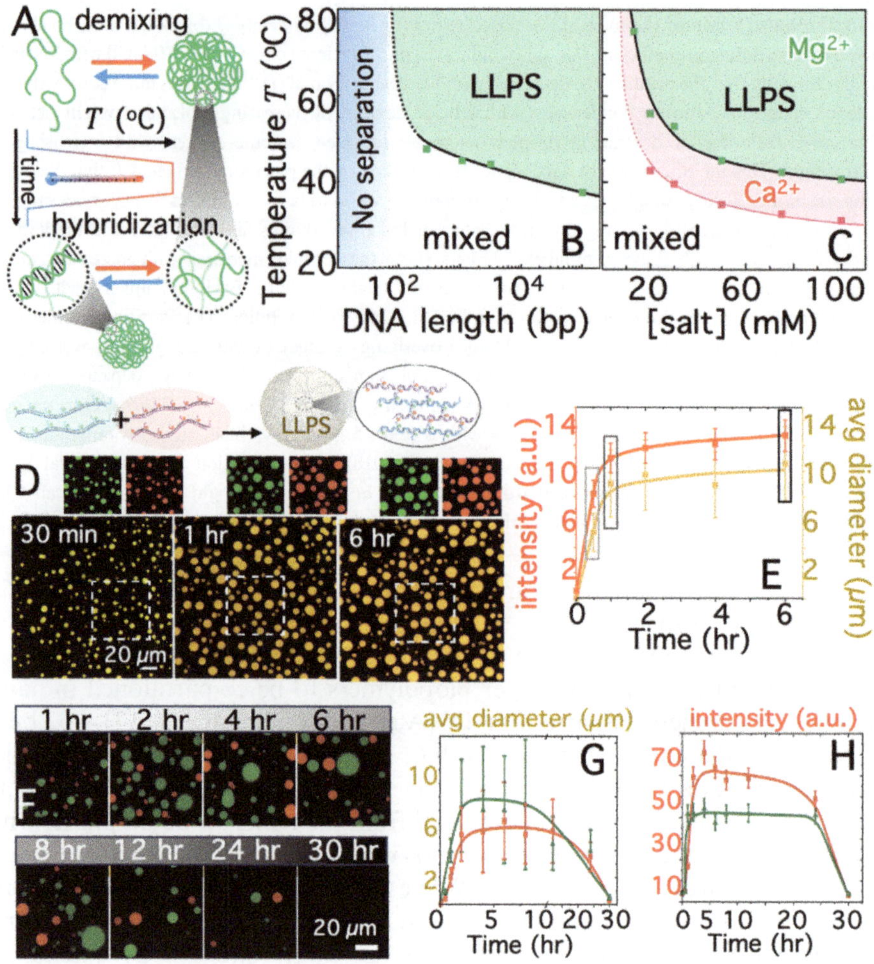

Figure 9.7. Liquid–liquid phase separation of single-stranded DNA. (A–C) Self-assembly of single-stranded DNA condensates using (A) temperature controlled de-mixing and hybridization can be tuned by varying the (B) length of the ssDNA constructs and (C) concentration of Mg^{2+} (green) or Ca^{2+} (red). (D and E) Complementary ssDNA constructs (red, green) co-condense into liquid-like droplets via hybridization (D) to form metastable droplets that (E) grow rapidly in diameter (gold, right axis) and fluorescence intensity, i.e., density (red, left axis), over the first 1 hour, after which they reach a metastable state that persists for >6 hours. Data in E enclosed by rectangles correspond to data in D. (F–G) Including two orthogonal hybridization pairs (red and green) allows for the (F) formation of two distinct condensate populations to form (top row) and then dissolve (bottom row) via ATP-fueled enzymatic reactions, as quantified by the time-dependent (G) average diameter and (H) fluorescence intensity of both green and red condensates over the course of 30 hours. (A–C) Adapted from Merindol *et al* (2018) Copyright (2018), with permission from Springer Nature. (D–H) Adapted from Deng and Walther (2020) Copyright (2020), with permission from Elsevier.

sticky overhangs and allowing polymerization and binding of oligos (figures 9.7(D)–(H)) (Deng and Walther 2020). In this system, LLPS of these 'sequence-defined functionalized nucleic acid polymers' (SfNAPs) requires an interaction length and separation distance of the side groups of $\geqslant$8 bp and $\leqslant$38 bp, respectively, and equilimolar oligo concentrations of $\geqslant$10 μM (Deng and Walther 2020). LLPS onset was set by SfNAP polymerization and multivalency, with droplets forming after $\sim$30 min, when sufficient polymerization ($\sim$1 kbp, valence of $\sim$26) was reached, and growing over the course of $\sim$1 hour, until reaching a steady-state average diameter of $\sim$10.5 μm (figures 9.7(D) and (E)). This technology was also shown to be able to self-assemble two different condensate populations in one sample, and trigger dissolution following droplet formation via ATP-driven enzymatic reactions (figures 9.7(F)–(H)).

9.7 Structurally heterogeneous condensates

The LLPS systems described so far have exhibited largely homogeneous organization within droplets. However, by tuning biopolymer properties and condensate self-assembly methods, heterogeneous structures can emerge with distinct hierarchy and patterns (Merindol *et al* 2018, Nguyen *et al* 2019, Deng and Walther 2020, Erkamp *et al* 2023).

For example, the system of DNA nanostars and strongly-linking DNA strands I discuss above (figure 9.6(F)) (Nguyen *et al* 2019) was shown to exhibit nested droplets of linkers and nanostars, with small, linker-rich droplets forming and coalescing within larger linker-poor droplets of nanostars (figure 9.8(A)) (Nguyen *et al* 2019). This hierarchical structure was also often bordered by a shell of linkers localizing to the droplet periphery (figures 9.6(E) and 9.8(A)). Similar shell-core structures have been assembled by combining two independent condensate-forming systems (Merindol *et al* 2018, Kaur *et al* 2021) (figures 9.8(B)–(E)). Such realizations include combining two types of kinetically-trapped ssDNA condensates with orthogonal hybridization schemes (figure 9.8(B)) (Merindol *et al* 2018), as well as simultaneous self-assembly of homotypic prion-like polypeptide (PLP) condensates and heterotypic condensates of arginine-rich-polypeptides and RNA (RRP-RNA) (figures 9.8(C)–(E)) (Kaur *et al* 2021).

Similar structural nesting of small droplets engulfed by larger ones (figure 9.8(A)) was also observed in co-condensates of Poly-rA RNA and PEG, in which 'dilute' droplets, poor in both Poly-rA and PEG, assembled within polymer-rich condensates due to dynamic arrest during phase separation (figures 9.8(F)–(H)) (Erkamp *et al* 2023). The formation of internal droplets was shown to be temperature dependent and reversible, forming at 20 °C, progressively becoming smaller and disappearing as temperature increased to 55 °C, then re-emerging and growing as the condensates were cooled back to 20 °C (figures 9.8(F) and (G)). However, the prevalence of interior dilute phase droplets was markedly reduced at lower cooling/heating rates (<1 °C min^{-1}) and for smaller condensates ($\lesssim$15 μm radius), further suggesting that this phenomenon is kinetically driven, due to dynamic arrest of the dense phase, rather than a thermodynamic process (Erkamp *et al* 2023). Similar to the interior droplets in the nanostar-linker condensates, interior polymer-poor droplets were observed to coalesce over time at similar rates as dense-phase coacervates, causing the number and size of internal droplets to shrink and grow, respectively, over time (figure 9.8(H)). The time-dependent reduction of interior droplets was also facilitated by absorption of interior droplets into the exterior dilute phase when they reached the condensate boundary, suggesting that interior and exterior dilute phases and interfaces have similar properties (Erkamp *et al* 2023).

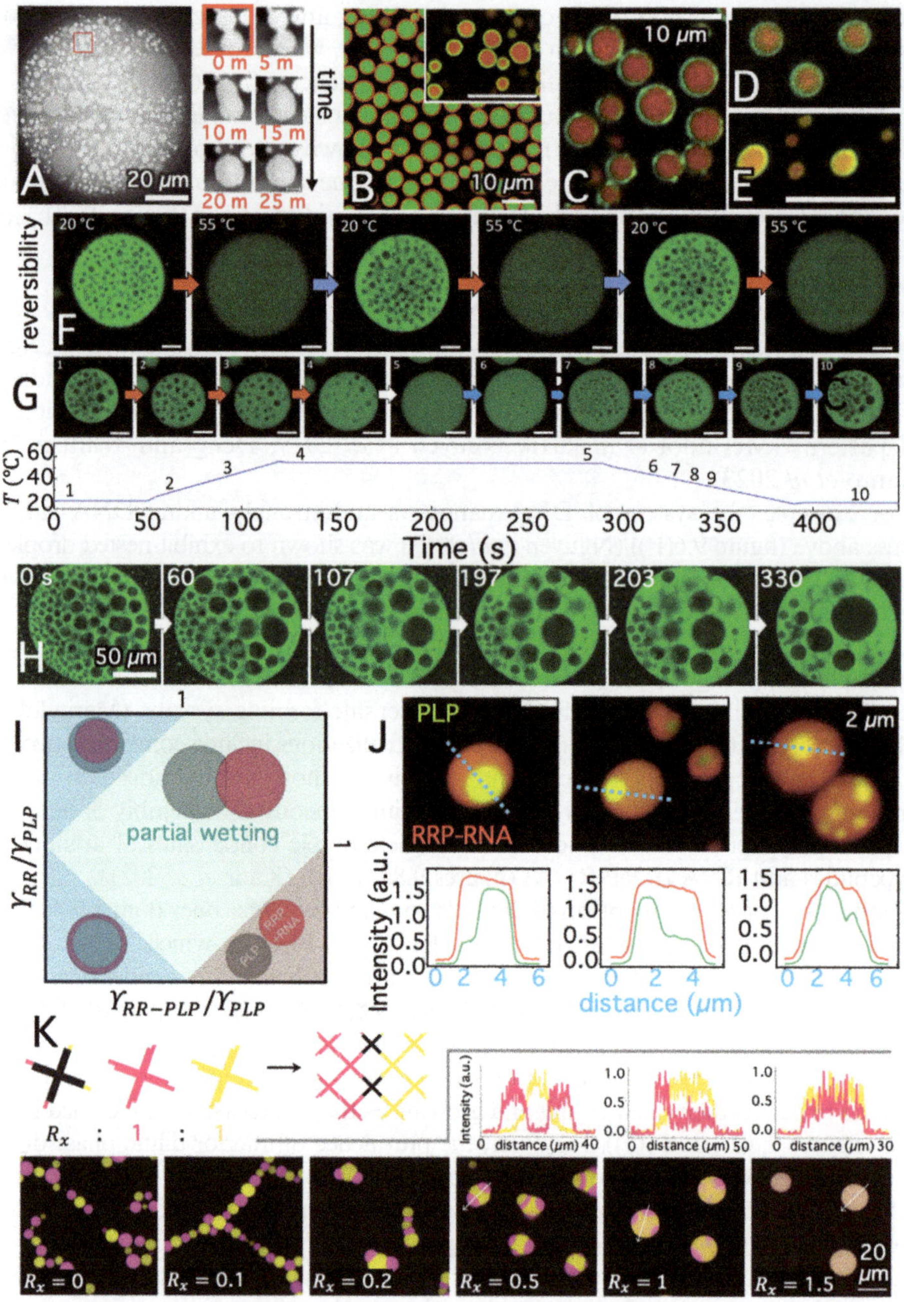

Figure 9.8. Heterogeneous structures can be programmed into the liquid–liquid phase separation pathway. (A) Condensates of 4-arm DNA nanostars and strongly-binding DNA linker strands (labeled in the image) form small linker-rich (higher intensity) droplets nested inside of a larger nanostar-rich droplet with very few linkers. A linker-rich shell surrounds the larger droplet. (Right) The pair of linker-rich droplets in the red box in the left image undergo coalescence over the course of 25 min, demonstrating their liquid-like properties. (B) Temperature controlled annealing and hybridization of two different ssDNA populations can form shell-core droplets with either

population serving as core and shell. (C–E) Co-condensation of homotypic condensates of prion-like polypeptides (PLP) and heterotypic condensates of argine-rich-polypeptide (PLP) and RNA (RRP-RNA) form similar shell-core structures that depend on the specific PLP: EWS (C), FUS (D), or BRG1 (E). (F–H) Co-condensation of poly-rA RNA and PEG form polymer-poor droplets nested in polymer-rich condensates that can be (F) repeatedly dissolved and reformed by increasing the temperature to 55 °C then returning to 20 °C, with the (G) time-resolved details of one assembly and dissolution cycle and the corresponding temperature ramp shown. (H) Over time (left to right) the interior dilute droplets coalesce and fuse with the exterior bulk dilute phase to cause the number of interior droplets to shrink and their diameters to increase. (I and J) Predicted state diagram (I) and examples of nested droplets (J) of PLP (green/grey) and RRP-RNA (RR, red). (I) Simulations predict regimes of complete wetting of PLP in RRP-RNA and vice versa, observed as nesting (blue); partial wetting, resulting in metastable fusion of droplets (green); and no wetting or interactions (red). These different regimes depend on the interfacial surface tension of RR droplets γ_{RR} (y-axis) and the RR-PLP interface γ_{RR-PLP} (x-axis) compared to that of PLP droplets γ_{PLP}. (J) The fluorescence intensities of the RR (red) and PLP (green) phases along the dashed cyan lines show the larger RR droplets completely engulfing smaller PLP droplets. (K) Mixing of two orthogonal species of 4-arm DNA nanostars at 1:1 molar ratio with crosslinker nanostars that can co-link the two species, at varying ratios R_x, form diverse two-phase structures that vary from chains of loosely-connected droplets to complete co-mixing of the two species as R_x increases (left to right). Intensity profiles plotted above the corresponding image show the intensities across the lines drawn, for examples of (left to right) partial wetting, complete wetting, and complete mixing. (A) Adapted with permission from Nguyen *et al* (2019). Copyright (2019) American Chemical Society. (B) Adapted from Merindol *et al* (2018) Copyright (2018), with permission from Springer Nature. (C–E, I, J) Adapted with permission from Kaur *et al* (2021). CC BY 4.0. (F–H) Adapted from Erkamp *et al* (2023). CC BY 4.0. (K) Adapted with permission from Jeon *et al* (2020). Copyright (2020) American Chemical Society.

More generally, the presence of interior 'dilute' droplets, analogous to vacuoles, suggests complete wetting of the two phases, and have been shown to be a generic feature of many LLPS systems due to kinetic arrest of droplet constituents that slows their structural response to chemical disassembly triggers (Banerjee *et al* 2017, Chen *et al* 2020, Deng and Walther 2020, Freibaum *et al* 2021, Kaur *et al* 2021, Gouveia *et al* 2022, Erkamp *et al* 2023).

Another ubiquitous multi-component phenomenon in LLPS systems is the fusing of droplets of different species, i.e., partial wetting, which is controlled by the relative surface tensions of each phase (figures 9.8(I)–(K)) (Jeon *et al* 2020, Kaur *et al* 2021, Gouveia *et al* 2022). For comparable surface tensions, stable fused structures form, whereas a strong mismatch leads to complete enveloping of one phase by the other (figures 9.8(I) and (J)) (Kaur *et al* 2021). DNA nanostar condensates have also been shown to exhibit fused, enveloped, and mixed structures of two populations of droplets by combining two orthogonal DNA nanostar constructs with a population of nanostar crosslinkers (figure 9.8(K)) (Jeon *et al* 2020). In these studies, the molar ratio of the two types of nanostars were matched while the ratio of crosslinkers to nanostars was varied from $R_x = 0$ to $R_x = 1.5$, showing increased fusing and mixing of the two populations with increasing R_x (figure 9.8(K)) (Jeon *et al* 2020).

9.8 Active and dynamic liquid–liquid phase separation

LLPS systems are generally considered out of equilibrium—aging, coalescing and coarsening over time—en route to thermodynamic equilibrium or metastable states.

However, incorporating enzymes and other energy transducing chemical reactions into LLPS systems have been shown to push LLPS off of this free energy minimizing path to engineer 'active' coacervates that actively change shape, size, and stiffness (Zwicker *et al* 2015, Deng and Walther 2020, Donau *et al* 2020, Saleh *et al* 2020). Fueling coacervates have also been shown to suppress Ostwald ripening, stabilize droplets from growing and coalescing (Zwicker *et al* 2015), and even cause droplets to divide (Zwicker *et al* 2017).

For example, incorporating a single-cutter restriction endonuclease, SmaI, into the DNA nanostar LLPS systems discussed above (figures 9.6 and 9.8(A) and (K)), has been shown to activate droplet dissolution dependent on the hybridization strength and valence of the nanostar arms (figures 9.9(A–C)) (Saleh *et al* 2020). SmaI bluntly cuts 3 of the 4 arms of the nanostars, resulting in DNA fragments that can dissolve into the dilute phase to facilitate dissolution. For strongly-binding nanostars, SmaI was unable to penetrate the droplet so dissolution proceeded by enzymatic degradation at the surface that continuously shrunk the droplet (figure 9.9(A)). Alternatively, weakly-binding nanostars, which are inherently less stable, allowed SmaI to penetrate the droplet and fragment the DNA in local regions throughout the coacervate volume. This volumetric degradation led to the formation and dissolution of transient and dynamic interior vacuoles, similar to Erkamp *et al* (2023), that appeared as bubbling events (figures 9.9(B) and (C)) (Saleh *et al* 2020).

Incorporating a single-cutter restriction endonuclease BsaI and ATP-fueled T4 ligase into the SfNAP LLPS system described above (Deng and Walther 2020) has also been shown to produce active, energy-dissipating coacervates of SfNAPs undergoing continuous ligation, polymerization, bond-breakage, and depolymerization (figures 9.7(F)–(H)) (Deng and Walther 2020). Programmable competition between ATP-fueled ligation, via T4 ligase, and depolymerization, via BsaI-mediated cleavage of side groups, was shown to either dissolve droplets that were otherwise metastable in the passive state (figures 9.7(F)–(H)), or prolong the coacervate lifetime. These active processes led to larger droplets as compared to passive condensates with lifetimes that scaled linearly with ATP concentration (Deng and Walther 2020). Incorporating two other complementary SfNAPs into the system before inducing LLPS led to the formation of two distinct populations of condensates, sorted by their SfNAP pairs (figures 9.7(F)–(H)) (Deng and Walther 2020).

Active droplets of polyU-RNA and engineered peptides that self-assemble via chemically fueled RNA-peptide association, and disassemble via spontaneous hydrolysis of the peptide have been realized, with stability and lifetime programmed by the reaction kinetics (Donau *et al* 2020). Specifically, LLPS of 4.1 mM RNA and 23 mM peptide is achieved by fueling the solution with $\geqslant$7.5 mM EDC (1-ethyl-3-(3-(dimethylaminopropyl)-carbodiimide) that converts the aspartate of the peptide to its anhydride via its hydrolysis to urea (figure 9.9(D)) (Donau *et al* 2020). Subsequent droplet dissolution, following fusion and vacuole formation, occurs as EDC is depleted and anhydride spontaneously hydrolyzes (figure 9.9(D)) (Donau *et al* 2020). These dynamic droplets, with kinetics that were synced with the reaction kinetics, could be made metastable by increasing EDC concentration to $\geqslant$40 mM, leading to droplets that persisted well after EDC depletion due to kinetic arrest (Donau *et al* 2020). Metastability could also be achieved by lowering RNA

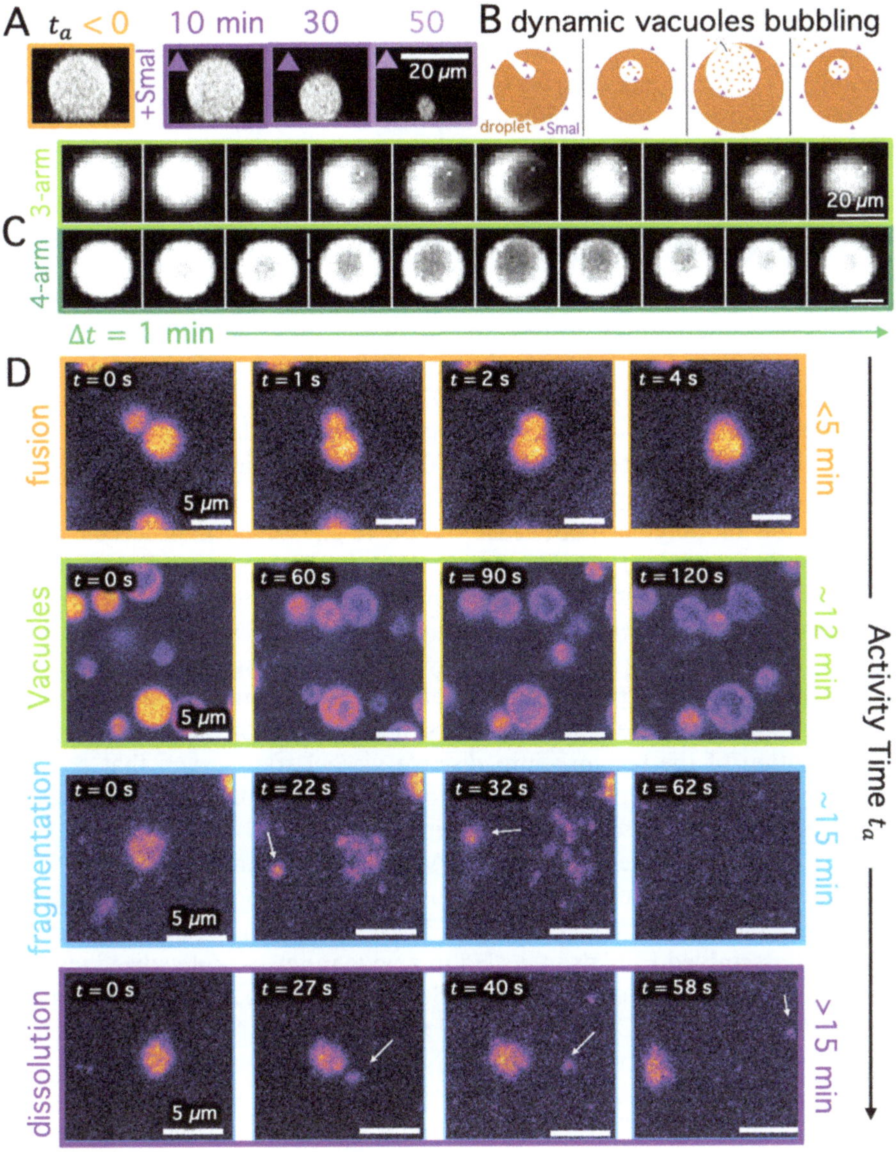

Figure 9.9. Active droplets undergoing self-assembly, shrinkage, and bubbling driven by enzymatic activity or chemical fuel. (A–C) Condensates of DNA nanostars in the presence of restriction enzyme SmaI that breaks bonds between 3 of the 4 nanostar arms. (A) A condensate with strong bonds shrinks and dissolves under the action of SmaI by breaking bonds at the droplet surface. (B and C) Droplets with weaker bonds allow SmaI to penetrate the droplet to create vacuoles, and dissolve the droplet from the interior, as depicted in (B) and shown for (C) droplets of 3-arm and 4-arm nanostars over the course of 9 min, with each image separated by $\Delta t = 1$ min. (D) False color confocal images of active droplets of polyU-RNA (labeled) and peptides, fueled by EDC, undergoing (top to bottom) fusion (orange), vacuole formation (green), fragmentation (blue), and dissolution (purple). The start time of each time-lapse series relative to the addition of EDC t_a is listed to the right of the corresponding row. Times listed in each image are relative to the initial image shown. Arrows show fragments that persist for several seconds before dissolving. (A)–(C) Adapted from Saleh *et al* (2020) with permission of PNAS. (D) Adapted from Donau *et al* (2020). CC BY 4.0.

concentration, thereby increasing the peptide:RNA ratio, which increases the barrier to disassemble both kinetically and thermodynamically. Finally, dynamic droplets were shown to immediately take up RNA, nucleate, grow, and coalesce upon EDC activation. However, when deactivation kinetics were faster than self-assembly kinetics, droplets expelled RNA into the dilute phase, formed RNA-poor vacuoles, and often broke apart (figure 9.9(D)).

9.9 Viscoelastic phase separation (VPS)

A phenomenon related to LLPS that emerges in composite biopolymer networks is viscoelastic phase separation (VPS), in which the condensates adopt viscoelastic properties that allow for the formation of a percolated network of condensates (figure 9.10) (Fare *et al* 2021, Ma *et al* 2021, Wiedner and Giudice 2021, Tanaka 2022). In contrast, liquid-like LLPS droplets ripen and coalesce into larger droplets, preventing dynamic arrest of connected droplets. VPS in systems in which the volume fraction of the biopolymer-rich 'slow' phase (e.g., RNA or IDPs) is much lower than the biopolymer-poor 'fast' phase (e.g., solvent), proceeds by initial formation of discrete liquid-like droplets, followed by solvent expulsion and droplet shrinkage that leads to condensates comprising highly entangled biopolymer gels that connect to form a network of condensates (figure 9.10(A)). Conversely, in dense conditions, the slow VPS phase forms a system-spanning gel that is punctured by discrete holes of the fast phase and undergoes coarsening and shrinkage, which expands the footprint of the holes and alters their morphology. This process leads to either dissolution of the network into discrete viscoelastic clusters that continue to shrink, or dynamic arrest from crosslinking or substantial entanglements that stabilize a percolated sponge-like viscoelastic structure (figure 9.10(B)) (Tanaka 2022).

Recent experiments have demonstrated VPS in the ubiquitous FUS LLPS system with the addition of RNA of varying lengths, sequences, and higher order structures (figures 9.10(C) and (D)) (Ma *et al* 2021). These studies showed that the uptake of RNA by self-assembled FUS droplets led to a wide range of co-localized viscoelastic networks, aggregates, and droplets of FUS and RNA, depending on the properties of the RNA (figure 9.10(C)). For example, disordered RNA was shown to form viscoelastic percolated networks while RNA with more ordered structure led to more liquid-like FUS-RNA droplets (figure 9.10(D)) (Ma *et al* 2021).

Notably, an important feature of VPS (as well as LLPS), which is distinct from motor-driven aggregation of biopolymers, is their reversibility upon changing the chemical environment to lower the phase separation driving force, which may allow for repeatable activity and programmability (Lin *et al* 2015, Nguyen *et al* 2019, Erkamp *et al* 2023).

9.10 Considerations and outlook

The last decade has witnessed an explosion of discovery and work on liquid–liquid phase separation of biopolymers, motivated by their relevance to membrane-less organelles as well as intracellular compartmentalization, sequestration, transport, and co-localization. The majority of this work, as briefly summarized above, has focused

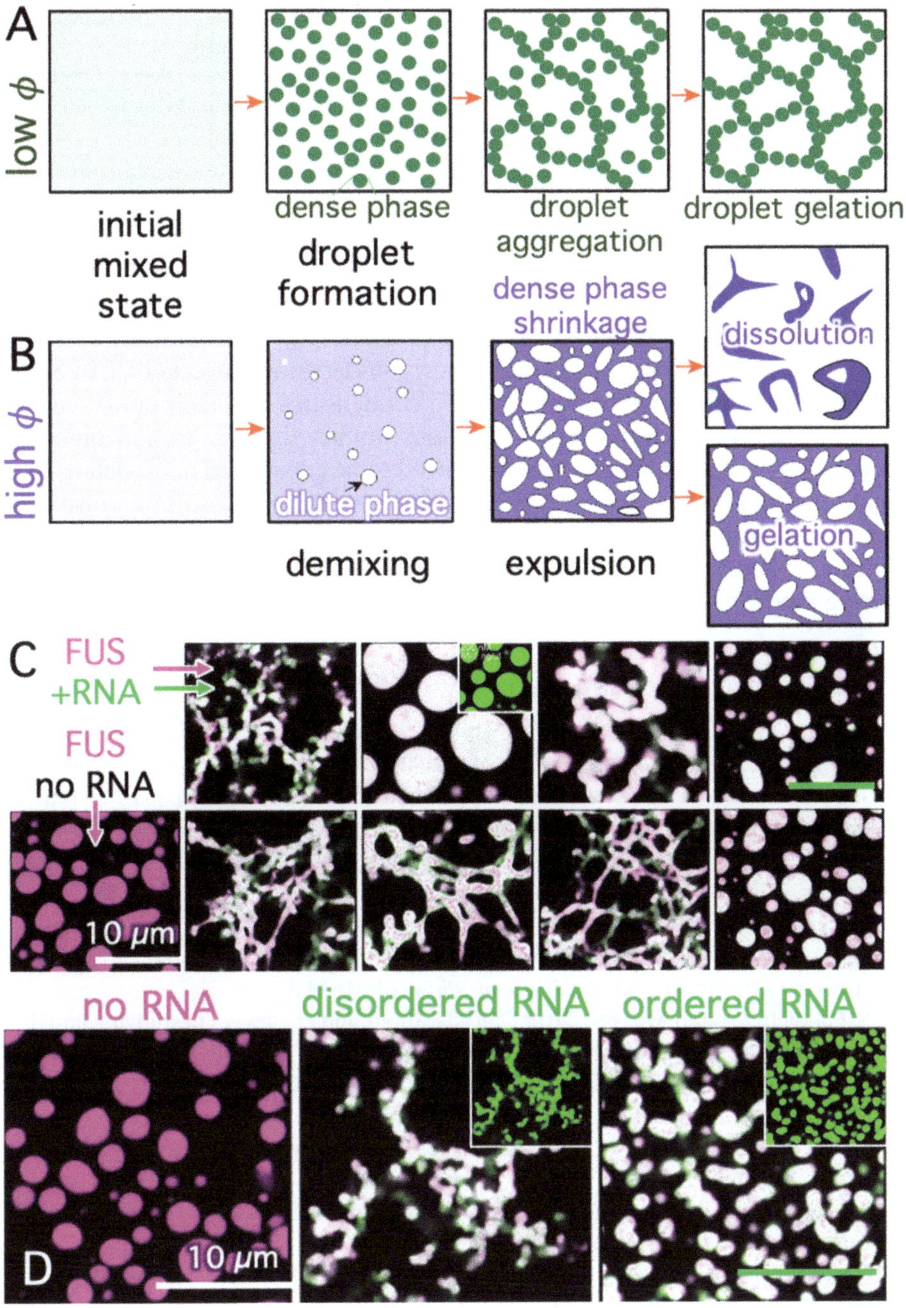

Figure 9.10. Principles and examples of viscoelastic phase separation of biopolymers. (A) Cartoon description of viscoelastic phase separation in the limits of low (A, green) and high (B, purple) volume fractions ϕ of the phase-separating polymer. Both limits can lead to percolation and gelation with sufficient entanglements or crosslinking between polymers. (C and D) Liquid-like condensates of the disordered FUS protein (magenta) form various types of viscoelastic networks and aggregates of droplets with the addition of different lengths and types of polyU-RNA (green). All images are merged FUS and RNA channels, with white indicating

co-localization. Insets show RNA channel for the corresponding merged image. (C) Different types of viscoelastic networks and droplets form with the addition of RNA of different lengths and sequences. (D) FUS droplets (left) form viscoelastic networks (middle) or fused droplets (right) with disordered or ordered RNA. (A, B) Adapted from Tanaka (2022). CC BY 4.0. (C, D) Adapted from Ma *et al* (2021). CC BY 4.0.

on identifying LLPS systems, mapping the corresponding state diagram and criteria for LLPS, and characterizing the properties of the self-assembled condensates. More recently, researchers have turned to incorporating programmability and activity into LLPS systems. These efforts to engineer 'designer' condensates will likely prove to reveal new emergent properties that may shed light on the role of LLPS in cells, and how LLPS may be harnessed for industrial applications in sequestration, filtration, chaperoning, etc. Other important, still poorly understood, aspects of LLPS include the aging process, how the properties of the condensates and their constituents vary over time, and how environmental conditions impact this maturation process. The extent to which viscoelasticity and gelation need to be considered in modeling LLPS at different stages of self-assembly, ripening, maturation, and dissolution also requires further investigation. Finally, the dynamics and properties of the biopolymers comprising condensates need to be better characterized to fully understand the underlying mechanisms driving LLPS of different systems.

References

Aarts D G A L, Lekkerkerker H N W, Guo H, Wegdam G H and Bonn D 2005 Hydrodynamics of droplet coalescence *Phys. Rev. Lett.* **95** 164503

Abyzov A, Blackledge M and Zweckstetter M 2022 Conformational dynamics of intrinsically disordered proteins regulate biomolecular condensate chemistry *Chem. Rev.* **122** 6719–48

Abyzov A, Salvi N, Schneider R, Maurin D, Ruigrok R W H, Jensen M R and Blackledge M 2016 Identification of dynamic modes in an intrinsically disordered protein using temperature-dependent NMR relaxation *J. Am. Chem. Soc.* **138** 6240–51

Adhikari S, Leaf M A and Muthukumar M 2018 Polyelectrolyte complex coacervation by electrostatic dipolar interactions *J. Chem. Phys.* **149** 163308

Alberti S, Gladfelter A and Mittag T 2019 Considerations and challenges in studying liquid–liquid phase separation and biomolecular condensates *Cell* **176** 419–34

Alvarado J, Sheinman M, Sharma A, MacKintosh F C and Koenderink G H 2013 Molecular motors robustly drive active gels to a critically connected state *Nat. Phys.* **9** 591–7

André A A M and Spruijt E 2020 Liquid–liquid phase separation in crowded environments *Int. J. Mol. Sci.* **21** 5908

Babinchak W M and Surewicz W K 2020 Liquid–liquid phase separation and its mechanistic role in pathological protein aggregation *J. Mol. Biol.* **432** 1910–25

Banani S F, Lee H O, Hyman A A and Rosen M K 2017 Biomolecular condensates: organizers of cellular biochemistry *Nat. Rev. Mol. Cell Biol.* **18** 285–98

Banerjee P R, Milin A N, Moosa M M, Onuchic P L and Deniz A A 2017 Reentrant phase transition drives dynamic substructure formation in ribonucleoprotein droplets *Angew Chem. Int. Ed.* **56** 11354–9

Bauer T, Lunkenheimer P and Loidl A 2013 Cooperativity and the freezing of molecular motion at the glass transition *Phys. Rev. Lett.* **111** 225702

Berezney J, Goode B L, Fraden S and Dogic Z 2022 Extensile to contractile transition in active microtubule–actin composites generates layered asters with programmable lifetimes *Proc. Natl. Acad. Sci.* **119** e2115895119

Biffi S, Cerbino R, Bomboi F, Paraboschi E M, Asselta R, Sciortino F and Bellini T 2013 Phase behavior and critical activated dynamics of limited-valence DNA nanostars *Proc. Natl. Acad. Sci.* **110** 15633–7

Biswas N, Ichikawa M, Datta A, Sato Y T, Yanagisawa M and Yoshikawa K 2012 Phase separation in crowded micro-spheroids: DNA–PEG system *Chem. Phys. Lett.* **539–540** 157–62

Boeynaems S *et al* 2018 Protein phase separation: a new phase in cell biology *Trends Cell Biol.* **28** 420–35

Borcherds W, Bremer A, Borgia M B and Mittag T 2021 How do intrinsically disordered protein regions encode a driving force for liquid–liquid phase separation? *Curr. Opin. Struct. Biol., Theory Simul. Comput. Methods. Macromol. Assemblies* **67** 41–50

Brady J P *et al* 2017 Structural and hydrodynamic properties of an intrinsically disordered region of a germ cell-specific protein on phase separation *Proc. Natl. Acad. Sci.* **114** E8194–203

Brangwynne C P, Tompa P and Pappu R V 2015 Polymer physics of intracellular phase transitions *Nat. Phys.* **11** 899–904

Burke K A, Janke A M, Rhine C L and Fawzi N L 2015 Residue-by-residue view of *in vitro* FUS granules that bind the C-terminal domain of RNA polymerase II *Mol. Cell.* **60** 231–41

Caragine C M, Haley S C and Zidovska A 2018 Surface fluctuations and coalescence of nucleolar droplets in the human cell nucleus *Phys. Rev. Lett.* **121** 148101

Castelnovo M and Joanny J-F 2001 Complexation between oppositely charged polyelectrolytes: beyond the random phase approximation *Eur. Phys. J.* E **6** 377–86

Chang L-W, Lytle T K, Radhakrishna M, Madinya J J, Vélez J, Sing C E and Perry S L 2017 Sequence and entropy-based control of complex coacervates *Nat. Commun.* **8** 1273

Chen N, Zhao Z, Wang Y and Dimova R 2020 Resolving the mechanisms of soy glycinin self-coacervation and hollow-condensate formation *ACS Macro Lett.* **9** 1844–52

Choi J-M, Holehouse A S and Pappu R V 2020 Physical principles underlying the complex biology of intracellular phase transitions *Annu. Rev. Biophys.* **49** 107–33

Choi U B, McCann J J, Weninger K R and Bowen M E 2011 Beyond the random coil: stochastic conformational switching in intrinsically disordered proteins *Structure* **19** 566–76

Conrad N, Chang G, Fygenson D K and Saleh O A 2022 Emulsion imaging of a DNA nanostar condensate phase diagram reveals valence and electrostatic effects *J. Chem. Phys.* **157** 234203

Conrad N, Kennedy T, Fygenson D K and Saleh O A 2019 Increasing valence pushes DNA nanostar networks to the isostatic point *Proc. Natl. Acad. Sci.* **116** 7238–43

Das S, Amin A N, Lin Y-H and Chan H S 2018a Coarse-grained residue-based models of disordered protein condensates: utility and limitations of simple charge pattern parameters *Phys. Chem. Chem. Phys.* **20** 28558–74

Das S, Eisen A, Lin Y-H and Chan H S 2018b A lattice model of charge-pattern-dependent polyampholyte phase separation *J. Phys. Chem.* B **122** 5418–31

de Gennes P P-G 1979 *Scaling Concepts in Polymer Physics* (Ithaca, NY: Cornell University Press)

de Jong H G B and Kruyt H R 1930 Koazervation *Kolloid-Z* **50** 39–48

Delarue M *et al* 2018 mTORC1 controls phase separation and the biophysical properties of the cytoplasm by tuning crowding *Cell* **174** 338–349.e20

Deng J and Walther A 2020 Programmable ATP-fueled DNA coacervates by transient liquid–liquid phase separation *Chem.* **6** 3329–43

Donau C *et al* 2020 Active coacervate droplets as a model for membraneless organelles and protocells *Nat. Commun.* **11** 5167

Eggers J, Lister J R and Stone H A 1999 Coalescence of liquid drops *J. Fluid Mech.* **401** 293–310

Elson E L 2011 Fluorescence correlation spectroscopy: past, present, future *Biophys. J.* **101** 2855–70

Erkamp N A, Sneideris T, Ausserwöger H, Qian D, Qamar S, Nixon-Abell J, St George-Hyslop P, Schmit J D, Weitz D A and Knowles T P J 2023 Spatially non-uniform condensates emerge from dynamically arrested phase separation *Nat. Commun.* **14** 684

Fare C M, Villani A, Drake L E and Shorter J 2021 Higher-order organization of biomolecular condensates *Open Biol.* **11** 210137

Feric M, Vaidya N, Harmon T S, Mitrea D M, Zhu L, Richardson T M, Kriwacki R W, Pappu R V and Brangwynne C P 2016 Coexisting liquid phases underlie nucleolar subcompartments *Cell* **165** 1686–97

Fitzpatrick R, Michieletto D, Peddireddy K R, Hauer C, Kyrillos C, Gurmessa B J and Robertson-Anderson R M 2018 Synergistic interactions between DNA and actin trigger emergent viscoelastic behavior *Phys. Rev. Lett.* **121** 257801

Fonin A V, Antifeeva I A, Kuznetsova I M, Turoverov K K, Zaslavsky B Y, Kulkarni P and Uversky V N 2022 Biological soft matter: intrinsically disordered proteins in liquid–liquid phase separation and biomolecular condensates *Essays Biochem.* **66** 831–47

Freibaum B D, Messing J, Yang P, Kim H J and Taylor J P 2021 High-fidelity reconstitution of stress granules and nucleoli in mammalian cellular lysate *J. Cell Biol.* **220** e202009079

Fu J and Schlenoff J B 2016 Driving forces for oppositely charged polyion association in aqueous solutions: enthalpic, entropic, but not electrostatic *J. Am. Chem. Soc.* **138** 980–90

Ghosh A, Kota D and Zhou H-X 2021 Shear relaxation governs fusion dynamics of biomolecular condensates *Nat. Commun.* **12** 5995

Ghosh A, Mazarakos K and Zhou H-X 2019 Three archetypical classes of macromolecular regulators of protein liquid–liquid phase separation *Proc. Natl. Acad. Sci.* **116** 19474–83

Gorczyca S M, Chapman C D and Robertson-Anderson R M 2015 Universal scaling of crowding-induced DNA mobility is coupled with topology-dependent molecular compaction and elongation *Soft Matter* **11** 7762–8

Gouveia B, Kim Y, Shaevitz J W, Petry S, Stone H A and Brangwynne C P 2022 Capillary forces generated by biomolecular condensates *Nature* **609** 255–64

Guo Y E *et al* 2019 Pol II phosphorylation regulates a switch between transcriptional and splicing condensates *Nature* **572** 543–8

Guseva S, Schnapka V, Adamski W, Maurin D, Ruigrok R W H, Salvi N and Blackledge M 2023 Liquid–liquid phase separation modifies the dynamic properties of intrinsically disordered proteins *J. Am. Chem. Soc.* **145** 10548–63

Harmon T S, Holehouse A S, Rosen M K and Pappu R V 2017 Intrinsically disordered linkers determine the interplay between phase separation and gelation in multivalent proteins *eLife* **6** e30294

Henkin G, DeCamp S J, Chen D T N, Sanchez T and Dogic Z 2014 Tunable dynamics of microtubule-based active isotropic gels *Philos. Trans. Royal Soc. A: Math., Phys. Eng. Sci.* **372** 20140142

Hyman A A, Weber C A and Jülicher F 2014 Liquid–liquid phase separation in biology *Annu. Rev. Cell Dev. Biol.* **30** 39–58

Ijavi M *et al* 2021 Surface tensiometry of phase separated protein and polymer droplets by the sessile drop method *Soft Matter* **17** 1655–62

Jawerth L M, Ijavi M, Ruer M, Saha S, Jahnel M, Hyman A A, Jülicher F and Fischer-Friedrich E 2018 Salt-dependent rheology and surface tension of protein condensates using optical traps *Phys. Rev. Lett.* **121** 258101

Jeon B, Nguyen D T, Abraham G R, Conrad N, Fygenson D K and Saleh O A 2018 Salt-dependent properties of a coacervate-like, self-assembled DNA liquid *Soft Matter* **14** 7009–15

Jeon B, Nguyen D T and Saleh O A 2020 Sequence-controlled adhesion and microemulsification in a two-phase system of DNA liquid droplets *J. Phys. Chem.* B **124** 8888–95

Kashchiev D 2000 *Nucleation* (Amsterdam: Elsevier)

Kaur T, Alshareedah I, Wang W, Ngo J, Moosa M M and Banerjee P R 2019 Molecular crowding tunes material states of ribonucleoprotein condensates *Biomolecules* **9** 71

Kaur T, Raju M, Alshareedah I, Davis R B, Potoyan D A and Banerjee P R 2021 Sequence-encoded and composition-dependent protein-RNA interactions control multiphasic condensate morphologies *Nat. Commun.* **12** 872

Kayitmazer A B 2017 Thermodynamics of complex coacervation *Adv. Colloid Interface Sci.* **239** 169–77

Khanal P, Peddireddy K R, Marfai J, McGorty R and Robertson-Anderson R M 2022 DNA topology dictates emergent bulk elasticity and hindered macromolecular diffusion in DNA-dextran composites *J. Rheol.* **66** 699–715

Lytle T K and Sing C E 2018 Tuning chain interaction entropy in complex coacervation using polymer stiffness, architecture, and salt valency *Mol. Sys. Design Eng.* **3** 183–96

Koenderink G H and Paluch E K 2018 Architecture shapes contractility in actomyosin networks *Curr. Opinion Cell Biol., Cell Archit.* **50** 79–85

Kudlay A and Olvera de la Cruz M 2003 Precipitation of oppositely charged polyelectrolytes in salt solutions *J. Chem. Phys.* **120** 404–12

Lee D S W, Strom A R and Brangwynne C P 2022 The mechanobiology of nuclear phase separation *APL Bioeng.* **6** 021503

Lee T, Do S, Lee J G, Kim D-N and Shin Y 2021 The flexibility-based modulation of DNA nanostar phase separation *Nanoscale* **13** 17638–47

Li L, Srivastava S, Andreev M, Marciel A B, de Pablo J J and Tirrell M V 2018 Phase behavior and salt partitioning in polyelectrolyte complex coacervates *Macromolecules* **51** 2988–95

Lin Y, Protter D S W, Rosen M K and Parker R 2015 Formation and maturation of phase-separated liquid droplets by RNA-binding proteins *Mol. Cell* **60** 208–19

Liu Y, Momani B, Winter H H and Perry S L 2017 Rheological characterization of liquid-to-solid transitions in bulk polyelectrolyte complexes *Soft Matter* **13** 7332–40

Lu T and Spruijt E 2020 Multiphase complex coacervate droplets *J. Am. Chem. Soc.* **142** 2905–14

Lyon A S, Peeples W B and Rosen M K 2021 A framework for understanding the functions of biomolecular condensates across scales *Nat. Rev. Mol. Cell Biol.* **22** 215–35

Lytle T K and Sing C E 2017 Transfer matrix theory of polymer complex coacervation *Soft Matter* **13** 7001–12

Ma W, Zhen G, Xie W and Mayr C 2021 *In vivo* reconstitution finds multivalent RNA–RNA interactions as drivers of mesh-like condensates *eLife* **10** e64252

Manning G S 2003 Limiting laws and counterion condensation in polyelectrolyte solutions I. colligative properties *J. Chem. Phys.* **51** 924–33

Marfai J, McGorty R J and Robertson-Anderson R M 2023 Cooperative rheological state-switching of enzymatically-driven composites of circular DNA and dextran *Adv. Mater.* **35** 2305824

Marianelli A M, Miller B M and Keating C D 2018 Impact of macromolecular crowding on RNA/spermine complex coacervation and oligonucleotide compartmentalization *Soft Matter* **14** 368–78

Martin E W, Holehouse A S, Peran I, Farag M, Incicco J J, Bremer A, Grace C R, Soranno A, Pappu R V and Mittag T 2020 Valence and patterning of aromatic residues determine the phase behavior of prion-like domains *Science* **367** 694–9

McCarty J, Delaney K T, Danielsen S P O, Fredrickson G H and Shea J-E 2019 Complete phase diagram for liquid–liquid phase separation of intrinsically disordered proteins *J. Phys. Chem. Lett.* **10** 1644–52

McGorty R J *et al* 2023 Kinesin and myosin motors compete to drive rich multiphase dynamics in programmable cytoskeletal composites *PNAS Nexus* **2** pgad245

Merindol R, Loescher S, Samanta A and Walther A 2018 Pathway-controlled formation of mesostructured all-DNA colloids and superstructures *Nat. Nanotech.* **13** 730–8

Miyagi A, Tsunaka Y, Uchihashi T, Mayanagi K, Hirose S, Morikawa K and Ando T 2008 Visualization of intrinsically disordered regions of proteins by high-speed atomic force microscopy *Chem. Phys. Chem.* **9** 1859–66

Molliex A, Temirov J, Lee J, Coughlin M, Kanagaraj A P, Kim H J, Mittag T and Taylor J P 2015 Phase separation by low complexity domains promotes stress granule assembly and drives pathological fibrillization *Cell* **163** 123–33

Murthy A C, Dignon G L, Kan Y, Zerze G H, Parekh S H, Mittal J and Fawzi N L 2019 Molecular interactions underlying liquid−liquid phase separation of the FUS low-complexity domain *Nat. Struct. Mol. Biol.* **26** 637–48

Narayanan A, Meriin A, Andrews J O, Spille J-H, Sherman M Y and Cisse I I 2019 A first order phase transition mechanism underlies protein aggregation in mammalian cells *eLife* **8** e39695

Ndlec F J, Surrey T, Maggs A C and Leibler S 1997 Self-organization of microtubules and motors *Nature* **389** 305–8

Nguyen D T, Jeon B, Abraham G R and Saleh O A 2019 Length-dependence and spatial structure of DNA partitioning into a DNA liquid *Langmuir* **35** 14849–54

Nguyen D T and Saleh O A 2017 Tuning phase and aging of DNA hydrogels through molecular design *Soft Matter* **13** 5421–7

Nott T J *et al* 2015 Phase transition of a disordered nuage protein generates environmentally responsive membraneless organelles *Mol. Cell* **57** 936–47

Overbeek J T G and Voorn M J 1957 Phase separation in polyelectrolyte solutions. Theory of complex coacervation *J. Cell Comp. Physiol.* **49** 7–26

Pan Q, Sun D, Xue J, Hao J, Zhao H, Lin X, Yu L and He Y 2021 Real-time study of protein phase separation with spatiotemporal analysis of single-nanoparticle trajectories *ACS Nano* **15** 539–49

Peddireddy K R, Michieletto D, Aguirre G, Garamella J, Khanal P and Robertson-Anderson R M 2021 DNA conformation dictates strength and flocculation in DNA–microtubule composites *ACS Macro Lett.* **10** 1540–8

Priftis D, Laugel N and Tirrell M 2012 Thermodynamic characterization of polypeptide complex coacervation *Langmuir* **28** 15947–57

Protter D S W, Rao B S, Treeck B V, Lin Y, Mizoue L, Rosen M K and Parker R 2018 Intrinsically disordered regions can contribute promiscuous interactions to RNP granule assembly *Cell Rep.* **22** 1401–12

Qin J and de Pablo J J 2016 Criticality and connectivity in macromolecular charge complexation *Macromolecules* **49** 8789–800

Radhakrishna M, Basu K, Liu Y, Shamsi R, Perry S L and Sing C E 2017 Molecular connectivity and correlation effects on polymer coacervation *Macromolecules* **50** 3030–7

Ray S *et al* 2020 α-Synuclein aggregation nucleates through liquid–liquid phase separation *Nat. Chem.* **12** 705–16

Record M T Jr, Anderson C F and Lohman T M 1978 Thermodynamic analysis of ion effects on the binding and conformational equilibria of proteins and nucleic acids: the roles of ion association or release, screening, and ion effects on water activity *Q. Rev. Biophys.* **11** 103–78

Riback J A, Zhu L, Ferrolino M C, Tolbert M, Mitrea D M, Sanders D W, Wei M-T, Kriwacki R W and Brangwynne C P 2020 Composition-dependent thermodynamics of intracellular phase separation *Nature* **581** 209–14

Rosowski K A, Sai T, Vidal-Henriquez E, Zwicker D, Style R W and Dufresne E R 2020 Elastic ripening and inhibition of liquid–liquid phase separation *Nat. Phys.* **16** 422–5

Rubinstein M and Colby R H 2003 *Polymer Physics* (Oxford: Oxford University Press)

Rubinstein M, Liao Q and Panyukov S 2018 Structure of liquid coacervates formed by oppositely charged polyelectrolytes *Macromolecules* **51** 9572–88

Rumyantsev A M and de Pablo J J 2019 Liquid crystalline and isotropic coacervates of semiflexible polyanions and flexible polycations *Macromolecules* **52** 5140–56

Sahu S, Chauhan P, Lumen E, Moody K, Peddireddy K, Mani N, Subramanian R, Robertson-Anderson R, Wolfe A J and Ross J L 2023 Interplay of self-organization of microtubule asters and crosslinking protein condensates *PNAS Nexus* **2** pgad231

Saleh O A, Jeon B and Liedl T 2020 Enzymatic degradation of liquid droplets of DNA is modulated near the phase boundary *Proc. Natl. Acad. Sci.* **117** 16160–6

Salehi A and Larson R G 2016 A molecular thermodynamic model of complexation in mixtures of oppositely charged polyelectrolytes with explicit account of charge association/dissociation *Macromolecules* **49** 9706–19

Schuster B S, Reed E H, Parthasarathy R, Jahnke C N, Caldwell R M, Bermudez J G, Ramage H, Good M C and Hammer D A 2018 Controllable protein phase separation and modular recruitment to form responsive membraneless organelles *Nat. Commun.* **9** 2985

Shakya A, Girard M, King J T and Olvera de la Cruz M 2020 Role of chain flexibility in asymmetric polyelectrolyte complexation in salt solutions *Macromolecules* **53** 1258–69

Shimobayashi S F, Ronceray P, Sanders D W, Haataja M P and Brangwynne C P 2021 Nucleation landscape of biomolecular condensates *Nature* **599** 503–6

Shin Y and Brangwynne C P 2017 Liquid phase condensation in cell physiology and disease *Science* **357** eaaf4382

Shin Y, Chang Y-C, Lee D S W, Berry J, Sanders D W, Ronceray P, Wingreen N S, Haataja M and Brangwynne C P 2018 Liquid nuclear condensates mechanically sense and restructure the genome *Cell* **175** 1481–1491.e13

Shusharina N P, Zhulina E B, Dobrynin A V and Rubinstein M 2005 Scaling theory of diblock polyampholyte solutions *Macromolecules* **38** 8870–81

Silva M S E, Depken M, Stuhrmann B, Korsten M, MacKintosh F C and Koenderink G H 2011 Active multistage coarsening of actin networks driven by myosin motors *PNAS* **108** 9408–13

Sing C E 2017 Development of the modern theory of polymeric complex coacervation *Adv. Colloid Interface Sci.* **239** 2–16

Sing C E and Perry S L 2020 Recent progress in the science of complex coacervation *Soft Matter* **16** 2885–914

Spruijt E 2023 Open questions on liquid–liquid phase separation *Commun. Chem.* **6** 5

Spruijt E, Cohen Stuart M A and van der Gucht J 2013 Linear viscoelasticity of polyelectrolyte complex coacervates *Macromolecules* **46** 1633–41

Spruijt E, Sprakel J, Lemmers M, Stuart M A C and van der Gucht J 2010 Relaxation dynamics at different time scales in electrostatic complexes: time-salt superposition *Phys. Rev. Lett.* **105** 208301

Stam S, Freedman S L, Banerjee S, Weirich K L, Dinner A R and Gardel M L 2017 Filament rigidity and connectivity tune the deformation modes of active biopolymer networks *Proc. Natl. Acad. Sci.* **114** E10037–45

Stetefeld J, McKenna S A and Patel T R 2016 Dynamic light scattering: a practical guide and applications in biomedical sciences *Biophys. Rev.* **8** 409–27

Strom A R and Brangwynne C P 2019 The liquid nucleome—phase transitions in the nucleus at a glance *J. Cell Sci.* **132** jcs235093

Tanaka H 2022 Viscoelastic phase separation in biological cells *Commun. Phys.* **5** 12

Taylor N O, Wei M-T, Stone H A and Brangwynne C P 2019 Quantifying dynamics in phase-separated condensates using fluorescence recovery after photobleaching *Biophys. J.* **117** 1285–300

Tiebackx F W 1911 Gleichzeitige ausflockung zweier kolloide *Zeitschr f Chem. Ind. Kolloide* **8** 198–201

Vega I E, Umstead A and Kanaan N M 2019 EFhd2 affects tau liquid–liquid phase separation *Front. Neurosci.* **13** 00845

Vieregg J R, Lueckheide M, Marciel A B, Leon L, Bologna A J, Rivera J R and Tirrell M V 2018 Oligonucleotide–peptide complexes: phase control by hybridization *J. Am. Chem. Soc.* **140** 1632–8

Wang J *et al* 2018 A molecular grammar governing the driving forces for phase separation of prion-like RNA binding proteins *Cell* **174** 688–699.e16

Wang J and McGorty R 2019 Measuring capillary wave dynamics using differential dynamic microscopy *Soft Matter* **15** 7412–9

Wang Q and Schlenoff J B 2014 The polyelectrolyte complex/coacervate continuum *Macromolecules* **47** 3108–16

Wang Z and Rubinstein M 2006 Regimes of conformational transitions of a diblock polyampholyte *Macromolecules* **39** 5897–912

Wei M-T, Elbaum-Garfinkle S, Holehouse A S, Chen C C-H, Feric M, Arnold C B, Priestley R D, Pappu R V and Brangwynne C P 2017 Phase behaviour of disordered proteins underlying low density and high permeability of liquid organelles *Nat. Chem.* **9** 1118–25

Weirich K L, Dasbiswas K, Witten T A, Vaikuntanathan S and Gardel M L 2019 Self-organizing motors divide active liquid droplets *PNAS* **116** 11125–30

Wiedner H J and Giudice J 2021 It's not just a phase: function and characteristics of RNA-binding proteins in phase separation *Nat. Struct. Mol. Biol.* **28** 465–73

Yanagisawa M, Nigorikawa S, Sakaue T, Fujiwara K and Tokita M 2014 Multiple patterns of polymer gels in microspheres due to the interplay among phase separation, wetting, and gelation *PNAS* **111** 15894–9

Yang P *et al* 2020 G3BP1 is a tunable switch that triggers phase separation to assemble stress granules *Cell* **181** 325–345.e28

Zeng X, Holehouse A S, Chilkoti A, Mittag T and Pappu R V 2020 Connecting coil-to-globule transitions to full phase diagrams for intrinsically disordered proteins *Biophys. J.* **119** 402–18

Zhang R and Shklovskii B I 2005 Phase diagram of solution of oppositely charged polyelectrolytes *Phys. A: Stat. Mech. App. Phys. Appl. Biol. Syst.* **352** 216–38

Zwicker D, Hyman A A and Jülicher F 2015 Suppression of ostwald ripening in active emulsions *Phys. Rev.* E **92** 012317

Zwicker D, Seyboldt R, Weber C A, Hyman A A and Jülicher F 2017 Growth and division of active droplets provides a model for protocells *Nat. Phys.* **13** 408–13

Part V

What now?

Chapter 10

Past, present, and future: perspectives from the community

This chapter summarizes the previous chapters and discusses the big open questions in the field. Rather than my own perspective, I showcase the wisdom of prominent researchers and rising stars in the field to provide a community perspective on the foundational works, open questions, and challenges in the field. I also highlight community voices describing the need to come together as researchers to advance knowledge and promote collaboration, resource-sharing, and training; and ideas about and how we may achieve these goals.

10.1 What we have learned

I started this monograph with an introduction to biopolymers and their networks (**chapter 1**), followed by an overview of polymer physics concepts used to describe and understand the dynamics of biopolymer networks (**chapter 2**), as well as key experimental tools used to measure biopolymer network properties (**chapter 3**) and computational analysis techniques to characterize and interpret data (**chapter 4**). I followed with a foundational chapter describing the dynamics, structure, and rheology of single-component networks of key linear biopolymers: DNA, actin, microtubules, and intermediate filaments (**chapter 5**), opening the door to discussing more complex systems that are of current widespread interest and investigation (chapters 6–9), with many mysteries still needing to be solved.

10.2 What we are still learning

The complexity and diversity of biopolymer networks leave many open questions that researchers are actively investigating. One such topic, which I discussed in **chapter 6**, is the role of polymer topology. Biopolymers are unique in the broad diversity of topologies and conformations they can adopt, including relaxed rings and supercoiled circular constructs; branched, star-like, and bottlebrush configurations; and higher-order

doi:10.1088/978-0-7503-5037-2ch10

structures that contain loops, hairpins, kinks, folds, knots, and sticky patches (Matthews 1992, Blanchoin *et al* 2000, Cloutier and Widom 2004, Espeli and Marians 2004, Bikard *et al* 2010, Honda *et al* 2010, Choi *et al* 2011, Chapman *et al* 2012, Rogers *et al* 2014, Gorczyca *et al* 2015, Li *et al* 2015, Mai and Schroeder 2016, Dong *et al* 2020, Smrek *et al* 2021, Khanal *et al* 2022). Groups of biopolymers can also form larger-scale structures such as bundles, sheets, and concatemers (Shin *et al* 2004, Krajina *et al* 2018, Klotz *et al* 2020, Lenz 2020, Abyzov *et al* 2022). The effects of these various topologies on the rheology and dynamics of the networks they comprise remain a topic of intense investigation.

Another frontier area of biopolymer network research, that I discussed in **chapter 7**, is understanding the properties and underlying mechanisms of composite systems comprising two or more distinct biopolymers (Fitzpatrick *et al* 2018, Ricketts *et al* 2018, Dogterom and Koenderink 2019, Francis *et al* 2019, Lopez-Menendez and Gonzalez-Torres 2019, Michieletto *et al* 2019, Shen 2020, Peddireddy *et al* 2021, 2022, Schaedel *et al* 2021, Shen *et al* 2021, Khanal *et al* 2022, Marfai *et al* 2023). Many previous works have shown that composites exhibit emergent mechanical properties that cannot be predicted by the properties of the corresponding single-component systems (Jensen *et al* 2014, Fitzpatrick *et al* 2018, Francis *et al* 2019, Lopez-Menendez and Gonzalez-Torres 2019, Khanal *et al* 2022). However, predicting the parameter space and network designs that give rise to emergent properties, and understanding the underlying physics, remain fervent areas of research.

Moreover, as I discussed in **chapter 8**, understanding the behavior and properties of non-equilibrium 'active' biopolymer networks is of critical importance to the burgeoning field of active matter research and understanding the multitude of cellular processes that are driven by various forms of free-energy transduction processes (Mogilner and Oster 1996, Pollard *et al* 2001, Sanchez *et al* 2012, Merindol and Walther 2017, Voth 2017, Needleman and Dogic 2017, Alvarado *et al* 2019, Burkholder and Brady 2019, Burla *et al* 2019, Banerjee *et al* 2020). Biopolymer networks can be pushed out of equilibrium by, e.g., externally triggered changes to their environment, energy-consuming motors that do mechanical work on the comprising polymers, or enzymatic changes to polymer topology or structure (Bertrand *et al* 2012, Nakamura *et al* 2014, Linsmeier *et al* 2016, Nguyen and Saleh 2017, Gurmessa *et al* 2018, 2021, Bacca *et al* 2019, Jahnke *et al* 2020, Ricketts *et al* 2020, Michieletto *et al* 2022, Lemma *et al* 2023, Marfai *et al* 2023, McGorty *et al* 2023, Lee *et al* 2021). Biopolymer networks are facile systems to engineer and interrogate such non-equilibrium behavior to reveal new emergent phenomena and test growing theoretical models to describe active matter phenomenon (Lenz 2014, Ronceray and Lenz 2015, Fodor *et al* 2016, Alvarado *et al* 2017, Ramaswamy 2017, Burkholder and Brady 2019).

Finally, liquid–liquid phase separation, which I discussed in **chapter 9**, is perhaps the most rapidly growing and active area of biopolymer network research, with many new phases of biological matter being discovered that raise new questions that require interdisciplinary investigations to answer (Hyman *et al* 2014, Brangwynne *et al* 2015, Shin and Brangwynne 2017, Jeon *et al* 2018, Alberti *et al* 2019, Kaur *et al* 2019, 2021, McCarty *et al* 2019, Deng and Walther 2020, Riback *et al* 2020,

Sing and Perry 2020, Shimobayashi *et al* 2021, Conrad *et al* 2022, Gouveia *et al* 2022, Sahu *et al* 2023).

To make progress in these frontier research areas of biopolymer networks, new methods are needed that can connect mechanical properties to macromolecular dynamics and network structure. In these complex systems, understanding the relaxation dynamics and rearrangements of biopolymers that give rise to bulk rheological properties is not straightforward, demanding improved methods to simultaneously measure both dynamics and rheology across different scales. In parallel, advancing modeling approaches to build in more complexity and extend the spatiotemporal scales that can be accessed to match experimental scales is essential to directly comparing experiment and theory. Finally, biopolymer networks that comprise multiple species (i.e., blends and composites), topologically complex polymers (e.g., ring, supercoiled, branched), or networks undergoing non-equilibrium processes, often display spatiotemporally heterogeneous and/or hierarchical structural and rheological properties. This complexity requires measurements that can probe network properties from the level of single biopolymers to the bulk; and, importantly, determine how the properties vary in the mesoscopic regime that bridges microscopic and macroscopic scales. How polymers distribute and propagate local stress and strain throughout the network is a rich question applicable to cell biology, polymer physics, and materials engineering.

10.3 Who 'we' are and what we think

To give a proper perspective on the past, present, and future of research in biopolymer networks, it is important to recognize how diverse and interdisciplinary the researchers that work in this field are, and the unique perspectives they bring. Many of the groundbreaking discoveries and advances in the field have only been possible through collaborations between researchers with a broad range of disciplinary expertise, backgrounds, perspectives and skillsets, including physicists, chemists, biologists, engineers and mathematicians. Participation from students and early career researchers, ranging from high school students to postdocs, has likewise elevated the field and provided robust training opportunities for the next generation of interdisciplinary scientists. Given the richness of the community and diversity of perspectives, to be able to paint an inclusive picture of the open questions, needs, and foundational works in the field, I turn to both leaders and rising stars in the field to answer the questions entitling the following sections. Each quote is from a different researcher with a unique story and perspective. I am indebted to those who contributed, listed below, who have taught me so much through the years and continue to inspire me daily.

Full Professors
Moumita Das, Rochester Institute of Technology
Zvonimir Dogic, University of California, Santa Barbara
Gijsje Koenderink, Delft University of Technology
Sarah Köster, University of Göttingen
Michael Rubinstein, Duke University

Omar A. Saleh, University of California, Santa Barbara
Charles Schroeder, University of Illinois at Urbana-Champaign
Ken Schweizer, University of Illinois at Urbana-Champaign

Associate Professors
Ronit Freeman, The University of North Carolina—Chapel Hill
Vernita D. Gordon, University of Texas at Austin
Michael Murrell, Yale University
Alison Sweeney, Yale University

Assistant Professors
Alexander R. Klotz, California State University, Long Beach
Sara M. Hashmi, Northeastern University
Danielle J. Mai, Stanford University
Nathan John Oldenhuis, University of New Hampshire
Alison Patteson, Syracuse University

10.4 What are the big open questions in the field of biopolymer networks?

'How can we generate completely synthetic mimics that recapitulate the structural organization, mechanical behavior, and dynamic properties of natural biopolymers?'

'How do biopolymers in nature work together to form functional, adaptable, active materials?'

'How can we learn from nature and rebuild the astonishing properties of biopolymers, networks, and materials?'

'What are the design principles that enable biopolymer networks to be versatile and multifunctional, often combining apparently conflicting properties?

'When do networks display rubber mechanical elasticity versus isostatic (rigidity-controlled) mechanics?'

'How can we understand the physics of entanglements in different biopolymer networks?'

'How do the topology and mechanics of a network influence interactions with proteins and other biomacromolecules?'

'How do we integrate the broad mechanical features found in biopolymer networks into synthetic materials?'

'How can we leverage the richness of protein function to expand the possible functions of protein-based networks?'

'Recent efforts in synthetic polymer networks focus on mechanical properties: stretchability, flexibility, mechanical strength, shape memory, actuation, etc: How might we recapitulate these properties in biopolymer networks and then go a step further to introduce new functions?'

'What functions are well-suited for biopolymers instead of synthetic polymers (e.g. tissue mimicry, programmed degradation, novel actuation mechanisms)?'

'How can we understand and harness adaptive control and physical learning in biopolymer networks? How has biology honed these features?'

'How can we design active and autonomous biopolymer networks and their composites that can be programmed to have desired structural and dynamic properties?'

'How can we predict material responses from thermodyamic equilibrium?'

'Can we think about biofilms as polymer networks? If so, how can we use that perspective to think about how to treat harmful biofilms, so that they're more easily cleared by the immune system, and how to engineer 'good' biofilms to do what we want?'

'We still do not have a good understanding of the mechanics response and dynamics of biopolymer films subject to flow. How do we couple elasto-hydrodynamics, mixed transport modes, reaction kinetics, and concentration fluxes with fluid dynamics?'

'How can we improve *in situ* measurements of rheology to better understand mechanics and dynamics in flowing systems?'

'How can we incorporate network analysis, such as that now being employed in colloidal gels and networks, to understand biopolymer networks? For example, to learn about both hidden and structural nodes in these networks and methods of 'communication' within the networks.'

'How can we develop better understanding of systems far from thermodynamic equilibrium?'

'What are the fundamental physical mechanisms underlying the nonlinear rheological response of biopolymer networks under different protocols (creep, continuous shear, startup response, steady-state response)? How does this response couple to the structure of the fundamental units?'

'How do the roles of topological entanglements, as well as different attractive and repulsive forces known to be crucial in nanoparticle and colloid rheology, impact the nonlinear rheological response of biopolymer networks?'

'Why are there three cytoskeletal networks? What are the properties of these three networks together?'

'What are the differences between the rheological behavior of flexible and semiflexible entropic networks (e.g., gelatin and actin) and stiff enthalpic (e.g., fibrin) networks?'

'How does biopolymer network structure impact chemical signaling in cells?'

'How do cytoskeletal networks impact nuclear shape from the outside?'

'What kinds of new materials can we design using intermediate filaments that are resilient and resistant to breakage and promote wound healing?'

'Are there general rules for the structure–function relationships of polysaccharide networks? And what role does physical confinement play in generating network function in living systems?'

'The coarse-grained hydrodynamic description of soft active matter is capable of explaining diverse experimental observations. However, we still lack robust multi-scale quantitative understanding of the phenomena.'

'How do we start with known dynamics of active microscopic constituents and predict the emergent large-scale dynamics?'

'How can we determine if active stresses will be extensile or contractile?'

'So far, the active stresses generated by reconstituted materials is very meek, e.g., of the order of tens of mPa for microtubule-based active fluids. There is a fundamental mismatch of several orders of magnitude between such active stresses and the passive stresses of other soft materials, which precludes formation of active soft composites. How do we generate protocols and networks that can magnify the magnitude of active stresses?'

'How can we design biopolymer networks with desired functionality and targeted mechanical properties? For example, electrically conductive biopolymer networks (or hybrid biopolymer networks) that can self-heal, change shape, or show time-dependent mechanical properties depending on an external stimulus.'

'When will this field turn towards applications or more serious biology?'

'Do the findings from biopolymer physics research actually have biological relevance? By studying these biopolymer dynamics and interactions can we learn something about how cells behave, about the origins of life, about treating and preventing disease?'

'How can we use biopolymers to produce sustainable materials?'

'The last century we spent mapping the atom. The century before mapping the world. This century we are mapping the cell. How can research on biopolymer networks advance this goal?'

10.5 What is needed in the research community to make advances in the field?

The responses to this question from the community focused largely on four main topics: Collaboration, Synthesis, Theory, Experimental Methods.

10.5.1 Collaboration

'While many groups work on their specific 'favorite' biopolymer, we will benefit from more attempts to derive design rules common across classes of biopolymers, to inform engineering and technology development.'

'Mainly collaboration and exchange of ideas with other fields (for example, computer science and cell biology) so that there is always a fresh infusion of ideas.'

'Collaborations amongst teams of physicists, engineers, and biologists.'

'This is a niche field that needs to interact more with the bigger fields that surround it. Polymer materials people still need convincing that a single DNA molecule tells them something useful; biologists who study the cytoskeleton need convincing that knowing the rheological properties of actin networks tells them something useful.'

'Interdisciplinary training of students.'

'A common language between theory and experiment and between physics, biology, chemistry, and mathematics.'

'Theories and experiments that bridge scales from molecules to tissues and organisms.'

'Physical scientists need the humility to realize that biology is hard and they should be open to listening to biological and medical researchers.'

'Everyone needs to be better at data sharing and transparency.'

'More collaborations between fields.'

10.5.2 Synthesis

'Sustainable synthesis of biopolymer networks.'

'Increasing the throughput of biopolymer synthesis, including faster molecular design, recombinant protein expression and purification methods, and high-throughput screening that is straightforward to scale up to make enough material to sweep the parameter space of network properties and function.'

'Molecular design and synthesis, facilitated by close collaboration of materials chemists with physical chemists and soft materials researchers.'

'Well-controlled and well-characterized model experimental systems with systematically tunable sets of key parameters.'

'Effective sharing and access of soft active materials of biological origin. This challenge is hindering physics-oriented groups from embarking on research in this general area.'

10.5.3 Theory

'Development of constitutive equations for active matter systems.'

'Theoretical frameworks from network science might be currently under-leveraged, and will bring a unique perspective to understanding biopolymer networks.'

'Idea development in statistical mechanics that is predictive and microscopic, and includes viscoelastic effects.'

'We need a fundamental understanding of how things like mechanics, porosity, charge sign, spatial heterogeneity, and other physical properties matter in naturally occurring biopolymer networks.'

'Polysaccharides have a primary and secondary sequence analogous to proteins, but it is clear that their network assembly rules are very different. Orthogonal thinking to develop new theory in this area is needed.'

'Multiscale modeling from molecule to material and ever closer convergence of different disciplines.'

10.5.4 Methods

'Experiments that measure bulk response and more local dynamics either directly in real space-time or via some form of microrheology.'

'More rigor in terms of structural measurements and of biochemistry.'

'Characterization and simulation of network heterogeneity across lengthscales.'

'Improvements in *in situ* measurement techniques for rheology and microrheology to better understand mechanics and dynamics in flowing systems.'

10.6 What is a 'must-read' for anyone interested in learning more about the field?

Future progress in the field relies on a firm understanding of the phenomenal work that has been done over the last several decades to advance our understanding of biopolymer networks. Everyone in the field has their favorite foundational papers that they have read thousands of times for understanding and inspiration. Now that you have finished your journey through this book, here are some favorite papers and books that the voices in this chapter have suggested to continue your voyage.

PG de Gennes. *Scaling Concepts in Polymer Physics* Cornell University Press (1979).

TT Perkins, DE Smith, S Chu. Direct observation of tube-like motion of a single polymer chain *Science* **264** 819–22 (1994). (Perkins *et al* 1994).

JF Marko, ED Siggia. Stretching DNA *Macromolecules* **28** 8759–70 (1995). (Marko and Siggia 1995).

M Rubinstein, AN Semenov. Thermoreversible gelation in solutions of associative polymers. 2. Linear dynamics *Macromolecules* **31** 1386–97 (1998). (Rubinstein and Semenov 1998).

ML Gardel *et al.* Elastic behavior of cross-linked and bundled actin networks *Science* **304** 1301–05 (2004). (Gardel *et al* 2004).

JH Shin, ML Gardel, L Mahadevan, P Matsudaira, DA Weitz. Relating microstructure to rheology of a bundled and cross-linked F-actin network *in vitro* *Proc. Natl. Acad. Sci.* **101** 9636–9641 (2004). (Shin *et al* 2004).

C Storm, JJ Pastore, FC MacKintosh, TC Lubensky, PA Janmey. Nonlinear elasticity in biological gels *Nature* **435** 191–4 (2005). (Storm *et al* 2005).

CP Broedersz, X Mao, TC Lubensky, FC MacKintosh. Criticality and isostaticity in fibre networks *Nature Phys.* **7** 983–88 (2011). (Broedersz *et al* 2011).

T Sanchez, DTN Chen, SJ DeCamp, M Heymann, Z Dogic. Spontaneous motion in hierarchically assembled active matter *Nature* **491** 431–4 (2012). (Sanchez *et al* 2012).

CP Broedersz, FC MacKintosh. Modeling semiflexible polymer networks *Rev. Modern Phys.* **86** 995 (2014). (Broedersz and MacKintosh 2014).

J Prost, F Jülicher, J-F Joanny. Active gel physics *Nat. Phys.* **11** 111–17 (2015). (Prost *et al* 2015).

L Dooling, DA Tirrell. Engineering the dynamic properties of protein networks through sequence variation *ACS Central Sci.* **2** 812–19 (2016). (Dooling and Tirrell 2016).

Y Zhou, B Li, S Li, HAM Ardoena, WL Wilson, JD Tovar, CM Schroeder. Concentration-driven assembly and sol–gel transition pi-conjugated oligopeptides *ACS Central Sci.* **3** 986–94 (2017). (Zhou *et al* 2017).

R Freeman *et al.* Reversible self-assembly of superstructured networks *Science* **362** 808–13 (2018). (Freeman *et al* 2018)

F Burla, Y Mulla, BE Vos, A Aufderhorst-Roberts, GH Koenderink. From mechanical resilience to active material properties in biopolymer networks *Nat. Phys. Rev.* **1** 249–63 (2019). (Burla *et al* 2019).

ER Jira, K Shmilovich, TS Kale, A Ferguson, JD Tovar, CM Schroeder, Effect of core oligomer length on the phase behavior and assembly of pi-conjugated peptides *ACS Appl. Mater. Interfaces* **12** 20722–32 (2020). (Jira *et al* 2020).

M Das, CF Schmidt, M Murrell. Introduction to active matter *Soft Matter* **16** 7185–90 (2020). (Das *et al* 2020).

C Scheibner, A Souslov, D Banerjee, P Surowka, WTM Irvine, V Vitelli. Odd elasticity *Nat. Phys.* **16** 475–80 (2020) (Scheibner *et al* 2020).

P Stewart. Biophysics of biofilm infection *Pathogens Dis.* **70** 212–18 (2014). (Stewart 2014).

AE Patteson, RJ Carroll, DV Iwamoto, PA Janmey. The vimentin cytoskeleton: when polymer physics meets cell biology *Phys. Biol.* **18** 011001 (2021). (Patteson *et al* 2020).

M Chang, W Huang, DJ Mai. Monomer-scale design of functional protein polymers using consensus repeat sequences *J. Polym. Sci.* **59** 2644–64 (2021). (Chang *et al* 2021).

K Pogoda. Unique role of vimentin networks in compression stiffening of cells and protection of nuclei from compressive stress *Nano Lett.* **22** 4725–32 (2022). (Pogoda *et al* 2022).

KR Peddireddy, R Clairmont, P Neill, RJ McGorty, RM Robertson-Anderson. OpTiDDM (Optical Tweezers integrating Differential Dynamic Microscopy) maps the spatiotemporal propagation of nonlinear stresses in polymer blends and composites *Nat. Commun.* **13** 5180 (2022).

Y Li, Y Li, E Prince, JI Weitz, S Panyukov, A Ramachandran, M Rubinstein, E Kumacheva. Fibrous hydrogels under biaxial confinement *Nat. Commun.* **13** 1–6 (2022). (Li *et al* 2022).

DB Hill, B Button, M Rubinstein, RC Boucher. Physiology and pathophysiology of human airway mucus *Physiol. Rev.* **102** 1757–1836 (2022). (Hill *et al* 2022).

MA Morris *et al.* Democratizing the rapid screening of protein expression for materials development *Mol. Syst. Design Eng.* **8** 227–39 (2023). (Morris *et al* 2023).

Thanks for joining me on this adventure.

References

Abyzov A, Blackledge M and Zweckstetter M 2022 Conformational dynamics of intrinsically disordered proteins regulate biomolecular condensate chemistry *Chem. Rev.* **122** 6719–48

Alberti S, Gladfelter A and Mittag T 2019 Considerations and challenges in studying liquid-liquid phase separation and biomolecular condensates *Cell* **176** 419–34

Alvarado J, Cipelletti L and Koenderink G H 2019 Uncovering the dynamic precursors to motor-driven contraction of active gels *Soft Matter* **15** 8552–65

Alvarado J, Sheinman M, Sharma A, MacKintosh F C and Koenderink G H 2017 Force percolation of contractile active gels *Soft Matter* **13** 5624–44

Bacca M, Saleh O A and McMeeking R M 2019 Contraction of polymer gels created by the activity of molecular motors *Soft Matter* **15** 4467–75

Banerjee S, Gardel M L and Schwarz U S 2020 The actin cytoskeleton as an active adaptive material *Annu. Rev. Condens. Matter Phys.* **11** 421–39

Bertrand O J N, Fygenson D K and Saleh O A 2012 Active, motor-driven mechanics in a DNA gel *Proc. Natl. Acad. Sci.* **109** 17342–7

Bikard D, Loot C, Baharoglu Z and Mazel D 2010 Folded DNA in action: hairpin formation and biological functions in prokaryotes *Microbiol. Mol. Biol. Rev.* **74** 570–88

Blanchoin L, Pollard T D and Mullins R D 2000 Interactions of ADF/cofilin, Arp2/3 complex, capping protein and profilin in remodeling of branched actin filament networks *Curr. Biol.* **10** 1273–82

Brangwynne C P, Tompa P and Pappu R V 2015 Polymer physics of intracellular phase transitions *Nat. Phys.* **11** 899–904

Broedersz C P and MacKintosh F C 2014 Modeling semiflexible polymer networks *Rev. Mod. Phys.* **86** 995–1036

Broedersz C P, Mao X, Lubensky T C and MacKintosh F C 2011 Criticality and isostaticity in fibre networks *Nat. Phys.* **7** 983–8

Burkholder E W and Brady J F 2019 Fluctuation-dissipation in active matter *J. Chem. Phys. ACTV2019* **150** 184901

Burla F, Mulla Y, Vos B E, Aufderhorst-Roberts A and Koenderink G H 2019 From mechanical resilience to active material properties in biopolymer networks *Nat. Rev. Phys.* **1** 249–63

Chang M P, Huang W and Mai D J 2021 Monomer-scale design of functional protein polymers using consensus repeat sequences *J. Polym. Sci.* **59** 2644–64

Chapman C D, Shanbhag S, Smith D E and Robertson-Anderson R M 2012 Complex effects of molecular topology on diffusion in entangled biopolymer blends *Soft Matter* **8** 9177–82

Choi U B, McCann J J, Weninger K R and Bowen M E 2011 Beyond the random coil: stochastic conformational switching in intrinsically disordered proteins *Structure* **19** 566–76

Cloutier T E and Widom J 2004 Spontaneous sharp bending of double-stranded DNA *Mol. Cell* **14** 355–62

Conrad N, Chang G, Fygenson D K and Saleh O A 2022 Emulsion imaging of a DNA nanostar condensate phase diagram reveals valence and electrostatic effects *J. Chem. Phys.* **157** 234203

Das M, Schmidt F, Murrell C and M 2020 Introduction to active matter *Soft Matter* **16** 7185–90

Deng J and Walther A 2020 Programmable ATP-fueled DNA coacervates by transient liquid-liquid phase separation *Chem.* **6** 3329–43

Dogterom M and Koenderink G H 2019 Actin–microtubule crosstalk in cell biology *Nat. Rev. Mol. Cell Biol.* **20** 38–54

Dong Y, Yao C, Zhu Y, Yang L, Luo D and Yang D 2020 DNA functional materials assembled from branched DNA: design, synthesis, and applications *Chem. Rev.* **120** 9420–81

Dooling L J and Tirrell D A 2016 Engineering the dynamic properties of protein networks through sequence variation *ACS Cent. Sci.* **2** 812–9

Espeli O and Marians K J 2004 Untangling intracellular DNA topology *Mol. Microbiol.* **52** 925–31

Fitzpatrick R, Michieletto D, Peddireddy K R, Hauer C, Kyrillos C, Gurmessa B J and Robertson-Anderson R M 2018 Synergistic interactions between DNA and actin trigger emergent viscoelastic behavior *Phys. Rev. Lett.* **121** 257801

Fodor É, Nardini C, Cates M E, Tailleur J, Visco P and van Wijland F 2016 How far from equilibrium is active matter? *Phys. Rev. Lett.* **117** 038103

Francis M L, Ricketts S N, Farhadi L, Rust M J, Das M, Ross J L and Robertson-Anderson R M 2019 Non-monotonic dependence of stiffness on actin crosslinking in cytoskeleton composites *Soft Matter* **15** 9056–65

Freeman R *et al* 2018 Reversible self-assembly of superstructured networks *Science* **362** 808–13

Gardel M L, Shin J H, MacKintosh F C, Mahadevan L, Matsudaira P and Weitz D A 2004 Elastic behavior of cross-linked and bundled actin networks *Science* **304** 1301

Gorczyca S M, Chapman C D and Robertson-Anderson R M 2015 Universal scaling of crowding-induced DNA mobility is coupled with topology-dependent molecular compaction and elongation *Soft Matter* **11** 7762–8

Gouveia B, Kim Y, Shaevitz J W, Petry S, Stone H A and Brangwynne C P 2022 Capillary forces generated by biomolecular condensates *Nature* **609** 255–64

Gurmessa B J, Bitten N, Nguyen D T, Saleh O A, Ross J L, Das M and Robertson-Anderson R M 2018 Triggered disassembly and reassembly of actin networks induces rigidity phase transitions *Soft Matter* **15** 1335–44

Gurmessa B J, Rust M J, Das M, Ross J L and Robertson-Anderson R M 2021 Salt-mediated stiffening, destruction, and resculpting of actomyosin network *Front. Phys.* **9** 760340

Hill D B, Button B, Rubinstein M and Boucher R C 2022 Physiology and pathophysiology of human airway mucus *Physiol. Rev.* **102** 1757–836

Honda S, Yamamoto T and Tezuka Y 2010 Topology-directed control on thermal stability: micelles formed from linear and cyclized amphiphilic block copolymers *J. Am. Chem. Soc.* **132** 10251–3

Hyman A A, Weber C A and Jülicher F 2014 Liquid-liquid phase separation in biology *Annu. Rev. Cell Dev. Biol.* **30** 39–58

Jahnke K, Weiss M, Weber C, Platzman I, Göpfrich K and Spatz J P 2020 Engineering light-responsive contractile actomyosin networks with DNA nanotechnology *Adv. Biosyst.* **4** 2000102

Jensen M H, Morris E J, Goldman R D and Weitz D A 2014 Emergent properties of composite semiflexible biopolymer networks *BioArchitecture* **4** 138–43

Jeon B, Nguyen D T, Abraham G R, Conrad N, Fygenson D K and Saleh O A 2018 Salt-dependent properties of a coacervate-like, self-assembled DNA liquid *Soft Matter* **14** 7009–15

Jira E R, Shmilovich K, Kale T S, Ferguson A, Tovar J D and Schroeder C M 2020 Effect of core oligomer length on the phase behavior and assembly of π-conjugated peptides *ACS Appl. Mater. Interfaces* **12** 20722–32

Kaur T, Alshareedah I, Wang W, Ngo J, Moosa M M and Banerjee P R 2019 Molecular crowding tunes material states of ribonucleoprotein condensates *Biomolecules* **9** 71

Kaur T, Raju M, Alshareedah I, Davis R B, Potoyan D A and Banerjee P R 2021 Sequence-encoded and composition-dependent protein-RNA interactions control multiphasic condensate morphologies *Nat. Commun.* **12** 872

Khanal P, Peddireddy K R, Marfai J, McGorty R and Robertson-Anderson R M 2022 DNA topology dictates emergent bulk elasticity and hindered macromolecular diffusion in DNA-dextran composites *J. Rheol.* **66** 699–715

Klotz A R, Soh B W and Doyle P S 2020 Equilibrium structure and deformation response of 2D kinetoplast sheets *Proc. Natl. Acad. Sci.* **117** 121–7

Krajina B A, Zhu A, Heilshorn S C and Spakowitz A J 2018 Active DNA olympic hydrogels driven by topoisomerase activity *Phys. Rev. Lett.* **121** 148001

Lee G, Leech G, Rust M J, Das M, McGorty R J, Ross J L and Robertson-Anderson R M 2021 Myosin-driven actin-microtubule networks exhibit self-organized contractile dynamics *Sci. Adv.* **7** eabe4334

Lemma L M, Varghese M, Ross T D, Thomson M, Baskaran A and Dogic Z 2023 Spatio-temporal patterning of extensile active stresses in microtubule-based active fluids *PNAS Nexus* **2** pgad130

Lenz M 2020 Reversal of contractility as a signature of self-organization in cytoskeletal bundles *eLife* **9** e51751

Lenz M 2014 Geometrical origins of contractility in disordered actomyosin networks *Phys. Rev.* X **4** 041002

Li Y, Hsiao K-W, Brockman C A, Yates D Y, Robertson-Anderson R M, Kornfield J A, Francisco M J S, Schroeder C M and McKenna G B 2015 When ends meet: circular DNA stretches differently in elongational flows **48** 5997–6001

Li Y, Li Y, Prince E, Weitz J I, Panyukov S, Ramachandran A, Rubinstein M and Kumacheva E 2022 Fibrous hydrogels under biaxial confinement *Nat. Commun.* **13** 3264

Linsmeier I, Banerjee S, Oakes P W, Jung W, Kim T and Murrell M P 2016 Disordered actomyosin networks are sufficient to produce cooperative and telescopic contractility *Nat. Commun.* **7** 12615

Lopez-Menendez H and Gonzalez-Torres L 2019 A theory to describe emergent properties of composite F-actin and vimentin networks *J. Mech. Phys. Solids* **127** 208–20

Mai D J and Schroeder C M 2016 Single polymer dynamics of topologically complex DNA *Curr. Opin. Colloid Interface Sci.* **26** 28–40

Marfai J, McGorty R J and Robertson-Anderson R M 2023 Cooperative rheological state-switching of enzymatically-driven composites of circular DNA and dextran **35** 2305824

Marko J F and Siggia E D 1995 Stretching DNA *Macromolecules* **28** 8759–70

Matthews K S 1992 DNA looping *Microbiol. Rev.* **56** 123–36

McCarty J, Delaney K T, Danielsen S P O, Fredrickson G H and Shea J-E 2019 Complete phase diagram for liquid–liquid phase separation of intrinsically disordered proteins *J. Phys. Chem. Lett.* **10** 1644–52

McGorty R J *et al* 2023 Kinesin and myosin motors compete to drive rich multiphase dynamics in programmable cytoskeletal composites *PNAS Nexus* **2** pgad245

Merindol R and Walther A 2017 Materials learning from life: concepts for active, adaptive and autonomous molecular systems *Chem. Soc. Rev.* **46** 5588–619

Michieletto D, Fitzpatrick R and Robertson-Anderson R M 2019 Maximally stiffening composites require maximally coupled rather than maximally entangled polymer species *Soft Matter* **15** 6703–17

Michieletto D, Neill P, Weir S, Evans D, Crist N, Martinez V A and Robertson-Anderson R M 2022 Topological digestion drives time-varying rheology of entangled DNA fluids *Nat. Commun.* **13** 4389

Mogilner A and Oster G 1996 Cell motility driven by actin polymerization *Biophys. J.* **71** 3030–45

Morris M A, Bataglioli R A, Mai D J, Yang Y J, Paloni J M, Mills C E, Schmitz Z D, Ding E A, Huske A C and Olsen B D 2023 Democratizing the rapid screening of protein expression for materials development *Mol. Syst. Des. Eng.* **8** 227–39

Nakamura M, Chen L, Howes S C, Schindler T D, Nogales E and Bryant Z 2014 Remote control of myosin and kinesin motors using light-activated gearshifting *Nat. Nanotechnol.* **9** 693–7

Needleman D and Dogic Z 2017 Active matter at the interface between materials science and cell biology *Nat. Rev. Mater.* **2** 1–14

Nguyen D T and Saleh O A 2017 Tuning phase and aging of DNA hydrogels through molecular design *Soft Matter* **13** 5421–7

Patteson A E, Carroll R J, Iwamoto D V and Janmey P A 2020 The vimentin cytoskeleton: when polymer physics meets cell biology *Phys. Biol.* **18** 011001

Peddireddy K R, Clairmont R, Neill P, McGorty R and Robertson-Anderson R M 2022 Optical-tweezers-integrating-differential-dynamic-microscopy maps the spatiotemporal propagation of nonlinear strains in polymer blends and composites *Nat. Commun.* **13** 5180

Peddireddy K R, Michieletto D, Aguirre G, Garamella J, Khanal P and Robertson-Anderson R M 2021 DNA conformation dictates strength and flocculation in DNA–microtubule composites *ACS Macro Lett.* **10** 1540–8

Perkins T T, Smith D E and Chu S 1994 Direct observation of tube-like motion of a single polymer chain *Science* **264** 819–22

Pogoda K *et al* 2022 Unique role of vimentin networks in compression stiffening of cells and protection of nuclei from compressive stress *Nano Lett.* **22** 4725–32

Pollard T D, Blanchoin L and Mullins R D 2001 Cell science at a glance *J. Cell Sci.* **114** 3–4

Prost J, Jülicher F and Joanny J-F 2015 Active gel physics *Nat. Phys.* **11** 111–7

Ramaswamy S 2017 Active matter *J. Stat. Mech: Theory Exp.* **2017** 054002

Riback J A, Zhu L, Ferrolino M C, Tolbert M, Mitrea D M, Sanders D W, Wei M-T, Kriwacki R W and Brangwynne C P 2020 Composition-dependent thermodynamics of intracellular phase separation *Nature* **581** 209–14

Ricketts S N, Khanal P, Rust M J, Das M, Ross J L and Robertson-Anderson R M 2020 Triggering cation-induced contraction of cytoskeleton networks via microfluidics *Front. Phys.* **8** 596699

Ricketts S N, Ross J L and Robertson-Anderson R M 2018 Co-entangled actin-microtubule composites exhibit tunable stiffening and power-law stress relaxation **115** 1055–67

Rogers S A, Calabrese M A and Wagner N J 2014 Rheology of branched wormlike micelles *Curr. Opin. Colloid Interface Sci.* **19** 530–5

Ronceray P and Lenz M 2015 Connecting local active forces to macroscopic stress in elastic media *Soft Matter* **11** 1597–605

Rubinstein M and Semenov A N 1998 Thermoreversible gelation in solutions of associating polymers. 2. linear dynamics *Macromolecules* **31** 1386–97

Sahu S, Chauhan P, Lumen E, Moody K, Peddireddy K, Mani N, Subramanian R, Robertson-Anderson R, Wolfe A J and Ross J L 2023 Interplay of self-organization of microtubule asters and crosslinking protein condensates *PNAS Nexus* **2** pgad231

Sanchez T, Chen D T N, DeCamp S J, Heymann M and Dogic Z 2012 Spontaneous motion in hierarchically assembled active matter *Nature* **491** 431–4

Schaedel L, Lorenz C, Schepers A V, Klumpp S and Köster S 2021 Vimentin intermediate filaments stabilize dynamic microtubules by direct interactions *Nat. Commun.* **12** 3799

Scheibner C, Souslov A, Banerjee D, Surówka P, Irvine W T M and Vitelli V 2020 Odd elasticity *Nat. Phys.* **16** 475–80

Shen Y 2020 Microrheology of actin-vimentin-microtubule composite cytoskeletal networks *Biophys. J.* **118** 440a

Shen Y *et al* 2021 Effects of vimentin intermediate filaments on the structure and dynamics of *in vitro* multicomponent interpenetrating cytoskeletal networks *Phys. Rev. Lett.* **127** 108101

Shimobayashi S F, Ronceray P, Sanders D W, Haataja M P and Brangwynne C P 2021 Nucleation landscape of biomolecular condensates *Nature* **599** 503–6

Shin J H, Gardel M L, Mahadevan L, Matsudaira P and Weitz D A 2004 Relating microstructure to rheology of a bundled and cross-linked F-actin network *in vitro Proc. Natl. Acad. Sci.* **101** 9636–41

Shin Y and Brangwynne C P 2017 Liquid phase condensation in cell physiology and disease *Science* **357** eaaf4382

Sing C E and Perry S L 2020 Recent progress in the science of complex coacervation *Soft Matter* **16** 2885–914

Smrek J, Garamella J, Robertson-Anderson R and Michieletto D 2021 Topological tuning of DNA mobility in entangled solutions of supercoiled plasmids *Sci. Adv.* **7** eabf9260

Stewart P S 2014 Biophysics of biofilm infection *Pathog. Dis.* **70** 212–8

Storm C, Pastore J J, MacKintosh F C, Lubensky T C and Janmey P A 2005 Nonlinear elasticity in biological gels *Nature* **435** 191–4

Voth G A 2017 A multiscale description of biomolecular active matter: the chemistry underlying many life processes *Acc. Chem. Res.* **50** 594–8

Zhou Y, Li B, Li S, Ardoña H A M, Wilson W L, Tovar J D and Schroeder C M 2017 Concentration-driven assembly and sol–gel transition of π-conjugated oligopeptides *ACS Cent. Sci.* **3** 986–94

Glossary of symbols, abbreviations, and acronyms

Chapter 1

Abbreviation	Quantity (typical units used in the text)
F	force (pN)
η	viscosity (Pa-s)
v	speedm (μm s^{-1})
σ	stress (Pa)
γ	strain (unitless)
A	area perpendicular to applied force (μm^2)
$\dot{\gamma}$	strain rate (s^{-1})
G	shear modulus (Pa)
d	polymer diameter (nm)
L	contour length (μm)
l_p	persistence length (nm–mm)
$\frac{Q}{L}$	linear charge density (e nm^{-1})
bp	basepair
kbp	kilobasepair
ABP	actin binding protein

doi:10.1088/978-0-7503-5037-2ch11

MAP	microtubule associated protein
MT	microtubule
Taxol	paclitaxel, microtubule stabilizing agent
IF	intermediate filament
ULF	unit length filament
PTS	pyrene-threonine-serine
IDP	intrinsically disordered protein

Chapter 2

FJC	freely jointed chain
$l_k = 2l_p$	Kuhn length
$N = L/l_k$	number of monomers, i.e., Kuhn lengths, comprising a polymer
$\langle R_0^2 \rangle^{1/2} = l_k\sqrt{N}$	root-mean-square end-to-end distance of a linear polymer (nm)
R_0	short-hand for root-mean-square end-to-end distance (nm)
COM	center-of-mass
$R_G = \frac{1}{\sqrt{6}}\langle R_0^2 \rangle^{1/2}$	radius of gyration, i.e., mean distance of a Kuhn segment from polymer center-of-mass (nm)
SAW	self-avoiding random walk
ν	Flory exponent: $\nu = 0.5$ in theta solvent, $\nu = 0.588$ in good solvent)
$R_H \simeq k_B T/6\pi\eta_s D$	hydrodynamic radius: $R_G = 1.6R_H$ (good solvent), $R_G = 1.5R_H$ (theta solvent)
D	diffusion coefficient (μm^2 s^{-1})
η_s	solvent viscosity (Pa-s)
$c^* \simeq \left(\frac{M}{N_A}\right)/\left(\frac{4}{3}\pi R_G^3\right)$	polymer overlap concentration (mg mL^{-1})
c_e	critical entanglement concentration (mg mL^{-1})
M_w	polymer molecular weight = monomer molecular weight × number of monomers (kDa)
l_e	polymer length between entanglements (nm)

$N_e = l_e / l_k$	unitless length between entanglements, number of Kuhn lengths per entanglement
$d_T \approx l_k N_e^{1/2}$	diameter of reptation model confinement tube (nm)
$L_0 \approx d_T L / l_e$	primitive path length, i.e., length of entanglement tube (μm)
$\xi_T \approx l_k n_T^{1/2}$	thermal blob size (nm)
n_T	number of Kuhn lengths per thermal blob
D_0	dilute limit or tracer diffusion coefficient ($\mu m^2\ s^{-1}$)
ζ	friction coefficient ($kg\ s^{-1}$)
τ_Z	Zimm time, time for polymer to diffuse a distance R_0 (ms)
$\tau_{R1} \approx \frac{2NR_G^2}{\pi^2 D_0}$	Rouse time for a single linear polymer (ms)
$\tau_R \simeq \tau_{R1}(c/c^*)^{\frac{2-3\nu}{3\nu-1}}$	Rouse time in semidilute solutions (ms - s)
$D_{R1} \simeq k_B T N_e / \zeta N^2$	reptation model diffusion coefficient in melt phase ($\mu m^2\ s^{-1}$)
$D_R \simeq D_{R1}(c/c^*)^{-\frac{(2-\nu)}{(3\nu-1)}}$	reptation model diffusion coefficient in semidilute solutions ($\mu m^2\ s^{-1}$)
$Z = \frac{N}{N_e}$	number of entanglement segments per polymer
$\tau_D \simeq \frac{12NR_G^4}{\pi^2 d_T^2 D_0}$	disengagement time, time for an entangled polymer to reptate out of its tube (s)
$\frac{\tau_D}{\tau_R} \simeq \frac{3N}{N_e} = 3Z$	relation between disengagement time and Rouse time
$\tau_e \simeq \frac{d_T^4}{6NR_G^2 D_0} \simeq \frac{d_T^4}{D_0 l_k^2}$	entanglement time, time for a polymer segment to diffuse the width of the tube
$\frac{\tau_R}{\tau_e} \simeq Z^2$	relation between Rouse time and entanglement time
$\frac{\tau_D}{\tau_e} \simeq Z^3$	relation between disengagement time and entanglement time
CR	constraint release
$\tau_{CR} \approx \tau_{DT} Z^2$	constraint release relaxation timescale (s)
τ_{DT}	disengagement time of polymers surrounding a test chain (s)
CLF	contour length fluctuations
$L_{CLF} \approx L_0(1 - X/\sqrt{Z})$	primative path length taking into account contour length fluctuations with X a constant of order unity (μm)

$\tau_{D\_CLF} \approx \tau_D\left(1 - \frac{X}{\sqrt{Z}}\right)^2$	reduced disengagement time due to contour length fluctuations (s)
$\dot{\gamma}$	strain rate (s^{-1})
$G'(\omega)$	storage modulus, elastic modulus (Pa)
$G''(\omega)$	loss modulus, viscous modulus (Pa)
$\lvert G^*(\omega)\rvert = (G'(\omega)^2 + G''(\omega)^2)^{1/2}$	magnitude of complex modulus
$\eta^*(\omega) = \frac{\lvert G^*(\omega)\rvert}{\omega}$	complex viscosity (Pa-s)
$\tan\delta(\omega) = \frac{G''(\omega)}{G'(\omega)}$	loss tangent
$\omega_c \simeq 2\pi/\tau_D$	crossover frequency at which $G'(\omega)$ becomes larger than $G''(\omega)$ (rad s^{-1})
G^0	plateau modulus where $G'(\omega) \sim \omega^0$ and $G''(\omega)$ is a local minimum
$\omega_e \simeq 2\pi/\tau_e$	crossover frequency at which $G''(\omega)$ becomes larger than $G'(\omega)$ (rad s^{-1})
U_T	entanglement tube potential k_BT
$\xi \simeq 1/\sqrt{c_N a}$	mesh size for network of biopolymers with monomer size a (nm)
$l_e \simeq (l_p\xi^2)^{1/3}$	entanglement length predicted from worm-like chain model (nm–μm)
$d_T \approx \xi^{6/5} l_p^{-1/5}$	tube diameter for a semiflexible polymer (nm)
$l_e \approx \xi^{4/5} l_p^{1/5}$	entanglement length for a semiflexible polymer (nm)
$G^0 \approx k_BT/\xi^2 l_e$	plateau modulus for a semiflexible polymer (Pa)
$\tau_\xi \approx \left(\frac{\zeta}{k_BT}\right)\xi^4 l_p$	mesh time: time for a polymer segment of length ξ to relax (ms)
$\tau_p \approx \left(\frac{\zeta}{k_BT}\right)\xi^{\frac{8}{5}} l_p^{\frac{7}{5}}$	persistence length relaxation time, time for a polymer segment of length l_p to relax (ms)
$\tau_L \approx \left(\frac{\zeta}{k_BT}\right)L^2\xi^{\frac{8}{5}} l_p^{-\frac{3}{5}}$	tube length relaxation time, time for a polymer segment of length $L_0 \simeq L$ to relax (s)
$\tau_b \approx \left(\frac{\epsilon}{l_p k_BT}\right)\left(\frac{2L}{3\pi}\right)^4$	relaxation time associated with bending modes for semiflexible polymers (s)
$\epsilon = \frac{4\pi\eta_S}{\ln\left(\frac{2\xi}{a}\right)}$	perpendicular drag coefficient that hinders filament bending (Pa-s)

$\zeta_{\parallel} = \frac{2\pi\eta_s L}{\ln\left(\frac{L}{d}\right)}$	drag coefficient along the long axis of a rigid rod (Pa-s)
$\zeta_{\perp} = 2\zeta_{\parallel}$	drag coefficient along the short axis of a rigid rod (Pa-s)
$D_{0,\parallel} = 2D_{0,\perp}$	dilute limit diffusion coefficients for motion along the long and short axis of a rigid rod ($\mu m^2\ s^{-1}$)
ϵ_b	bending modulus of a crosslinked semiflexible polymer (pN μm^2)
κ	elastic spring constant of a crosslinked semiflexible polymer
$l_b \approx \left(\frac{\epsilon_b}{\kappa}\right)^{\frac{1}{2}}$	bending lengthscales for a crosslinked network (μm)
l_c	length between crosslinkers in a crosslinked polymer networks (nm)
$\lambda_{NA} \approx l_c\left(\frac{l_b}{l_c}\right)^{\frac{1}{4}}$	non-affinity lengthscales (nm)
$L_{RP} \simeq Pl_c$	polymer length required to achieve rigidity percolation with $P \simeq 2.53$–5.9
$K'(\gamma) = \frac{d\sigma}{d\gamma}$	differential modulus (Pa)
$\sigma_R(t)$	time-dependent relaxation stress following cessation of strain (Pa)
CCR	convective constraint release

Chapter 3

NA	numerical aperture
CMOS	complementary metal-oxide semiconductor
EMCCD	electron multiplying charge-coupled device
FOV	field-of-view
fps	frames per second
GSER	generalized Stokes–Einstein relation
LSCM	laser scanning confocal microscopy
PMT	photomultiplier tube
TIRF	total internal reflection fluorescence

PEG	polyethylene glycol
LSM	light-sheet microscopy
OT	optical tweezers
k_{OT}	optical trap stiffness (pN V^{-1})
OTM	optical tweezers microrheology
PTM	particle-tracking microrheology
$\zeta^{*}=\frac{\eta}{\eta^{*}(\omega)}\zeta$	generalized drag coefficient in terms of Newtonian drag ζ, viscosity η, and complex viscosity $\eta^{*}(\omega)$
$\widetilde{G}(s)$	Laplace transform of complex modulus G^{*}
$\pi(\Delta t) = \frac{\langle(\Delta r(\Delta t))^2\rangle}{2\langle(\Delta r)^2\rangle}$	normalized mean-squared displacement
$\lvert x_0 \rvert$	OTM oscillatory position amplitude (μm)
$\lvert F_0 \rvert$	OTM oscillatory force amplitude (pN)
δ	angular phase difference between oscillatory position (or strain) and force (or stress)
F_R	force measured during relaxation phase of nonlinear OTM (pN)
c_i	fractional amplitude of exponential decay term where $\sum c_i = 1$
f_R	fractional force relaxation
MTM	magnetic tweezers microrheology
AFM	atomic force microscopy
DLS	dynamic light scattering
I	pixel intensity
g_2	second-order intensity correlation measured in DLS
g_1	first-order intensity correlation measured in DLS
Γ	characteristic DLS intensity correlation decay time (s)
q	wave vector (μm^{-1})

Chapter 4

α	anomalous transport coefficient in $\langle(\Delta\bar{r})^2\rangle \sim (\Delta t)^{\alpha}$
$G(\Delta x, \Delta t)$	van Hove particle displacement distribution
G_1	Gaussian peak of van Hove displacement

λ_{NG}	characteristic decay length of exponential van Hove distributions
Ω	scaling exponent relating decay length of exponential van Hove distribution and lag time: $\lambda_{NG}(\Delta t) \sim (\Delta t)^{\Omega}$
EB	ergodicity breaking parameter
NG	non-Gaussianity parameter
$\overline{(\Delta x)^2(\Delta t)}$	time-averaged MSD (different than the ensemble-averaged MSD $\langle(\Delta x)^2\rangle$)
$\vec{R}_{\max}$	major axis of spheroidal polymer conformation (e.g., random coil)
$\vec{R}_{\min}$	minor axis of spheroidal polymer conformation (e.g., random coil)
R_{coil}	average coil size determined from $R_{\max}$ and $R_{\min}$
$\theta_{\max}$	angular orientation of major axis vector $\vec{R}_{\max}$
$\theta_{\min}$	angular orientation of minor axis vector $\vec{R}_{\min}$
D_{θ}	rotational diffusion coefficient
E	eccentricity parameter
$\langle(\Delta\tilde{r})^2(\omega)\rangle$	Fourier transform of $\langle(\Delta r)^2(\Delta t)\rangle$
$\alpha(\omega)$	local logarithmic slope of $\langle(\Delta r)^2(\Delta t)\rangle$
MPM	multiple particle microrheology (2-point microrheology)
$D_{rr}(\rho, \Delta t)$	cross-correlation of the motion of pairs of particles separated by a radial distance ρ
$\langle(\Delta r)^2(\Delta t)\rangle_2$	two-particle mean-squared displacement determined from D_{rr}
PIV	particle image velocimetry
$p_x \times p_y$	pixel dimensions of an image
$n_x \times n_y$	dimensions of PIV grid
$p_x/n_x \times p_y/n_y$	dimensions of PIV interrogation window
$\nabla\vec{v}$	divergence of velocity
$\vec{u}(T)$	local displacement field from integrating the PIV velocity field from $t = 0$ to $t = T$
$\varepsilon_{xy}(T)$	accumulated strain at time T determined from $\vec{u}(T)$
$\frac{d\varepsilon}{dt} = \nabla\vec{v}$	strain rate determined from PIV
ε_1, ε_2	principal components of strain field

$T = \|\varepsilon_1 - \varepsilon_2\|/2$	shear strain from PIV
$\sigma_r(r)$	radial stress for a contracting system
$\nabla \times \vec{v}$	curl of the velocity
$I(\vec{x})$	2D image as a matrix of intensity values in real space
$\vec{q} = 2\pi/\vec{x}$	wave vector
$I(\vec{q})$	2D image in Fourier space
$\Delta I(\vec{x}, \Delta t)$	Image difference for a given lag time Δt
$\Delta \tilde{I}(\vec{q}, \Delta t)$	Fourier transform if image difference
$D(\vec{q}, \Delta t)$	DDM image structure function
$f(q, \Delta t)$	intermediate scattering function
$\tau(q)$	DDM density fluctuation decay time (s)
ϑ	generalized transport coefficient
β	dynamic exponent in power-law relation $\tau \sim q^{-\beta}$
$s(q)$	stretching exponent in the exponential that describes $f(q, \Delta t)$
$C(q)$	DDM ergodicity breaking parameter
$D(q_1, q_2, \Delta t)$	generalized 2D DDM image structure function
$D_i(\vec{q}, \Delta t, t)$	instantaneous image structure function
A_F	alignment factor
$G(D_i)$	distribution of instantaneous image structure functions
S_K	distribution skewness
κ_D	distribution kurtosis
$g(\Delta\vec{x})$	2D spatial image autocorrelation function
$F(I(\Delta\vec{x}))$	2D fast Fourier transform of $I(\vec{x})$
$F(I(r))$	one-dimension Fourier transform as a function of radial separation r between to pixels
$F^*(I(r))$	complex conjugate of $F(I(r))$
$g(r)$	1D spatial image autocorrelation function as a function radial separation r
ξ	structural correlation length
g_∞	long-range structural correlation factor

Chapter 5

$U_{\perp}(y)$	confining potential associated with tube confinement of an entangled polymer
$P_{\perp}(y)$	probability distribution of displacements of entangled polymer segments transverse to the local orientation of the primitive path and tube of the polymer
c_e	critical entanglement concentration (mg mL^{-1})
d^*	effective DNA diameter that accounts for negatively charged backbone and counterion charge screening
$\eta^* \sim \omega^{-x}$	shear thinning with thinning exponent x
Wi	Weissenberg number
c_A	molar concentration of actin (μM)
ρ_A	mass concentration of actin (mg mL^{-1})
c_G	molar concentration of gelsolin (μM)
c_p	critical molar concentration for polymerization (μM)
d'_T	dilated tube diameter
τ'_D	shortened disengagement time associated with dilated tube diameter
R	molar ratio of crosslinker (e.g. ABP) to biopolymer subunits (e.g. actin monomers)
b-actin	biotinylated actin monomer
NA	NeutrAvidin
χ	scaling exponent relating the elastic modulus to R for crosslinked networks ($G^0 \sim R^{\chi}$)
$K = dF/dx$	network stiffness computed from the force $F(x)$ measured in nonlinear OTM, analogous to differential modulus K' in bulk rheology measurements but with different units (pN μm^{-1})
γ_c	critical strain for onset of nonlinear stiffening
p	bond occupation probability
F_T	terminal force retained following relaxation phase of OTM measurements
c_T	molar concentration of tubulin (μM)
ρ_T	mass concentration of tubulin (mg mL^{-1})

Δx_F	displacement of magnetic probe in response to force F applied in MTM measurements
$K = F/\Delta x_F$	network stiffness computed from the applied force F and measured probe displacement Δx_F, analogous to bulk differential modulus K' and OTM stiffness K (pN μm^{-1})
K_0	linear regime stiffness measured in MTM
b	scaling exponent relating K_0 to c and G^0 to ρ: $K_0 \sim G^0 \sim c^b \sim \rho^b$
Δx_R	distance that magnetic probe recoils back towards its starting position following the cessation of force
υ_p	poroelastic draining rate (Hz)
$\vartheta = MSD/\Delta t^{\alpha}$	generalized transport coefficient ϑ that equates to the diffusion coefficient when $\alpha = 1$
y	scaling exponent relating G^0 to mass concentration R: $G^0 \sim \rho^y$
R_{2+}	molar ratio of divalent salt (e.g., Mg^{2+}, Ca^{2+}) to intermediate filaments
$\mho$	scaling exponent relating G^0 to R_{2+}: $G^0 \sim R_{2+}^{\mho}$
σ_c	critical stress for onset of nonlinear stiffening
$\sigma_{\max}$	max stress achieved during stiffening phase before yielding, rupturing or softening; equates to σ_y in the case of yielding

Chapter 6

$R_{G,\,L}$	radius of gyration of a linear polymer
$R_{G,\,R}$	radius of gyration of a ring (relaxed circular) polymer
$R_{G,\,S}$	radius of gyration of a supercoiled polymer
$R_{H,\,L} = k_B T/6\pi\eta D_{0,\,L}$	hydrodynamic radius of a linear polymer
$R_{H,\,R}$	hydrodynamic radius of a linear polymer
$R_{H,\,S}$	hydrodynamic radius of a supercoiled polymer
L_R	extended length of a ring polymer $\left(=\frac{1}{2}L\right)$
$U_\perp(y)$	confining potential associated with tube confinement of an entangled polymer
$F_\perp(y)$	force resisting motion of a polymer transverse to its contour
K	stiffness associated with transverse confinement

PPR	pom-pom ring
DFLA	double-folded lattice animal
FLG	fractal loopy globule
$L_{0,p}$	primitive path length of the central trunk of a tree-like or amoeba-like conformation of a ring polymer
υ	scaling exponent in the PPR model with $\upsilon \simeq 0.3$ for DNA in good solvent
n_l	number of pom-poms or loops along the central trunk in the PPR model
L_l	length of loops in PPR model
$R_{0,p}$	mean end-to-end distance of the central trunk or primitive path
d_f	global fractal dimension of polymer conformation
d_p	fractal dimension of the primitive path
A_{ms}	minimal surface area of circular polymer conformation
σ	degree of supercoiling
σ_c	critical degree of supercoiling
n_{th}	number of threadings per polymer
T2	Topoisomerase II
L_T	trunk length for a branched polymer
L_B	branch length for a branched polymer
n_B	number of branches per branched polymer
τ_f	longest relaxation timescale of branched polymer
μ	electrophoretic mobility

Chapter 7

$\phi_L = \rho_L/[\rho_L + \rho_R]$	mass fraction of linear polymer in ring-linear polymer blend
ϕ_{DNA}	mass fraction of DNA in DNA-dextran composites
Φ_A	mass fraction of actin in DNA-actin and DNA-IF composites
ϕ_A	molar fraction of actin in actin-vimentin networks
ϕ_T	molar fraction of tubulin in actin-microtubule composites

G_N	initial ($t = 0$) stress relaxation modulus
$C_x(\Delta t)$	conformational autocorrelation of a stretched polymer chain
s	maximum strain distance in OTM (the distance the probe is moved through the sample)
$\lambda = 2\pi q^{-1}$	lengthscales associated with a given wave vector q in DDM
$\xi_C \backsimeq (\xi_A^{-3} + \xi_B^{-3})^{-1/3}$	mesh size for a composite of polymer A and polymer B determined from their respective single-component network mesh sizes (nm)
$\Delta f_R = (F_{R,0} - F_{R,\infty})/F_{R,0}$	fractional force relaxation following strain
σ_y	yield stress (Pa)
γ_y	yield strain

Chapter 8

c_m	molar concentration of myosin
R_m	molar ratio of myosin to actin
CPK	creatine phosphokinase
ℓ	size of clusters or foci in contracting actomyosin networks
ℓ_1	size of largest cluster
ℓ_2	size of second largest cluster
v_p	speed at the periphery of a globally contracting network
f_m	force generated by motors
σ_{cr}/γ_{cr}	critical stress/strain for the onset of nonlinearity
σ_{ext}	external stress applied to a material
σ_{int}	internal stress generated by molecular motors
σ_{max}	rupture stress
δ	filament curvature
κ_b	filament bending rigidity
N	number of myosin heads per minifilament
Ω_m	planar motor density
∇v	divergence of the PIV velocity field

$\dot{\varepsilon}$	strain rate computed from PIV flow field
t_a	myosin activation time
$\varepsilon_{\max}$	maximum strain computed from PIV flow field
n_{Hill}	Hill coefficient or cooperativity parameter in the Hill equation
τ_t	actin turnover time
τ_x	elastic crossover time
R_k	molar ratio of kinesin to tubulin
k401-b	biotinylated kinesin-401 dimer
k365-b	biotinylated kinesin-365 monomer
ξ_v	correlation length of flow with speed v
PCR1	protein regulator of cytokinesis 1
T_A	active lifetime of network
iLID	improved light-induced dimer
t_a	motor/enzyme/fuel activity time
S	enzyme:DNA stoichiometry
$[E]$	enzyme concentration
l_f	DNA fragment length after digestion
$P_2(f)$	probability to be in state 2 of a 2-state system that depends on the system parameter f
$\mathscr{F}_s$	characteristic value of f at which $P_2 = P_1 = 0.5$ in the Hill function
τ_s	switching time associated with time-dependent switch from state 1 to state 2

Chapter 9

LLPS	liquid–liquid phase separation
IDP	intrinsically disordered protein
Δf	change in free energy between mixed and demixed states
ϕ	volume fraction of polymer in solution
χ_P	interaction term associated with polymer–polymer interactions
χ_{PS}	interaction term associated with polymer–solvent interactions

$\Delta p = 2Y/R$	capillary pressure across the interface of a condensate of radius R
Y	surface tension
$\Delta\hat{f} = \frac{\Delta f}{k_B T}$	free energy density difference between the condensed and bulk phases
R_c	critical radius of droplet to form condensate
ϕ_{sat}	minimum polymer volume fraction for condensate nucleation
ϕ_{max}	maximum polymer volume fraction able to sustain LLPS
T_{max}	LLPS dissolution temperature
η_d	viscosity in the dense phase of a phase separated system
η_c	viscosity of a liquid-like condensate
$v_c = Y/\eta$	coalescence speed
$\tau_c = \eta R_c/Y$	coalescence timescale
ϕ_{gel}	minimum polymer volume fraction for gelation
N_{st}	number (valence) of stickers along a polymer chain modeled as a series of stickers and spacers
$\|\Delta G\|$	Gibbs free energy for nanostar overhang hybridization
V_{mol}	volume a nanostar occupies in the bulk phase of the condensate interior
SfNAP	sequence-defined functionalized nucleic acid polymers
R_x	ratio of crosslinkers to DNA nanostars
PLP	prion-like polypeptide
RRP	arginine-rich polypeptide
EDC	1-ethyl-3-(3-(dimethylaminopropyl)-carbodiimide
VPS	viscoelastic phase separation

www.ingramcontent.com/pod-product-compliance
Ingram Content Group UK Ltd.
Pitfield, Milton Keynes, MK11 3LW, UK
UKHW051907100926
8556IPUK00005B/797

9 780750 350358